CLINICAL HANDBOOK OF SCHIZOPHRENIA

CLINICAL HANDBOOK OF SCHIZOPHRENIA

Edited by
KIM T. MUESER
DILIP V. JESTE

THE GUILFORD PRESS
New York   London

© 2008 The Guilford Press
A Division of Guilford Publications, Inc.
72 Spring Street, New York, NY 10012
www.guilford.com

Printed in the United States of America

This book is printed on acid-free paper.

Last digit is print number: 9 8 7 6 5 4 3 2 1

The authors have checked with sources believed to be reliable in their efforts to provide
information that is complete and generally in accord with the standards of practice that
are accepted at the time of publication. However, in view of the possibility of human
error or changes in medical sciences, neither the authors, nor the editor and publisher,
nor any other party who has been involved in the preparation or publication of this
work warrants that the information contained herein is in every respect accurate or
complete, and they are not responsible for any errors or omissions or the results
obtained from the use of such information. Readers are encouraged to confirm the
information contained in this book with other sources.

Library of Congress Cataloging-in-Publication Data

Clinical handbook of schizophrenia / edited by Kim T. Mueser, Dilip V. Jeste.
        p. ; cm.
    Includes bibliographical references and index.
    ISBN 978-1-59385-652-6 (hardcover : alk. paper)
    1. Schizophrenia—Handbooks, manuals, etc.   I. Mueser, Kim Tornvall.
II. Jeste, Dilip V.   III. Title.

    [DNLM: 1. Schizophrenia. WM 203 C641153 2008]
    RC514.C564 2008
    616.89′8—dc22

                                                              2007033713

ABOUT THE EDITORS

Kim T. Mueser, PhD, is a licensed clinical psychologist and a Professor in the Departments of Psychiatry and Community and Family Medicine at the Dartmouth Medical School in Hanover, New Hampshire. He was on the faculty of the Psychiatry Department at the Medical College of Pennsylvania in Philadelphia until 1994, when he moved to Dartmouth Medical School and joined the Dartmouth Psychiatric Research Center. Dr. Mueser's clinical and research interests include psychiatric rehabilitation for persons with severe mental illnesses, intervention for co-occurring psychiatric and substance use disorders, and the treatment of posttraumatic stress disorder. His research has been supported by the National Institute of Mental Health (NIMH), the National Institute on Drug Abuse, the Substance Abuse and Mental Health Services Administration, and the National Alliance for Research on Schizophrenia and Depression (NARSAD). He has served on numerous editorial boards, has published many journal articles and book chapters, and has coauthored 10 books. In 2007 his book *The Complete Family Guide to Schizophrenia* (with Susan Gingerich) received the National Alliance on Mental Illness NYC Metro Ken Book Award for outstanding contributions to better understanding of mental illness.

Dilip V. Jeste, MD, is the Estelle and Edgar Levi Chair in Aging, Director of the Sam and Rose Stein Institute for Research on Aging, and Distinguished Professor of Psychiatry and Neurosciences, University of California, San Diego (UCSD) and VA San Diego Healthcare System. He is also the Director of the NIMH-funded Advanced Center for Interventions and Services Research at UCSD focusing on psychosis in late life, and of the John A. Hartford Center of Excellence in Geriatric Psychiatry. Dr. Jeste was a research fellow, and later, Chief of the Units on Movement Disorders and Dementias at NIMH before moving to San Diego. He is the Principal Investigator on several research and training grants; has published 8 books and over 500 articles in peer-reviewed journals and books; and is the Editor-in-Chief of the *American Journal of Geriatric Psychiatry*. He is a member of the Institute of Medicine of the National Academy of Sciences, and of the National Advisory Mental Health Council of the National Institutes of Health. Dr. Jeste is a past President of the American Association for Geriatric Psychiatry (AAGP) and the West Coast College of Biological Psychiatry, and Founding President of the International College of Geriatric Psychoneuropharmacology. His numerous awards include NIMH's MERIT Award; the Society of Biological Psychiatry's A. E. Bennett Neuropsychiatric Research Award; AAGP's Senior Investigator Award; the American Psychiatric Association's Research Award; Most Distinguished Physician Teacher/Researcher Award from the American Association of Physicians of Indian Origin; Asian Heritage Award for Excellence in Science, Technology, and Research; American College of Psychiatrists' Geriatric Research Award; and Distinguished Investigator Award from NARSAD.

CONTRIBUTORS

Donald Addington, MD, Department of Psychiatry, Foothills Hospital, Calgary, Alberta, Canada

Jean Addington, PhD, Department of Psychiatry, University of Toronto, and PRIME Clinic, Centre for Addiction and Mental Health, Toronto, Ontario, Canada

Britton Ashley Arey, MD, private practice, Costa Mesa, California

Christine Barrowclough, PhD, Academic Division of Clinical Psychology, School of Psychiatry and Behavioural Sciences, Wythenshawe Hospital, Manchester, United Kingdom

Stephen J. Bartels, MD, Department of Psychiatry, New Hampshire–Dartmouth Psychiatric Research Center, Dartmouth Medical School, Concord, New Hampshire

Paul Bebbington, MD, Department of Mental Health Sciences, Royal Free and University College Medical School, London, United Kingdom

Deborah R. Becker, MEd, Department of Psychiatry, New Hampshire–Dartmouth Psychiatric Research Center, Dartmouth Medical School, Concord, New Hampshire

Alan S. Bellack, PhD, Department of Psychiatry, University of Maryland School of Medicine, Baltimore, Maryland

Jonathan Bindman, MD, PhD, Lambeth Hospital, London, United Kingdom

Gary R. Bond, PhD, Department of Psychology, Indiana University–Purdue University Indianapolis, Indianapolis, Indiana

Catherine Briand, PhD, Faculty of Medicine, University of Montreal, Montreal, Quebec, Canada

Tyrone D. Cannon, PhD, Departments of Psychology and Psychiatry and Biobehavioral Sciences, University of California, Los Angeles, Los Angeles, California

William T. Carpenter, Jr., MD, Departments of Psychiatry and Pharmacology and Maryland Psychiatric Research Center, University of Maryland School of Medicine, Baltimore, Maryland

David J. Castle, MD, Mental Health Research Institute, University of Melbourne, Parkville, Victoria, Australia

Robin E. Clark, PhD, Center for Health Policy and Research, University of Massachusetts Medical School, Shrewsbury, Massachusetts

Carl I. Cohen, MD, Division of Geriatric Psychiatry, State University of New York Downstate Medical Center, Brooklyn, New York

Marc Corbière, PhD, Institute of Health Promotion Research, University of British Columbia, Vancouver, British Columbia, Canada

Patrick W. Corrigan, PsyD, Institute of Psychology, Illinois Institute of Technology, Chicago, Illinois

John G. Cottone, PhD, Stony Brook Psychotherapy and Wellness, Stony Brook, New York

Gary S. Cuddeback, PhD, Department of Social Work, Cecil G. Sheps Center for Health Services Research, University of North Carolina at Chapel Hill, Chapel Hill, North Carolina

Larry Davidson, PhD, Program on Recovery and Community Health, School of Medicine and Institution for Social and Policy Studies, Yale University, New Haven, Connecticut

Kenneth L. Davis, MD, Department of Psychiatry, Mount Sinai School of Medicine, New York, New York

Natalie L. DeLuca, PhD, National Center for Organizational Development, VA Healthcare System of Ohio, Cincinnati, Ohio

Lisa Dixon, MD, MPH, Division of Health Services Research, University of Maryland School of Medicine, Baltimore, Maryland

Christian R. Dolder, PharmD, Wingate University School of Pharmacy, Wingate, North Carolina

Jonathan Downar, MD, PhD, Department of Psychiatry, University of Toronto, Toronto, Ontario, Canada

Robert E. Drake, MD, PhD, Department of Psychiatry, New Hampshire–Dartmouth Psychiatric Research Center, Dartmouth Medical School, Concord, New Hampshire

Lauren M. Ellman, PhD, New York State Psychiatric Institute, Columbia University, New York, New York

Lisa T. Eyler, PhD, Department of Psychiatry, University of California, San Diego, La Jolla, California

Walid K. H. Fakhoury, PhD, Unit for Social and Community Psychiatry, Newham Centre for Mental Health, London, United Kingdom

Roger D. Fallot, PhD, Community Connections, Washington, DC

Alan Felix, MD, Department of Psychiatry, College of Physicians and Surgeons, Columbia University, New York, New York

Richard B. Ferrell, MD, Department of Psychiatry, Dartmouth–Hitchcock Medical Center, Dartmouth Medical School, Lebanon, New Hampshire

Bernard A. Fischer IV, MD, Department of Psychiatry, University of Maryland School of Medicine, Baltimore, Maryland

Frederick J. Frese III, PhD, Summit County Recovery Project, Akron, Ohio

Matthew A. Fuller, PharmD, Pharmacy Service, Louis Stokes Cleveland Department of Veterans Affairs Medical Center, Brecksville, Ohio

Susan Gingerich, MSW, private practice, Philadelphia, Pennsylvania

Stephen J. Glatt, PhD, Department of Psychiatry, University of California, San Diego, La Jolla, California

Richard J. Goscha, MSW, School of Social Welfare, University of Kansas, Lawrence, Kansas

Gillian Haddock, PhD, Academic Division of Clinical Psychology, University of Manchester, Manchester, United Kingdom

Heinz Häfner, PhD, Schizophrenia Research Unit, Central Institute of Mental Health, Mannheim, Germany

Wolfram an der Heiden, DiplPsych, Schizophrenia Research Unit, Central Institute of Mental Health, Mannheim, Germany

Marnin J. Heisel, PhD, Departments of Psychiatry and Epidemiology and Biostatistics, Schulich School of Medicine and Dentistry, University of Western Ontario, London, Ontario, Canada

Dan Herman, DSW, Department of Clinical Epidemiology, Mailman School of Public Health, Columbia University, New York, New York

Mustafa M. Husain, MD, Department of Psychiatry, University of Texas Southwestern Medical Center at Dallas, Dallas, Texas

Dilip V. Jeste, MD, Institute for Research on Aging and Departments of Psychiatry and Neurosciences, University of California, San Diego, and VA San Diego Healthcare System, La Jolla, California

Shitij Kapur, MD, PhD, Centre for Addiction and Mental Health and Department of Psychiatry, University of Toronto, Toronto, Ontario, Canada

David J. Kavanagh, PhD, Department of Psychiatry, University of Queensland, Brisbane, Australia

Alex Kopelowicz, MD, San Fernando Mental Health Center, Granada Hills, California

Elizabeth Kuipers, PhD, Department of Psychology, Institute of Psychiatry, Kings College London, London, United Kingdom

Sanjiv Kumra, MD, Department of Psychiatry, University of Minnesota, Minneapolis, Minnesota

Eric C. Kutscher, PharmD, Department of Pharmacy Practice, South Dakota State University College of Pharmacy, Brookings, South Dakota; Department of Psychiatry, Sanford School of Medicine, University of South Dakota School of Medicine, Vermillion, South Dakota; Department of Psychiatry, Avera Behavioral Health Center, Sioux Falls, South Dakota

Jonathan E. Larson, PhD, Rehabilitation Psychology Faculty, Institute of Psychology, Illinois Institute of Technology, Chicago, Illinois

Helen Lavretsky, MD, MS, Department of Psychiatry and Behavioral Sciences, University of California, Los Angeles, Los Angeles, California

William B. Lawson, MD, PhD, Department of Psychiatry, Howard University Hospital, Washington, DC

Tania Lecomte, PhD, Department of Psychology, University of Montreal, Montreal, Quebec, Canada

Robert Paul Liberman, MD, Department of Psychiatry and Behavioral Sciences, University of California, Los Angeles, Los Angeles, California

Fiona Lobban, PhD, Academic Division of Clinical Psychology, School of Psychiatry and Behavioural Sciences, University of Manchester, Manchester, United Kingdom

James B. Lohr, MD, Department of Psychiatry, University of California, San Diego, La Jolla, California

Subramoniam Madhusoodanan, MD, St. John's Episcopal Hospital, Far Rockaway, New York; Department of Psychiatry, State University of New York Downstate Medical Center, Brooklyn, New York

Stephen R. Marder, MD, Semel Institute for Neuroscience and Human Behavior and Department of Psychiatry, David Geffen School of Medicine, University of California, Los Angeles, Los Angeles, California

Thomas W. McAllister, MD, Department of Psychiatry, Dartmouth–Hitchcock Medical Center, Dartmouth Medical School, Lebanon, New Hampshire

Shawn M. McClintock, PhD, Department of Psychiatry, University of Texas Southwestern Medical Center at Dallas, Dallas, Texas

John R. McQuaid, PhD, Department of Psychiatry, University of California, San Diego, La Jolla, California

Thomas W. Meeks, MD, Department of Psychiatry, University of California, San Diego, La Jolla, California

Matthew R. Merrens, PhD, New Hampshire–Dartmouth Psychiatric Research Center, Dartmouth Medical School, Lebanon, New Hampshire

Alexander L. Miller, MD, Department of Psychiatry, University of Texas Health Science Center at San Antonio, San Antonio, Texas

Laura Miller, MD, Department of Psychiatry, University of Illinois at Chicago, Chicago, Illinois

David J. Moore, PhD, Department of Psychiatry, University of California, San Diego, La Jolla, California

Vera Morgan, MA, School of Psychiatry and Clinical Neurosciences, University of Western Australia, Perth, Australia

Anthony P. Morrison, PhD, Department of Clinical Psychology, Mental Health Services, Manchester, United Kingdom

Joseph P. Morrissey, PhD, Departments of Health Policy and Administration and Psychiatry and Cecil G. Sheps Center for Health Services Research, University of North Carolina at Chapel Hill, Chapel Hill, North Carolina

Lorna L. Moser, MS, Department of Psychology, Indiana University–Purdue University Indianapolis, Indianapolis, Indiana

Kim T. Mueser, PhD, Department of Psychiatry, New Hampshire–Dartmouth Psychiatric Research Center, Dartmouth Medical School, Concord, New Hampshire

Barnaby Nelson, PhD, The PACE Clinic, ORYGEN Youth Health, Parkville, Victoria, Australia

Joanne Nicholson, PhD, Department of Psychiatry and Community Health Center for Mental Health Services Research, University of Massachusetts Medical School, Worcester, Massachusetts

Thomas O'Hare, MSW, PhD, Graduate School of Social Work, Boston College, Boston, Massachusetts

Fred C. Osher, MD, Health Systems and Services Policy Justice Center, Council of State Governments, Bethesda, Maryland

Barton W. Palmer, PhD, Department of Psychiatry, University of California, San Diego, La Jolla, California

Roger H. Peters, PhD, Department of Mental Health Law and Policy, Louis de la Parte Florida Mental Health Institute, University of South Florida, Tampa, Florida

Stefan Priebe, PhD, Unit for Social and Community Psychiatry, Newham Centre for Mental Health, London, United Kingdom

Najeeb Ranginwala, MD, Department of Psychiatry, University of Texas Southwestern Medical Center at Dallas, Dallas, Texas

Charles A. Rapp, MSW, PhD, School of Social Welfare, University of Kansas, Lawrence, Kansas

Priscilla Ridgway, PhD, Connecticut Mental Health Center, Yale University, New Haven, Connecticut

David Roe, PhD, Department of Community Mental Health, Faculty of Social Welfare and Health Studies, University of Haifa, Haifa, Israel

Stanley D. Rosenberg, PhD, Department of Psychiatry and Dartmouth Trauma Intervention Research Center, Dartmouth Medical School, Lebanon, New Hampshire

Abraham Rudnick, MD, PhD, Departments of Psychiatry and Philosophy, University of Western Ontario, London, Ontario, Canada

Ingrid B. Rystedt, MD, PhD, Department of Community and Family Medicine, New Hampshire–Dartmouth Psychiatric Research Center, Dartmouth Medical School, Lebanon, New Hampshire

Martha Sajatovic, MD, Department of Psychiatry, Case Western Reserve University School of Medicine, Cleveland, Ohio

Mihail Samnaliev, PhD, Center for Health Policy and Research, University of Massachusetts Medical School, Shrewsbury, Massachusetts

Antonio M. Santos, PhD, private practice, La Jolla, California

Gauri N. Savla, MA, MS, Department of Psychiatry, University of California, San Diego, La Jolla, California

Mary V. Seeman, MD, Centre for Addiction and Mental Health, University of Toronto, Toronto, Ontario, Canada

Jennifer J. Shaw, MD, Guild Lodge Medium Secure Unit, Lancashire, United Kingdom

Pattie B. Sherman, BA, Department of Psychology, University of South Florida, Tampa, Florida

Margaret V. Sherrer, MSW, Department of Psychology, Lyndon State College, Lyndonville, Vermont

Mounir Soliman, MD, Department of Psychiatry, University of California, San Diego, La Jolla, California

Daniel G. Stewart, MD, Department of Psychiatry, Mount Sinai School of Medicine, New York, New York

Donald Stolar, PhD, Department of Psychiatry, University of California, Los Angeles, Los Angeles, California

Ezra Susser, MD, Department of Epidemiology, Mailman School of Public Health, Columbia University, New York, New York

Wendy N. Tenhula, PhD, Department of Psychiatry, University of Maryland School of Medicine, Baltimore, Maryland

Graham Thornicroft, MD, PhD, Institute of Psychiatry, King's College London, London, United Kingdom

Ipsit V. Vahia, MD, Sam and Rose Stein Institute of Research for Aging, University of California, San Diego, La Jolla, California

Vihang N. Vahia, MD, Department of Psychiatry, Dr. R. N. Cooper Hospital and Seth G. S. Medical College, Mumbai, India

Dawn I. Velligan, PhD, Department of Psychiatry, University of Texas Health Science Center at San Antonio, San Antonio, Texas

Charles Weijer, MD, PhD, Department of Philosophy, Talbot College, University of Western Ontario, London, Ontario, Canada

Karen Wohlheiter, PhD, Department of Psychiatry, University of Maryland School of Medicine, Baltimore, Maryland

Til Wykes, PhD, Institute of Psychiatry, King's College London, London, United Kingdom

Alison Yung, MD, Department of Psychiatry, University of Melbourne, Parkville, Victoria, Australia

PREFACE

Schizophrenia is arguably the most serious major psychiatric disorder, usually developing in late adolescence or early adulthood, and often having a profound effect over the lifetime on daily functioning. People with schizophrenia frequently have difficulties living independently and caring for themselves, working or attending school, fulfilling parental or other role obligations, and enjoying close relationships and rewarding leisure activities (American Psychiatric Association, 2000). Although schizophrenia develops in about 1 in 100 individuals, it accounts for a disproportionate share of treatment costs and, according to the World Health Organization, is ranked as the second highest contributor to overall burden of diseases, behind cardiovascular disease (Murray & Lopez, 1996).

Despite the severity of schizophrenia, in recent years there has been enormous progress in our understanding of the illness, and the treatment for it is a rapidly evolving field. Two to three decades ago only a few treatments had been shown to be effective for schizophrenia, and most people with the illness continued to be substantially disabled throughout their lives. Although no "cure" for schizophrenia is currently known, a growing number of treatments, both pharmacological and psychosocial, have been shown to be effective. Of equal or greater importance, there has been a sea change in how the treatment, course, and outcome of schizophrenia are conceptualized. Whereas treatment used to focus primarily on a reduction or containment of psychopathology, traditional concepts of medical recovery have been challenged and recently have given way to new and more meaningful definitions of recovery that emphasize improved functioning, client self-direction, empowerment, and hope (Anthony, 1993; Bellack, 2006; Deegan, 1988). There are now solid grounds for optimism in the treatment of schizophrenia, and the potential to help individuals with this disorder lead rewarding and productive lives. The change in the perception about schizophrenia (although still quite limited in the public mind) may be exemplified by two films that won the Oscar for the best film of the year: *One Flew over the Cuckoo's Nest* in 1976 versus *A Beautiful Mind* in 2002. The former depicted prevalent treatment of serious mental illnesses within a rigid, authoritarian, impersonal chronic mental institution, whereas the latter focused on a person with schizophrenia who not only had a remission of his illness, but also received a Nobel Prize for his earlier scientific work.

Because knowledge about schizophrenia and its treatment has grown at an exponential rate in recent years, clinicians have a critical need to keep abreast of the latest developments, within the constraints of limited time, resources, and their own expertise. Specifically, clinicians require access to authoritative information and recommended resources, written in nontechnical language and covering a broad range of topics related to schizophrenia and its treatment. The *Clinical Handbook of Schizophrenia* is designed to meet these practical needs of clinicians working with individuals with schizophrenia and their families.

Each chapter in the *Handbook* has been written by a world authority on the topic, in plain language with minimal (or no) references in the text, and a resource list of references and recommended readings at the end. All of the chapters on treatment are aimed at providing not only guidelines to clinicians about implementing specific treatment approaches or working with particular populations but also succinct reviews of the research literature supporting these methods. The major "take-home" messages on each topic are summarized in a series of "Key Points" at the end of each chapter. The selection of topics, the writing style, the emphasis on briefly summarizing research findings rather than exhaustively reviewing the scientific literature, and the focus on providing practical clinical recommendations are intended to make the *Handbook* an interesting and useful resource for clinicians. In addition, the comprehensive yet accessible nature of this book will be of interest to students in the health professions (e.g., clinical psychology, psychiatry, general medical practice or family medical practice, psychiatric rehabilitation, social work, nursing, occupational therapy, family and marital counselors), mental health administrators and policymakers, relatives and other support persons, and individuals with schizophrenia themselves.

The *Handbook* is divided into eight different sections, each covering a variety of topic areas. Part I focuses on *Core Science and Background Information* on schizophrenia. The section begins with a chapter on the history of the concept of schizophrenia, followed by chapters on epidemiology, biological theories, brain imaging, neuropathology, genetics, and pre- and perinatal influences on the development of the illness. This section also includes chapters on psychosocial factors in schizophrenia, psychopathology, cognitive functioning, and the course and outcome of the disease.

Part II addresses practical issues related to *Assessment and Diagnosis* of schizophrenia. The first chapter in this section addresses clinical methods for the diagnosis of schizophrenia and related schizophrenia spectrum disorders (e.g., schizoaffective disorder and schizophreniform disorder), which are of critical importance considering symptom overlap in schizophrenia and major mood disorders. The second chapter addresses the assessment of medical comorbidity, which is now recognized as the most important factor contributing to premature mortality for individuals with schizophrenia (Jeste, Gladsjo, Lindamer, & Lacro, 1996). A third chapter addresses the assessment of psychosocial functioning—a crucial topic considering that impaired social functioning is a hallmark of schizophrenia. The final chapter in this section provides a framework for treatment planning and ongoing monitoring of outcomes.

Part III addresses the *Somatic Treatment* of schizophrenia. The primary focus of this section is on pharmacological approaches, which are widely accepted as the "mainstay" in the treatment of schizophrenia. Although not everyone with schizophrenia benefits from medication, the vast majority do, and effective pharmacological treatment makes it possible for many individuals to participate in psychosocial treatment. This section also includes a chapter on the use of electroconvulsive therapy for schizophrenia, a frequently misunderstood but potentially useful treatment approach for a small proportion of individuals with intractable symptoms.

Part IV addresses the *Psychosocial Treatment* of schizophrenia. Extensive research in recent years has demonstrated the effectiveness of a variety of different approaches to psychosocial treatment and self-help for schizophrenia. The chapters in this section reflect the broad range of psychosocial interventions for schizophrenia, including the incorporation of environmental supports into individuals' lives to facilitate medication adherence and improve daily functioning, family intervention to educate relatives about schizophrenia and the principles of its management, cognitive-behavioral therapy for psychosis, social skills training, cognitive rehabilitation, vocational rehabilitation, and training in illness self-management skills. In addition, the specific application of psychosocial treatments in a group format is covered in one chapter, whereas another describes the principles of supported housing. The final chapter in this section addresses the role of self-help in promoting coping and recovery from schizophrenia.

Part V focuses on *Systems of Care* for delivering treatment to people with schizophrenia. The initial chapter in this section is devoted to the role of clinical case management in coordinating mental health treatment, followed by chapters on strengths-based case management and the assertive community treatment (ACT) model. In addition, one chapter addresses treatment in emergency room, inpatient, and residential settings, whereas another describes the treatment of schizophrenia in jails and prisons, a topic of major interest considering the dramatic and distressing growth in recent years of individuals with severe mental illness in the criminal justice system (Torrey, 1995).

Part VI addresses a range of *Special Populations and Problems* among the broad group of individuals with schizophrenia. The first chapter describes the treatment of the first episode of schizophrenia, a topic that has garnered a great deal of interest over the past decade. The second addresses the treatment of the prodromal phase of schizophrenia, a new and promising area of research. The third chapter describes the treatment of schizophrenia in older individuals, also a growing topic of interest considering the rapidly growing population of people over age 50 with the illness. This section also contains chapters on common problems experienced by individuals with schizophrenia, including aggression and violence, housing instability and homelessness, medical comorbidity, intellectual disability, trauma and posttraumatic stress disorder, and substance abuse. Finally, one chapter describes the treatment of individuals with schizophrenia who are parents, and strategies for ensuring that their children's needs are met. This is a topic of considerable importance, especially for women with schizophrenia who have children, but frequently have difficulty fulfilling their parental obligations (Apfel & Handler, 1993). Another chapter describes the treatment of schizophrenia in children and adolescents. This section concludes with a chapter on suicide.

Part VII addresses *Policy, Legal, and Social Issues* related to the treatment of schizophrenia. One chapter in this section discusses the economics of schizophrenia, including estimates of the direct and indirect costs of the illness. Two chapters deal with legal aspects of the care of people with schizophrenia, including involuntary commitment to treatment and treatment in jail and prison settings. One chapter in this section addresses the vexing problem of stigma, including both social rejection and fear of people with the illness, and the dispiriting effects of self-stigma, or the integration of social beliefs about the illness into one's self-concept. Another chapter addresses implementation of evidence-based practices for the treatment of schizophrenia. This topic is of particular importance, because research has shown that a wide range of treatments are effective for schizophrenia, but there has been an unacceptably long delay between the discovery of effective treatments and access to them in public mental health care settings (Drake et al., 2001; Lehman & Steinwachs, 1998). The final chapter in this section addresses schizophrenia in developing nations, a topic that has been the focus of increasing attention in recent years.

Part VIII is devoted to *Special Topics* related to the treatment of schizophrenia. The section begins with a chapter defining criteria for remission of schizophrenia, followed by a chapter on growth and recovery that addresses the paradigm shift from approaching schizophrenia mainly in terms of psychopathology and impairment to exploring the potential of individuals with the illness to achieve personally meaningful recovery and to continue to grow as people. The next chapter in this section addresses issues related to gender, followed by a chapter that considers the topic of quality of life, including both subjective and objective approaches to the issue. Two chapters in this section address the topics of religion (and spirituality) and sexuality, both of paramount importance in the lives of many people with and without mental illness, but frequently neglected in books and guidelines describing the treatment of schizophrenia. One chapter addresses the topic of schizophrenia in African Americans; the extensive research by this chapter's author and his group may have important and useful implications for understanding the complex interrelationships between schizophrenia and race/ethnicity. This section concludes with a chapter on ethics, an increasingly complex topic in both research and clinical practice as treatment options multiply, and the importance of engaging and empowering individuals with schizophrenia in making decisions about their own treatment is now recognized.

The treatment of schizophrenia has now evolved to the point that clinicians, individuals with the illness, and their loved ones have numerous choices, and a more hopeful future. However, to take advantage of the latest developments in the causes and the treatment of schizophrenia, the people interested in this topic need an authoritative yet accessible guide. We hope that our readers will find the *Clinical Handbook of Schizophrenia* a valuable resource in furthering their understanding of schizophrenia, and in guiding their treatment decisions. Ultimately, broad dissemination of scientifically accurate and clinically relevant information is the best means of reducing social stigma against serious mental illnesses such as schizophrenia.

KIM T. MUESER
DILIP V. JESTE

REFERENCES

American Psychiatric Association. (2000). *Diagnostic and statistical manual of mental disorders* (4th ed., text rev.). Washington, DC: Author.

Anthony, W. A. (1993). Recovery from mental illness: The guiding vision of the mental health service system in the 1990s. *Psychosocial Rehabilitation Journal, 16*, 11–23.

Apfel, R. J., & Handler, M. E. (1993). *Madness and the loss of motherhood: Sexuality, reproduction, and long-term mental illness.* Washington, DC: American Psychiatric Press.

Bellack, A. S. (2006). Scientific and consumer models of recovery in schizophrenia: Concordance, contrasts, and implications. *Schizophrenia Bulletin, 32*, 432–442.

Deegan, P. E. (1988). Recovery: The lived experience of rehabilitation. *Psychosocial Rehabilitation Journal, 11*, 11–19.

Drake, R. E., Goldman, H. H., Leff, H. S., Lehman, A. F., Dixon, L., Mueser, K. T., et al. (2001). Implementing evidence-based practices in routine mental health service settings. *Psychiatric Services, 52*, 179–182.

Jeste, D. V., Gladsjo, J. A., Lindamer, L. A., & Lacro, J. P. (1996). Medical comorbidity in schizophrenia. *Schizophrenia Bulletin, 22*(3), 413–430.

Lehman, A. F., & Steinwachs, D. M. (1998). Patterns of usual care for schizophrenia: Initial results from the Schizophrenia Patient Outcomes Research Team (PORT) client survey. *Schizophrenia Bulletin, 24*, 11–20.

Murray, C. J. L., & Lopez, A. D. (Eds.). (1996). *The global burden of disease: A comprehensive assessment of mortality and disability from diseases, injuries, and risk factors in 1990 and projected to 2020.* Cambridge, MA: Harvard School of Public Health, on behalf of the World Health Organization and the World Bank, Harvard University Press.

Torrey, E. F. (1995). Jails and prisons: American's new mental hospitals [Editorial]. *American Journal of Public Health, 85*, 1611–1613.

CONTENTS

I. CORE SCIENCE AND BACKGROUND INFORMATION

II. ASSESSMENT AND DIAGNOSIS

III. SOMATIC TREATMENT

IV. PSYCHOSOCIAL TREATMENT

VII. POLICY, LEGAL, AND SOCIAL ISSUES

VIII. SPECIAL TOPICS

PART I

CORE SCIENCE AND BACKGROUND INFORMATION

CHAPTER 1

HISTORY OF SCHIZOPHRENIA AS A PSYCHIATRIC DISORDER

HELEN LAVRETSKY

HISTORY OF CLINICAL DIAGNOSIS OF SCHIZOPHRENIA

Schizophrenia is one of the most serious psychiatric disorders. It carries a lifetime risk of approximately 1%. The symptoms of schizophrenia remain perhaps the most mysterious form of human psychological experience. The early onset of the disease, most often occurring between ages 15 and 30 years, and its chronic course make this a particularly disabling disorder for patients and their families. Chronic disability results primarily from the negative and cognitive symptoms, whereas acute relapses result from exacerbations of the positive psychotic symptoms, such as delusions and hallucinations. The social and economic impact of the disorder on society and families is enormous.

Despite extensive research, the international psychiatric community still lacks diagnostic precision, clarity of etiology, and knowledge of underlying pathophysiology of schizophrenia. Disputes over concepts and appropriate models of mental illness extend back to classical times. Reports of schizophrenia-like illness can be found even in ancient literature. However, the first comprehensive description dates to the beginning of the 18th century. Schizophrenia was defined as an early dementia in the 19th century. French psychiatrist, Benedict Augustine Morel (1809–1873), coined the term *dementia praecox*, or "precocious dementia."

The modern concept of schizophrenia was first formalized by the German psychiatrist Émil Kraepelin (1856–1927), who integrated contemporary descriptions of catatonia by Kahlbaum (1863), and hebephrenia by Hecker (1871), and his own "dementia paranoia" into a single disorder with an early onset, poor prognosis, and 36 "psychic" symptoms and 19 "bodily" or physical symptoms. Among the most common psychic symptoms were hallucinations occurring in all sensory modalities, but most commonly "hallucinations of hearing." Although Kraepelin defined dementia praecox on the basis of the characteristic course and outcome of a cluster of symptoms and signs, he also stated that it was a disorder with a specific neuroanatomical pathology and etiology. This statement generated an early and continuing interest in the anatomy of the central nervous system underlying schizophrenic process. The sixth edition of Kraepelin's *Textbook of Psychiatry* (1899/1990) distinguished between dementia praecox and manic–depressive disorder. He described one group of patients whose clinical picture was dominated by disordered mood and who followed a cyclical pattern of relapse and relative remission; for this condition, Kraepelin coined the term *manic depressive insanity*. Another group of patients had a deteriorating illness characterized by an acute onset of psychosis in adolescence, with a prolonged course marked by profound social and functional disability; this he called dementia praecox.

Kraepelinian concepts profoundly influenced European and American psychiatry. These diagnostic categories continue to guide our clinical practice and research in the 21st century, despite the fact that Kraepelin himself recognized their limitations, such as the existence of late-onset disorders and the possibility of reasonable functional remission in some individuals.

Kraepelin's (1899/1990) diagnostic concept of dementia praecox was expanded with the inclusion of Magnan and Legrain's (1895) notion of *délire chronique*. By the time of the seventh edition of Kraepelin's (1904) textbook, his concept embraced all disorders with a course leading to psychic invalidism of varying severity. Subsequently, however, he separated paranoid deteriorations (paraphrenias) with prevalent delusions, but without emotional and volitional psychopathology, from the paranoid form of dementia praecox. Then, he identified 10 different forms of dementia praecox: dementia simplex, silly deterioration (replacing the term *hebephrenia*), depressive deterioration, depressive deterioration with delusional manifestations, circular, agitated, periodic, catatonic, paranoid, and schizophasia. Finally, in the eighth edition of his textbook, Kraepelin (1913) described 10 different end states of the disease: cure; cure with defect; simple deterioration; imbecility with confusion of speech; hallucinatory deterioration; hallucinatory insanity; paranoid deterioration; flighty, silly deterioration; and dull, apathetic dementia. In the same edition, he defined *dementia praecox* as a series of clinical states that have as their common characteristic a peculiar destruction of the internal connections of the psychic personality, with the most marked damage to the emotional and volitional life. In 1959, Kurt Schneider further defined a list of relatively easily and reliably identified first-rank symptoms that were considered to be most consistent with the diagnosis of schizophrenia: audible thoughts; arguing or commenting voices; feeling controlled or influenced by an external force; thought withdrawal; diffusion of thought; and delusions.

The Swiss psychiatrist Eugen Bleuler coined the term *schizophrenia* in 1911, and that term rapidly replaced dementia praecox. Although Bleuler subtitled his book on dementia praecox *The Group of Schizophrenias*, his major argument was that the concept of schizophrenia was unified by a single defining phenotype that was present in all patients with the illness. Bleuler thought of schizophrenia in psychological rather than in neuropathological terms. He chose the name *schizophrenia* because it meant literally "a mind that is torn asunder." He developed a hierarchy that distinguished between fundamental and accessory symptoms. *Fundamental symptoms* were shared by all schizophrenia subtypes as a common endophenotype, and included "fragmented" disturbed associations, or what we now term *cognitive disturbances*. Psychic schisis or split, ambivalence, cognitive features of "loose associations," avolition, inattention, autism, and incongruent features signified primary deficits for Bleuler, whereas florid psychotic symptoms of delusions and hallucinations were conceptualized as secondary or *accessory* to the core cognitive disturbances. Bleuler's advanced cognitive theory of schizophrenia was ahead of its time, and difficult to prove and define reliably due to a lack of measurement tools, particularly for the "softer" concepts of "simple" or" latent" types of schizophrenia that addressed personality characteristics of "odd individuals." It required another 100 years of neurocognitive research to narrow down the fundamental schizophrenic deficit of cognitive dysmetria, which Bleuler hypothesized as a disruption of the fluid, coordinated sequences of thought and action that are the hallmark of normal cognition (Andreasen, 1999).

The conceptual confusion at the beginning of the 20th century was compounded by clinical heterogeneity of schizophrenia, lack of clear prognostic features, and failure to discover any definitive pathological abnormalities. Bleuler's approach led to an expansion of the diagnostic concept of schizophrenia that incorporated many other neuropsychiatric disorders, particularly, in the United States during the early development of the *Diagnostic and Statistical Manual of Mental Disorders* (DSM-I and II) through the 1970s, and in the former Soviet Union.

Another prominent influence on the concept of schizophrenia in the United States was provided by the theories of Adolph Meyer, who emphasized the impact of the individual history of each particular patient on the schizophrenia syndrome (Peteres, 1991). Other important broad diagnostic concepts included schizoaffective psychosis (Kasanin, 1933), ambulatory schizophrenia (Zilboorg, 1956), and "pseudoneurotic schizophrenia" (Hoch & Polatin, 1949). DSM-II (American Psychiatric Association, 1968) presented schizophrenia in its broadest interpretation. In 1966, the World Health Organization sponsored the International Pilot Study of Schizophrenia (IPSS; 1973), which investigated the illness in several centers around the world and found a high degree of consistency in the clinical features of schizophrenia when using strict diagnostic criteria. This finding led to the critical revision of diagnostic categories during the 1970s in the United States, with narrowing of its definitions and development of the core symptoms criteria. DSM-III became a turning point for U.S. psychiatry, reintroducing a neo-Kraepelinian approach toward the diagnosis of mental disorders that brought U.S. and European concepts closer. Further revisions of both DSM (III-R and IV) and the *International Classification of Diseases* (ICD-10) brought these systems even closer. Both systems identify a number of subtypes of schizophrenia, and both use only cross-sectional disease status for diagnostic purposes. These diagnostic systems differ only in the affective categorization of psychosis, with mood-incongruent features subsumed under affective psychosis in DSM-IV, and under schizophrenias in the ICD-10.

In addition to the improved clinical diagnostic boundaries, major advances have been made in the psychopharmacological and psychosocial treatments of schizophrenia, providing new hope for improved outcomes of this disabling disease.

HISTORY OF TREATMENT OF SCHIZOPHRENIA

For decades following Kraepelin's seminal description of schizophrenia there was no effective medical treatment. Unfortunate patients were treated with some "desperate" methods, such as prolonged barbiturate-induced sleep therapy, insulin coma, or psychosurgery (Valenstein, 1986). Insulin coma involved creating a hypoglycemic state through administration of large doses of insulin that resulted in loss of consciousness and seizures. A few reports suggested that a series of such insulin shocks might reduce patients' psychotic episodes. However, the technique was never carefully evaluated, and posed risks of heart attack and stroke.

Frontal lobotomies, or leukotomies, involved neurosurgery that cut the nerve tracts of the frontal lobes, thereby reducing agitation and impulsive behavior, but causing additional cognitive impairment. Large numbers of patients underwent the operation, with little demonstrable benefit and little concern for ethical requirements such as informed consent for treatment.

Limited therapeutic options and prospects during the first half of the 20th century meant that thousands of patients with schizophrenia were warehoused in huge psychiatric hospitals. By the mid-1950s, the United States and Canada alone had over 500,000 psychotic inpatients who were hospitalized indefinitely. Despite the efforts of the pioneers of psychiatry to address treatment of schizophrenia, patients' quality of life did not improve. Modern psychopharmacology was started serendipitously. A French naval surgeon, Henry Laborit, was testing a new drug, promethazine, to determine its effect on autonomic nervous system. He was looking for a treatment for circulatory shock after surgeries. However, the secondary properties of the drug included drowsiness, reduced pain, and feelings of euphoria. Laborit published observations of the psychotropic effects of promethazine that stimulated interest of researchers at the laboratories of the firm Rhone-Poulenc. They, in turn, modified the promethazine formula, resulting in the creation of the first effective antipsychotic drug, chlorpromazine. The initial observations of promethazine and chlorpromazine in psychiatric patients reflected the drugs' short-term antipsychotic and sedating effects. Later, a number of clinical trials, especially those by Delay, Deniker, and Harl (1952), and Sigwald and Bouttier (1953) in Europe, Lehmann and Hanrahan (1954) in Canada, and finally, the large, collaborative National Institute of Mental Health (NIMH; Cole, Goldberg, & Klerman, 1964) study in the United States, demonstrated the efficacy of new medications. Chlorpromazine reduced agitation and mood disturbance, as well as positive psychotic symptoms of delusions, hallucinations, and thought disorder, and even some negative symptoms. Patients who received this medication spent less time in the hospital, had fewer relapses, and showed enhanced life functioning compared to untreated patients.

Although psychopharmacological interventions revolutionized care for patients with chronic schizophrenia and changed the cost of care for society, they did not provide a cure. A minority of patients responded poorly to antipsychotic drugs, and even responsive patients had to deal with unpleasant and occasionally disabling side effects. Many patients relapsed, if the drug was discontinued. In addition, even in improved patients, a lack of occupational and daily living skills or social support undermined successful functioning after discharge from the hospital. Such services were not available to a vast majority of chronically mentally ill patients. Deinstitualization of patients with severe mental illness, beginning in the mid-1950s, without adequate follow-up care resulted in a social drift to poverty and stigma despite improvement in treatment outcomes.

The main form of psychotherapy used for schizophrenia in the United States and the United Kingdom until the early 1960s was psychoanalysis or dynamically oriented psychotherapy. The NIMH-sponsored 1964 study showed that such psychotherapy (as well as electroconvulsive therapy) was significantly less effective than antipsychotic drugs. At the same time, it became clear that the medications were only useful for reducing severity of symptoms and for preventing relapse. Supportive psychotherapy was therefore considered an essential adjunct to pharmacotherapy. Subsequently, other forms of psychosocial interventions, such as cognitive-behavioral therapy (CBT), social skills training, supported employment, and family intervention programs, were developed and tested for usefulness in people with schizophrenia. It is now well accepted that medications alone are inadequate for management of schizophrenia, and that a combined psychopharmacological–psychosocial approach is a must for improving long-term outcome in persons with schizophrenia.

PSYCHOPHARMACOLOGY AND NEUROSCIENCE OF SCHIZOPHRENIA

The revolution in psychopharmacology and biological psychiatry started by the introduction of chlorpromazine provided the first effective treatment for schizophrenia, as well as ideas and evidence about the pathophysiology of the illness. There is evidence for a variety of neurochemical abnormalities, ranging from excessive to deficient concentrations of dopamine, serotonin, and glutamate, in studies comparing patients with schizophrenia and controls.

Dopamine

The early 1960s implicated monoamines in the effects of the antipsychotic drugs and in the pathophysiology of schizophrenia and related drug side effects. Dopamine was one of the approximately 10 neurotransmitters distributed diffusely throughout the brain considered for pathophysiology of schizophrenia. The strongest support for a connection between dopamine function and schizophrenia came from studies showing that the clinical efficacy of drugs depends on their ability to block dopamine receptors, especially the dopamine D_2 receptor subtype. These studies, carried out in the 1970s, used postmortem brain tissue samples. The studies of dopamine metabolites in the cerebrospinal fluid and dopamine receptor binding that used *in vivo* functional neuroimaging provided additional evidence for dopamine abnormalities in schizophrenia.

Serotonin

In 1943, Swiss chemist Albert Hoffman ingested a new chemical compound—an ergot derivative called lysergic acid diethylamide (LSD). He experienced psychotic delusions and vivid hallucinations. That experience led him to the studies of drugs that produce psychotic symptoms. LSD seemed to enhance and potentiate the effects of serotonin in the brain. This finding initiated interest in the role of serotonin in schizophrenia, which was rekindled in the late 1980s and early 1990s with the development of atypical antipsychotic drugs, starting with clozapine and risperidone. These compounds appeared to work by blocking both dopamine D_2 and serotonin S_2 receptors. This dual activity distinguished these newer, atypical antipsychotics from the older, typical antipsychotics that only blocked dopamine receptors. The serotonin-blocking action seemed to be an important part of the demonstrated efficacy for positive and, to some extent, negative symptoms of schizophrenia, as well as a reduction in the risk of tardive dyskinesia with atypical compared with typical antipsychotics. Other, newer atypical antipsychotic agents developed since then, such as olanzapine, quetiapine, ziprasidone, and aripiprazole, share this dual neurotransmitter action. However, direct evidence for a primary role of serotonin in the pathophysiology of schizophrenia remains less convincing compared to that for dopamine.

Glutamate

The search for other altered neurotransmitter systems involved in the pathophysiology of schizophrenia continues. Glutamate is a principal excitatory neurotransmitter distributed in the brain structures implicated in schizophrenia, such as the frontal cortex, hippocampus, and entorhinal cortex. Dopamine antagonizes the glutamate system, reducing glutamate release. The most suggestive evidence for the role of glutamate comes from the effects of a drug of abuse, phencyclidine (PCP), which serves as one of the putative neurochemical models for schizophrenia (Kornhuber, 1990). PCP binds to a specific site on the N-methyl-D-aspartate (NMDA) receptor and blocks the action of glutamate, which is considered to be responsible for its analgesic, anesthetic, and physiological effects. Supportive evidence comes from postmortem neuropathological studies reporting reduction in the glutamate transmitter binding in brains of people with schizophrenia. Deficient glutamate neurotransmission may be a primary or secondary, underlying mechanism in schizophrenia.

Other candidate neurotransmitters include aspartate, glycine, and gamma-aminobutyric acid (GABA), collectively dominating excitatory and inhibitory neurotransmission. Eventually, we might discover that dysregulation of several neurotransmitter systems is the unifying underlying mechanism of the disease. Brain imaging studies of receptor densities in young adults and children, or in patients with first-episode schizophrenia may be helpful in identifying early vulnerability factors.

HISTORY OF THE NEUROSCIENCE OF SCHIZOPHRENIA

Over the last two decades, with the rapid development of the neurosciences, new hope and confidence have arisen that schizophrenia will soon be cured or, at least, that its outcome will be dramatically improved. It is our hope that knowledge of the structure and function of the brain yields breakthroughs in science and treatment.

In 1989, the U.S. Congress declared the coming "Decade of the Brain," in expectation of a major victory in conquering serious mental illness by the new millennium. The resulting "explosion" of neuroscience and drug development research did lead to improved schizophrenia treatment portfolios, but unfortunately failed to lead to dramatic changes in the disease course and long-term outcomes. The failure to achieve this goal reflects the complexity of schizophrenia and the limitations of our conceptual understanding of its pathophysiology and diagnostic classification, as well as the limitations of new technologies and research methodology.

For these reasons, in the recent years, schizophrenia research has expanded the search for markers to include behavior, neuroanatomy, neuropathology, and most recently, genetics to define vulnerability to the disease. A genuine marker must be prevalent and occur at high frequency in patients with the disease, and at very low frequencies in people with other disorders or in healthy controls. Next, we review the major historical milestones in schizophrenia research that have led toward identification of biological markers.

Neuroanatomy and Structural Neuroimaging

Since the time of Émil Kraepelin and Alois Alzheimer (who first described what is now considered the most common form of dementia), many investigators have examined neuropathological and neuroanatomical brain changes in schizophrenia. The initial work in this area concerned coarse brain structure, and reported lower brain weight, frontal atrophy, lacunae, pyknotic neuronal atrophy, focal demyelination, and metachromatic bodies. However, the relative lack of gliosis in patients' brains has generated considerable interest, supporting the idea of the neurodevelopmental origin of schizophrenia. Abnormalities in neuronal distribution, cell size, and laminar density in schizophrenic brain tissue have been reported. At the same time, a frequent absence of consistency in findings and small effect sizes have diminished enthusiasm about histopathological findings.

The next technological development, pneumoencephalography, an early precursor of the modern structural neuroimaging techniques, by the American neurosurgeon Dandy in 1919 was applied to the studies of neuroanatomical brain changes in schizophrenia. The main findings were cortical atrophy and ventricular enlargement in patients compared to controls. Pneumoencephalography is a complex, invasive procedure with enormous variations in technical details and potentially serious adverse effects due to the draining of the different amounts of cerebrospinal fluid, and volume-for-volume exchange with air. This technique was replaced with noninvasive computerized axial tomography (CAT) developed in the early 1970s.

CAT findings have supported those of pneumoencephalography, reporting increased cortical atrophy and lateral ventricular enlargement, as well as increased ventricle-to-brain ratio. The effects of medications and other somatic treatments were not examined. Although CAT was a great improvement in neuroimaging tools, with its gradual enhancement of resolution, it did not allow for distinction between gray and white matter, thus precluding precision in localizing pathology and standardization of procedures during rescanning.

In 1984, the first magnetic resonance imaging (MRI) scan study in schizophrenia was published. The images were much clearer than those with CAT, and allowed differentiation of the white and gray matter. MRI studies of schizophrenia consistently reported ventricular enlargement, decreased cortical volume, and disproportionate volume loss in the temporal lobe.

Neuroimaging studies of schizophrenia are limited by their use of convenience clinical samples that are generally small and a lack of specificity of findings (compared to those of other serious mental illnesses). Despite these limitations, the MRI techniques brought an understanding of the neuroanatomical substrates of schizophrenia in sight. Newer MRI techniques, such as magnetic resonance proton spectroscopy, or magnetization transfer and diffusion tensor imaging (DTI) continue to improve the range of investigation from white matter tract connectivity to biochemical changes in the brain, approaching the goals of *in vivo* functional imaging. Enhanced by the new computational brain atlases and statistical algorithms, the morphometric methods offer an advantage of mapping structural abnormalities and correlating them with any other functional, metabolic, spectroscopic, and architectonic data. Furthermore, cortical mapping can also identify deficit patterns associated with genetic risk for schizophrenia, which may provide researchers with the neuroimaging-defined rather then pure clinical endophenotypes.

Functional Neuroimaging

Functional MRI

The first report by Belliveau and colleagues (1991) of localized changes in cerebral blood oxygenation in the occipital cortex following visual stimulation in humans was of seminal importance to neuropsychiatric research. This technological development enabled noninvasive visualization of *in vivo* human brain function (based on investigation of changes in oxyhemoglobin) in response to specific cognitive tasks in patients with schizophrenia compared to age-matched controls. The techniques have the advantage of optimal spatial resolution, and (in comparison to the functional imaging techniques described below) lower cost.

Functional MRI (fMRI) research in schizophrenia has explored a broad range of cognitive functioning, especially executive function, attention, working memory, psychomotor function, and basic sensory processing. fMRI studies further define the hypothesized hypofrontality in the activation studies of schizophrenia, evaluating the subject performance on the executive cognitive tasks. The fMRI approach is well suited for use in the within-subject longitudinal design evaluating changes over time and the effects of treatment and for developing more disease-specific cognitive probes.

Single Photon Emission Computed Tomography and Positron Emission Tomography

The reconstruction of three-dimensional images deriving from radiotracer distribution in the human brain was achieved by Kuhl and Edwards (1964). This achievement gave birth to both single photon emission computed tomography (SPECT) and positron emission tomography (PET).

Functional neuroimaging studies with PET and SPECT have demonstrated three patterns of abnormal cerebral blood flow in schizophrenia. First, abnormal blood flow and glucose utilization in the dorsolateral prefrontal cortex (DLPFC) have been associated with impaired executive functions and working memory. Second, dysfunction of temporal–limbic circuits has been associated with disinhibition of subcortical dopamine release and the manifestation of positive symptoms. Third, positive symptoms, such as auditory hallucinations, have been associated with increased blood flow in subcortical, medial temporal, and limbic brain areas. These findings support the 19th-century theory of Hughling Jackson, the renowned English neurologist. According to this hypothesis, the evolution of the brain increases vulnerability of the frontal or temporal–limbic cortex to the disease. The resulting loss of neuronal function is thought to cause negative symptoms. As a result, evolutionarily older brain areas may become disinhibited, leading to a manifestation of positive symptoms, such as hallucinations and delusions.

PET and SPECT are powerful techniques that enable exploration of the neurochemistry of the living brain. They have been instrumental in testing the hyperdopaminergic theory of schizophrenia, as well as the dopaminergic occupancy theory of antipsychotic drugs. PET and SPECT have also proven to be invaluable tools for measuring drug occupancy at D_2 and other receptors *in vivo*, and exploring relationships between occupancy and clinical measures. This observation presents a clear opportunity for drug development and for further understanding of the psychopharmacological effects of antipsychotic medications and the pathophysiology of schizophrenia.

The development of new and exciting technologies of neuroimaging advances our understanding of the pathophysiological substrates of schizophrenia, generally supporting earlier clinical–neuropathological observations. However, a pattern of brain dysfunction that would serve as a biological trait marker or predict treatment response has not emerged to date. A combination of genetics, cognitive neuropsychology, and multimodal structural–functional neuroimaging can further elucidate vulnerability factors and help define endophenotypes. Despite great advances in technology, neuroimaging remains a research tool for schizophrenia, with no utility for clinical practice at the present time.

Cognitive Neuroscience

While psychoanalysts theorized about psychological causes of schizophrenia, suggesting psychotherapy to resolve infantile traumas and early rejection experiences believed to cause the disease, the search continued for behavioral vulnerability markers. Stemming from the ideas of Bleuler and Kraepelin, it is increasingly believed that impaired cognitive processing may be a marker of vulnerability to schizophrenia, including deficits in attention and concentration, in sustained mental effort, and in selecting and processing information. Physiological indicators can be used as objective markers of cognitive disturbances.

Since the turn of the 20th century, theories of frontal dysfunction have provided a framework that may be helpful in understanding the consequences of injury to the brain. Neuropsychological tests serve as probes of brain dysfunction. The extent to which schizophrenia is a disorder of executive dysfunction remains an object of extensive investigation. Structural and functional imaging, combined with neuropsychological testing, can improve the precision of the search for markers.

Genetics

The first theory about the role of heredity in mental illness was proposed by Morel (1857). He postulated that insanity was the result of an innate biological defect, and that the severity of mental syndromes increased in lineal descents. Morel's theory of hereditary brain degeneration remained in mainstream psychiatry for several decades. Its proponents included Krafft-Ebing (1868) in Austria, Maudsley (1870) in England, Magnan and Legrain (1895) in France, and many others. In the eighth edition of his textbook, Kraepelin (1919/1971) noted that about 70% of his patients with dementia praecox at the Heidelberg Clinic (1891–1899) had family histories of psychosis. His findings set the stage for research in the genetics of the disease. Findings in family studies are consistent with a genetic etiology of schizophrenia. The risk of developing schizophrenia was found to be consistently higher in the relatives of patients with schizophrenia than in the general population, with greater risk for first-degree relatives than for second-degree relatives. In Zerbin-Rudin's (1967) pooled data, the risk for children with one parent with schizophrenia was nearly 15 times greater (12.3%) than that in the general population (0.85%); with siblings and parents, about 10 times greater (8.5% and 8.2%, respectively); and with uncles and aunts (2%), nephews and nieces (2.2%), grandchildren (2.8%), and half-siblings (3.2%), roughly three times greater than the general population rate.

Recent research has identified genetic variations associated with schizophrenia. The primary goal of modern genetic research is first to characterize how genes associated with schizophrenia affect brain development and function, and second, to see how this translates into the clinical manifestation of the disorder. This will ultimately have implications for the prevention and treatment of the disease. The goal has become more immediate as we witness a shift in psychiatric genetics from mapping illness loci to identifying gene effects on information processing in the brain.

Genomic approaches to schizophrenia are also becoming increasingly feasible as data from the Human Genome Project accumulate. However, studies aiming to identify susceptibility genes for schizophrenia and other complex psychiatric disorders are faced with confounds of subjective clinical criteria, commonly occurring phenocopies, significant between-subject variability of candidate traits, and a likelihood of allelic and locus heterogeneity.

Over the past couple of years, several specific genes have been shown to be associated with schizophrenia risk in a number of populations around the world. Some of the genes that have been studied more extensively include catechol-O-methyltransferase (COMT; chromosome 22q), dysbindin-1 (chromosome 6p), neuregulin 1 (chromosome 8p), metabotropic glutamate receptor 3 (GRM-3; chromosome 7q), glutamate decarboxylase 1 (chromosome 2q), and disrupted-in-schizophrenia 1 (DISC1; chromosome 1q). A functional polymorphism in the COMT gene, which affects prefrontal cortical function by changing dopamine signaling in the prefrontal cortex, has probably been studied most extensively. Data suggest that these susceptibility genes influence the cortical information processing that characterizes the schizophrenic phenotype.

Taken together, the new and improved methods of neuroscience are dazzling in their ability to display the biology of the brain. They offer new avenues for developing transgenic animal models of the disease and further advancing our understanding of the pathophysiology of the disease. Genetic influence on neurobiological mechanisms of schizophrenia may be a key to developing future prevention strategies and new "individualized" treatments. The next decade is shaping up to become the "Decade of Translational Neuroscience."

KEY POINTS

- The history of schizophrenia as a psychiatric disorder represents the history of modern neuropsychiatry, neuropsychopharmacology, and neuroscience.
- French psychiatrist Benedict Augustine Morel (1809–1873) coined the term *dementia praecox*, describing clinical features of schizophrenia and postulating that insanity was the result of an innate biological defect, and that the severity of mental syndromes increased in lineal descents as a sign of "degeneration."
- Émil Kraepelin (1856–1927) integrated the contemporary concept of dementia praecox on the basis of the characteristic course and outcome of a cluster of symptoms and signs, but also stated that the disorder had a specific neuroanatomical pathology and etiology.
- The Swiss psychiatrist, Eugen Bleuler, coined the term *schizophrenia* in 1911. Bleuler developed a hierarchy that distinguished between *fundamental* and *accessory* symptoms; fundamental symptoms were shared by patients with schizophrenia and included "fragmented," disturbed associations or neurocognitive disturbances; positive psychotic symptoms were conceptualized as "accessory" symptoms—a product of fundamental symptoms.
- In 1966 the World Health Organization sponsored the International Pilot Study of Schizophrenia, which suggested a high degree of consistency in the clinical features of schizophrenia across the world and led to the critical revision of U.S. diagnostic categories during the 1970s, with narrowing of definitions and development of the core symptom criteria in DSM-III.
- By the end of the 20th century, major advances in neuroscience, neuroimaging, and psychopharmacological and psychosocial treatments of the disease provided new hope for improved outcomes.
- However, a lack of precision of clinical endophenotypes of schizophrenia continues to impede further advances in the development of novel psychopharmacological agents and in disease prevention.
- The new and improved scientific methods combining genetic, neuroimaging, and neurocognitive approaches offer exciting avenues for developing transgenic animal models and advancing our understanding of the pathophysiology of the disease, potentially, leading to the development of new "individualized" treatments.

ACKNOWLEDGMENT

This work was supported by Grant No. K23-MH01948 to Helen Lavretsky.

REFERENCES AND RECOMMENDED READINGS

Amador, X. F., & David A. S. (Eds.). (2004). *Insight and psychosis: Awareness of illness in schizophrenia and relate disorders.* Oxford, UK: Oxford University Press.

American Psychiatric Association. (1968). *Diagnostic and statistical manual of mental disorders* (2nd ed.). Washington, DC: Author.

Andreasen, N. C. (1999). A unitary model of schizophrenia: Bleuler's "fragmented phrene" as schizencephaly. *Archives of General Psychiatry, 56,* 781–787.

Ban, T. A. (2004). Neuropsychopharmacology and the genetics of schizophrenia: A history of the diagnosis of schizophrenia. *Progress in Neuropsychopharmacology and Biological Psychiatry, 28,* 753–762.

Belliveau, J. W., Kennedy, D. N. Jr., McKinstry, R. C., Buchbinder, B. R., Weisskoff, R. M., Cohen, M. S., et al. (1991). Functional mapping of the human visual cortex by magnetic resonance imaging. *Science, 254*, 716–719.

Cohen, C. I. (Ed.). (2003). *Schizophrenia into later life: Treatment, research, and policy.* Washington, DC: American Psychiatric Press.

Cole, J. O., Goldberg, S. C., & Klerman, G. L. (1964). National Institute of Mental Health Psychopharmacology Service Center Collaborative Study Group: Phenothiazine treatment in acute schizophrenia. *Archives of General Psychiatry, 10*, 246–261.

Delay, J., Deniker, P., & Harl, J. M. (1952). Utilisation en thérapeutique psychiatrique d'une phénothiazine d'action centrale élective. *Annales médico-psychologiques, 110*(2), 112–117.

Fleishman, M. (2005). *The casebook of a residential care psychiatrist: Psychopharmacosocioeconomics and the treatment of schizophrenia in residential care facilities.* New York: Haworth Clinical Practice Press.

Hecker, E. (1871). Die Hebephrenie. *Archiv fur Pathologische Anatomic und Physiologic und fur clinische Medizin, 25*, 394–429.

Heinrichs, W. R. (2001). *In search of madness: Schizophrenia and neuroscience.* Oxford, UK: Oxford University Press.

Hoch, P. N., & Polatin, J. (1949). Pseudoneurotic forms of schizophrenia. *Psychiatric Quarterly, 23*, 248–278.

Horrobin, D. F. (2001). *The madness of Adam and Eve: How schizophrenia shaped humanity.* London: Bantam.

Jackson, D. D. (1960). *The etiology of schizophrenia.* New York: Basic Books.

Kahlbaum, K. L. (1863). *Die Gruppierung der psychischen Krankheiten und die Einteilung der Seelenstoerungen.* Danzig, Germany: AW Kafemann.

Kasanin, J. (1933). The acute schizoaffective psychoses. *American Journal of Psychiatry, 90*, 97–126.

Kingdon, D. G., & Turkington, D. (2005). *Cognitive therapy of schizophrenia.* New York: Guilford Press.

Kornhuber, J. (1990). Glutamate and schizophrenia. *Trends of Pharmacological Science, 11*(9), 357.

Kraepelin, E. (1971). *Dementia praecox and paraphrenia.* Huntington, NY: Krieger. (Original work published 1919)

Kraepelin, E. (1990). *Psychiatry: A textbook for students and physicians* (J. Quen, Ed.) (H. Metoui & S. Ayed, Trans.). Canton, MA: Science History Publications. (Original work published 1899)

Kraft-Ebing, R. (1868). *Lehrbuch der Psychiatrie* (2nd ed.). Stuttgart, Germany: Enke.

Kuhl, D. E., & Edwards, R. Q. (1964). Cylindrical and section radioisotope scanning of the liver and brain. *Radiology, 83*, 926–936.

Lavretsky, H. (1998). The Russian concept of schizophrenia: A review of the literature. *Schizophrenia Bulletin, 24*, 537–557.

Lawrie, S. M., Weinberger, D. R., & Johnstone, E. C. (2004). *Schizophrenia: From neuroimaging to neuroscience.* Oxford, UK: Oxford University Press.

Lehmann, H. D., & Hanrahan, G. E. (1954). Chlorpromazine: New inhibiting agent for psychomotor excitement and manic states. *Archives of Neurology and Psychiatry, 71*, 227–237.

Magnan, V., & Legrain, V. (1895). *Des degeneres.* Paris: Rueff.

Maudsley, H. (1870). *Body and mind.* London: MacMillan.

Peteres, U. H. (1991). The German classical concept of schizophrenia. In J. G. Howells (Ed.), *The concepts of schizophrenia: Historical perspectives* (pp. 59–75). Washington, DC: American Psychiatric Press.

Sigwald, J., & Bouttier, D. (1953). Utilization of the neuroplegic properties of chloro-3-(dimethylamino-3'-propyl)-10-phenothiazine hydrochloride (R.P. 4560) in neuropsychiatric therapy. *Presse Medicine, 61*, 607–609.

Valenstein, E. S. (1986). *Great and desperate cures: The rise and decline of psychosurgery and other radical treatments for mental illness.* New York: Basic Books.

Weinberger, D. R. (2005). Genetic mechanisms of psychosis: *In vivo* and postmortem genomics. *Clinical Therapeutics, 27* (Suppl. A), S8–S15.

World Health Organization. (1973). *The International Pilot Study of Schizophrenia and Related Health Problems* (Vol. 1). Geneva: Author.

Zerbin-Rudin, E. (1967). [What are the implications of the current findings in twins for schizophrenia research?] *Deutsche medizinische Wochenschrift, 17*, 2121–2122.

Zilboorg, G. (1956). The problem of ambulatory schizophrenia. *American Journal of Psychiatry, 113*, 519–525.

CHAPTER 2

EPIDEMIOLOGY

DAVID J. CASTLE
VERA MORGAN

This chapter reviews the epidemiology of schizophrenia, covering rates across different settings and over time, and particularly populations that appear to be at high risk. We consider gender differences in schizophrenia, as well as late-onset schizophrenia. We also cover risk factors, both genetic and environmental, and attempt to integrate findings in those domains. Finally, we turn to the longitudinal course of schizophrenia and describe factors that may impact upon outcomes for people with this disorder. But first, we ask how common schizophrenia is.

HOW COMMON IS SCHIZOPHRENIA?

Studies that have attempted to determine rates of schizophrenia are bedevilled by a number of methodological problems that include the following:

- *Definition of illness*. There is still no truly valid definition of the disease entity we call schizophrenia. Indeed, definitions have changed over time, dependent upon the prevailing view of what constitutes this putative disorder, and this can have profound implications for estimates of rates. For example, different duration criteria (anything from 2 weeks to 6 months of symptoms) and age cutoffs (anything from age 40 years to no age limit) result in differential proportions of potential cases being excluded from epidemiological samples.
- *The failure to use valid diagnostic interview schedules*. Many early studies simply applied clinical or "best-guess" diagnoses, with an inevitable lack of consistency across raters. More modern studies have tended to use diagnostic interview schedules or applied operational definitions to case record material. Some such schedules produce diagnoses that correlate well with operational definitions, for example, the Structured Clinical Interview for DSM (SCID), which generates *Diagnostic and Statistical Manual of Mental Disorders* (DSM) diagnoses, and the Diagnostic Interview for Psychoses (DIP; Castle et

al., 2006), which generates, among others, International Classification of Diseases (ICD) and DSM diagnoses. However, others, such as the lay interviewer–administered Diagnostic Interview Schedule (DIS; Robins, Helzer, Croughan, & Ratcliff, 1981) used in the U.S. Epidemiologic Catchment Area (ECA) study (Regier et al., 1984), tends to overdiagnose schizophrenia, producing higher rates than those found in studies using clinician-rated scales.

• *Different methods of case ascertainment.* Many studies have relied solely on inpatient admission data, but this approach undoubtedly misses some cases. Case registers that record all contacts with psychiatric services are a better reflection of true rates, though in some settings a proportion of cases seek help from agencies other than mental health services. To address this problem in its two incidence studies of schizophrenia in a number of countries across the globe, the World Health Organization (WHO) attempted to ascertain all persons with schizophrenia in contact with any treating agency, including traditional healers where appropriate (Jablensky et al., 1992). General population sampling is another approach (mostly for prevalence studies), but this is expensive and the low rates of schizophrenia in the general population require that a very large sample be screened. Using clinicians for this task is not feasible, and lay interviewers, even if trained in the use of structured interview schedules, tend to be inaccurate in case ascertainment (as discussed earlier).

Despite these problems, a number of more recent studies have sufficient rigor to give us a good sense of prevalence and incidence rates of schizophrenia across diverse settings.

Prevalence

Prevalence refers to the number of cases of schizophrenia is a given population at a particular point in time (point prevalence) or over a stipulated period (period prevalence). Because it is a relatively rare disease, but one that tends to be chronic, prevalence studies are generally easier to perform than incidence studies (see below) requiring less ascertainment time to accumulate sufficient numbers of cases for meaningful analysis. However, methodological issues remain, notably those that have to do with sampling frames: In a general population sample, for example, the relatively few cases found would require screening of very large samples to detect any sizable number of schizophrenia cases. Also, the validated brief screening instruments that have been created tend to lose their positive predictive power in samples with low proportions of cases.

An example of a population-based study is the ECA study (Regier et al., 1984), which used lay interviewers to assess cases of mental illness across five sites in the United States. The aggregated point prevalence estimate for schizophrenia was 7.0 per 1,000 population at risk; lifetime risk was 15.0. However, as already mentioned, there were concerns about the validity of diagnosis in this study, suggesting an overestimation of cases.

Another approach is to use an enriched sample, which is likely to contain a higher proportion of cases, enhancing the efficacy of screening instruments. An example is the Australian National Survey of Low Prevalence (Psychotic) Disorders (Jablensky et al., 2000), which ascertained treated cases of psychosis across four geographical catchments with a total population of some 1,000,000. Supplementary estimates were made of patients solely in contact with either their family doctors or a private psychiatrist, as well as those out of contact with services altogether. Point prevalence rates ranged from 3.1 to 5.9 per 1,000.

This finding of relatively little variation in rates across different settings has been largely upheld by other studies. Suggestions that rates were particularly high in Western

Ireland and Yugoslavia have largely been put down to methodological issues, such as inclusion criteria used. However, it does seem that certain settings do have markedly higher rates of schizophrenia. This might be due to a high aggregation of highly genetic cases in inbred communities (e.g., northern Sweden), or drift into urban areas (and perhaps a "toxic" effect of growing up in big cities), leading to higher rates in more urbanized settings. There is also evidence of higher rates in areas with high proportions of migrants or of those ethnic minorities found to be at heightened risk of schizophrenia (see below).

Incidence

Incidence refers to the number of new cases with the onset of the disorder over a certain time period. Landmark incidence studies were conducted by the WHO in a range of developed and developing countries (Jablensky et al., 1992). Case ascertainment was rigorous (discussed earlier), and diagnoses were made according to the CATEGO algorithm linked to the Present State Examination (PSE; Wing, Cooper, & Sartorius, 1974). Rates ranged from 1.6 per 10,000 population at risk (ages 15–54 years) in Honolulu, to 4.2 in a rural Indian site. When a stricter definition of schizophrenia was applied (so-called S+ under CATEGO), rates varied far less, with the lowest being 0.7 (in Denmark) and the highest 1.4 (in Nottingham, United Kingdom). In a recent review of the world literature that included 55 studies, the distribution of rates was much broader, with some studies with higher rates skewing the distribution. The median rate was 15.2 per 100,000, and the central 80% of rates ranged from 7.7 to 43.0 per 100,000. This suggests greater variability in rates than might usually be assumed.

Variations in rates can be influenced (though not entirely accounted for) by a number of the methodological considerations we addressed earlier. One issue is definition of illness. The extent of variation in rates consequent to vagaries of illness definition has been shown clearly in the Camberwell Register First Episode Study (Castle, Wessely, Van Os, & Murray, 1998), where all patients who used psychiatric services in a defined area of southeast London were rediagnosed according to a range of diagnostic criteria. Use of broad ICD-9 criteria (akin to a clinical diagnoses of schizophrenia or related disorders) gave a rate of 19.2 per 100,000 population per year for males, and 17.6 for females; more stringent DSM-III criteria produced rates of 13.9 for males and 6.3 for females; and the rates using very stringent Feighner criteria were 14.8 and 6.0 for males and females, respectively.

These data also point to the fact that males are more vulnerable to schizophrenia than females, and that this difference is more marked when more stringent criteria are applied. This has been confirmed in an analysis of data from 55 studies from around the globe that showed a median male:female risk ratio of 1.4. It is also clear that males with schizophrenia tend to have an onset of illness later than their female counterparts. This, along with the findings of poorer premorbid adjustment and premorbid IQ, and overall worse outcome for males with schizophrenia, has led to the conclusion that males might be differentially susceptible to a severe early-onset form of the illness consequent to neurodevelopemental deviance. Another consideration has been the potential ameliorating effect of endogenous estrogens in females with schizophrenia, leading to a more benign outcome, but also leaving women at risk for a later onset, menopause-related surge in incidence of schizophrenia.

In the controversy about whether the rates of schizophrenia have been declining over the last few decades, studies supporting such a notion are generally from developed countries and have relied on treated incidence statistics, which might be biased expressly by changes over time in treatment service provision models. Furthermore, studies using case registers in a defined setting (e.g., the previously discussed Camberwell Register), have not generally found any decline in rates: indeed, in Camberwell, the rates rose over the two decades from the mid-1980s, in part at least due to an influx of African Caribbeans, who are at a high risk for developing the disorder (see below).

Immigrants and Ethnic Minorities

The literature is replete with evidence to support immigrants' particularly high risk of developing schizophrenia. Most consistently this has been shown for African Caribbean migrants to the United Kingdom. A number of studies using different methodologies and different sets of diagnostic criteria have found that both first-generation migrants and their offspring are at higher risk of developing schizophrenia than native-born white inhabitants.

A recent meta-analysis (Cantor-Graae & Selten, 2005) of 18 studies of migrants from a number of different ethnic backgrounds (one from Australia, and the others from the United Kingdom, the Netherlands, Denmark, and Sweden) yielded a mean weighted relative risk for first-generation migrants (40 effect sizes) of 2.7 (95% confidence interval [CI], 2.3–3.2). For second-generation migrants, the mean relative risk was 4.5 (95% CI, 1.5–13.1). Diagnostic issues did not explain these differences, an important consideration given that some authors have suggested that immigrants are particularly vulnerable to brief psychotic episodes that do not meet stringent criteria for schizophrenia.

There was, however, a positive association between risk of schizophrenia and lower socioeconomic status of region of birth (i.e., those immigrants from developing countries had higher rates than those from developed countries). There was also a significant association with skin color, in that immigrants from countries with a majority of black inhabitants had a relative risk of schizophrenia of 4.8 (95% CI, 3.7–6.2), clearly higher than all migrants combined. The elevated relative risk was found for both males and females.

Thus, it seems clear that migrants have a higher risk of developing schizophrenia than native-born individuals in their own or their adoptive countries. The offspring of migrants also appear to be at heightened risk, though there is more spread in those results. The reasons for this increased vulnerability are complex and may encompass differential migration of vulnerable individuals, and/or biological–social risk factors in the adopted countries. For example, researchers have found an association between rates of schizophrenia and the perception of discrimination in the adopted country.

IS THERE A LATE-ONSET FORM OF SCHIZOPHRENIA?

Kraepelin's original view of dementia praecox was of an early-onset disorder (all individuals under age 40 years, and most under age 25). More recently, DSM-III stipulated that onset of the disorder could not occur after age 45, but this constraint was scrapped in later revisions of the criteria. The European tradition has tended to "allow" an onset of schizophrenia at any age, and there is good evidence for a late "peak" in onsets, predominantly among women, after the age of 60. This group of individuals has been labeled variably "late paraphrenia" and "paraphrenia" (in ICD-9), and most recently "late-onset schizophrenia-like psychosis" (by the International Late-Onset Schizophrenia Working Group). The features are usually of florid and well systematized delusional systems; mostly of a persecutory nature; and auditory, visual, olfactory, and somatic hallucinations in the absence of formal thought disorder or negative symptoms.

What remains somewhat controversial is whether late-onset cases represent the same disease entity, or whether alternative etiological processes are occurring. Some of the risk factors associated with early-onset disorder (see below) are not common in late-onset cases, but a family history of psychosis still bestows an elevated risk (albeit less than that in younger patients). Some researchers have suggested etiological links with mood disorders, and there is good epidemiological and clinical evidence that increased risk is associated with poor premorbid social (but not occupational) adjustment, premorbid paranoid and schizoid personality traits, uncorrected sensory impairment (visual and auditory), and social isolation.

RISK FACTORS

The genetic contribution to schizophrenia is well-documented in tables of morbid risk of the disease for relatives of affected probands, as outlined elsewhere (Glatt, Chapter 6) in this volume. The morbid risk in the monozygotic twin of a proband is estimated to be 48% compared to 1% for the general population. However, transmission within families does not follow a simple Mendelian pattern, and it is likely that schizophrenia is caused by many genes of small effect in combination with stochastic factors, as well as environmental risk factors, that exert their impact independently or interactively with genetic risk.

Although no major environmental risk factor has been definitively demonstrated, a number have been proposed. Unfortunately, at this stage, none of the putative risk factors are specific to schizophrenia or meet all the epidemiological criteria for causality proposed by Mervyn Susser, including strength of association; specificity of cause and of effect; consistency in replicability and in survivability; predictive performance; and theoretical, factual, biological, and statistical coherence.

Obstetric Complications and the Neurodevelopmental Hypothesis of Schizophrenia

There is good evidence that neurodevelopmental deviance contributes to the pathophysiology of schizophrenia. Neuropathological evidence for a neurodevelopmental basis to schizophrenia includes the following:

- Ventricular enlargement already present at the time of onset of symptoms.
- An absence of gliosis in postmortem brain tissue.
- Evidence for cytoarchitectural abnormalities, including neuronal disarray.
- Neuronal malpositioning (possibly as a result of aberrant neuronal migration).

Other evidence for the neurodevelopmental hypothesis comes from elevated levels of minor physical anomalies and abnormal dermatoglyphics in persons with schizophrenia, indicative of neuronal disruption *in utero*. In addition, developmental delays and other motor, social, and cognitive deficits in childhood, apparent well before illness onset, are also important pointers. Further evidence is to be found in the increased risk of pregnancy, birth, and neonatal complications in persons who later develop the disorder, with estimates ranging from a two- to a seven-fold increased risk depending on the study design and the manner in which obstetric complications have been operationalized.

Specific complications that have been significantly associated with later onset of schizophrenia include the following:

- Measures of fetal growth retardation, including measures of small-for-gestational-age births and reduced head circumference.

- Intrauterine infections such as influenza, Coxsackie B, rubella, and toxoplasmosis.
- Malnutrition (specifically, exposure to famine in the northern Netherlands in the winter of 1944–1945 following German blockade of the region).
- Nutritional deficiencies, such as hypovitaminosis D.
- Placentation abnormalities.
- Rhesus factor (RH) incompatibility.

Increasingly, however, researchers are developing more sophisticated frameworks for identifying homogeneous, etiologically plausible obstetric insults, and positive associations have been observed for preeclampsia, fetal distress, low Apgar scores, as well as composite markers of neonatal hypoxic encephalopathy, birth asphyxia, and other hypoxic–ischemic complications. In addition, there is less reliance on crudely summated, generalized scales to measure obstetric complications, and one of the most refined scales currently in use, the McNeil–Sjöström Scale, takes into account the biological plausibility of the obstetric insult, including its potential effect on the developing central nervous system, its severity, and its timing in pregnancy.

The period of greatest vulnerability appears to be the second trimester *in utero*, when one would expect more subtle sequelae to adverse exposures, with consequences for neuronal migration, glial–neuronal interactions, and resultant cortical connectivity. By contrast, there is less evidence of gross organogenic and structural abnormalities in the brain that one might find following first trimester insult, whereas the absence of gliosis provides limited evidence that the impact of exposure was prior to the third trimester. Nonetheless, critical development of the brain is still taking place in the first few years of life and the impact of insults at later stages of development should not be underestimated. The impact is not limited to physical insults, and rearing environment and childhood stressors have also been associated with later schizophrenia.

Season of Birth

Interest in the seasonality of births of individuals who develop schizophrenia has persisted since the results of the first systematic study of the association between season of birth and schizophrenia, published in 1929, showing an excess of winter births among Swiss inpatients. A comprehensive review of the literature in 1997 uncovered over 250 studies of seasonality of births in schizophrenia and affective psychoses. Studies of birth seasonality in the northern hemisphere have consistently shown a winter–spring excess of 5–8% in schizophrenia. The findings in southern hemisphere studies have not been as consistent and, where positive, have tended to show smaller effect sizes. Correlations have been found between season of birth and parameters including sociodemographic factors, family history, and obstetric complications; and between season of birth and specific subtypes, symptoms, and signs in schizophrenia. Explanatory models for seasonal variation in births in schizophrenia cover the following:

- Genetic factors.
- Obstetric complications, particularly those that impact the developing central nervous system, some of which may be environmentally determined (e.g., exposure to viral and bacterial agents).
- External environmental factors, such as variation in light and external toxins, including cigarette smoke, nutritional deficiencies, temperature, and other climatic effects.
- Different procreational habits in the parents of high-risk children.

There is no strong evidence for age-incidence and age-prevalence effects in the findings.

Paternal Age

Recent studies have found an association between schizophrenia and paternal, but not maternal, age, with older fathers more likely to have children who later develop the disorder. This association persists even after researchers control for potential confounders. The association is stronger in nonfamilial cases of schizophrenia, and there appears to be a dose-dependent effect with increasing paternal age. It is suggested that sporadic de novo mutations in male germ cells, which increase with increasing age, may be modifying the expression of the paternal gene.

Urbanicity and Other Social Risk Factors

Urbanicity (generally constructed as urban dwelling but sometimes operationalized as urban birth) is associated with schizophrenia. For the most part, researchers have concentrated on two potential mechanisms underlying this association. On the one hand, the breeder (or causation) hypothesis proposes that urban environments contribute to causation of psychosis through increased exposure to infections, toxins, poverty, stress, and the like. On the other hand, the urban drift (or selection) hypothesis maintains that the increase is due to the drift of affected persons into urban centers. These mechanisms are not mutually exclusive, and both may underlie the association between urbanicity and schizophrenia. There is some evidence that the causation hypothesis may be exerting a stronger impact than the selection hypothesis, and more recent studies suggest that the effect may be genetically mediated.

In utero exposure to maternal stressors (e.g., maternal exposure to the 5-day invasion of the Netherlands in 1940; death of a spouse during the pregnancy period; unwanted pregnancy) has been implicated in schizophrenia. Childhood stressors, such as separation from a parent, death of a parent through suicide, and sexual abuse in childhood, have also been reported as independent risk factors for schizophrenia. It has been proposed that the increased risk of schizophrenia in immigrants (2.7 times higher than in the general population) may be a result of broader social risk factors related to social isolation (discussed previously) or "social defeat."

Burden of Disease, Morbidity, and Mortality

Schizophrenia is one of the top 10 causes of years lived with disability (YLD) worldwide for all ages, and is one of the leading causes of disability adjusted life years (DALY) for 15- to 44-year-olds. A major Australian national survey of the prevalence of schizophrenia and the other psychoses revealed a disturbing picture of disability and reduced quality of life for affected persons. Persons with schizophrenia were more likely than the general population not to have completed secondary education (56.1%) and to be currently unemployed, broadly defined to include formal employment, study, and home duties (77.5%), with a very large proportion (90.6%) reliant on welfare benefits as their main source of income. Over half of the schizophrenia sample (55.5%) reported a chronic course of illness, with 33.1% experiencing a significant clinical deterioration over time. Another one-third of the total (36.9%) described a remittent pattern of illness. Levels of disability and impairment across the entire range of variables assessed were high. Overall, 52.9% of the interviewed sample with schizophrenia experienced serious or major dysfunction in social or occupational functioning, including dysfunction in capacity for self-care (35.3%), participation in daily household activities (50.0%), and ability to socialize (61.2%) and to maintain intimate relationships (48.4%).

The physical health of people with schizophrenia is poor, and detection and treatment rates in this group are notoriously low. Lifestyle factors (poor nutrition, lack of exercise, and high rates of smoking and nonmedical use of drugs) underlie myriad poor health outcomes. In addition, use of antipsychotic medications is associated with an increased risk of a range of conditions, including diabetes and the metabolic syndrome. Smoking, in particular, is a likely contributory factor for the spectrum of morbidity and mortality outcomes related to cardiovascular and cerebrovascular disease.

An excess of HIV and hepatitis, diseases associated with substance abuse, has also been found and is not unexpected given the high levels of drug and alcohol comorbidity in this group. One surprising finding, in view of the high rates of smoking among persons with schizophrenia, has been the reported reduction in cancer incidence and mortality in this population. Some recent studies have not found this association, although one Danish study using national registers confirmed the findings for tobacco-related cancers, including lung cancer, in males but not females. It is posited that age cohort effects may explain some of the inconsistencies and that one may expect to find increased incidence of cancer in younger cohorts who are more likely to be exposed to smoking risks than older, institutionalized cohorts. Although it has been suggested that the reduction in non-smoking-related cancers found in some studies may be due to the protective action of neuroleptic medication, the evidence is not conclusive.

Overall mortality from both natural and unnatural causes is increased in schizophrenia when standardized by sex and age group. The excess in natural causes of mortality covers the range of conditions including cardiovascular disease, cerebrovascular disease, respiratory disease, digestive disease, and genitourinary disease. Moreover, there is compelling evidence from population-based register linkage studies that persons with schizophrenia are underdiagnosed and undertreated for ischemic heart disease but overrepresented in mortality statistics for ischemic heart disease. However, the single largest cause of excessive mortality in schizophrenia is suicide, with suicide rates elevated above not only population rates but also rates for other psychiatric disorders. The risk of suicide is significantly increased in the first year after discharge following inpatient admission, but especially in the first few weeks after discharge.

Marital Status, Fertility, and Fecundity

Social isolation in schizophrenia is pervasive. It is therefore not surprising that, compared to the general population, persons with schizophrenia are less likely to marry or to enter into long-term conjugal relationships. They are also less likely to have children, and if they do have children, they have fewer children. In the Australian National Prevalence Survey across a catchment of 1.1 million persons ages 18–64, a large proportion of the study sample with schizophrenia was single, separated, divorced, or widowed (72.7%). Only a small proportion had children (27.1%). The findings were different for men and women, with women more likely than men to be in long-term relationships and to be parents.

Data from epidemiological studies on fertility and fecundity in schizophrenia challenge researchers to explain why schizophrenia persists, with incidence rates relatively stable over time and place, despite the reported reduction in "reproductive fitness" in persons with the disorder. Some of the hypotheses put forward include the following:

- That low rates of fertility and fecundity in women with schizophrenia are offset by high rates in men with schizophrenia.
- That fertility and fecundity are increased among unaffected family members, who pass on the unexpressed genetic liability.
- That unaffected family members benefit from evolutionary physiological advantages, such as resistance to infection or injury.
- That an increase over time in environmental causal factors, such as obstetric complications, compensates for a reduction over the same time in genetic risk.

However, the supporting evidence for any of these theories is poor, with inconsistent findings and little resolution of the contradictions that arise. Furthermore, it has been proposed that in a model of schizophrenia that includes multiple genes and latent carriers, the impact of lowered reproductive fitness leading to loss of susceptibility alleles would be negligible.

LONGITUDINAL COURSE

The Kraepelinian notion that schizophrenia (actually dementia precox, a severe early-onset subtype of schizophrenia as we know it today) was a disease with an inevitably poor outcome has been challenged by more recent longitudinal studies.

Problems with research in this area include the following:

- *Differences in sample selection.* For example, including only long-term hospitalized cases, inevitably biasing toward a poor outcome.
- *Incomplete ascertainment of cases.* It would be expected that patients lost to follow-up would more likely be those with a good outcome, who no longer required active treatment.
- *Varying duration of follow-up.* Most decline in psychosocial functioning occurs in the first 5 years of the illness and later flattens out or even shows some degree of improvement.
- *Lack of consistency in defining outcome, with various parameters being considered.* For example, symptom alleviation (mostly positive symptoms), social outcome, occupational outcome, "quality of life," and service utilization.

Factors robustly associated with a poorer longitudinal illness course include being male, early onset of illness, poor premorbid social and occupational adjustment, low premorbid IQ, a predominance of negative symptoms, and a lack of affective symptoms. It has been argued that this reflects a particular subtype of schizophrenia consequent to neurodevelopmental deviance (discussed earlier).

A number of other factors serve to perpetuate a poor outcome. These include delayed, suboptimal, or intermittent treatment with antipsychotic medication and ongoing illicit substance use. There is also a strong association between poor outcome and a family environment characterized by so-called high expressed emotion (EE). High EE is a construct that encompasses critical comments, hostility, and/or overinvolvement of family members with nominally more than 72 hours per week of face-to-face contact with the individual. Clinical interventions have been shown to be effective in reducing EE in family members and enhancing outcomes for patients.

KEY POINTS

- Schizophrenia appears in all known human societies at a rate of around 0.5%, though there is variation according to definition of illness and geographical setting.
- Immigrants are at higher risk of developing schizophrenia, as are ethnic minorities.
- Schizophrenia is largely a disorder of young adulthood (expressly in males), but it can manifest for the first time even very late in life.
- The most powerful know risk factor for schizophrenia is genetic, but a number of environmental factors, expressly those afflicting early neurodevelopment, also serve to increase the risk of developing the disorder.
- Social risk factors for schizophrenia include urban birth and upbringing, and being an ethnic migrant.
- Schizophrenia often has a chronic longitudinal course, expressly if the onset of the illness is early in life, insidious in onset, and dominated by negative symptoms.
- Substance abuse is common among people with schizophrenia and is associated with a worse longitudinal course of illness.
- Schizophrenia is often associated with significant psychosocial disability, relationship problems, isolation, and lack of gainful employment.
- People with schizophrenia are at high risk for certain medical problems, including cardiovascular risk factors, that are often underdiagnosed and undertreated, leading to increased mortality.

REFERENCES AND RECOMMENDED READINGS

Brown, S. (1997). Excess mortality of schizophrenia. *British Journal of Psychiatry, 171,* 502–508.

Cantor-Graae, E., & Selten, J.-P. (2005). Schizophrenia and migration: A meta-analysis and review. *American Journal of Psychiatry, 162,* 12–24.

Castle, D. J., Jablensky, A., McGrath, J., Carr, V., Morgan, V., Waterreus, A., et al. (2006). The diagnostic Interview for Psychoses (DIP): Development, reliability and applications. *Psychological Medicine, 36,* 69–80.

Castle, D. J., & Murray, R. M. (1993). The epidemiology of late onset schizophrenia. *Schizophrenia Bulletin, 19,* 691–700.

Castle, D. J., Wessely, S., Der, G., & Murray, R. M. (1991). The incidence of operationally defined schizophrenia in Camberwell, 1965–1984. *British Journal of Psychiatry, 159,* 790–794.

Castle, D. J., Wessely, S., & Murray, R. M. (1993). Sex and schizophrenia: Effects of diagnostic stringency, and associations with premorbid variables. *British Journal of Psychiatry, 162,* 658–664.

Castle, D. J., Wessely, S., Van Os, J., & Murray, R. M. (1998). *Psychosis in the inner city: The Camberwell First Episode Study.* Hove, UK: Psychology Press.

Eaton, W. W. (1991). Update of the epidemiology of schizophrenia. *Epidemiologic Reviews, 13,* 320–328.

Jablensky, A. V., & Kalaydjieva, L. V. (2003). Genetic epidemiology of schizophrenia: Phenotypes, risk factors, and reproductive behavior. *American Journal of Psychiatry, 160,* 425–429.

Jablensky, A., Sartorius, N., Ernberg, G., Anker, M., Korten, A., & Cooper, J. E. (1992). Schizophrenia: Manifestations, incidence, and course in different cultures: A World Health Organization ten-country study. *Psychological Medicine Monograph Supplement 20,* 1–97.

Jablensky, A., McGrath, J., Herrman, H., Castle, D., Gureje, O., Morgan, V., et al. (2000). Psychotic disorders in urban areas: An overview of the methods and findings of the Study on Low Prevalence Disorders, National Survey of Mental Health and Well-Being 1996–1998. *Australian and New Zealand Journal of Psychiatry, 34,* 221–236.

Jones, P., & Cannon, M. (1998). The new epidemiology of schizophrenia. *Psychiatric Clinics of North America, 21,* 1–25.

McGrath, J. J. (2005). Myths and plain truths about schizophrenia epidemiology—the NAPE lecture 2004. *Acta Psychiatrica Scandinavica, 111,* 4–11.

Morgan, V. A., Mitchell, P. B., & Jablensky, A. V. (2005). The epidemiology of bipolar disorder: Sociodemographic, disability and service utilization data from the Australian National Study of Low Prevalence (Psychotic) Disorders. *Bipolar Disorder, 7,* 326–337.

Murray, J. L., & Lopez, A. D. (Eds). (1996). *The global burden of disease.* Geneva: World Health Organization, Harvard School of Public Health, and World Bank.

Regier, D. A., Myers, J. K., Kramer, M., Robins, L. N., Blazer, D. G., Hough, R. L., et al. (1984). The NIMH Epidemiologic Catchment Area Program: Historical context, major objectives, and population characteristics. *Archives of General Psychiatry, 41,* 934–941.

Robins, L. N., Helzer, J. E., Croughan, J., & Ratcliff, K. (1981). The National Institute of Mental Health Diagnostic Interview Schedule. *Archives of General Psychiatry, 38,* 381–389.

Torrey, E. F., Miller, J., Rawlings, R., & Yolken, R. (1997). Seasonality of births in schizophrenia and bipolar disorder: A review of the literature. *Schizophrenia Research, 28,* 1–38.

Van Os, J., & Marcelis, M. (1998). The ecogenetics of schizophrenia: A review. *Schizophrenia Research, 32,* 127–135.

Wing, J. K., Cooper, J. E., & Sartorius, N. (1974). *The measurement and classification of psychiatric symptoms.* Cambridge, UK: Cambridge University Press.

CHAPTER 3

BIOLOGICAL THEORIES

JONATHAN DOWNAR
SHITIJ KAPUR

Despite more than a century of research, the cause of schizophrenia remains, in the words of Winston Churchill (1939), "a riddle wrapped in a mystery inside an enigma." In the last few years a long list of *in utero* risk factors and developmental abnormalities has been assembled, imaging technologies have produced a list of established macroscopic abnormalities, genetic studies have begun to reveal specific gene loci conferring a risk of disease, and tantalizing glimpses of microscopic abnormalities have also emerged. All of these pieces are beginning to come together, providing a sense of how nature and nurture interact to give rise to this enigma.

The story of the treatment of schizophrenia is somewhat clearer than the story of the disease itself. The era of effective antipsychotic drugs began more than 50 years ago, and over the last five decades we have developed a much more definitive understanding of antipsychotic drugs: We have learned what receptors they bind to, which brain regions they interact with, and what psychological processes they impact. However, in the absence of a clear picture of what is wrong in schizophrenia in the first place the two stories march in parallel.

In keeping with this state of knowledge, we first review the biological theories of schizophrenia, then describe the knowledge about the mechanism of action of currently available antipsychotic treatments. In the end we present a framework that may be helpful in linking the major aspects of the biology, phenomenology, and pharmacology of psychosis in schizophrenia.

BIOLOGICAL THEORIES OF SCHIZOPHRENIA

Early Theories of Schizophrenia

Early descriptions of schizophrenia focused on the phenomenology of the disease. In 1893, Kraepelin developed the diagnostic category of *dementia praecox*—premature dementia—to describe the rapid, early-onset development of cognitive dysfunction. Dementia praecox was initially subdivided into subforms: simple, paranoid, hebephrenic or "silly," and catatonic. In 1908, Bleuler replaced the term *dementia praecox* with the modern term *schizophrenia*. Basic symptoms included the "four A's" of loosened associations, inappropriate affect, ambivalence, and autism. These criteria were widely used for 50 years. In 1957, Schneider produced a new formulation that included "first-rank symptoms": audible thoughts, voices arguing or discussing or commenting, thought control or thought broadcasting, "made" acts and emotion, and delusional perceptions. These phenomenological descriptions have influenced the current diagnostic systems around the world. Current diagnostic approaches, such as the fourth edition of the *Diagnostic and Statistical Manual of Mental Disorders* (DSM-IV) and the 10th edition of the *International Classification of Diseases* (ICD-10), describe not only the positive symptoms of delusions, hallucinations, and disorganized behavior and speech, but also negative symptoms such as alogia, avolition, and flattened affect. The distinction between positive and negative symptoms becomes important for some neurobiological theories of schizophrenia.

Environmental Factors

Most of the identified risk factors for schizophrenia involve events occurring during pre- or perinatal rather than postnatal development. In rough order of strength, these include winter birth; urban birth; intrauterine infections (rubella in particular, but also influenza, polio, and respiratory and central nervous system [CNS] infections); maternal stressors (bereavement in particular, but also famine, flood, unwanted gestation, and depression); obstetric complications (neonatal CNS injury in particular, but also low birthweight, preeclampsia, hypoxia, and Rhesus factor incompatibility). At present, it is unknown what common "mechanism of injury" leads from these risk factors to the onset of schizophrenia, or why symptoms such as psychosis only appear decades later.

Postnatal environmental risk factors for schizophrenia are also beginning to be identified. Cannabis use, particularly in early adolescence, is associated with the development of psychosis. Certain individuals, comprising a "psychosis-prone" subpopulation, may be especially vulnerable. It remains controversial whether cannabis use actually causes psychosis, or whether the association merely reflects higher use of cannabis in the psychosis-prone subpopulation. One interpretation is that cannabis does not so much cause schizophrenia in otherwise healthy individuals as it "unmasks" schizophrenia in those with a genetic predisposition toward the disease.

Social and environmental stressors may have similar effects on individuals who are vulnerable to schizophrenia. A personal or family history of migration is an important risk factor, increasing the risk of schizophrenia threefold. Other environmental stressors associated with schizophrenia include urban residency, minority ethnicity, childhood trauma, and social isolation. It is suggested that discrimination, or other forms of social or economic adversity, may cause some individuals to develop a cognitive bias toward paranoid or delusional thinking. In addition, the stress of such experiences, like the pharmacological stress of cannabis, may provide a final push that tips vulnerable individuals into developing a dysregulated neurochemical state, with psychotic symptoms emerging as a result.

Neuroanatomical Abnormalities

Macroscopic Abnormalities

Computed tomography (CT) and magnetic resonance imaging (MRI) neuroimaging studies have identified abnormalities of brain structure in schizophrenia. Well-established findings include enlarged lateral ventricles and reduced volumes of the hippocampus, parahippocampal gyrus, and amygdala. Some studies have also shown smaller prefrontal cortex (in correlation with negative symptoms) and auditory cortex of the superior temporal gyrus (in correlation with hallucinations). In comparison studies of monozygotic twins, the affected sibling shows smaller whole-brain volume overall, enlarged third and lateral ventricles, and specific volume reduction in the hippocampus and frontal lobes.

The limitations of volumetric studies should be noted here. First, they do not specify the microscopic pathology present in a region of reduced volume. Second, they may fail to identify regions where subtle pathology exists without reducing overall volume (e.g., ectopy or miswiring). Third, it is currently unclear how the macroscopic abnormalities of schizophrenia lead to positive, negative, and cognitive symptoms. Nonetheless, all of the evidence leaves little doubt that schizophrenia is a "brain disorder," though none of these abnormalities at the moment are pathognomonic or diagnostic.

Microscopic Abnormalities

Microscopic abnormalities in schizophrenia have been suggested in several regions, including hippocampus and entorhinal cortex, anterior cingulate cortex, and prefrontal cortex. Changes in gross neuron size and number have been reported, as well as a variety of changes in neuronal organization and structure. The significance of these findings is currently uncertain.

There is more revealing evidence for developmental abnormalities of the cortex at the microscopic level. Neurons migrate into the cortex in an "inside-out manner" during development; early neurons form lower cortical layers, and later neurons migrate through these from below to form higher cortical layers. Studies of frontal cortex, entorhinal cortex, and limbic cortex show reduced numbers of certain neuronal types in higher cortical layers. Instead, these neurons appear in lower layers, or even in subcortical white matter, as if their migration had arrested too early. Because this stage of neural migration occurs during the second trimester of pregnancy, the timing is coincident with many known schizophrenia risk factors. Abnormal neural migration in schizophrenia is likely to be a promising area for future research.

Genetic Factors

Of all known risk factors for schizophrenia, family history is the most powerful. The heritability of schizophrenia, or total variability explained by all genetic factors, is 81%. Monozygotic twins are 40–50% concordant for schizophrenia compared to 10% for fraternal twins. The risk of schizophrenia survives adoption into families without schizophrenia. These findings indicate that the genome carries a substantial share of the burden of schizophrenia risk, but these findings do not specify which particular genes bear the brunt of the burden.

Recently, genomewide linkage and association studies have revealed a steadily growing set of candidate genes for schizophrenia risk. Their functions are diverse, but these genes fall into two broad categories: neurotransmission and neurodevelopment/plasticity.

In the neurotransmission category, risk-conferring genes include an overactive allele for the dopamine-metabolizing enzyme catechol-O-methyltransferase (COMT), proposed to cause dopamine deficiency resulting in prefrontal dysfunction leading to cognitive and negative symptoms; underactive alleles for *dysbindin*, which are proposed to interfere with glutamate neurotransmission at the postsynaptic level; underexpression of the gene *RGS4*, thought to interfere with the guanine nucleotide–binding protein (G-protein) signaling pathway used by dopamine and some glutamate receptors; dysfunctional alleles of the genes *G72* and *GRM3*, thought to alter glutamate neurotransmission in the hippocampus and prefrontal cortex, thereby giving rise to the cognitive abnormalities seen in schizophrenia.

In the neurodevelopment/plasticity category, a prominent risk-conferring gene is *neuregulin*, thought to regulate neuronal migration, axonal guidance, myelin formation, and synapse formation—events coincident with the prenatal–natal environmental risk factors for schizophrenia. Another is *DISC1* (disrupted-in-schizophrenia-1), which has an allele associated with schizophrenia, reduced hippocampal gray matter, and hippocampal function abnormalities in functional MRI (fMRI) studies. *DISC1*, like *neuregulin*, is thought be involved in neural development and plasticity through a variety of roles in neuron migration and development, as well as receptor turnover.

A wide variety of other genes, many thought to play supporting roles in the key functions described earlier, are being added to the list of schizophrenia risk factors. The emerging picture from these findings is that schizophrenia risk develops through a complex interaction between genes guiding development and plasticity, genes guiding neurotransmission, and their environmental context.

Neurochemical Hypotheses

The Dopamine Hypothesis

The dopamine hypothesis postulates that the symptoms of schizophrenia result from dysregulation of dopamine in the CNS. Four dopaminergic anatomical pathways are described in this model. The *mesolimbic pathway* projects from the ventral tegmental area (VTA) to limbic areas. Excessive mesolimbic dopamine may lead to positive symptoms of schizophrenia, such as delusions and hallucinations. The *mesocortical pathway* projects from VTA to cortex, particularly prefrontal cortex. *Low* mesocortical dopamine is proposed to cause the negative symptoms and cognitive deficits of schizophrenia. The *nigrostriatal pathway,* from the substantia nigra to the striatum, regulates movements; low nigrostriatal dopamine leads to Parkinsonian motor symptoms. The *tuberoinfundibular pathway* travels from the hypothalamus to the pituitary gland and inhibits prolactin secretion; blockade of tuberoinfundibular dopamine leads to elevated prolactin and resultant galactorrhea, amenorrhea, and decreased libido.

There remains some controversy over the role of excess mesolimbic dopamine in psychosis. On the one hand, drug effects support this model: Dopamine agonists such as amphetamines and cocaine provoke psychotic symptoms in normal subjects and those with schizophrenia; likewise, effective antipsychotic drugs bind and block the D_2 subtype of dopamine receptors. Early studies showed increased dopamine metabolites and dopamine receptors in schizophrenia. Positron emission tomography (PET) imaging studies confirm increased synthesis of dopamine, increased levels of synaptic dopamine, and increased dopamine release in response to stressors such as amphetamine challenge.

On the other hand, increased levels of mesolimbic dopamine and dopamine receptors have not been consistently shown across studies and remain controversial. Furthermore, many cases of schizophrenia are unresponsive to D_2 blockade. Finally, some antipsychotic drugs, such as the atypical agent clozapine, have relatively poor D_2 binding, which suggests that other neurotransmitters or receptors may be involved. On the whole, current evidence appears to support a central role for striatal D_2 receptors in acute psychosis.

The role of low mesocortical dopamine in negative and cognitive symptoms is also controversial. On the one hand, a correlation has been shown between low levels of dopamine metabolites in cerebrospinal fluid (CSF), low cortical dopamine, and the poor performance on working memory tasks are seen in schizophrenia. Likewise, dopamine agonists improve prefrontal activation and cognitive performance in schizophrenia. Yet postmortem studies have not clearly shown altered dopamine receptor levels in prefrontal cortex in patients with schizophrenia. PET studies have shown increased, decreased, or unchanged receptor levels, depending on the radiotracer used. It has been proposed that increases may actually reflect compensation for low prefrontal dopamine levels; this would make the significance of either an increase or decrease unclear.

It is possible that the ongoing controversies over the role of dopamine in positive and negative symptoms results in part from the crudeness of available measuring techniques. Dopamine is thought to help define and "sharpen" cortical representations of sensation and action, enhancing salient patterns and dampening nonsalient ones. Attempting to explain brain dysfunction in terms of simple increases or decreases in dopamine may therefore be as futile as trying to measure the accuracy of a drawing by how much ink it contains. Subtle *dysregulation* of dopamine, whether in prefrontal cortex or striatum, could cause major deficits in information processing without overall excess or lack of dopamine.

The Glutamate Hypothesis

The glutamate hypothesis proposes that dysfunction of the N-methyl-D-aspartate (NMDA) glutamate receptor is the primary deficit underlying all the positive, negative, and cognitive symptoms of schizophrenia. Glutamate is the major excitatory neurotransmitter in the CNS. The NMDA receptor plays key roles in attention, perception, and cognition. Importantly, this receptor also plays critical roles in developmental processes such as axonal guidance, synaptic pruning, and plasticity, both *in utero* and during adolescence. For these reasons, the NMDA receptor is an attractive target for schizophrenia research.

As with the dopamine hypothesis, the glutamate hypothesis originates in early findings of low glutamate levels in the CSF of patients with schizophrenia, and in the observation that the effects of NMDA antagonist drugs (ketamine, phencyclidine [PCP]) mimic some of the positive, negative, and cognitive features of schizophrenia. Postmortem studies show changes in the expression of NMDA receptors and their related proteins in schizophrenia. Many genes conferring schizophrenia risk appear to interact with the NMDA receptor in some way (such as *GRM3*, described earlier). Recent PET imaging also suggests reduced hippocampal NMDA receptor binding in schizophrenia.

Glutamate models may be able to accommodate existing dopamine-centered hypotheses on schizophrenia. In one model, reduced prefrontal glutamate neurotransmission leads to reduced prefrontal activity. This results in decreased mesocortical activity, causing negative and cognitive symptoms. It also results in a loss of regulation in the mesolimbic projections. This pathway becomes hyperresponsive to stress or pharmacological challenge, leading to acute episodes of psychosis. Of note here, cannabis reduces corticostriatal glutamate release, while D_2 receptor blockade increases glutamate release. Dopamine–glutamate models may be able to explain how cannabis and dopamine agonists provoke psychosis, and how D_2 antagonists improve positive symptoms.

Glutamate-centered theories offer a potential means of unifying genetic, developmental, neuropathological, and neurochemical understanding of schizophrenia. Lines of supporting evidence for NMDA-related dysfunction in schizophrenia are beginning to emerge. Research over the next few years should determine whether this trend continues, and whether the glutamate hypothesis can inspire new approaches to treatment.

MECHANISM OF ACTION OF ANTIPSYCHOTIC DRUGS
History of Antipsychotic Drugs

The first antipsychotic drugs were discovered serendipitously. In 1950, the French chemist Charpentier synthesized chlorpromazine as an intended surgical sedative. The surgeon Laborit noted that it induced a profound state of "indifference" to surroundings. He persuaded psychiatric colleagues Hamon and Delay to use the drug on patients with psychoses. In subsequent years its use became widespread. Chlorpromazine represented the first of a new class of so-called typical antipsychotic drugs. Subsequently, several other typical antipsychotics were developed, with similar pharmacology and clinical effects.

The history of atypical antipsychotics is almost as long. In 1958, Schmutz and colleagues synthesized clozapine. Though effective as an antipsychotic, clozapine not only failed to induce extrapyramidal symptoms in animal models but also showed the potentially fatal side effect of agranulocytosis. These factors initially slowed its adoption worldwide. However, in 1989 a large study showed clozapine to have superior efficacy over the typical antipsychotics. Subsequently, a second generation of atypical antipsychotics was developed. This class is now usually taken to include risperidone, olanzapine, quetiapine, and ziprasidone in addition to the older clozapine. Sertindole, aripiprazole, and amisulpride are sometimes included as well.

The usefulness of the commonly used distinction between "typical" and "atypical" antipsychotics is controversial. In general, typical antipsychotics are usually described as having a common mechanism of D_2 blockade, effectiveness against positive symptoms, a tendency toward extrapyramidal symptoms at high doses, a greater need for anticholinergic remedies to these symptoms, tardive dyskinesia with chronic use, and prolactinemia. Atypicals are usually described as having an effect on positive symptoms with fewer extrapyramidal side effects, a lesser need for anticholinergics, less prolactinemia, possible improvement in both negative and positive symptoms, and possible greater effectiveness in cases refractory to typical antipsychotics.

Of note, a recent large trial found no reduction in extrapyramidal side effects in the novel atypicals risperidone, olanzapine, ziprasidone, or quetiapine versus the typical perphenazine. The distinction between "typical" and "atypical" antipsychotics may become less useful with the development of still newer agents whose properties do not clearly match either category.

Typical Antipsychotics

Typical antipsychotics are proposed to act on positive symptoms by reducing activity in the mesolimbic pathway, as discussed earlier. Unwanted side effects may occur via blockade of the other pathways. Reductions in mesocortical activity may worsen cognitive and negative symptoms. Nigrostriatal blockade may lead to Parkinsonian symptoms, and tuberoinfundibular blockade may lead to elevated prolactin and resultant galactorrhea, amenorrhea, and sexual dysfunction.

The potency of typical antipsychotics correlates with their affinity for the D_2 receptor. *In vivo* PET studies show that therapeutic doses of most antipsychotics occupy 60–80% of D_2 receptors. Clinical response appears at a mean occupancy level of 65%. Hyperprolactinemia appears at a mean occupancy of 72%, and extrapyramidal symptoms appear at a mean occupancy of 78%. This also holds true for the majority of atypical antipsychotics, with the exception of clozapine and quetiapine. These atypical antipsychotics have clinical effects at merely 10–45% D_2 occupancy; the significance of this finding is discussed below.

Recent computer models of D_2 receptor structure suggest that receptor binding is far more complex than the "key-in-a-lock" description traditionally used. D_2 is a membrane-bound receptor whose structure contains seven helices spanning the membrane. Dopamine appears to bind in an epitope between helices 3, 4, 5, and 6, and acts by drawing together helices 3 and 5. D_2 agonists appear to bind in the same epitope with similar effects. In contrast, D_2 antagonists divide into two classes. Class I agents (e.g., clozapine, raclopride) bind to the same epitope as dopamine, but prevents 3–5 coupling. Class II agents (e.g., haloperidol, domperidone, spiperone, sulpiride) bind to an entirely different epitope formed between the midsections of helices 2, 3, 6, and 7. Here, in addition to preventing 3–5 coupling, they cause an entirely separate, strong coupling between helices 3 and 6.

These findings suggest that the process of D_2 antagonism may be more complex than simple "blockade" of a receptor site. Some D_2 antagonists may work by binding to the same site as dopamine, but without causing the necessary conformational changes for signal transduction. Others may bind at an entirely different site, causing a conformational change that prevents dopamine from binding to its usual epitope.

Atypical Antipsychotics

Atypical antipsychotics are generally considered to be effective against not only positive symptoms but also negative symptoms, with a lower incidence of Parkinsonian side effects and elevated prolactin. The most widely accepted model of how this occurs proposes that atypical antipsychotics act via a dual blockade of not only D_2 but also serotonin 5-HT_{2A} receptors. Serotonin inhibits dopamine release, but it does so to different degrees in different pathways. In the serotonin–dopamine antagonist hypothesis, 5-HT_{2A} blockade reverses the effects of dopamine blockade in the nigrostriatal pathway, leading to fewer Parkinsonian side effects. Similar reversals in the tuberoinfundibular and mesocortical pathways avoid the elevated prolactin and negative and cognitive side effects seen with typical agents. However, serotonin's inhibitory effect is considered minimal in the mesolimbic pathway. Hence, atypical agents still reduce mesolimbic activity and improve the symptoms of psychosis. In other words, adding 5-HT_{2A} blockade to D_2 blockade is proposed to confine the effects of atypical agents to the desired (mesolimbic) pathway alone, thereby achieving the desired effects while avoiding the unwanted side effects.

Objections have been raised to the 5-HT_{2A}–D_2 blockade theory of atypicality. First, there is no direct demonstration that adding 5-HT_{2A} antagonist agents to typical antipsychotic regimen results in atypicality. Second, many typical antipsychotics have a strong component of 5-HT_{2A} blockade in addition to D_2 blockade. Third, some atypical antipsychotics, such as risperidone, become "typical" (i.e., give rise to extrapyramidal side effects) at higher doses despite near total 5-HT_{2A} blockade. Fourth, agents that block 5-HT_{2A} without D_2 blockade are poorly effective as antipsychotics. Fifth, the degree of atypicality among agents is considered to be quetiapine > olanzapine > risperidone, whereas the order of 5-HT_{2A} to D_2 blockade ratios for these agents is the opposite. In summary, there are several lines of evidence that activity at 5-HT_{2A} is neither necessary nor sufficient to explain atypicality. The relevance of 5-HT_{2A} antagonism to atypicality remains a subject of ongoing debate.

An alternative account, known as the "fast-off" hypothesis, proposes that an agent's atypicality depends on its rate of dissociation from the D_2 receptor rather than its effects at other receptors. In this model, all antipsychotics must block the D_2 receptor to be effective against positive symptoms. Their degree of atypicality depends on how easily they can be displaced from the D_2 receptor by endogenous dopamine. In effect, they must be "strict" enough to block D_2 overactivity, but "permissive" enough to allow for some physiological signaling.

The fast-off proposal accommodates findings that clozapine and some other atypical antipsychotics have significantly lower D_2 binding than typical agents. It also accommodates the observation that low D_2 affinity is a better predictor of atypicality than high 5-HT_{2A}

affinity, or affinity at other receptors. However, the fast-off theory also has difficulties: Several of the atypical antipsychotics have rather high affinities and slow dissociation (e.g., risperidone, sertindole); several of the newer atypicals in development have even higher D_2 affinities and presumably slower dissociation (e.g., lurasidone, asenapine); the fast-off idea is focused mainly on the dopamine D_2 blockade properties, and may hence explain the anti-"psychotic" aspect of atypicals, but it does not address the negative symptom and cognitive deficit efficacy of the newer agents.

As is evident, a consensus on the mechanism of action of atypical antipsychotics has yet to emerge. To complicate matters, a so-called third generation of antipsychotic medications is now emerging. The clinical effects and receptor binding profiles of these new agents are distinct from either first-generation/typical antipsychotics or second-generation/atypical antipsychotics.

Third-Generation Antipsychotics

A number of recently developed antipsychotics have promising effects on negative and cognitive symptoms and refractory cases. These agents have receptor profiles that do not clearly fit with either 5-HT_{2A}–D_2 or a fast dissociation from D_2 as their primary mode of action.

An example of this new class is aripiprazole, which is a partial agonist rather than an antagonist at D_2. Partial agonists block the usual transmitter from binding. However, unlike antagonists, they also provide a partial degree of stimulation. Aripiprazole effectively behaves as a weakened version of dopamine at the D_2 receptor. Interestingly, the structure of aripiprazole falls within the Class II (e.g., haloperidol) rather than the Class I (e.g., clozapine) antagonists described previously. In other words, aripiprazole is structurally more similar to a typical antipsychotic, but clinically it acts as an atypical antipsychotic. Additional effects of aripiprazole at 5-HT_{2A} and 5-HT_{1A} complicate its pharmacology even further.

Another new agent in schizophrenia is amisulpride, which is a selective D_2 and D_3 antagonist acting on presynaptic autoreceptors at low doses and postsynaptically at high doses. The presynaptic effects result in enhancement rather than blockade of dopamine neurotransmission at low doses. Amisulpride shows particular promise for treating the negative symptoms of schizophrenia.

One final point is that the optimal pharmacological strategy for treating schizophrenia may not lie in searching for a single "one-size-fits-all" agent with a precisely optimized suite of dopamine, serotonin, and other receptor binding properties. Rather, it may be more effective to use a regimen of multiple complementary agents tailored toward treating the distinct positive, negative, and cognitive symptoms of each individual patient. The role of complementary nonpharmacological treatments may be equally important, as described in the next section.

LINKING BIOLOGY, PHENOMENOLOGY, AND PHARMACOLOGY

Patients with schizophrenia present to the emergency room complaining of delusions and hallucinations, not dopamine overload. The symptoms of psychosis are perceptual, behavioral, and cognitive, yet the predominant theories are neurochemical. How may this gap be bridged?

Perception, behavior, and cognition are functions of widespread, distributed networks of neurons operating across the brain. These networks link value-neutral sensory representations to value-laden representations of the internal milieu: homeostasis, basic drives, motivations, and emotional states. They add "salience," or subjective importance, to an otherwise unprioritized sensory world.

Dopamine can be considered a neurochemical "salience marker" for networks representing sensations and actions. If dopamine becomes dysregulated, features of the sensory world may become "aberrantly salient": subjectively important when they should not be, or vice versa. This may lead to the perceptual disturbances of schizophrenia: disproportionate significance of stimuli such as police cars, or particular numbers or letters. Ultimately these are incorporated into delusional beliefs: attempts to explain the perceptual disturbances via the brain's usual confabulatory mechanisms.

D_2 receptor blockade may dampen these aberrant saliences. This would stop further perceptual disturbances and remove the basis for further delusions. This process would occur relatively quickly, along the time course of the D_2 blockade. However, existing delusions would remain, and would need to be gradually extinguished—a lengthier process requiring cognitive or behavioral approaches.

One prediction of this hypothesis is that ideal treatment of psychosis has two components: pharmacological dopamine blockade to prevent new delusions from forming, and ongoing cognitive therapy to extinguish or reformulate existing delusions. A less encouraging prediction is that it may be difficult to block only aberrant saliences without also blocking the normal saliences that enable functional, goal-directed behavior. In other words, indifference may be the price of avoiding psychosis. As discussed earlier, the use of agents with less "strict" dopamine blockade might be one way of leaving room for some physiological signaling of salience. It remains to be seen whether these agents prove more advantageous in clinical practice.

KEY POINTS

- Despite extensive investigations, the etiology and pathophysiology of schizophrenia remain incompletely understood.
- A complex interaction of multiple genes guiding neurotransmission and neurodevelopment may create a vulnerability to environmental influences that lay the groundwork for schizophrenia before or at birth.
- Neurodevelopmental abnormalities may involve glutaminergic or gamma-aminobutyric acid (GABA)-ergic neurons, and may involve abnormal migration or pruning, possibly via the NMDA receptor.
- One result of the putative neurodevelopmental process is a dysregulated state of elevated dopamine in ventral striatum and possibly low dopamine in prefrontal cortex.
- Overactivity in the mesolimbic dopamine pathway may lead to psychosis. Correcting this state via blockade of dopamine D_2 receptors resolves the positive symptoms in most (but not all) cases.
- Underactivity or dysregulation in the mesocortical dopamine pathway may lead to negative and cognitive symptoms. Atypical antipsychotics may be more effective in correcting this state (and resolving negative symptoms) via blockade of D_1, $5-HT_{2A}$, or other receptors. However, this state and the associated negative symptoms remain more refractory to treatment than the positive symptoms.
- The brain may use dopamine as a neurochemical marker of the salience (i.e., subjective relevance) of events. Dopamine dysregulation may lead to the creation of dysfunctional "aberrant saliences," abnormally salient perceptions that ultimately coalesce into delusional beliefs.
- Optimal treatment of psychotic episodes may require two approaches: (1) treatment of mesolimbic overactivity with antipsychotic medication to prevent new aberrant saliences from forming and (2) ongoing cognitive therapy to extinguish or reformulate any aberrant saliences that have already formed during the psychotic episode.

- The heterogenous nature of schizophrenia is often lost in the current diagnostic approaches, which may be conflating several distinct pathologies with similar surface symptoms. Multiple pathological categories of schizophrenia may be delineated on neurochemical or other bases, and each category may have a different optimal treatment strategy.
- The ideal pharmacological treatment for schizophrenia ultimately may come not from a single "fix-all" compound with a particular receptor binding profile, but from a combination of agents, each targeted to different features of the disease on an individual-by-individual basis.

REFERENCES AND RECOMMENDED READINGS

Ban, T. A. (2004). Neuropsychopharmacolgy and the genetics of schizophrenia: A history of the diagnosis of schizophrenia. *Progress in Neuropsychopharmacology and Biological Psychiatry, 28*(5), 753–762.

Belsham, B. (2001). Glutamate and its role in psychiatric illness. *Human Psychopharmacology, 16,* 139–146.

Churchill, W. (1939, October). Radio broadcast. Retrieved June 6, 2007, from *www.phrases.org.uk/meanings/31000.html*

Harrison, P. J., & Weinberger, D. R. (2005). Schizophrenia genes, gene expression, and neuropathology: On the matter of their convergence. *Molecular Psychiatry, 10,* 40–68.

Kapur, S., & Mamo, D. (2003). Half a century of antipsychotics and still a central role for dopamine D_2 receptors. *Progress in Neuropsychopharmacology and Biological Psychiatry, 27*(7), 1081–1090.

Kapur, S. (2004). How antipsychotics become anti-"psychotic"—from dopamine to salience to psychosis. *Trends in Pharmacological Science, 25*(8), 402–406.

Laruelle, M., Frankle, W. K., Narendran, R., Kegeles, L. S., & Abi-Dargham, A. (2005). Mechanism of action of antipsychotic drugs: From dopamine D(2) receptor antagonism to glutamate NMDA facilitation. *Clinical Therapeutics, 27*(Suppl. A), S16–S24.

Lewis, D. A., & Levitt, P. (2002). Schizophrenia as a disorder of neurodevelopment. *Annual Review of Neuroscience, 25,* 409–432.

Meltzer, H. Y., Li, Z., Kaneda, Y., & Ichikawa, J. (2003). Serotonin receptors: Their key role in drugs to treat schizophrenia. *Progress in Neuropsychopharmacology and Biological Psychiatry, 27*(7), 1159–1172.

Naber, D., & Lambert, M. (2004). Aripiprazole: A new atypical antipsychotic with a different pharmacological mechanism. *Progress in Neuropsychopharmacology and Biological Psychiatry, 28*(8), 1213–1219.

Stahl, S. M. (2003). Describing an atypical antipsychotic: Receptor binding and its role in pathophysiology. *Journal of Clinical Psychiatry, 5*(Suppl. 3), 9–13.

Sullivan, P. (2005). The genetics of schizophrenia [Abstract]. *PLoS Medicine, 2*(7), e212.

Tamminga, C. A., & Holcomb, H. H. (2005). Phenotype of schizophrenia: A review and formulation. *Molecular Psychiatry, 10,* 27–39.

Van Os, J., Krabbendam, L., Myin-Germeys, I., & Delespaul, P. (2005). The schizophrenia envirome. *Current Opinion in Psychiatry, 18*(2), 141–145.

CHAPTER 4

BRAIN IMAGING

LISA T. EYLER

> ... in dementia praecox, partial damage to, or destruction of
> cells, of the cerebral cortex must probably occur ... which
> mostly brings in its wake a singular, permanent impairment of
> the inner life.
>
> —KRAEPELIN (1919/1971, p. 154)

Schizophrenia was first classified as a disorder in the early 1900s, during a time when unique neuropathological features were being discovered for other disturbances of thought and behavior, such as Alzheimer's dementia. Thus, it was expected that post mortem studies of the brains of patients with schizophrenia would also reveal characteristic abnormalities that were pathognomonic for the disorder. Unfortunately, very few consistent patterns were found based on initial qualitative investigations of the brains of patients with schizophrenia. Interest in exploring the neuropathology of schizophrenia consequently waned (coincident with increased interest in nonbiological theories of the cause of the disorder), and did not rise again until the 1970s, when several brain imaging modalities became available that allowed for *in vivo,* quantitative measurement of structure and function. These techniques made it possible to detect more subtle deficits across groups of patients and ushered in a new era of interest in brain abnormalities in schizophrenia. Since then, much has been learned about structural brain abnormalities using volumetric techniques such as computed tomography (CT) and magnetic resonance imaging (MRI), and neurochemical methods such as magnetic resonance spectroscopy (MRS). We have also learned a great deal about functional deficits of schizophrenia using electroencephalography (EEG), xenon blood flow techniques, positron emission tomography (PET), single photon emission computed tomography (SPECT), and functional magnetic resonance imaging (fMRI). This chapter reviews the relative strengths and weaknesses of these techniques, as well as general findings from studies that have used these tools to explore deficits associated with schizophrenia. Promising future directions for brain imaging in schizophrenia are also highlighted.

STRUCTURAL BRAIN IMAGING

Computed Tomography

CT was one of the earliest brain imaging techniques to be applied to the study of schizophrenia. In CT scanning, X-rays passing through the brain strike detectors that rotate slowly about the head. The differential absorption of X-rays by different tissue types creates contrast between gray matter, white matter, cerebrospinal fluid (CSF), and bone to create an image of the brain in multiple two-dimensional slices. Early *in vivo* studies of brain structure in schizophrenia used hand measurement or qualitative judgments based on CT scans, often on a predetermined single slice located by an anatomical landmark. In general, these studies found enlargement of the lateral ventricles of patients with schizophrenia compared to healthy participants. Although the finding of a mean difference between groups was fairly consistent, there was considerable overlap of the distribution of ventricular size between patients and comparison participants, and ventricular enlargement was also observed in other psychiatric conditions. The modest nature of the deficits revealed by using CT, combined with limitations of the technique as a research tool, such as poor gray–white matter contrast, artifacts due to bone, and concerns about repeated exposure to X-radiation, motivated a switch to the use of the newly developed MRI technique.

Magnetic Resonance Imaging

MRI creates images by capitalizing on the inherent magnetic properties of atoms in the body. The most abundant, and most commonly visualized, is the hydrogen atom. By altering the energy state of protons in the brain through a combination of (1) placement in a static magnetic field, (2) introduction of radiofrequency energy, and (3) recording as the protons relax back to their initial state after the energy pulse, the signals detected vary depending on the local environment. This allows for good visualization of tissue types that differ in their water concentration, such as gray matter, white matter, and CSF. The lack of ionizing radiation in this technique means that scans can be repeated, allowing for longitudinal studies of the course of brain abnormalities in schizophrenia. Magnet strengths of 1.5 Tesla are commonly available in most medical centers and allow for spatial resolution of 1 mm × 1 mm × 1 mm.

Initial psychiatric studies using MRI replicated the finding of ventriculomegaly in schizophrenia. Third ventricle enlargement has also been frequently observed. The promise of MRI, however, was more fully realized when it was used to examine the size of individual cortical and subcortical regions within the brain. The most consistent observation in this regard has been reduced temporal lobe volume. In particular, more than 80% of studies have found reduced volume of the hippocampus and superior temporal gyrus. Frontal lobe volume has also been frequently examined, and the majority of studies have found overall volume decrements in patients with schizophrenia compared to healthy individuals. Slightly less consistent results have been found in the smaller number of investigations of parietal lobe, occipital lobe, and cerebellar volumes. Among subcortical structures, the basal ganglia have most consistently shown volume reductions, although some evidence exists for abnormalities of the thalamus and corpus callosum.

Thus, the MRI evidence that patients with schizophrenia, on average, have larger ventricles and smaller subcortical and cortical structures, particularly in the temporal lobes, is strong. The widespread nature of the structural abnormalities has led to several theories about the etiology of these deficits. The theories commonly emphasize the idea of a disconnection between areas that are normally coordinated, and several postulate a neurodevelopmental origin to the disconnection and subsequent volume loss. There has yet to be strong evidence to support any single theory; however, investigations using newer techniques, such as functional neuroimaging and diffusion tensor imaging (DTI), which can be used to visualize integrity of white matter tracts, are likely to provide a more direct means of testing disconnection theories. The idea that structural deficits may be neurodevelopmental in origin is supported to some degree by the fact that MRI abnormalities have generally been found among both first-episode patients and chronically ill individuals. Longitudinal studies, however, suggest that there may also be additional factors that lead to patients' somewhat steeper decline in cortical volume with age compared to healthy individuals. Many studies of structural deficits in schizophrenia have attempted to relate these abnormalities to clinical and, particularly, cognitive features of the disorder. Although methodological inconsistencies between studies make it difficult to draw strong conclusions, it does appear that structure–function relationships are common to patients and controls (e.g., positive association between whole-brain volume and general cognitive ability, and between IQ and dorsal prefrontal cortex gray matter volume), and that some relationships are specific to schizophrenia (e.g., positive associations between cognitive flexibility and prefrontal cortex volume, and between language functioning and volumes of superior temporal gyrus and parahippocampal gyrus). Other important issues that deserve further study include the relationship of structural deficits to genetic risk for schizophrenia and whether volume deficits predict course or outcome. Recent imaging studies that have focused on individuals at high genetic risk or those showing prodromal symptoms of schizophrenia are promising first steps toward addressing both of these issues. In addition, not much is known about the potential effects of antipsychotic medication and the specificity of the findings to schizophrenia compared to other psychiatric disorders. As automated or semiautomated techniques to parcel the brain into regions of interest become more established, larger studies with the power to examine such questions should be feasible.

Magnetic Resonance Spectroscopy

Another method for examining the integrity of the brain involves examination of chemicals related to metabolic activity. MRS uses nuclear magnetic resonance principles to generate a spectrum of peaks related to the biochemical composition of a region of the brain. The most common form of MRS is sensitive to hydrogen protons and can measure levels of compounds such as amino acids and sugars. The strength of this technique is its unique ability to measure *in vivo* neurochemistry. The weaknesses include low spatial resolution compared to MRI, and, as yet, no ability to measure neurochemical change due to cognitive activity.

The majority of MRS studies in schizophrenia have focused on measuring levels of N-acetylaspartate (NAA), which is hypothesized to be a marker of neuronal integrity. NAA levels appear to be reduced in the hippocampus and in the gray and white matter of the frontal lobe among patients with schizophrenia. Fewer studies have examined phosphorus-containing metabolites, such as phosphomonoesters and phosphodiesters, but these studies have also revealed temporal lobe and frontal abnormalities in patterns that may be reflective of synaptic pruning failures.

FUNCTIONAL BRAIN IMAGING

The functional significance of the subtle but well-documented structural brain abnormalities in schizophrenia is not completely understood. Because the distribution of brain volumes and neurochemical levels among patients and healthy individuals seems to overlap, it is clear that some patients have clinical symptoms of schizophrenia in the absence of these deficits, and some healthy people have small volumes or MRS abnormalities but do not meet criteria for schizophrenia. In addition, volume measurements, even at the high resolution of modern MRI scanners, are a crude index of underlying neuropathology. For example, neuronal disarray and improper connections between neurons may not result in apparent volume loss at the level of millimeter resolution. Furthermore, neurotransmitter abnormalities may cause problems with the functioning of perfectly intact and properly connected neurons. If part of the "lesion" of schizophrenia is at the level of neuropharmacological interactions, as might be inferred by the clinical efficacy of substances that alter neurotransmission, then structural imaging may not be sensitive to this type of abnormality. In contrast, functional neuroimaging techniques were designed to assess the function of the brain *in vivo,* either by measuring metabolic activity, regional blood flow, neurotransmitter binding, regional blood oxygenation, or electrical or magnetic activity.

Positron Emission Tomography and Single Photon Emission Computed Tomography

The earliest functional imaging studies in schizophrenia were conducted in the mid-1970s and used a technique that measured blood flow by detecting levels of inhaled radio-labeled xenon gas. This method was eventually surpassed by the tomographic (*tomos,* slice; *graphia,* writing) techniques of PET and SPECT, which were able to collect images in multiple planes, or slices, through the brain. Areas of high concentration of radioactive tracers are localized by detecting single photons with a collimator (SPECT) or by detecting the coincidence of two photons traveling at a 180° angle from each other as a result of collisions between a positron and an electron (PET). Cerebral blood flow is measured by PET or SPECT by introducing a tracer attached to a molecule delivered by the blood to active areas of the brain, such as ^{15}O-labeled water (PET) or ethyl cysteinate dimer (ECD) labeled with technetium-99m (SPECT). PET can also measure glucose metabolism through use of ^{18}fluorodeoxyglucose (^{18}FDG), which is taken up by active neurons but is not broken down like standard glucose. Most recently, PET imaging with radioactively labeled agonists of neural receptors (e.g., ^{11}carbon-raclopride for dopamine D_2 receptors) has been used to study the *in vivo* neuropharmacology of schizophrenia. Modern scanners allow for 1 cm^3 spatial resolution, providing fairly good localization of regional blood flow, metabolism, or receptor affinity. Temporal resolution depends of the kinetics of the tracer used, and can vary from 30 to 90 seconds for ^{15}O-labeled water to 45 minutes for ^{18}FDG. PET is more expensive than SPECT, due to the need for an onsite cyclotron to synthesize the compounds with very short half-lives, but may still be preferred for research since it has better spatial resolution and is more repeatable. Both PET and SPECT use ionizing radiation, which increases risks to participants and limits the techniques' usefulness for longitudinal follow-up studies.

The earliest functional neuroimaging studies in schizophrenia aimed to measure whole-brain and regional cerebral blood flow or metabolism while the participant was at rest, that is, not actively engaged in a prescribed cognitive task. Flow or metabolism was measured in cortical and subcortical regions of interest, sometimes corrected for whole-brain measures. These studies were heterogeneous in their results, with the earliest reports finding lower blood flow or metabolism in the frontal cortex of patients with schizophrenia relative to controls, termed "hypofrontality," but an equal number of subsequent studies failing to find a significant difference. Overall, there appears to be a slight tendency for lower whole-brain flow and metabolism, as well as resting hypofrontality, but the size of the effect seems to depend on age and duration of illness (with more abnormality among older, more chronic patient groups), and whether patients are treated with neuroleptic agents (more abnormality among treated patient groups). A few researchers have suggested that the modest and sometimes contradictory nature of these findings also may be related to the unstructured nature of the behavioral state of patients at "rest." Thus, more recent studies have used cognitive challenge tasks to standardize cognitive activities during scanning and to stimulate particular brain systems that are hypothesized to be impaired. Many of the tasks have targeted cognitive challenge of the frontal cortex, and results from PET and SPECT studies again have been mixed but demonstrate a small overall hypofrontality effect.

Although there has been a focus on frontal lobe function, other regions have emerged as sites of functional abnormality based on PET studies of metabolism and blood flow. For example, lower metabolism among patients with schizophrenia has been shown for both the basal ganglia and temporal lobes. The function of the hippocampus has been of particular interest given the known structural abnormalities in this region and the putative role of the medial temporal lobe in memory deficits found in schizophrenia. Studies of patients at rest have been mixed, with metabolic studies often finding reduced values among patients, and blood flow studies finding hyperactivity. The PET literature on the response of the hippocampus to learning and retrieval challenge tasks is small, but again there are findings of both under- and overactivation of the region. The role of the level of performance deficits as a possible moderator of these effects deserves further study. PET studies have also been used to examine brain functioning related to hallucinations, either by comparing hallucinators to nonhallucinators or by examining blood flow or metabolism during self-reported hallucinations. Findings have been inconsistent, but there is some suggestion that hallucinations may be related to abnormalities of the function of speech perception areas in the superior temporal gyrus.

PET and SPECT studies using receptor ligands have examined *in vivo* evidence for the involvement of several neurotransmitter systems in the pathogenesis of schizophrenia. In general, these studies have confirmed the theory of hyperstimulation of dopamine D_2 receptors in the striatum among patients. The few studies that have tested directly for the existence of postulated deficits in D_1 receptor-modulated dopamine activity in the prefrontal cortex have had mixed results, however. PET receptor studies have also been used to examine mechanisms of treatment response. These investigations have confirmed that treatment with antipsychotic medications results in D_2 receptor blockade, and have found that although clinical response is optimal between 50 and 80% occupancy, there is no observable correlation between D_2 occupancy and response within that window. Imaging studies have also investigated the mechanism of action of second-generation antipsychotics, which seem to have slightly greater efficacy than first-generation agents and are preferred due to better side effect profiles. Many of these agents share a high ratio of serotonin $5-HT_{2A}$ receptor affinity to D_2 receptor affinity, but this does not appear to be directly related to their efficacy, since imaging studies have failed to find response at doses that led to maximal $5-HT_{2A}$ occupancy but suboptimal D_2 occupancy. Rather, imaging evidence suggests that incidental $5-HT_{1A}$ agonism from the combined antagonism of $5-HT_{2A}$ and D_2 receptors, by increasing prefrontal dopamine function, may lead to clinical efficacy. The role of glutamate also is of particular interest in schizophrenia, and new radiotracers are being developed to examine this neurotransmitter system *in vivo*.

Functional Magnetic Resonance Imaging

Although PET and SPECT imaging have contributed greatly to our knowledge about metabolic, cerebrovascular, and neuropharmacological abnormalities in schizophrenia, the advent of fMRI in the early 1990s was heralded as a welcome addition to the arsenal of functional imaging research techniques. fMRI takes advantage of naturally occurring phenomena to localize areas of neuronal activity. Specifically, when oxygen is delivered by the blood to working neurons, it is not immediately consumed. Thus, there is excess vascular oxygen in the area near the active neurons. Because hemoglobin that is bound to oxygen causes less magnetic disruption than deoxyhemoglobin, the local signal is stronger in the areas of high activity. This is the basis of the blood oxygen level–dependent (BOLD) signal most commonly measured in fMRI. fMRI has several advantages over PET and SPECT imaging, including better temporal and spatial resolution, greater repeatability, and ability to collect functional and structural images in the same apparatus. One disadvantage relative to PET is that BOLD fMRI cannot quantify blood flow in absolute units; rather, it relies on a contrasting signal between two conditions. Thus, BOLD fMRI studies typically compare brain response between a baseline condition and an experimental condition. Although there are fMRI techniques that permit absolute quantification of blood flow using arterial spin labeling, these methods have not yet been applied to the study of schizophrenia.

fMRI studies in schizophrenia to date have generally focused on frontal and temporal lobe function, and on brain response to executive, language, and working and episodic memory tasks. Two main issues make summarizing the results of such studies complicated. First, even within particular information-processing domains, the specific cognitive challenge tasks vary greatly in terms of stimuli, instructions, and difficulty level. Second, fMRI studies, as well as most recent PET and SPECT studies, generally analyze every volume element (voxel) in the brain and report the location and size of voxel clusters that reach a significant threshold in terms of volume and magnitude. Thus, if two studies both report clusters within the left prefrontal cortex, but in slightly different locations, it is difficult to know whether the studies are replicating the same finding or have identified two separate areas of abnormality. In the area of working memory, however, in which only a small number of similar tasks have been used, some summary statements can be made. Although many studies have found less response of the dorsolateral prefrontal cortex during working memory tasks in patients with schizophrenia compared to controls, others have either failed to find a difference or have found hyperactivity. There is some evidence that this may be partly due to discrepancies between studies in the difficulty (i.e., working memory load) of the task. If there is an inverted-U curve that relates prefrontal activation to working memory load and prefrontal deficits in schizophrenia result in a shift of this curve to the left relative to controls, then patient–control comparisons will yield different, even opposite, results depending on the load used. Although most working memory tasks have focused on findings in the prefrontal cortex, other regions are sometimes found to be involved and overactivated, such as the anterior cingulate cortex. The general finding that there are areas of both hypo- and hyperactivation relative to controls within a certain information-processing domain is frequently observed in fMRI studies in schizophrenia. This suggests that there may be abnormal functional connections between regions, but very few studies to date have used multivariate techniques to examine this hypothesis directly using fMRI data.

Electroencephalography and Magnetoencephalography

A major limitation of fMRI as a functional imaging technique is that it only measures the functioning of neurons indirectly, through the effects of activity on blood flow and/or subsequent blood oxygenation changes. This means that the temporal resolution of fMRI is necessarily limited by the sluggishness of the hemodynamic response to neural events. Because methods such as EEG and magnetoencephalography (MEG), which measure the electrical or magnetic signal resulting from coordinated firing of collections of neurons, do not have this problem, they are able to resolve much more precise timing of neural events. However, there is a trade-off in terms of spatial resolution and limits to the regions that can be sensitively measured, because measurements must be recorded at the scalp, with localization inferred statistically. MEG is quite sensitive to current flows oriented tangentially to the scalp and is less affected by the conductance of the brain, skull, and scalp than EEG, but it cannot detect radially oriented electrical current.

Most EEG and MEG studies of schizophrenia have examined the electrical potentials or magnetic fields that are evoked in response to a transient cognitive activity, referred to as event-related potentials (ERPs) or event-related fields (ERFs). The greatest body of evidence concerns a positive-going wave that is observed 300 ms after presentation of a novel stimulus, the P300, which may arise from several sources, including prefrontal, parietal and temporal cortex locations. Reduced P300 amplitudes consistently have been found among patients with schizophrenia, with some evidence for greater left-sided abnormalities. Although P300 abnormalities are also found in other psychiatric populations, the laterality effects may be more specific to schizophrenia. Another focus of schizophrenia ERP research has been on early, automatic responses, such as the P50 and mismatch negativity. Among healthy individuals, the P50 response, which may be generated in the auditory cortex, is suppressed to the second of two rapidly presented auditory stimuli. Patients with schizophrenia show less suppression, interpreted as a failure of sensory gating. In addition, the normal negative-going response to deviant stimuli, termed mismatch negativity and thought to be generated in prefrontal and superior temporal cortex, is diminished in amplitude among schizophrenia patients. The N400 response to semantic incongruity also has been shown to be longer in latency among patients. Tantalizing results from a handful of recent studies have linked electrophysiological deficits such as reduced P300 and mismatch negativity amplitudes to psychosocial outcome, but more work is needed to determine the specificity of these findings to schizophrenia.

Interpretative Challenges Common to Functional Imaging Techniques

In addition to the pitfalls inherent to particular functional imaging methods, there are also general challenges that must be considered in interpreting the results of functional imaging studies. First, there is the issue of generalizability. Because of the expense of data collection and analysis, functional imaging studies often employ small sample sizes. Although efforts are made to select a sample from the population in an unbiased manner, lack of representativeness is bound to occur, because of both the small samples and the demands of neuroimaging that may exclude some patients (e.g., the need to lie still, risks of claustrophobia, or fears about radiation). This makes it difficult to generalize from the conclusions in any single study and also confounds efforts to combine results across studies. Second, attempts to measure brain function are complicated by limitations in our knowledge of how mental activity influences neurophysiology. For example, the basic question of whether good task performance is related to more or less regional blood flow and oxygenation has not been thoroughly answered, although it likely depends on many factors. Studies of the "resting state," which attempt to circumvent this problem, are likely instead to reflect a complicated mix of mental activities with variable underlying patterns of brain activity. Requiring participants to engage in a particular cognitive challenge task may reduce the variability in brain response somewhat, but there are still individual differences in motivation, attention, strategy, performance, and response to failure or success. Many of these factors may differ systematically between patients and controls, and the neuroimaging investigator must decide which element(s) should be matched between groups. Once this is determined, there is the further challenge of figuring out how to control for group differences. For example, whereas some investigators have argued for statistical covariation of the effect of task performance, others have advocated for a priori matching of samples or testing both patients and controls at multiple levels of difficulty. A third interpretive challenge for functional neuroimaging is the possible confounding effect of antipsychotic medication. Although structural imaging studies share this challenge to some degree, the confound may be greater for functional imaging, because medications may affect both neural activity and hemodynamic factors measured as a proxy for neural activity. If functional neuroimaging is used to draw conclusions about the nature of underlying brain pathology in schizophrenia by comparing patients and healthy controls, the fact that most samples of patients include many people taking antipsychotic medications must be considered. Longitudinal treatment studies have shown that antipsychotic agents can increase cortical and subcortical blood flow among patients, so a finding of normal or increased activity compared to controls might be partly accounted for by medication effects. On the other hand, antipsychotic medications may also increase resting perfusion, which can decrease the amount of change in brain response due to challenge that can be observed with hemodynamic methods, thus biasing toward findings of less apparent neural activity. Because researchers are beginning to address all of these challenges, the quality of functional neuroimaging studies should improve in the future.

FUTURE DIRECTIONS

In addition to improvements in methods, several new directions of neuroimaging research hold great promise for leading to a better understanding of schizophrenia and its treatment. The first direction is toward greater integration between imaging modalities. Little is currently known, for instance, about how structural and neurochemical abnormalities relate to known deficits in functional brain response. Does a single process lead to both volume loss and poor brain response in the temporal cortex, or are there separate causes? Studies that combine careful structural measurements with spectroscopy and functional imaging could address this issue. Similarly, investigators are starting to combine fMRI and EEG in an effort to take advantage of fMRI's high spatial resolution and EEG's high temporal resolution. This should help to pinpoint the location and timing of functional abnormalities within the same study. The second future direction in functional imaging is a greater emphasis on techniques and analytical methods that examine the interaction between brain regions. Hypothesized abnormalities of structural and functional connectivity among patients with schizophrenia based on interpretations of previous findings have only recently been examined directly. As mentioned earlier, DTI can be used to measure the integrity of white matter tracts. In addition, multivariate statistical methods can be used to examine how brain areas vary together in both size and function. Since it is likely that the complex behavioral patterns in schizophrenia are generated by the interaction of multiple areas, measures of abnormal connectivity may be much better predictors of clinical and cognitive symptoms and functional outcome than size or response of single regions. A third future direction is the growing use of functional imaging measures in treatment studies. Functional brain response appears to be a fairly sensitive index of change with pharmacological treatment and can therefore shed light on the mechanism of improvement, as well as correlates of treatment response. Finally, an exciting new research area involves the combination of functional neuroimaging and measurement of genetic polymorphisms and gene products. These studies offer the promise of a better understanding of how genes influence brain function among patients with schizophrenia and may elucidate the pathway between liability for the disorder and its phenotypic expression.

KEY POINTS

- On average, patients with schizophrenia have bigger ventricles, smaller brains, and smaller temporal, parietal, and frontal lobes than healthy individuals, but the magnitude of this mean difference is modest.
- Volumetric deficits among patients may be related to cognitive deficits and clinical symptoms, but more research into the functional significance of structural abnormalities is needed.
- At rest, patients with schizophrenia tend to have mild deficits in frontal lobe blood flow and metabolism, and the degree of deficit may be related to age, duration of illness, and medication effects.
- Metabolic deficits of the basal ganglia and temporal lobes also are commonly observed among patients with schizophrenia.
- Cognitive challenge tests reveal abnormalities of frontal and temporal lobe functioning among patients with schizophrenia, but the nature and direction of these deficits may be related to task difficulty.
- Electrophysiological abnormalities during controlled and automatic processing are prevalent among patients with schizophrenia and may be related to functional outcome.
- Future directions for brain imaging in schizophrenia include integration between different imaging modalities, a focus on measurement of functional connectivity between regions, use of imaging in treatment studies, and a combination of imaging and genetic methods.

REFERENCES AND RECOMMENDED READINGS

Antonova, E., Sharma, T., Morris, R., & Kumari, V. (2004). The relationship between brain structure and neurocognition in schizophrenia: A selective review. *Schizophrenia Research, 70*(2–3), 117–145.

Buchsbaum, M. S., & Hazlett, E. A. (1998). Positron emission tomography studies of abnormal glucose metabolism in schizophrenia. *Schizophrenia Bulletin, 24*(3), 343–364.

Davis, C. E., Jeste, D. V., & Eyler, L. T. (2005). Review of longitudinal functional neuroimaging studies of drug treatments in patients with schizophrenia. *Schizophrenia Research, 78*(1), 45–60.

Ford, J. M. (1999). Schizophrenia: The broken P300 and beyond. *Psychophysiology, 36*(6), 667–682.

Hill, K., Mann, L., Laws, K. R., Stephenson, C. M., Nimmo-Smith, I., & McKenna, P. J. (2004). Hypofrontality in schizophrenia: A meta-analysis of functional imaging studies. *Acta Psychiatrica Scandinavica, 110*(4), 243–256.

Kraepelin, E. (1971). *Dementia praecox and paraphrenia.* Huntington, NY: Krieger. (Original work published 1919)

Light, G. A., & Braff, D. L. (1999). Human and animal studies of schizophrenia-related gating deficits. *Current Psychiatry Reports, 1*(1), 31–40.

Manoach, D. S. (2003). Prefrontal cortex dysfunction during working memory performance in schizophrenia: Reconciling discrepant findings. *Schizophrenia Research, 60*(2–3), 285–298.

Shenton, M. E., Dickey, C. C., Frumin, M., & McCarley, R. W. (2001). A review of MRI findings in schizophrenia. *Schizophrenia Research, 49*(1–2), 1–52.

Steen, R. G., Hamer, R. M., & Lieberman, J. A. (2005). Measurement of brain metabolites by (1)H magnetic resonance spectroscopy in patients with schizophrenia: A systematic review and meta-analysis. *Neuropsychopharmacology, 30*(11), 1949–1962.

Weinberger, D. R., & Berman, K. F. (1996). Prefrontal function in schizophrenia: Confounds and controversies. *Philosophical Transactions of the Royal Society of London: Series B, Biological Sciences, 351,* 1495–1503.

CHAPTER 5

NEUROPATHOLOGY

DANIEL G. STEWART
KENNETH L. DAVIS

Schizophrenia is a brain disease. Regardless of the theoretical stance from which one wants to view the terrain of schizophrenia symptomatology, etiology, and course, there remains little question that part of that terrain contains alterations to brain structure and brain function. Although arguments still persist as to the individual contributions of genetics and environment to the structural and functional pathology present in schizophrenia, our ever-increasing sophistication as a field has led us to begin to embrace the notion that neuropathology is both causal and resultant—that a neuroanatomical or neurochemical finding can be an upstream effect in one instance and a downstream effect in another, even within the same disease. The neuropathological findings and the symptom picture that emerge then, are the result of a complex interplay of genetic, environmental, and even stochastic forces that occur over time and within a context. The neuropathological findings in schizophrenia are often subtle, span brain regions and processes, share overlap with control populations, and are typically difficult to replicate in different samples of patients. These findings currently may be best seen in light of the endophenotype model. In other words, several different aberrations of brain structure and function likely converge in the symptom picture we call schizophrenia. And even if we ignore the divergent neuropathological and genetic findings, an examination of the myriad clinical presentations of the disease certainly suggests that multiple processes may be at work. The neuropathological data on schizophrenia are pieces of an explanation, awaiting assembly by what has been proven to be a rather elusive set of principles.

Because an exhaustive description of all the findings in the brains of patients with schizophrenia could easily be the topic of a book rather than a chapter, this chapter focuses on the major findings in schizophrenia brain research that are either well replicated or have particular importance for a basic understanding of schizophrenia. We begin with a brief discussion of the neurodevelopmental model of schizophrenia, then go on to discuss global and regional findings (summarized in Table 5.1). Other overarching issues are then examined briefly, including the disconnectivity model of schizophrenia, limitations of neuropathological investigation (summarized in Table 5.2), and the progressive versus static nature of some neuropathological findings.

TABLE 5.1. Summary of Major Findings in the Brains of Patients with Schizophrenia

Region	Findings
Global	• Decreased brain volume • Increased ventricular volume

Cortical	• Frontal lobe volume reduced, particularly in
	  • Dorsolateral prefrontal cortex
	  • Orbitofrontal and dorsomedial regions
	• Increased frontal lobe neuronal packing density
	• Temporal lobe volume reduced, particularly in
	  • Medial temporal lobe
	  • Superior temporal gyrus
	• Decreased asymmetry of planum temporale
	• Parietal lobe potentially with volume reduction
	• Cerebellar findings inconsistent

Subcortical	• Thalamic volume decreased • Decreased organization of thalamocortical pathways • Basal ganglia volume increased with typical antipsychotic medication treatment • Basal ganglia volume potentially decreased pretreatment

White matter	• Oligodendrocyte number reduced in schizophrenia
	• Coherence of white matter in various brain regions decreased, including
	  • Temporal lobe
	  • Frontal lobe
	  • Corpus callosum
	• White matter tracts in schizophrenia decreased in organization, including
	  • Thalamocortical tracts
	  • Uncinate fasciculus
	  • Arcuate fasciculus
	  • Cingulum bundle

THE NEURODEVELOPMENTAL MODEL OF SCHIZOPHRENIA

That schizophrenia has a neurodevelopmental component is essentially established. Various structural and functional abnormalities that are present at first break—that is, when an individual has his or her first formal psychotic episode—along with the absence of any gross neurodegenerative markers (i.e., gliosis), have led to the suggestion that at least some of the processes that predispose individuals to the disease are prenatal. However, this often accepted position, when considered in light of the evidence, may at best be only partially true. For example, the idea that gliosis must be present for there to be a neurodegenerative process taking place is an incomplete notion, probably limited by our knowledge of pathophysiology at the time of its inception. Several other insults that may be active and ongoing in the brains of patients who have or will develop schizophrenia, such as excessive pruning, inadequate supply of trophic factors to neurons, or poor functioning or even death of oligodendrocytes, could cause the loss of neurons over time without necessarily causing gliosis. Furthermore, any of these types of insults could predate the illness, yet not occur during intrauterine life. So the question becomes, what exactly is meant by the term *neurodevelopmental*? If one intends to suggest that this requires an intrauterine event, then this conclusion remains somewhat speculative. If however, one means a process that involves any aberration in the typical pattern of brain development, including not only neuronal development but also glial development (not to mention the hitherto unknown factors that regulate the timing of specific developmental milestones in

TABLE 5.2. Limitations on Neuropathological Investigation

Limitation	Affects postmortem studies	Affects imaging studies
Postmortem index	+	−
Variations in sample selection or delineation of region of interest	+	+
Differing methodologies for analysis	+	+
Small sample sizes	+	+

brain development across the lifespan), then little doubt exists that schizophrenia is at least partly neurodevelopmental.

GLOBAL BRAIN FINDINGS

Decreased Brain Volume

Early research into brain volumes in schizophrenia, at least partially driven by theories that brain volume was related to mental illness, cognitive deficits, and low socioeconomic status, reach as far back as the early 1800s. Using postmortem tissue, the brains of patients with schizophrenia have been found to be reduced in length, volume, and weight. In imaging studies, schizophrenia has been found to be associated with reduced global brain volumes; however, the majority of studies have not found significant differences between patients with schizophrenia and controls. There are several explanations for these discrepant findings, and it is likely that each plays a part in this inconsistency. First, global brain volume is a somewhat imprecise and gross measure in and of itself. Second, controlling for brain size differences related to variations in head size rather than to schizophrenia is difficult to do. Third, sample sizes in schizophrenia studies are typically small, and the volume changes themselves are likely to be small, thus increasing the likelihood that subtle brain volume differences will be missed. Fourth, many of these studies did not separate patients by differences in symptom severity, age, or disease course, and it is possible, if not likely, that patients whose disease has a particularly severe progression would have more profound brain changes than those who have a relatively good outcome. When these heterogeneous groups are examined together, those with good outcome—who might have less brain pathology—may wash out the findings that would be seen if patients with poor outcome were examined separately. Last, and perhaps most important, schizophrenia may be better characterized as a disorder with regional aberrations. It is important to note that few diseases that have a profound effect on global brain volume are not only consistent with life but also allow those afflicted to function in society. Even though the schizophrenia symptom picture is devastating and debilitating, one must keep in mind that these changes are subtle in the grand scheme of self-maintenance and self-preservation; consequently, they might be better explained by regional neuropathology or dysconnectivity (both discussed below). All this having been said, meta-analyses have demonstrated small but significant reductions in total brain volume in schizophrenia.

Ventricular Enlargement

There is enlargement of the ventricles in schizophrenia. Data come from both imaging and postmortem investigations. Areas typically noted to be enlarged in patients with schizophrenia include the lateral ventricles as a whole, the temporal horn portion of the lateral ventricular system (particularly on the left), and the third ventricle (which is of particular importance given its proximity to the thalamus, discussed below). Rather than use an absolute measurement, ventricular size is often measured by ventricule–brain ratio (VBR), which adjusts for differences in subjects' overall brain volumes. Schizophrenia has been associated with a wide range of increases in VBR, from 20 to 75%, with a recent review citing a median enlargement of 40%. Although estimates of the size of this increase remain somewhat variable, the enlargement of the ventricles in schizophrenia is a ubiquitous finding. There is a significant amount of overlap in VBR between subjects with schizophrenia and controls, so it is worth noting that VBR has no diagnostic or predictive ability. Although overall brain volumes have often been found to be reduced in schizophrenia as described earlier, this decrease has not been shown to correlate with the degree of VBR increase.

Not only is the increase in VBR a common finding, but twin studies also lend support to the idea that this may be partially a predisposing factor and partially a disease-specific finding. On the one hand, in monozygotic twins discordant for schizophrenia, the ventricles of the affected twin are larger than those of the unaffected sibling, along with reductions in cortical and hippocampal size. These findings suggest that increased VBR is part of a schizophrenia phenotype; in other words, this increase accompanies the presentation of the disease and does not merely reflect an underlying genetic vulnerability. On the other hand, family studies that examine patients with schizophrenia and their unaffected siblings demonstrate that unaffected siblings have smaller ventricles than their siblings with schizophrenia but larger ventricles than healthy controls who are not part of the family. This suggests, instead, that at least some aspect of ventricular size in schizophrenia may be under genetic influence.

CORTICAL FINDINGS

Prefrontal Cortex

The prefrontal cortex is a region of interest in schizophrenia, because it is believed to modulate many cognitive and behavioral tasks at which patients with schizophrenia are deficient. Postmortem studies have shown prefrontal abnormalities, and although imaging studies have not been as conclusive, the majority of such studies do find deficits in this region. Likely, the reason for the negative findings includes the fact that the frontal lobe has often been measured as a whole, and small regional abnormalities in these cases might be missed. Importantly, when white matter and gray matter are examined differentially, studies have shown that each is reduced. Furthermore, when the frontal cortex is subdivided, differences do appear in dorsolateral regions, as well as in orbitofrontal (in females) and dorsomedial (in males) regions. Investigations into subdivisions of the frontal lobe have also revealed correlations with performance tests of verbal recall, visual memory, semantic fluency, and negative symptoms, consistent with theories of schizophrenia's cognitive deficits residing in aberrations of frontal lobe structures.

Increased neuronal packing density has been reported over the entire frontal lobe, particularly in the dorsolateral prefrontal cortex (DLPFC). Although negative findings have been reported on this measure in these regions, the importance of the DLPFC in schizophrenia is largely accepted, because many of the symptom- and cognition-related findings have been associated with alterations in DLPFC functioning. Of note, the absolute number of neurons in the DLPFC has not been found to be altered in patients with schizophrenia.

The DLPFC has been shown to demonstrate a decrease in synaptophysin, a marker of postsynaptic density, and this finding is supplemented by a lower density of dendritic spines in this area in patients with schizophrenia. This may represent an excess of synaptic pruning in this area, but it may also reflect the loss of dendrites, with resultant increases in synaptic density due to some other aberrant process that divests these neurons of trophic or sustaining factors. Magnetic resonance spectroscopic (MRS) investigations have demonstrated a reduction in N-acetylaspartate (NAA), a marker of neuronal integrity, in the DLPFC, which is present at first break and is consistent with a reduction in synaptic and dendritic density. Furthermore, several studies have demonstrated a state of relative hypofunctioning in the frontal cortex in patients with schizophrenia, consistent with the notion that there is both functional and structural aberration in this region.

Temporal Lobe

Like all investigations into brain pathology in schizophrenia, investigations into the temporal lobe have produced conflicting results. Although the majority of studies demonstrate reductions in total temporal lobe volume, almost 40% report negative findings. However, like so much of schizophrenia research, these conflicting findings are likely due in part to methodological differences that impact the accuracy of measurement, differences in the definition of boundaries of the temporal lobe, and sample size limitations. As more studies have used more rigorous methods and better instruments, the number of positive studies in this area has been increasing. One might question whether the entire temporal lobe is a sufficiently specific region of interest to capture differences between patients with schizophrenia and controls. Subdividing the temporal lobe has revealed alterations in three structures within the temporal lobe in schizophrenia: the medial temporal lobe, the superior temporal gyrus, and the planum temporale.

The medial temporal lobe includes the amygdala (responsible for emotional valence) and the parahippocampal gyrus (involved in aspects of memory), and has been found to be reduced in volume in the vast majority of imaging studies in schizophrenia, consistent with postmortem findings in this region and with the common finding of increased volume of the temporal horn of the lateral ventricles, which surrounds the medial temporal lobe. Volume reductions in both substructures—amygdala–hippocampal complex and parahippocampal gyrus—are evident in chronic patients, but volume reductions in the amygdala–hippocampal complex are also present in first-episode patients. However, amygdala–hippocampal complex reductions are also present in mood disorders, some anxiety disorders, and as a function of aging, thus lacking specificity as an aspect of schizophrenia. And although the meaning of any lateralized differences remains unknown, it is common to find a left-greater-than-right separation between patients with schizophrenia and control subjects. Investigations into the hippocampus specifically, though, have yielded some intriguing results.

In healthy subjects, there is an anatomical asymmetry in the hippocampus, with the right hippocampus being somewhat larger. Functionally, the hippocampus is involved in memory: The right hippocampus is preferentially involved in spatial memory, whereas the left is concerned with verbal memory. Reductions in hippocampal size and alterations in hippocampal shape have both been demonstrated in patients with schizophrenia. Volume reductions in the hippocampus have generally been found to be greater on the left, which coincides with parahippocampal reductions being greater on the left, as well as volume increases in the left temporal horn of the lateral ventricle. The cross-sectional area of pyramidal neuron cell bodies has also been found to be reduced in patients with schizophrenia. Again, negative reports have been published as well. Hippocampal neuronal shape has been reported to be altered; pyramidal neurons of patients with schizophrenia are longer and thinner compared to those of controls. Conversely, the total number of hippocampal neurons appears to be unchanged in patients with schizophrenia. Smaller hippocampal volumes are present at first break, and twin studies suggest that this may be a genetic predisposition. These alterations may in fact represent an aberrant developmental process that occurs in early life; however, delineating whether these changes reflect a primarily genetic or environmental pattern is still a task for the future.

Neuronal packing density findings are inconsistent. Some findings show an increased packing density, others show a decreased packing density, and still others show no change in packing density. In contrast, there is some evidence that dendritic spines are decreased in density, with less apical arborization. Further support for these dendritic findings comes from *spinophilin*, a spine marker gene, which is also decreased in the hippocampus in patients with schizophrenia. These findings are consistent with and supported by the finding of decreased NAA—a biochemical marker of neuronal integrity—in the hippocampus of patients with schizophrenia, which incidentally is present at first break and across all stages of the disease. Functional imaging shows metabolic activation patterns that are altered in relation to symptoms. Ionotropic glutamate receptors appear to be altered as well, along with gamma-aminobutyric acid (GABA), nicotinic, and serotonin receptors, although the bulk of evidence exists for glutamatergic alteration.

The expression of synaptic proteins (particularly synaptophysin, SNAP-25, and synapsin) has consistently been reported as decreased in patients with schizophrenia, suggesting that synapses in the hippocampus are themselves involved in the disorder, although whether these changes are casual or resultant remains elusive. Two other synaptic proteins, complexin I and II, are altered in expression in the hippocampus in patients with schizophrenia and are involved in inhibitory and excitatory processes, respectively. Although both are altered in expression, there is some evidence that complexin II is more affected, suggesting that excitatory pathways may be more affected. Further supporting the idea of excitatory neuron involvement, glutamatergic neurons appear to be affected as well in this region, as evidenced by a decrease in expression of the vesicular glutamate transporter (VGLUT1). Be that as it may, GABA neurons, which are inhibitory, are apparently involved in this region as well. And changes in these glutamatergic and GABAergic markers over the course of the disease lend support to the idea that schizophrenia is a progressive disease.

The superior temporal gyrus (STG) contains primary auditory cortex within Heschl's gyrus. On the left, the STG contains Wernicke's area, which includes the planum temporale (PT). Investigations into the STG are some of the strongest findings in schizophrenia research, with volume reductions noted in upwards of 65% of studies. Interestingly, STG abnormalities have also been demonstrated in patients with schizophrenia spectrum disorders. Studies that compare schizophrenia and bipolar disorder are equivocal, with two studies showing decreased STG in patients with schizophrenia but not those with bipolar disorder, and one study showing the opposite. As discussed below, findings in the STG are associated with schizophrenia symptoms. The PT is within the boundary of the STG, but because of its role in language and speech processing has been a separate focus of investigation in schizophrenia. The usual left-greater-than-right PT asymmetry seen in control subjects is reduced and sometimes reversed in patients with schizophrenia, and because this asymmetry has been demonstrated in healthy subjects as early as the end of the second trimester of gestation, this loss of asymmetry has been hypothesized to reflect abnormal lateralization in neurodevelopment.

Although this chapter is not concerned with psychopathology per se, it is worth mentioning that some of the most robust associations between brain structure and schizophrenia symptoms have been with temporal lobe structures. Symptom severity has been associated with reductions in bilateral temporal lobe volume, along with decreased hippocampal and left STG volumes. The left anterior and left posterior STG have been strongly associated with the severity of both auditory hallucinations and thought disorder. Schneiderian symptom severity has been associated with volumes of the right posterior cingulate gray matter and left anterior parahippocampal gyrus. Positive symptoms are not the only ones related to temporal lobe findings. Negative symptoms have been correlated with decreases in left medial temporal lobe volumes (as well as prefrontal white matter volume). Investigations specifically directed at white matter in patients with schizophrenia (discussed below) have noted an association between the organization and coherence of white matter tracts in temporal lobe regions and impulsivity. Recently, the integrity of white matter tracts in the medial temporal lobe has been determined to relate to the severity of positive, negative, and general psychopathology symptom domains.

Parietal Lobe

Relatively few investigations have been directed at the parietal lobe in patients with schizophrenia, and most of those that have do not subdivide the parietal lobe into subregions. Nonetheless, the majority of studies directed at parietal lobe structures have shown some volume reductions. More recently, subdivisions of the parietal lobe on imaging studies have revealed reductions in the inferior parietal lobe and supramarginal gyrus. Perhaps most strikingly, correlations have been demonstrated between the inferior parietal lobe, prefrontal cortex, and temporal cortex, supporting the idea that connected brain structures, and perhaps even the connecting tracts themselves, may be critical to our understanding of schizophrenia.

Cerebellum

Although the cerebellum historically was relegated to the role of coordinating movement, recent evidence has suggested that it may play a role in higher cognitive functions. The cerebellum is highly connected to cortical association areas and limbic regions, and the notion has been put forth that the cerebellum may be associated with schizophrenia. Unfortunately, there have only been a handful of studies, and these studies have not yet consistently borne out any reliable findings. It should be noted, however, that these studies have varied widely in methodology, and little attempt has been made to subdivide the cerebellum into functionally discrete regions.

SUBCORTICAL FINDINGS

Thalamus

The thalamus is a relay station modulating input from cortical, limbic, and reticular activation areas, and it modulates sensory input and is involved in attention. The thalamus is also intimately connected to the prefrontal cortex, including the orbitofrontal and DLPFC with reciprocal connections.

The size of the thalamus has been demonstrated to be smaller in patients with schizophrenia. Subdivision of the thalamus in cytoarchitectural investigations seems particularly appropriate given that the thalamus receives input and sends output to a variety of cortical structures, each with potentially independent functions. The dorsomedial nucleus, which sends projections to the prefrontal cortex, has been shown to have a significantly decreased number of axons. The coherence of this thalamocortical pathway has also been demonstrated to be decreased in patients with schizophrenia, as measured by diffusion tensor imaging (DTI), a method by which the organization of white matter tracts can be determined (discussed below). The anteroventral nucleus, which projects largely to the prefrontal cortex, has also been found to have a decrease in the number of axons present. This is not to say that other areas of the thalamus do not have irregularities; rather, the lack of information regarding other thalamic nuclei reflects a paucity of investigation into these areas. Importantly, a reduction in synaptic protein rab3a has also been found in studies utilizing a substantial sample of subjects with schizophrenia.

Basal Ganglia

An increase in the volume of the basal ganglia has repeatedly been demonstrated in patients with schizophrenia. However, this increase has been determined to be largely a medication effect. Interestingly, it may be that typical neuroleptics are more responsible for this effect, because in one study, switching patients to an atypical neuroleptic for 1 year led to a decrease in caudate nucleus size. In contrast, medication-naive patients with schizophrenia have been shown to have reduced caudate size in several studies, although this finding is, of course, contradicted in a study that noted no significant size difference between basal ganglia volume in treated and never-treated patients. Finally, reduced volume of the basal ganglia has been demonstrated in patients with depression as well, making the specificity of this finding to schizophrenia somewhat suspect.

DYSCONNECTIVITY AND THE POSSIBLE ROLE OF WHITE MATTER IN SCHIZOPHRENIA

The theory of dysconnectivity suggests that the inability of different brain regions to communicate effectively with each other has a causal impact on the symptoms, course, and neuropathology of schizophrenia. Disorganized or poorly insulated neurotransmission may explain at least some of the observable psychophenomena of the disease. Proposed neuroanatomical consequences include the idea that areas that should receive ongoing, function-maintaining trophic signaling fall into disrepair when the tracts that connect these regions are not communicating optimally, and that this might explain some of the regional evidence we presented in earlier sections. In addition, if disconnectivity is part of the neuropathology of schizophrenia, then the components of these connections, particularly white matter, should be somehow aberrant in the brains of patients with schizophrenia.

Over the past several years, multiple lines of evidence have converged in support of the idea that, indeed, white matter—specifically oligodendrocytes and myelin—is involved in patients with schizophrenia. Increased cell density has been found in the deep white matter in patients with schizophrenia, along with maldistribution of neurons in white matter of the prefrontal cortex (PFC), although both of these findings have not been universally demonstrated. Microarray studies have found decreased expression of myelin-related genes in several brain regions, and quantification and qualification of oligodendrocytes in postmortem samples have found a deficit of close to 25% in the PFC of patients with schizophrenia, along with altered spacing and distribution. Other postmortem examinations have revealed abnormal changes in both myelin and oligodendrocytes in the PFC and caudate nucleus of patients with schizophrenia. DTI (a special type of MRI analysis that is well suited to the examination of white matter) has found decreased organization and coherence of white matter in widespread brain regions, including the PFC, temporoparietal and parieto-occipital regions, splenium, cingulum, posterior capsule, medial temporal cortex, and frontal white matter underlying the DLPFC and anterior cingulate. This evidence is buttressed by a finding of globally reduced fractional anisotropy (FA)—the output measure of the sum of vectors in a given brain region—in the brains of patients with schizophrenia. Relationships between symptoms of schizophrenia and decreased FA have been demonstrated as well. For example, decreased FA in the medial temporal lobe has been associated with increasing symptom severity, as has a relationship between decreasing FA in frontal white matter in patients with schizophrenia and the ability to live independently. Other associations between decreased FA in the cingulum bundle and executive function have been recently demonstrated in patients with schizophrenia, whereas decreased FA in the uncinate fasciculus has been associated with deficits in declarative–episodic memory. Interestingly, increased FA has been demonstrated in the arcuate fasciculus in patients with auditory hallucinations. These findings, which continue to accumulate, strongly support the idea of white matter involvement and dysconnectivity in schizophrenia, although the exact nature of the role white matter plays in the disease is still under investigation.

IS SCHIZOPHRENIA PROGRESSIVE?

Although debate about whether schizophrenia is a progressive disease still continues, there appears to be increasing evidence that, at least in some populations and in some neuroanatomical measures, schizophrenia is progressive. For example, increase in ventricular size has been shown to progress over time as patients with schizophrenia further diverge from controls as time with the disease lengthens, and patients with the largest ventricles have been demonstrated to have both the worst premorbid levels of functioning, and the worst prognoses and most severe symptoms. Temporal lobe and frontal lobe volume changes have been reported to progress with time as well. Further supporting the idea of schizophrenia as a progressive disease, in childhood-onset schizophrenia (COS), a rare but fairly well-characterized presentation, ventricles are enlarged and temporal volumes are decreased. But more importantly, patients with COS have a progression of brain pathology, with severe reductions in frontal and temporal lobes that by age 18 begin to resemble those of adult schizophrenia. Finally, patients with schizophrenia have been demonstrated to have a quickly progressing decline in cognitive function, beginning near age 65, despite years of stable cognitive performance over the course of their disease, highlighting the fact that cross-sectional evidence that argues for the static nature of the disease may require longitudinal confirmation.

LIMITATIONS ON NEUROPATHOLOGICAL INVESTIGATIONS IN SCHIZOPHRENIA

There are several problems with neuropathological investigations of schizophrenia (summarized in Table 5.2 on page 46). First, in postmortem investigations, the postmortem index (PMI) is a profound determinant of tissue integrity and, consequently, of the validity and generalizability of findings. The PMI is essentially a measure of the integrity of brain tissue at the time of fixation, and it includes numerous variables, including the time from death to fixation, the pH of brain tissue at the time of death, the exact nature of death (i.e., suicide vs. "natural causes"), and the presence of agonal events that could alter brain tissue. Second, the variable attention to stereological methods in sampling or sectioning brain tissue is comparable to different methods of regional differentiation in imaging studies. The lack of reliable methods in either instance can lead to inaccurate results, especially given the subtleties of the findings in schizophrenia. Third, different groups of investigators apply different methodologies to the analysis of data, even when using similar investigatory techniques and looking at presumably identical brain regions. This particular problem is to a certain extent due to the progress of knowledge in the field. The increasing specificity of investigation is partly the product of ongoing confirmation of more generalized findings, and partly the consequence of advances in investigational technology. In any event, the result is that comparing results or performing meta-analyses over time become problematic, because these variations make datasets unique and difficult to pool. Finally, small sample sizes remain problematic in schizophrenia research, increasing the likelihood of both false-positive and false-negative results.

FUTURE DIRECTIONS

We began this chapter by stating that schizophrenia is likely an endophenotype. After this cursory review of the neuropathology of schizophrenia, one can readily see the disparate and piecemeal nature of the evidence at hand. Subtle findings are the rule rather than the exception, and although conflicting results may represent technological differences, they may also reveal different processes that lead to the same gross symptom picture in people with schizophrenia. Research in this devastating disease is fraught with difficulty, from the vast variation in the nature of the clinical presentation to the current impossibility of dividing schizophrenia into more homogenous subgroupings that further delineate different brain processes that may have gone awry in a particular patient. Treatment development remains hampered by this limitation as well, because etiology-driven treatments remain on the horizon so long as the nature of the disease remains elusive. As technology advances in brain imaging, as well as in microscopic analysis, so will our understanding of how to partition schizophrenia in ways that propel our understanding forward, ultimately leading to advances in treatment and perhaps even prevention.

KEY POINTS

- Schizophrenia is likely an endophenotype, in which differences in disease presentation and course may reflect distinct but potentially interrelated neuropathological deficits.
- There are undoubtedly genetic and environmental contributions to the etiology of schizophrenia. The neurodevelopmental model of schizophrenia should be given substantial weight, and it should be noted that insults that occur early in life may not have consequences until young adulthood.
- The neuropathological findings in schizophrenia are subtle, and as technology progresses, we may find that many of the conflicts surrounding current findings are resolved more definitively.
- Increased ventricle size, reductions in temporal lobe and frontal lobe structures, along with thalamic abnormalities, reflect some of the most robust findings in schizophrenia research at this time.
- White matter has a place in the study of schizophrenia. Alterations in connectivity that may result from alterations in myelin and oligodendrocytes seem to be worthy of serious consideration by the field.
- At least portions of the neuroanatomical findings in schizophrenia research appear to be progressive.
- Both white matter and gray matter aberrations may make separate but intimately reciprocal contributions to the schizophrenia syndrome.

REFERENCES AND RECOMMENDED READINGS

Davis K. L., Stewart D. G., Friedman, J. I., Buchsbaum, M., Harvey, P. D., Hof, P. R., et al. (2003). White, matter changes in schizophrenia: Evidence for myelin-related dysfunction. *Archives of General Psychiatry, 60*(5), 443–456.

du Bois, T. M., Deng, C., & Huang, X. F. (2005). Membrane phospholipid composition, alterations in neurotransmitter systems and schizophrenia. *Progress in Neuropsychopharmacology and Biological Psychiatry, 29*(6), 878–888.

Frith, C. (2005). The neural basis of hallucinations and delusions. *Comptes Rendus Biologies, 328*(2), 169–175.

Harrison, P. J. (1999). The neuropathology of schizophrenia: A critical review of the data and their interpretation. *Brain, 122*(4), 593–624.

Hemsley, D. R. (2005). The development of a cognitive model of schizophrenia: Placing it in context. *Neuroscience and Biobehavioral Reviews, 29*(6), 977–988.

Konradi, C. (2005). Gene expression microarray studies in polygenic psychiatric disorders: Applications and data analysis. *Brain Research Reviews, 50*(1), 142–155.

Kubicki, M., McCarley, R., Westin C. F., Park, H.J., Maier, S., Kikinis, R., et al. (2005). A review of diffusion tensor imaging studies in schizophrenia. *Journal of Psychiatric Research, 41*, 15–30.

Shenton, M. E., Dickey, C. C., Frumin, M., & McCarley, R. W. (2001). A review of MRI findings in schizophrenia. *Schizophrenia Research, 49*(1–2), 1–52.

Shoval, G., & Weizman, A. (2005). The possible role of neurotrophins in the pathogenesis and therapy of schizophrenia. *European Neuropsychopharmacology, 15*(3), 319–329.

van den Buuse, M., Garner, B., Gogos, A., & Kusljic, S. (2005). Importance of animal models in schizophrenia research. *Australian and New Zealand Journal of Psychiatry, 39*(7), 550–557.

CHAPTER 6

GENETICS

STEPHEN J. GLATT

The goal of this text is to provide a concise, hands-on, up-to-date, authoritative book to assist clinicians in planning and delivering treatment for their clients with schizophrenia. As the title suggests, this chapter provides clinicians with an orientation to the subspecialty of psychiatry known as psychiatric genetics, and to the types of clinically relevant information that psychiatric genetic research can yield for the early identification of—and intervention in—schizophrenia. Psychiatric genetics is an area of research in which human behavior and mental phenomena are studied in relation to inherited factors, or genes. However, the term *psychiatric genetics* is actually shorthand for *psychiatric genetic epidemiology*, which more accurately reflects the discipline's alignment with the larger field of genetic epidemiology. *Genetic epidemiology* has been defined as "a science that deals with etiology, distribution, and control of disease in groups of relatives and with inherited causes of disease in populations" (Morton, 1982, Preface). Genetic epidemiologists examine the distribution of illness within families with the goal of finding genetic *and* environmental causes of illness. Thus, psychiatric genetic epidemiology, or psychiatric genetics, considers both environmental and genetic factors—and their interactions—to be on an equal footing and to have an equal likelihood of influencing a given behavior, until data indicate otherwise. These assumptions are then tested empirically, of course, and the relative environmental and genetic contributions to a behavior can be determined.

Psychiatric genetic research on a particular disorder such as schizophrenia (or any relevant "phenotype," including subthreshold psychopathology, biological traits, etc.) tends to follow a series of questions in a logical progression (Table 6.1). This sequence, which has been referred to as "the chain of psychiatric genetic research" (Faraone, Tsuang, & Tsuang, 1999), proceeds as follows: First we ask, "Is the phenotype familial?" or "Does it run in families?" Second, "What is the relative magnitude of genetic and environmental contributions to the phenotype?" Third, "How is the phenotype transmitted from generation to generation?" Fourth, "If genes mediate this transmission, where are they located?" Fifth, "What specific genes influence risk for the phenotype?" These are difficult questions to answer for any trait, but particularly so for phenotypes as complex as human behavior and psychiatric disorders. Fortunately, a wide variety of methods are available to help psychiatric genetic researchers resolve these issues. Those listed in Table

TABLE 6.1. The Chain of Psychiatric Genetic Research

Question	Appropriate methods
1. Does the phenotype run in families?	Family study
2. What are the contributions of genes and environment?	Twin study, adoption study
3. What is the mode of transmission?	Segregation analysis
4. Where are the genes located?	Linkage analysis
5. What are the responsible genes?	Association analysis

6.1 represent a sampling of the most popular and powerful methods available for answering these fundamental questions in the chain of psychiatric genetic research.

RESEARCH METHODS

Psychiatric genetics is a multidisciplinary field whose roots in psychiatry, human genetics, statistics, and epidemiology date back nearly 100 years. The earliest work on schizophrenia involved clinical and behavioral genetic methods such as family, twin, and adoption studies, and segregation analyses, which are effective for establishing whether, to what degree, and in what manner genetic factors influence the disorder (questions 1–3 in Table 6.1). Subsequently, the field branched out to include molecular genetic methods that could enable the isolation of chromosomal regions and identification of specific genes mediating familial transmission of schizophrenia through linkage and association analyses (questions 4 and 5 in Table 6.1).

Question 1: Is Schizophrenia Familial?

The first question that must be answered when attempting to delineate the genetic and environmental components of a disorder is, "Does the phenotype run in families?" or "Is this phenotype familial?" This question can be answered through the use of family studies. The basic design of the family study begins with the ascertainment of a group of subjects that is affected with schizophrenia (cases) and a comparable group of control subjects who do not have the disorder. Next, the biological relatives of these index subjects, or *probands*, are ascertained and evaluated for the presence of schizophrenia. The rate of the disorder among family members of affected probands is then compared to the rate of the disorder among family members of control probands to determine the familial risk, or relative risk. In a family study, or in any of the other genetic studies described in this chapter, it should be recognized that schizophrenia can be defined by the presence of formal diagnostic criteria or, for research purposes, alternative classification schemes (e.g., schizophrenia spectrum disorders) may be used to maximize inferential power.

If schizophrenia has a genetic etiology, then biological relatives of cases should have a higher likelihood than relatives of controls of carrying the gene or genes that influenced illness in their relative; thus, they should be at greater risk for the illness themselves. In addition, the risk to relatives of cases should be correlated with their degree of relationship to the proband, or the amount of genes they share in common. First-degree relatives, such as parents, siblings, and children, share 50% of their genes, on average, with the proband. Thus, first-degree relatives of cases should be at greater risk for the disorder than second-degree relatives (grandparents, uncles, aunts, nephews, nieces, and half-siblings), because second-degree relatives share only 25% of their genes with the proband.

Question 2: What Are the Relative Contributions of Genes and Environment?

Once a disorder has been established as familial, it becomes necessary to determine whether that pattern is attributable to the inheritance of genes or to shared familial and other environmental factors. It is also important to quantify the contribution that genes make relative to that made by environmental factors, because this may not only encourage or discourage future molecular genetic studies but also influence the decisions made by individuals seeking genetic counseling. These questions can be answered by both twin and adoption studies.

Twin Studies

In twin study designs, identical (monozygotic [MZ]) and fraternal (dizygotic [DZ]) twin pairs are included if at least one pair member is affected with schizophrenia. Twin pairs are deemed "concordant" if both members of the pair have schizophrenia, and discordant if only one member of the pair is affected. The ratio of concordant:discordant MZ twin pairs is then compared to the ratio of concordant:discordant DZ twin pairs.

MZ twins are derived from the same zygote and share 100% of their genetic material. In contrast, DZ twins result from separate fertilizations and share, on average, 50% of their genes—no more or less than any other pair of siblings. Thus, a typical MZ twin pair will have 50% more genes in common than a typical DZ twin pair. The degree of similarity in environmental exposures between members of an MZ twin pair should be no different than that between members of a DZ twin pair, however. Thus, any difference in concordance for schizophrenia between the two types of twin pairs can be attributed to the effects of the additional gene sharing in the MZ twins. In other words, sharing 50% more genes in common can be attributed as the sole factor responsible for any increased phenotypic similarity among MZ twin pairs relative to DZ twin pairs.

Concordance for schizophrenia that is higher for MZ twin pairs than for DZ twin pairs is a good indication that there is a genetic contribution to the disorder; if MZ and DZ twin pairs have approximately equal concordance rates, environmental factors are more strongly implicated. Frequently, concordance rates in twin pairs are used to estimate the *heritability* of a disorder, which is the degree to which genetic factors influence variability in the manifestation of the phenotype. Heritability in the broad sense is the ratio of genetic to phenotypic variances, or the proportion of variance in schizophrenia risk that is accounted for by variability in genetic factors. A heritability of 1.0 indicates that all variability in the phenotype is due to genetic factors alone. In contrast, a heritability of zero attributes all phenotypic variation to environmental factors.

Adoption Studies

An alternative to the twin method for parsing the genetic and environmental contributions to schizophrenia is the adoption study, in which ascertainment targets individuals with schizophrenia who were involved in an adoption, either as an adoptee or as an adoptive or biological parent of an adoptee. Next, the biological and adoptive relatives of these probands are ascertained and evaluated for the presence of the disorder. The rate of schizophrenia among the biological relatives of probands is then compared to the rate of the disorder among adoptive relatives of the probands.

Children adopted at an early age have a genetic relationship to their biological parents and an environmental relationship to their adopted parents. Thus, adoption studies can determine whether biological or adoptive (environmental) relationships account for the familial transmission of schizophrenia. If genes are important, then the familial transmission of the illness should occur in the biological family but not in the adoptive family. In contrast, if culture, social learning, or other sources of environmental transmission cause schizophrenia, familial transmission should occur in the adoptive family but not in the biological family.

Question 3: What Is the Mode of Transmission?

Once twin and/or adoption studies demonstrate that the familial transmission of a disorder is due at least in part to genetic factors, it becomes necessary to identify the manner in which those genetic factors exert their influence. The mode of transmission of schizophrenia through multiply affected families can be modeled statistically through the use of segregation analysis. A model of familial transmission translates assumptions about genetic and environmental causes into mathematical equations. These equations are then used to predict the distribution of a disorder that we observe in pedigrees. If the pattern of disorder predicted by a given model is close to what we observe, then this provides evidence in favor of that model. In contrast, if the predicted pattern of disorder differs from what is observed in the pedigree, then we reject the model and seek another mechanism of transmission.

Segregation analysis is a flexible procedure that can test various known and hypothesized modes of genetic transmission; the familiar Mendelian model of single-gene transmission of a trait is only one of many transmission mechanisms that can be tested. In general, these alternative models can be assigned to three classes: single major gene, oligogenic, and multifactorial polygenic models. The word *major* indicates that one gene can account for most of the genetic transmission of a disorder, while other genes and environmental conditions may play minor roles in modifying the expression of the disease. In contrast, an oligogenic model assumes that the combined actions of several genes cause illness. These genes may combine in an additive fashion, such that the probability of illness is a function of the number of pathogenic genes; alternatively, the mechanism may be interactive. The multifactorial polygenic (MFP) model proposes that a large, unspecified number of genes and environmental factors combine in an additive fashion to cause schizophrenia. The difference between oligogenic and polygenic models is one of degree; the former test for effects of "several" genes (e.g., less than 10), whereas the latter evaluate a "large number" of genes (e.g., 100).

Although the MFP model posits that many genes and environmental factors contribute additively to development of a disorder, these individual factors are not directly modeled. According to the model, liability toward developing the disorder is normally distributed, and individuals above a certain threshold on the liability scale manifest the illness. More than one threshold may be placed along the liability continuum, representing varying degrees of severity. Thus, individuals beyond the threshold may develop a severe form of the disorder; those under the threshold may have minor problems or be unaffected; and those whose liability falls between the two thresholds may have an intermediate form of the disorder.

Question 4: Where are the Genes Located?

Knowing the manner in which a heritable psychiatric disorder is transmitted through families is useful for designing optimal molecular genetic studies to reveal the chromosomal location. To identify regions of chromosomes that have a high likelihood of harboring risk genes for schizophrenia, linkage analysis is a highly appropriate strategy. Families are ascertained for linkage analysis through a proband affected with schizophrenia. Each individual in the family is then genotyped at a series of DNA markers (not necessarily in genes) spaced evenly throughout the genome, and the cosegregation of these DNA markers with schizophrenia is tracked in each pedigree. Evidence for cosegregation at each marker locus is summed across pedigrees to derive an index of the likelihood of the obtained patterns of marker–phenotype cosegregation given the sampled pedigree structures.

Linkage analysis is a more powerful method of establishing the genetic etiology of psychiatric disorders than the statistical methods of segregation analysis. Segregation analysis can only show that the pattern of disease is consistent with a specific genetic model, whereas linkage analysis can actually determine where the gene is located on the human genome. Linkage analysis is made possible by the "crossing over" that takes place between two homologous chromosomes during *meiosis*, the process whereby gametes are created. Genetic transmission occurs because we inherit one member of each pair of chromosomes from our mother and one from our father; however, these inherited chromosomes are not identical to any of the original parental chromosomes. During meiosis, the original chromosomes in a pair cross over each other and exchange portions of their deoxyribonucleic acid (DNA). After multiple crossovers, the resulting two chromosomes each comprise a new and unique combination of genes.

The probability that two genes on the same chromosome will recombine during meiosis is a function of their physical distance from one another. We say that two loci on the same chromosome are "linked" when they are so close to one another that crossing over rarely or never occurs between them. Closely linked genes usually remain together on the same chromosome after meiosis is complete. The greater the distance between loci on the same chromosome, the more likely it is that they will recombine.

Although the DNA markers used for linkage analysis are not presumed to be actual risk genes for the disorder, they are numerous and dense enough to ensure that their coinheritance with a nearby (but unobserved) risk gene could be inferred with reasonable certainty based on the coinheritance of the marker with the phenotype that is influenced by that risk gene. In this design, the disorder serves as a proxy for the risk gene; thus, DNA markers that cosegregate commonly with the disorder are presumed to cosegregate commonly with its underlying risk gene. Because the probability of cosegregation of two pieces of DNA is inversely proportional to the distance between them, the regularity of the cosegregation of the DNA marker and schizophrenia gives an indirect indication of the genetic distance between the DNA marker and the unobserved risk gene.

The possible outcomes of a linkage analysis varies based on the structure of families ascertained for analysis. For example, linkage analysis can be performed with affected sibling pairs, with other affected relative pairs, with small nuclear families, or with large extended pedigrees. Regardless of which family structure is the principal unit of analysis, the common output across methods is some index of the degree of phenotypic similarity of family members and the degree of genotypic similarity between those individuals at each DNA marker. These indices are summed across families to determine the overall evidence for linkage at a given locus in the full sample. If a given DNA marker cosegregates with schizophrenia through families more often than would be expected by chance, then this indicates that the marker is "linked" (i.e., is in relatively close physical proximity) to a risk gene that influences expression of the disorder.

Question 5: What Are the Responsible Genes?

Once regions of certain chromosomes have been implicated by linkage analysis as harboring a risk gene for a disorder, the next step is to identify what specific gene is segregating through families to give rise to that linkage signal. A gene can be selected for such analysis subsequent to linkage analysis as a means to follow up on evidence for increased genetic similarity at a locus among affected individuals in a family (i.e., a "positional candidate gene" approach). Alternatively, specific genes can be examined in the absence of linkage information if there is some compelling reason to suspect that the gene influences risk for a given disorder (i.e., a "functional candidate gene" approach). For example, dopamine system genes, such as receptors and transporters, are commonly examined as functional candidates for schizophrenia. In contrast to linkage analysis, which uses random DNA markers as proxies for nearby risk genes, genetic association analysis is the appropriate method for determining whether a particular gene variant has a direct effect on risk for schizophrenia, or is very tightly linked to such a gene.

If a gene influences risk for schizophrenia, then this should be detectable as an increased frequency of the risk allele of the gene (or a tightly linked marker allele in a nearby gene) in cases relative to controls. Within the context of the family, this would be detectable as an increased likelihood of a patient with schizophrenia receiving the risk allele of the gene from his or her parent, even when both the risk and normal forms of the gene were present in the parent and could have been transmitted with equal frequency and likelihood.

In a case–control association study, we simply count the number of each type of allele of a gene that is found in cases and compare these counts with the allele distribution seen in the control group (this process can also be performed for genotypes). A simple statistical test can then be used to determine whether the distribution of alleles observed in the group of cases is different from that seen in the control group. If it is different, then we have found evidence for a genetic association with schizophrenia, where the allele that is overrepresented in the group of cases is considered the risk allele. The degree of overrepresentation of the risk allele in cases relative to controls can be used to derive an odds ratio, which gives a numeric indication of an individual's chance of being affected by a disorder if he or she possesses the risk allele. In family-based studies, we can use analogous statistics to determine whether any difference from the expected equal inheritance of risk and normal alleles of a gene is detected in affected probands who could have received either allele from their parent. In a family-based study, the odds ratio estimates the haplotype relative risk, which represents the increase in the probability of the affected offspring receiving the risk allele relative to the normal allele.

MAJOR FINDINGS

Family Studies

The results of many family studies of schizophrenia strongly support the hypothesis that schizophrenia has a genetic etiology. Anecdotal evidence of the familial nature of schizophrenia was first offered more than a century ago by Kraepelin, who noted that as many as 70% of his patients with *dementia praecox* were familial cases. It was not until 1916, however, that the first systematic assessment of familial patterns of schizophrenia was undertaken by Rüdin (1916). In this first of many family studies of schizophrenia, the close relatives of an affected individual were found to have a sixfold increase in risk for developing the illness themselves. Subsequent reports routinely replicated a pattern of higher schizophrenia prevalence among the relatives of patients with schizophrenia. A quantitative review of 40 family studies of schizophrenia revealed a consistent pattern of elevated risk among relatives of affected individuals, with the degree of risk contingent upon the degree of biological relation to the patient. It is noteworthy, however, that this relationship was not linear: The risk to first-degree relatives was more than twice that to second-degree relatives despite the mere doubling of biological relation to the individual with schizophrenia. Furthermore, it was noted that the risk to offspring of two parents with schizophrenia, from whom the affected offspring received all of their genes, was not absolute (~46%).

Consistent with modern conceptualizations of schizophrenia as a continuous rather than discrete entity, most evidence suggests that family members of an affected patient are at a heightened risk for schizophrenia spectrum conditions, in addition to their increased liability to schizophrenia. For example, approximately 9% of the relatives of a patient with schizophrenia will have a psychotic disorder that does not meet criteria for schizophrenia (e.g., schizoaffective disorder or psychosis not otherwise specified). Aggregation of schizotypal personality disorder is also frequently observed in families affected by schizophrenia, with an incidence as high as 14.6% in relatives of a patient with schizophrenia.

Despite this powerful evidence, it is important to recognize that familiality does not necessarily establish heritability. For example, religion and language are familial traits, because all members of the same family often practice the same religion and speak the same language. These facts do not reflect the transmission of "religion genes" or "language genes" through the family, but rather the common environment and upbringing that those family members share.

Twin and Adoption Studies

Most of the twin studies of schizophrenia have supported a genetic contribution to the disorder. The best evidence from these studies suggests a concordance rate of approximately 46–53% for MZ twins and 14–15% for DZ twins. It is interesting to note that the concordance rate of MZ twins is not twice that of DZ twins, despite the fact that on average the former share twice the genetic material of the latter. Instead, the best available evidence indicates that MZ twins are more than three times more likely than DZ twins to exhibit concordance for schizophrenia, suggesting the possibility of gene–gene interactions (epistasis) in the etiology of the disorder. Furthermore, MZ twins are not 100% concordant for the disease. In fact, based on the differences in schizophrenia concordance between MZ and DZ twin pairs, the heritability of the disorder has been estimated at between 60 and 70%, whereas most of the remaining liability for the disorder is acquired through environmental factors that are unique to the individual rather than shared by family members. In the most compelling adoption study of schizophrenia, Kety, Rosenthal, Wender, and Schulsinger (1968) examined 5,483 Danish children who were adopted between 1923 and 1947, and found that more adoptees who were separated from a biological parent with schizophrenia developed schizophrenia or a related disorder than did control adoptees (8.7 and 1.9%, respectively). Thus, it appears that genetic transmission of schizophrenia risk genes is the major contributor to the familial aggregation of the disorder; however, these observations also highlight the important role of environmental factors in its development and expression.

Segregation Analyses

The complexity of schizophrenia inheritance was suggested by the observations of incomplete MZ twin concordance and less than complete transmission of the illness from two parents with schizophrenia to their offspring, along with the nonlinear relationship between risk and degree of biological relationship to a patient with schizophrenia. The clearest finding from analyses of the segregation of schizophrenia through extended pedigrees is that the disorder is not transmitted in a Mendelian fashion. For example, if a single dominant gene caused schizophrenia, 50% of individuals with one parent with schizophrenia would develop the disorder themselves; yet only 13% of such individuals actually become affected. Alternatively, if the disorder were caused by a single recessive gene, every individual with two affected parents would develop schizophrenia, but less than 50% of these individuals actually do.

It is also quite clear that, unlike Huntington's disease or other diseases caused by mutations in a single gene, schizophrenia has multiple genetic determinants. Models that posit a single major locus for schizophrenia are unable to predict accurately the incidence of the disorder in the parents, siblings, MZ twins, and DZ twins of a patient with schizophrenia. Through the analysis of segregation of schizophrenia through families, such a mode of inheritance has been rejected in favor of polygenic and multifactorial models. The evidence to support this etiological model is substantial. For example, such a model can account for varying degrees of severity of the disorder and, thus, the inheritance of subthreshold schizophrenia spectrum conditions in schizophrenia pedigrees. Furthermore, the risk for schizophrenia is related to both the number of cases and the severity of schizophrenia among an individual's relatives. The nonlinearity of the relationship between risk and biological relation to a patient with schizophrenia observed in family and twin studies is also strong evidence for a polygenic mechanism. A multifactorial polygenic explanation of this finding is strengthened further by allowing for epistasis among the putative risk genes.

Linkage Analyses

The results of no less than 18 independent genomewide linkage analyses have been published to date. Each of these studies has identified at least one chromosomal region in which some evidence for linkage between a marker and a putative schizophrenia-related gene was observed. Although the findings from these genomewide linkage scans do not entirely overlap, this is not unexpected given the methodological differences between the studies, including the regional distribution and lineage of ascertained target populations, the type and spacing of genotyped markers, and the various phenotypic definitions of schizophrenia applied to subjects. To narrow down the search for genetic linkage with schizophrenia, Badner and Gershon (2002) performed a meta-analysis of all previous genomewide linkage scans. The results of this pooled analysis identified loci on chromosomes 8p, 13q, and 22q as the best candidates to harbor schizophrenia-relevant risk genes. Other promising regions included chromosomes 1q, 2q, 6q, and 15q, but evidence for linkage at these loci was weaker, indicating a need for further replication. The results of these genome scans, and especially the more powerful meta-analysis, should inform subsequent efforts to examine linkage within finite, densely mapped regions of individual chromosomes. The alleles of specific genes that may eventually be identified from such methods can then be tested directly for association with the disorder.

Association Analyses

Many genes have been tested for an association with schizophrenia, because they either code for proteins thought to be involved in the pathology of the disorder or map to a chromosomal region implicated in the disorder by linkage analysis. In the former group, several genes have been verified in large, pooled samples to have a small but reliable influence on risk for the disorder. Some of these include the genes coding for the serotonin

2A receptor (*HTR2A*) and the dopamine D_2 (*DRD2*) and D_3 (*DRD3*) receptors. Genes coding for disrupted-in-schizophrenia 1 (*DISC1*), dystrobrevin-binding protein 1 (*DTNBP1*), neuregulin 1 (*NRG1*), and regulator of G-protein signaling 4 (*RGS4*) have emerged as the strongest positional candidate risk genes for schizophrenia, but these findings require verification. The identification of numerous risk genes of varying effect on the liability toward developing schizophrenia may ultimately make it possible to create a genetic risk profile that is predictive of future onsets of the disorder. Such a genetic risk profile may also be used in genetic counseling settings to help potential parents understand the risk of schizophrenia to their unborn child and to make decisions based on this information. Most relevant for the treatment of schizophrenia, several genes, including *DRD2* and *HTR2A*, have also been reported to influence the outcome of psychopharmacological interventions. As the relationships between these genes and specific aspects of favorable or unfavorable response to antipsychotic medications become further characterized, these too may attain clinical utility in the development and administration of genetically tailored, personalized medication management of schizophrenia. We must emphasize, however, that such uses of genetic data are not possible at this time and may not be possible for some time.

KEY POINTS

- Schizophrenia is a familial disorder, and the risk of schizophrenia to relatives of an affected individual increases as their degree of biological relationship increases.
- The familial nature of schizophrenia is largely due to the transmission of genetic risk factors through families; however, a sizable portion of the risk for the disorder is also influenced by environmental factors.
- The patterns of inheritance of schizophrenia through multiply affected families are not consistent with the effects of a single gene; rather, a multifactorial polygenic etiology is supported, in which multiple genetic and environmental factors each have a small effect on overall risk for the disorder.
- Genetic linkage analysis has revealed several "hot spots" that may harbor genes that influence the risk for schizophrenia.
- Functional candidate genes have been identified that have small effects on risk for schizophrenia; however, positional candidate genes of as yet unknown function may have even stronger influences.
- The major contributions of psychiatric genetic research to clinical psychiatry currently remain unrealized, but such research may ultimately be used to reduce uncertainty in formulating primary and differential diagnoses, to provide individually tailored pharmacotherapy and disease management, to enable early identification and intervention leading to better prognoses, and ultimately to inspire effective prevention programs.

REFERENCES AND RECOMMENDED READINGS

Badner, J. A., & Gershon, E. S. (2002). Meta-analysis of whole-genome linkage scans of bipolar disorder and schizophrenia. *Molecular Psychiatry, 7*(4), 405–411.

Faraone, S. V., Tsuang, M. T., & Tsuang, D. W. (1999). *Genetics of mental disorders: What practictioners and students need to know.* New York: Guilford Press.

Kety, S. S., Rosenthal, D., Wender, P. H., & Schulsinger, F. (1968). The types and prevalence of mental illness in the biological and adoptive families of adopted schizophrenics. *Journal of Psychiatric Research, 1*(Suppl.), 345–362.

Kraepelin, É. (1971). *Dementia praecox and paraphrenia* (R. M. Barclay, Trans.). Huntington, NY: Krieger. (Original work published 1919)

McGue, M., Gottesman, I. I., & Rao, D. C. (1983). The transmission of schizophrenia under a multifactorial threshold model. *American Journal of Human Genetics, 35* 1161–1178.

McGue, M., Gottesman, I. I., & Rao, D. C. (1985). Resolving genetic models for the transmission of schizophrenia. *Genetic Epidemiology, 2,* 99–110.

Morton, N. E. (1982). *Outline of genetic epidemiology.* Basel: Karger.

O'Rourke, D. H., Gottesman, I. I., Suarez, B. K., Rice, J., & Reich, T. (1982). Refutation of the general single-locus model for the etiology of schizophrenia. *American Journal of Human Genetics, 34,* 630–649.

Rüdin, E. (1916). *Zur Vererbung und Neuentstehung der Dementia Praecox* [Studies on the inheritance and origin of mental illness]. Berlin: Springer.

Tsuang, M. T., Stone, W. S., & Faraone, S. V. (1999). Schizophrenia: A review of genetic studies. *Harvard Review of Psychiatry, 7,* 185–207.

CHAPTER 7

ENVIRONMENTAL PRE- AND PERINATAL INFLUENCES IN ETIOLOGY

LAUREN M. ELLMAN
TYRONE D. CANNON

In the search for the causes of schizophrenia, the preponderance of evidence suggests that genes play a substantial role in the etiology of the disorder. Based on the results from twin, family, and adoption studies, genetic influences account for approximately 80% of the disorder's etiology. Although schizophrenia appears to be a highly heritable disorder, it is clear that environmental factors also are involved. Many environmental influences have been investigated as potential contributors to the disorder, such as family environment, socioeconomic status, and substance abuse; however, a repeatedly demonstrated environmental predictor of schizophrenia has been a history of obstetric complications (OCs). OCs constitute a fairly broad class of events, including any deviation from the normal course of pregnancy, labor–delivery, and the early neonatal period, such as low birthweight, prenatal maternal infection, and many others (discussed below). Such complications are relatively common, occurring in the histories of approximately 20–30% of patients with schizophrenia and approximately 5–10% of the population overall. In this chapter, we provide an overview of the various OCs that have been linked to schizophrenia, discuss different explanatory models of how OCs operate within the etiology of the disorder, and discuss the potential mechanisms underlying two main classes of OCs associated with schizophrenia: prenatal infection and fetal oxygen deprivation.

HOW DO OCs OPERATE WITHIN THE ETIOLOGY OF SCHIZOPHRENIA?

An array of models has been proposed to explain how OCs contribute to the causes of schizophrenia. We cover the most prominent models in schizophrenia research and discuss which model is best supported by empirical research.

Some theorists have proposed that there may be a subgroup of patients with schizophrenia who acquire the disorder from entirely nongenetic origins. According to this model, an obstetric insult could cause schizophrenia independently of genetic contributions. If this model were correct, then exposure to OCs (with a given degree of severity and during a sensitive period of gestation) would lead to expression of schizophrenia with a fair degree of reliably. The prevailing evidence suggests that this model is unlikely, because the rate of OCs in the general population is far higher than the rate of schizophrenia (approximately 1% of the population). Even if OCs during particularly critical periods of gestation only were considered, there would likely still be a much higher rate of schizophrenia in the population if OCs were the sole cause of the disease onset. Therefore, there currently is little support for the idea that OCs alone can produce schizophrenia.

Another model, the gene–environment covariation model, posits that OCs are associated with the genes for the disorder, but OCs do not exert any etiological role in the disease. This model predicts an increase in the number of OCs in individuals who carry genes associated with schizophrenia, regardless of whether they develop the disorder. The main support for the gene–environment covariation model comes from studies that found increased birth complications in offspring of mothers with schizophrenia (who carry the disease-producing genes given that they express the disorder phenotypically), but it is inconsistent with the finding that unaffected siblings of patients with schizophrenia do not differ from the general population in the incidence of OCs. Siblings of patients with schizophrenia would be expected to share some of the disease-promoting genes, therefore leading to increased risk of OCs, if the gene–environment covariation model were correct. In addition, interpretation of increases in OCs among mothers with schizophrenia is complicated by the elevated occurrence of health-risk behaviors during pregnancy among this cohort. Specifically, women with schizophrenia are less likely to receive prenatal care, more likely to be polydrug users, more likely to drink alcohol, more likely to be on psychiatric medications, and more likely to smoke cigarettes than women without schizophrenia, all of which have been associated with increases in OCs. Moreover, discontinuation of antipsychotic medication has been associated with a worsening of symptoms, often leading to psychotic episodes in relatively asymptomatic women. The onset of a psychotic episode likely has many consequences for prenatal health, including increased stress, poor nutrition, poor self-care, suicide attempts, attempts at premature delivery, and other risky behaviors that could lead to deleterious pregnancy and birth outcomes. Given the limitations of the available data, findings that support the gene–environment covariation model are difficult to interpret.

Most studies support the gene–environment interaction model, which asserts that obstetric influences depend on the presence of disease-promoting genes in the etiology of schizophrenia. According to this model, the occurrence of an OC in a genetically vulnerable individual would increase the likelihood of that individual developing the disorder. Support for this model comes from studies in which a history of OCs differentiated between siblings with and without schizophrenia, suggesting that this early insult interacted with disease-producing genes to cause the disorder. It also is possible that genetic and obstetric risk factors for schizophrenia occur independently of each other but additively influence risk for disease expression (additive influence model). Both the gene–environment interaction model and the additive influences model predict a relative increase in the rate of OCs among individuals who develop schizophrenia; therefore, the two models are often difficult to separate. Specifically, it is very difficult to examine directly gene–environment interactions or gene–environment aggregations. To do this, it is necessary to measure the environmental influence, as well as the gene, or genes. This may be more feasible now, with the recent availability of serological data from pregnancy and the identification of candidate genes involved in schizophrenia. Nevertheless, only a handful of candidate genes have been identified, and schizophrenia is not caused by one gene, which further complicates the ease of directly testing gene–environment interactions and aggregations. For our purposes in this chapter, we refer to the gene–environment interaction model, but many of the findings may also fit into the additive influences model.

Last, it is possible that multiple models are correct and operate simultaneously within the disorder. This possibility has not been explored as extensively, but it will likely gain more attention with the virtual explosion of studies investigating specific genetic variations among patients with schizophrenia, termed polymorphisms, as well as increasing attempts to map out molecular pathways implicated in the disorder. For instance, a genetic polymorphism associated with a magnified inflammatory response has been linked to schizophrenia (discussed further in section on prenatal infection). In the presence of infection, this genetic polymorphism leads to increased inflammation (gene–environment interaction), the consequences of which are discussed more extensively below. Interestingly, this polymorphism also is associated with increased incidence of certain OCs, such as preterm delivery (gene–environment covariation); therefore, we can see that a gene associated with schizophrenia could have multiple functions, some others of which may serve to play a role in the causes of the disorder and others of which may be unrelated to the etiology. The relatively new opportunity to investigate directly gene–environment interactions at a molecular level will certainly shed considerable light on how OCs operate within the disorder.

WHAT TYPES OF OCs ARE ASSOCIATED WITH SCHIZOPHRENIA?

OCs have been linked to the etiology of schizophrenia since the 1960s when Lane and Albee (1966) first observed that birthweights of 52 patients with schizophrenia were lower than those of their siblings without schizophrenia. Despite the fact that the differences were relatively small (about 175 grams), and few of the schizophrenia patients had birthweights that were less than 2,500 grams (the criterion for low birthweight), this study raised the possibility that events during the very early stages of life may have long-lasting neurobiological effects, potentially contributing to the causes of schizophrenia.

Since the 1960s dozens of articles have linked aberrant events during the pre- and perinatal periods to schizophrenia. Investigations into this area have taken many forms, such as following genetically at-risk individuals (e.g., offspring of patients with schizophrenia and unaffected siblings of patients with schizophrenia), comparing the prevalence of OCs in patients with schizophrenia and controls (often using maternal recall), and, last, taking advantage of population databases and registries containing detailed information about the pre- and perinatal periods, as well as information regarding psychiatric statuses. Given the variety of study procedures, the conflicting results from many of the investigations exploring the role of obstetric events in the etiology of schizophrenia are not surprising. For this reason, studies using population registries (e.g., in Scandinavia) have been especially useful in providing detailed, prospective obstetric information, in addition to having large enough samples to detect meaningful results. Recent findings from population-based studies have had the added advantage of exploring molecular pathways in schizophrenia by examining stored maternal blood sera from the pre- and perinatal periods. For our purposes in this chapter, we briefly summarize the types of OCs that have been associated with schizophrenia; however, we focus on the more recent, population-based results, especially those using serological data.

Many OCs have been linked to schizophrenia and can grossly be divided into categories of complications during pregnancy, fetal and neonatal underdevelopment, and birth complications. A meta-analysis of eight population-based studies found that diabetes during pregnancy, birthweight less than 2,000 grams, emergency caesarean section, congenital malformations, uterine atony, rhesus variables (comprising rhesus [Rh] incompatibility, Rh-negative mother, Rh antibodies), fetal asphyxia, bleeding during pregnancy, birthweight less than 2,500 grams, preeclampsia, placental abruption, head circumference less than 32 cm, and nonspontaneous delivery all were associated with increased risk of schizophrenia. Beyond these eight studies, a large body of research has linked multiple infections during pregnancy and maternal stress to schizophrenia outcome in offspring.

Given the vast number of OCs linked to schizophrenia, the question arises as to whether any insult in a genetically vulnerable individual could lead to schizophrenia outcome, or whether some underlying mechanisms link these obstetric events to each other. Two pathways have been linked to many of the obstetric abnormalities associated with schizophrenia: (1) decreased oxygen to the fetus, termed *fetal hypoxia* or *asphyxia*, and (2) maternal immune responses to infection and other insults during pregnancy.

Fetal Hypoxia

There have now been multiple reviews (see References and Recommended Readings) that show that fetal hypoxia is likely involved in a variety of OCs associated with schizophrenia. Specifically, OCs associated with schizophrenia, such as emergency caesarian section, bleeding during pregnancy, and preeclampsia, have all been associated with fetal hypoxia. To test the strength of the relationship between hypoxia-associated OCs and schizophrenia onset in offspring, two studies used a hypoxia-associated OCs scale, including both indirect and direct indicators of hypoxia. Direct hypoxia-associated complications included events such as blue at birth, required resuscitation, neonatal cyanosis, and neonatal apnea. Indirect complications were selected based on validation with direct measures of hypoxia from previous studies and included abnormalities of fetal heart rate or rhythm, umbilical cord knotted or wrapped tightly around neck, third trimester bleeding, placental hemorrhaging or infarcts, an excessive amount of amniotic fluid (polyhydramnios), meconium[1] in amniotic fluid, and breech presentation. Both studies found that hypoxia-associated OCs were associated with schizophrenia outcome in offspring, especially when patients exhibited disease onset at an early age.

Hypoxia-associated OCs also have been found to differentiate between siblings with and without schizophrenia, suggesting that in the presence of a common genetic background (i.e., sibship), fetal hypoxia increases the likelihood of later developing schizophrenia. Nevertheless, fetal hypoxia is unlikely to lead to schizophrenia on its own; therefore, a genetic factor associated with schizophrenia likely renders the fetal brain particularly vulnerable to the effects of hypoxia. This hypothesis is supported by brain imaging studies, in which hypoxia-associated OCs predicted ventricular enlargement in patients with schizophrenia but not among their unaffected siblings and controls at low genetic risk for schizophrenia. Similarly, one study compared hippocampal volumes of patients with schizophrenia, their unaffected siblings, and nonschizophrenia comparison subjects, and found a stepwise decrease in hippocampal volumes with increased genetic liability for the disorder. A history of hypoxia-associated OCs led to further reductions in

---

[1] A dark-green fecal material that accumulates in the fetal intestines and is discharged at or near the time of birth.

hippocampal volumes among patients with schizophrenia, suggesting that genetic contributions to hippocampal volume reductions in patients with schizophrenia were worsened by a history of fetal hypoxia. The aforementioned studies support a gene–environment interaction model, in which an early hypoxic event adds to or interacts with a genetic vulnerability for schizophrenia, leading to a form of schizophrenia characterized by earlier age of onset and greater neuroanatomical abnormalities.

Independently of a genetic liability for schizophrenia, fetal hypoxia has been found to affect many of the same neural substrates implicated in schizophrenia, depending on the severity and duration of the hypoxic event, as well as the period of gestation. In sheep, fetal hypoxia has been found to disrupt neuronal development and connections in the hippocampus, cerebellum, and visual cortex. When the duration of the hypoxia was increased to 20 days during late gestation, abnormalities were found in the cerebellum, as well as white matter lesions. Shorter periods of hypoxia during midgestation were associated with reductions in cortical white matter, as well as hippocampal density reductions. Brains of rat pups exposed to perinatal hypoxia during the last day of gestation showed myelination deficits in multiple brain regions, including the hippocampus and cerebellum, suggesting that hypoxia may also affect neuronal signal speed. In addition, findings from rat studies have linked perinatal oxygen insufficiency with dopamine abnormalities in the prefrontal cortex, nucleus accumbens, and striatum.

In humans, fetal hypoxia has been linked to a series of motor and cognitive deficits in children. Children exposed to mild fetal hypoxia exhibited no detectable motor or cognitive deficits later in childhood; however, exposure to moderate fetal hypoxia led to speech, language, motor, verbal, and overall cognitive deficits. Furthermore, survivors of moderate hypoxia were more likely to be behind more than one grade level compared to children in their age group. The more severe cases of fetal hypoxia often lead to neonatal death or cerebral palsy. Thus, infants exposed to moderate and severe fetal hypoxia are at risk for physical and mental impairment, as well as worsened school performance even in the absence of a genetic vulnerability for schizophrenia.

Infection during Pregnancy

The role of prenatal infection in the etiology of schizophrenia has been repeatedly documented through a series of epidemiological and, more recently, serological studies. Season of birth, especially during winter–spring months, has been consistently linked with schizophrenia outcome, and these months are typically associated with a higher incidence of infection. Among epidemiological studies, various prenatal infections, including influenza and rubella exposure, have been linked to schizophrenia outcome, although there have been some conflicting findings.

More recently, serological data confirming maternal infection during pregnancy have emerged in schizophrenia research. These studies provide major methodological advancements over previous investigations, given that biological indicators of infection can provide a better estimation of positive cases, as well as assess the timing and severity of the infection. These data have come from banked maternal sera from two large birth cohort studies in the United States that followed women throughout the prenatal period and subsequently followed their offspring during the 1950s and 1960s. Among these studies, herpes simplex virus–2 (HSV-2), influenza, maternal genital and reproductive infection (including endometritis, cervicitis, pelvic inflammatory disease, vaginitis, syphilis, condylomata, "venereal disease," and gonorrhea) antibodies have been linked to schizophrenia spectrum disorders. Prenatal exposure to the parasitic infection *Toxoplasma gondii* was linked to schizophrenia in one study, but another study failed to replicated this finding, which may have been due to a relatively small sample size (including 27 psychotic off-spring, only 13 of whom were diagnosed with schizophrenia).

With the exception of the parasite *T. gondii*, viral infections rarely cross the placenta; therefore, the damaging effects of fetal exposure to most viral infections likely involve multiple molecular pathways, a primary one being the mother's immune response to viral infections. During pregnancy, many immunological changes to protect the fetus from the mother mounting an immune response to a genetically dissimilar entity. Many of these changes involve signaling proteins called *cytokines*, which are considered the hormones of the immune system and, among other functions, are essential in combating infections. Although there are exceptions, there seems to be a shift in immune functioning during pregnancy, with preferential production of helper T cell (Type 2) T_h2 cytokines, such as interleukin–4 (IL-4), interleukin–5 (IL-5), and interleukin–10 (IL-10), that are mainly involved in the stimulation of B cells and antibody responses. The relative increase in T_h2 cytokines during pregnancy has been associated with a down-regulation of T_h1 cytokines, such as interferon-gamma (IFN-gamma), tumor necrosis factor-alpha (TNF-alpha) and interleukin–2 (IL-2), which are involved in cell-mediated immunity and inflammation (proinflammatory cytokines), thereby potentially decreasing the mother's ability to respond to viral infection.

In addition to the possibility that the fetus is more vulnerable to infection due to a shift in maternal immune functioning, studies suggest that the maternal antiviral response may contribute directly to the neuronal abnormalities found in offspring exposed prenatally to infection, with particular importance placed on the role of proinflammatory cytokines. Pregnant mice injected with a sham virus, capable of producing an antiviral reaction, had offspring with cognitive deficits similar to those found among patients with schizophrenia, such as deficits in prepulse inhibition (thought to be a measure of sensorimotor gating). In concert with these findings, rats prenatally exposed to proinflammatory cytokines have a multitude of brain abnormalities similar to those found among patients with schizophrenia, such as abnormalities in the hippocampus and cortex. In humans, exposure to elevated cytokines during pregnancy has been associated with neurodevelopmental damage, such as periventricular leukomalacia, cerebral palsy, and mental retardation. In summary, these findings suggest that neuronal abnormalities associated with prenatal infection may be related to elevated proinflammatory cytokine production, even in the absence of a genetic diathesis for schizophrenia.

In addition to the direct neurotoxic effects of proinflammatory cytokines, growing evidence suggests a causal relationship between inflammation and multiple OCs found in the histories of patients with schizophrenia, including preterm delivery, preeclampsia, and fetal oxygen deprivation (hypoxia). As discussed earlier, fetal hypoxia leads to a series of neuronal abnormalities found among patients with schizophrenia, even in the absence of infection and in individuals at low genetic risk for schizophrenia. Therefore, fetal neuronal damage following exposure to inflammation may be in part a result of the damaging effects of fetal hypoxia.

Given the aforementioned studies, it is not surprising that investigators have begun to explore the possible relationship between fetal exposure to proinflammatory cytokines and schizophrenia outcome. This area of research is somewhat complicated by the dynamic nature of the immune system. Specifically, cytokines typically aggregate around the site of infection and/or injury; therefore, cytokine levels in blood serum typically do not accurately reflect either the constantly changing state of the immune system or the interactions between the mother's immune system and the developing fetus. Nevertheless, two studies have linked markers of inflammation from maternal serum to psychotic outcome in offspring. Specifically, interleukin-8 (IL-8) during second and third trimesters and TNF-alpha at the time of birth (both proinflammatory cytokines) have been linked to increased incidence of psychosis in offspring.

In addition to the direct neurotoxic effects of fetal exposure to proinflammatory cytokines, emerging evidence suggests that genetic polymorphisms found in schizophrenia populations may make certain individuals more susceptible to the negative effects of infection and inflammation. TNF-a (promoter region A2) and IL-1 complex [IL-1-alpha (-889) allele 2, IL-1-beta (-511) allele 1, and IL-1RA allele 1] genetic polymorphisms have been associated with schizophrenia outcome. These polymorphisms typically lead to both production of proinflammatory cytokines without any known infection (i.e., basal levels) and overproduction of proinflammatory cytokines in response to infection. Although individuals with these polymorphisms do not always develop schizophrenia, they appear to be more vulnerable to multiple diseases and infections. Therefore, it is possible that carriers of genetic polymorphisms associated with inflammation could be more vulnerable to the damaging effects of prenatal infection, thus increasing the likelihood of psychotic onset in adulthood; however, no studies have directly tested this gene–environment interaction.

Cumulatively, studies implicate a series of prenatal infections in the etiology of schizophrenia. Nevertheless, it appears as though the deleterious effects of exposure to prenatal infection may be more related to maternal immune responses to infection than to the direct effects of the pathogen, given that most pathogens do not cross the placenta. Specifically, prenatal exposure to maternal proinflammatory cytokines has been found to alter multiple areas of the brain that have been implicated in schizophrenia, and these cytokines have been linked to psychotic outcome in offspring. In addition, genetic polymorphisms associated with overproduction of proinflammatory cytokines have been found in patients with schizophrenia, suggesting that individuals who later develop schizophrenia may be particularly vulnerable to infection and other prenatal insults. Last, both infection and proinflammatory cytokines have been linked to increased fetal hypoxia, which has been associated with schizophrenia and many of the brain abnormalities linked to the disorder. The availability of studies using serological data and the possibility of examining direct gene–environment interactions likely will lead to a much better understanding of the molecular pathways linking OCs to schizophrenia outcome, which is the starting point for developing treatment and early intervention strategies.

THE NEURODEVELOPMENTAL MODEL OF SCHIZOPHRENIA

The neurodevelopmental model of schizophrenia provides a framework for understanding how OCs interact with the developing brain to increase the likelihood of schizophrenia in late adolescence and early adulthood. In normal development, connections in the brain (referred to as *synaptic density*) increase until an individual is approximately 2 years of age, which slowly decline during childhood, then decline steeply during late childhood and early adolescence. Many of these connections are unnecessary and will be eliminated in the mature brain. During adolescence, a sharp increase in a process called *synaptic pruning*, which involves the elimination of superfluous connections, coincides with the emergence of abilities to solve abstract and complex problems. According to the neurodevelopmental model, patients with schizophrenia may have too many, too few, or unnecessary synaptic connections that are eliminated during adolescence, which results in the onset of psychotic symptomatology. According to one model, schizophrenia would occur due to an abnormally aggressive synaptic pruning process, leading to a reduction in synaptic connectivity beyond a psychosis threshold, resulting in a fragmented or disconnected brain. This lack of neural connectivity throughout the brain reflects the challenges faced by patients with schizophrenia, with deficits in most areas, including cognitive, social, emotional, and perceptual difficulties. Moreover, this model is supported by postmortem studies that have found reduced neuropil without neuronal loss, in which decreased neuropil represents a loss of connections between neurons.

Early environmental insults, such as OCs, would fit within this neurodevelopmental model by reducing the amount of synaptic pruning necessary to cause psychotic symptomatology. This would lead to an earlier age of onset and possibly portend a worsened clinical outcome. As we have seen, this is precisely what occurs in individuals with a history of hypoxia-associated OCs, who typically have an earlier age of onset and more pronounced neuroanatomical abnormalities.

Viewing schizophrenia as a developmental disorder encourages exploration into possible early intervention and prevention strategies in individuals who are genetically susceptible. The emergence of candidate disease genes, as well as the advances in mapping out molecular pathways involved in schizophrenia, will likely pave the road to understanding and treating an incredibly serious and debilitating disorder.

KEY POINTS

- OCs have been found to be repeatedly associated with schizophrenia outcome, occurring in the histories of 20–30% of patients with schizophrenia and 5–10% of the overall population.
- Of the prevailing explanatory models, the majority of evidence supports the gene–environment interaction model, which asserts that OCs interact with genes associated with schizophrenia to increase risk for the disorder.
- Many OCs have been associated with schizophrenia, including complications during pregnancy, fetal and infant underdevelopment, and birth complications.
- Lack of oxygen to the fetus, termed *fetal hypoxia*, likely is involved in many OCs associated with schizophrenia.
- A history of hypoxia-associated OCs differentiates between patients with schzophrenia and their nonschizophrenic siblings, and leads to a form of schizophrenia characterized by earlier age of onset and greater neuroanatomical abnormalities.
- Infection during pregnancy has been repeatedly associated with schizophrenia in offspring. More recent studies using serological confirmation of infection have found an association between HSV-2, influenza, genital and reproductive infection, and *T. gondii* exposure during pregnancy and schizophrenia spectrum disorders in offspring.
- Most prenatal infections do not cross the placenta; therefore, the damaging effects to the fetus seem to be partially related to the mother's immune response to infection, particularly involving inflammation.
- Genetic polymorphisms that amplify the inflammatory response to infection have been found among patients with schizophrenia, suggesting that genetic factors may confer heightened sensitivity to infection and other prenatal insults.
- Both infection and proinflammatory cytokines have been linked to increased fetal hypoxia, which has been associated with schizophrenia and many of the brain abnormalities linked to the disorder.
- Some theorists propose that schizophrenia arises due excessive reduction in the connections throughout the brain (synaptic pruning), leading to problems in most areas of functioning. OCs fit within this model by further reducing the amount of connections in the brain, leading to an earlier age of onset and worsened clinical outcome.

REFERENCES AND RECOMMENDED READINGS

Boin, F., Zanardini, R., Pioli, R., Altamura, C. A., Maes, M., & Gennarelli, M. (2001). Association between -G308A tumor necrosis factor alpha gene polymorphism and schizophrenia. *Molecular Psychiatry, 6*(1), 79–82.

Brown, A. S., Begg, M. D., Gravenstein, S., Schaefer, C. A., Wyatt, R. J., Bresnahan, M., et al., (2004). Serologic evidence of prenatal influenza in the etiology of schizophrenia. *Archives of General Psychiatry, 61*(8), 774–780.

Brown, A. S., Cohen, P., Harkavy-Friedman, J., Babulas, V., Malaspina, D., Gorman, J. M., et al. (2001). A. E. Bennett Research Award: Prenatal rubella, premorbid abnormalities, and adult schizophrenia. *Biological Psychiatry, 49*(6), 473–486.

Buka, S. L., Tsuang, M. T., Torrey, E. F., Klebanoff, M. A., Bernstein, D., & Yolken, R. H. (2001). Maternal infections and subsequent psychosis among offspring. *Archives of General Psychiatry, 58*(11), 1032–1037.

Buka, S. L., Tsuang, M. T., Torrey, E. F., Klebanoff, M. A., Wagner, R. L., & Yolken, R. H. (2001). Maternal cytokine levels during pregnancy and adult psychosis. *Brain, Behavior, and Immunity, 15*(4), 411–420.

Cannon, M., Jones, P. B., & Murray, R. M. (2002). Obstetric complications and schizophrenia: Historical and meta-analytic review. *American Journal of Psychiatry, 159*(7), 1080–1092.

Cannon, T. D. (1997). On the nature and mechanisms of obstetric influences in schizophrenia: A review and synthesis of epidemiologic studies. *International Review of Psychiatry, 9,* 387–397.

Cannon, T. D., Rosso, I. M., Hollister, J. M., Bearden, C. E., Sanchez, L. E., & Hadley, T. (2000). A prospective cohort study of genetic and perinatal influences in the etiology of schizophrenia. *Schizophrenia Bulletin, 26*(2), 351–366.

Cannon, T. D., van Erp, T. G., Rosso, I. M., Huttunen, M., Lonnqvist, J., Pirkola, T., et al. (2002). Fetal hypoxia and structural brain abnormalities in schizophrenic patients, their siblings, and controls. *Archives of General Psychiatry, 59*(1), 35–41.

Feinberg, I. (1982). Schizophrenia: Caused by a fault in programmed synaptic elimination during adolescence? *Journal of Psychiatric Research, 17*(4), 319–334.

Gilmore, J. H., Jarskog, L. F., Vadlamudi, S., & Lauder, J. M. (2004). Prenatal infection and risk for schizophrenia: IL-1beta, IL-6, and TNFalpha inhibit cortical neuron dendrite development. *Neuropsychopharmacology, 29*(7), 1221–1229.

Lane, E. A., & Albee, G. W. (1966). Comparative birth weights of schizophrenics and their siblings. *Journal of Psychology, 64*(2), 227–231.

McGlashan, T. H., & Hoffman, R. E. (2000). Schizophrenia as a disorder of developmentally reduced synaptic connectivity. *Archives of General Psychiatry, 57,* 637–647.

Rapoport, J. L., Addington, A. M., Frangou, S., & Psych, M. R. (2005). The neurodevelopmental model of schizophrenia: Update 2005. *Molecular Psychiatry, 10*(5), 434–449.

Torrey, E. F., & Yolken, R. H. (2003). Toxoplasma gondii and schizophrenia. *Emerging Infectious Diseases, 9*(11), 1375–1380.

Van Erp, T. G., Saleh, P. A., Rosso, I. M., Huttunen, M., Lonnqvist, J., Pirkola, T., et al. (2002). Contributions of genetic risk and fetal hypoxia to hippocampal volume in patients with schizophrenia or schizoaffective disorder, their unaffected siblings, and healthy unrelated volunteers. *American Journal of Psychiatry, 159*(9), 1514–1520.

CHAPTER 8

PSYCHOSOCIAL FACTORS

PAUL BEBBINGTON
ELIZABETH KUIPERS

In this chapter, we review the different ways in which social factors may impact on the process of schizophrenia, and draw out possible implications for managing people with the condition.

INSTITUTIONAL ENVIRONMENTS AND SOCIAL REACTIVITY

The earliest scientific demonstration that schizophrenia symptoms were socially responsive was carried out in long stay hospitals in England by Wing and Brown (1970), starting in the 1950s. These hospitals provided very little in the way of social stimulation. Wing and Brown were able to show that the level of hospital patients' negative symptoms was related to the degree of impoverishment in their social environment. They also demonstrated that enriching the environment improved patients' psychiatric conditions. However, it was also apparent that if patients underwent too much stress in a rehabilitation program, they ran the risk of worsening their *positive* symptoms. There seemed to be an optimum balance between too much and too little social stimulation. This led Wing and Brown to apply for the first time to schizophrenia new methodologies for evaluating stress, thus weakening the prevalent idea that schizophrenia was purely a biological condition.

LIFE EVENTS AND SCHIZOPHRENIA

There are a number of ways to research the link between life events and the onset of schizophrenia relapse. One way is to examine the effect of a single type of life event in a cohort of people undergoing it. An excellent early example of this was carried out by

Steinberg and Durell (1968), who 40 years ago studied the effects of recruitment into the army for the purposes of national service. Following this, they plotted the emergence of schizophrenia in their cohort of recruits and were able to show that the rate of breakdown was significantly higher in the few months immediately after recruitment.

However, much of the work on life events and schizophrenia has involved reactions to a wide range of potential events. Of the considerable methodological problems associated with this approach, one of the most important is having an objective way to assess the impact of events given that different types of events are unlikely to have equivalent impacts. Moreover, several different dimensions relating to the impact of events might be measured. Another crucial but difficult requirement is to establish as clearly as possible the date of both the psychosocial event in question and the illness event (onset or relapse). This is essential for inferences about causal direction.

Several designs can be used to establish links between life events and onset or relapse in schizophrenia. Retrospective, within-patient designs compare the experience of life events in a defined period before onset with a more distant period in the same person's life. This raises problems of recall but gets around the difficulty that people with schizophrenia may choose lifestyles that reduce their exposure to events, but at the same time may be abnormally sensitive to the life events they do experience. Thus, although the event rate before onset may be no more marked than that in someone without schizophrenia, it is still elevated in relation to the individual's own normal event rate.

Retrospective case–control designs compare the life experience of patients before onset with an equivalent period in controls. Clearly the control group requires careful selection. *Prospective designs* involving recent events are for all practical purposes concerned with relapse rather than onset. This enables identification of a group of people at risk of increasing symptoms. The participants may be interviewed, say, every 1 or 2 months. At these times their history of life events and symptom exacerbations are evaluated for the preceding period.

Studies published for the last 40 years, dating from the classic case–control study of Brown and Birley (1968), provide solid evidence for a link between recent stressful events and the onset of episodes of schizophrenia, although there have been a few negative results. There is also emerging evidence of an excess of life events in the period immediately preceding the *first onset* of schizophrenia symptoms. However, the impact of stressful events is not limited to schizophrenia; it applies to other psychiatric conditions (in particular, depression) and also to some physical disorders. Thus, the relationship demonstrated so far has not been specific to schizophrenia, and the necessary specificity is delegated to the concept of vulnerability. In other words, people who develop schizophrenia in response to a life event seem to be prone to doing so because of a putative underlying propensity, usually framed as a biological predisposition.

Recently, attempts have been made to explain the life event–schizophrenia link by investigating more specific "demand characteristics" of the events themselves. One promising candidate is the attribute of *intrusiveness*. Events of this type involve apparent close control of the individual by people who are, relatively speaking, strangers. When events can be characterized in this way, it appears that the link with onset or recurrence of schizophrenia symptoms is appreciably strengthened. There is even tentative evidence that intrusive events link with some specificity to persecutory ideation. There is some dispute concerning the period over which recent events can have an effect in inducing the emergence of schizophrenia symptoms. Some authors have found that this period is limited to just a few weeks; others have found that events can exert an influence over several months. The concept of a prior vulnerability has now led to an interest in the impact of events occurring much earlier in people's lives, years rather than months before onset.

The underlying conceptualization is that these early events might *sensitize* the person experiencing them, such that later events would trigger an episode of schizophrenia. The current view is that the early events might change an individual's propensity to interpret the world in an adverse way (i.e., might instill negative schemas about the self and others—the world being a dangerous place, for instance). These early events often involve victimization, such as child sexual abuse and bullying at school. There is certainly growing evidence for links between distant traumatic events and the later onset of schizophrenia. However, the interaction between early and more recent events has not yet been demonstrated. Thus, it has not clearly been shown that early environmental events confer vulnerability or whether this is primarily biological, cognitive or emotional, or an interaction effect. However, early life events do seem to increase later risk.

Again, we are faced with the problem of specificity. Child sexual abuse is also common in people with anxiety, depression, substance abuse, and personality disorder, although some studies have indicated the association may be particularly strong in schizophrenia. Studies of mechanism may help here. The mechanism of the association between early events, particularly sexual abuse, and later schizophrenia may involve processes similar, but certainly not identical, to those involved in the generation of posttraumatic stress disorder (PTSD). Thus, people with schizophrenia who have experienced child sexual abuse or other violent trauma tend to have more hallucinations than those without such experiences; *hallucinations* are defined as intrusive mental events with some similarities to reexperiencing phenomena in PTSD.

Some psychosocial contexts may not only increase the risk of certain types of events but also influence the interpretation of events and, indeed, of ordinary social interactions. One example is the position of immigrants, particularly if they are illegal or seeking asylum. Such people have often experienced horrible events due to war or political oppression in their country of origin, and arrive in the host country with vulnerabilities already set up. This may be *confirmed* by the experience of being treated with suspicion by local people and with ill-disguised scorn from officialdom. In these circumstances, a degree of paranoia may indeed be adaptive, and a Forrest Gump–like openness or naivete might be disastrous. Given this scenario, it is hardly surprising that disadvantaged immigrant groups seem to have much higher rates of psychosis than the host population. There are a number of possible explanations for this finding, but increasing credence is currently accorded to psychosocial interpretations based on empirical research (i.e., that adverse environments rather than biological differences are a key feature).

SOCIAL NETWORKS

Other psychosocial contexts may affect the way individuals interpret their environment. People with schizophrenia commonly have impaired social networks—small primary groups and inadequate social support. This has generally been interpreted as a direct consequence of either their disorder or its prodromal features, such as social withdrawal. However, one of the key functions of social networks, particularly confiding relationships, is that of cognitive triangulation: People try out their ideas in conversation with friends and confidantes. This usually leads to the pruning of their more bizarre ideas. In other words, within limits, conversation keeps them sane, and social isolation does the opposite. The first emergence of delusional ideation often occurs in the context of a period of isolation, whether other- or self-imposed. The possibility that isolation is associated with delusion formation and the emergence of anomalous experiences requires longitudinal studies. At present we just have the evidence that isolation in terms of sensory deprivation can increase anomalous experiences, and that it is associated with reduced insight.

FAMILY STUDIES IN SCHIZOPHRENIA

A further aspect of the environment that has been studied empirically to great effect relates to the family setting. Most of this work follows from the development of a specific measure of family interaction, *expressed emotion* (EE), based on prosodic aspects of speech. The need for this measure arose from an observation many decades ago that people with schizophrenia who returned from the hospital to live with relatives had a surprisingly high relapse rate compared to those who lived on their own, for instance, in a rental room in a private residence. It looked as though these relapses might result from difficult or intrusive family relationships. EE, a measure of this conflict, involves an interview with a main relative or a caregiver, usually shortly after a relapse. The semistructured interview is audiotaped and analyzed for the presence of negative aspects: emotional overinvolvement, hostility, and critical comments, all defined operationally and reliably identified by trained raters. Above a certain level, these features lead to people being rated as high on EE. Living with a high-EE relative has consistently been found to result in a much higher relapse rate (about 2.5 times higher) over the next year or so than living with a low-EE relative. Unfortunately, this has emphasized again the importance of negative relationships for poor outcomes in schizophrenia. Positive measures of EE (warmth) have not been found to be predictive, unless there are no negative relationships.

This research has had the added value of leading to the development of a particular style of family intervention, because it was possible to evaluate complex family relationship outcomes with the EE measure. Family intervention is now well-established as effective in reducing relapse in schizophrenia. Thus, not only is a particular negative psychosocial context associated with increased relapse but intervening to try to modify it has also been shown to reduce relapse rates considerably and improve patient and caregiver outcomes.

HOW DOES PSYCHOSOCIAL STRESS WORK?

If it is accepted that psychosocial stress has some level of causal influence in the development of psychotic symptoms, then there are two main hypotheses about its mode of action. The first carries with it the disadvantage of nonspecificity, in that it postulates that the phenomena of schizophrenia are more likely to emerge if the individual becomes psychologically and mentally aroused. Such arousal has been demonstrated in people who have recently experienced negative life events, or who are in the presence of relatives with whom their relationship is strained. It is also well established that people with schizophrenia are very likely to have comorbid anxiety disorders. Recently, anxiety has been implicated in some of the psychosocial processes that underlie the development of schizophrenia symptoms. Thus, there does appear to be a nonspecific role of anxiety, but by its very nature, anxiety is unable to explain why people develop schizophrenia rather than other mental health problems.

The other route postulated to link stressful events and contexts to the development of schizophrenia involves cognition. In other words, adverse experiences may change the way people think about themselves, their world, and the other people in it. Contextless arousal is far from universal, and content is necessary for the diagnosis of several anxiety disorders—specific phobias, agoraphobia, and social phobia. When people become anxious they have already begun to think differently, and this is sometimes in relation to social circumstances. It is perhaps via this route that the specific relationships between stressful events, stressful situations, and schizophrenia may be found.

The links between social phobia and paranoia are of particular interest. Why are some people anxious about the demands of social interaction, attributing their physical state to their own inadequacies (social anxiety), whereas others attribute their anxiety to the machinations of others (paranoia)? Researchers have begun to explore this issue in nonclinical and prodromal samples using virtual reality inhabited by computer-generated characters called *avatars*. The use of a virtual reality scenario with avatars (a library scene was used in one study) allows for control of the environment, while still eliciting realistic emotional reactions (as TV shows such as *The Simpsons* are able to do). We have found that such situations, which by definition are not threatening, can elicit paranoid reactions in some participants.

Another aspect of cognition that relates to the experience of social stress is self-esteem, which is very frequently diminished in people with schizophrenia. Moreover, they are very likely to have experienced events that virtually guaranteed diminution of their self-esteem. The work described earlier linking intrusive events specifically to schizophrenia is a further example of how the characteristics of events, in terms of their capacity to arouse particular patterns of thought, may account for their capacity to elicit responses with the typical features of schizophrenia, such as persecutory ideas.

Although it remains likely that some of the specificity of a schizophrenia response in many people lies in processes determined outside the person/social–environmental interaction, it is difficult to be sure. Social anxiety and paranoia are also distinguished because people prone to paranoia have a greater capacity for *anomalous experiences*. Is this capacity wired into the brain as a result of genetic and other biological processes? It is possible, but it may equally be caused by the impact of particular types of stress. For example, severe traumatic events can also elicit or exaggerate the likelihood of experiencing subsequent intrusive thoughts.

In conclusion, there is now good evidence that stressful events and circumstances form part of the causal nexus for the emergence of schizophrenia. A history of such experiences is not apparent in everyone with schizophrenia, but neither is a family history of the disorder. It seems likely that schizophrenia is caused by a range of influences, none of which is either necessary or sufficient in the individual case. These social influences then also operate to impede recovery.

MECHANISMS

Although we have discovered these relationships, we have not yet disentangled the specific mechanisms or how they may perhaps interact to cause initial episodes and relapses. We have made some progress with models of vulnerability, probably genetic, but also, plausibly, brought on by early adverse environments, such as emotional neglect, isolation, or specific trauma. Later, triggered by stresses such as negative life events or negative relationships, individuals may experience an increasing cascade of cognitive and perceptual anomalies that, together with emotional reactions, lead them to conclude not that this is a "bad day," but that external agents are conspiring against them (i.e., paranoia). Once triggered, recovery from such an episode also depends on a wide range of cognitive, emotional, and social factors, and their interaction determines outcome and future course.

This model of cognitive, emotional, and social process in schizophrenia is currently being tested.

CLINICAL MANAGEMENT

It is clear that social reactivity is often a central feature of schizophrenia: either too much or too little stimulation. Too little input on the one hand and we have evidence that people with schizophrenia (as do others) have increasing amounts of negative symptoms, such as reduced motivation. Too much stimulation, on the other hand, particularly if anxiety provoking, appears to be able to trigger renewed symptoms. Some of the life event literature adds to this by suggesting that, for some people with schizophrenia, events, particularly those with an intrusive content, might be particularly likely to lead to symptoms of paranoia over a relatively short time period.

The first-line treatment for schizophrenia is medication, which is discussed in detail in Chapters 16–19, this volume. One of the functions of medication is probably to dampen down social reactivity (i.e., the interaction of the cognitive and emotional processing of stresses in those vulnerable to episodes of schizophrenia). Given that stress and life events cannot readily be eliminated, use of medication in effect to reduce this social sensitivity may be an effective alternative.

In addition to medication (which is often incompletely effective), there is evidence for the effectiveness of psychological interventions.

If there are foreseeable life events, monitoring someone's reaction to events and discussing them can be helpful in reducing negative appraisals. Extra medication and support are indicated until emotional reactions have subsided.

Events that are particularly upsetting because they trigger preexisting cognitions, negative schemas, or emotional vulnerabilities can be explored and reviewed, as in treatments for depression. Cognitions such as "I am useless"; "The world is an evil place"; and "I'm never going to recover" can be evaluated and the evidence for them reexamined. If possible, forthcoming events should be thought through or minimized, if there is a choice, for instance, about taking a trip or making a life-changing decision. However, it may be argued that a life free of events or stress is not much of a life, and that people should be supported, if possible, through events and their possible negative reactions, rather than totally avoiding them.

COGNITIVE-BEHAVIORAL THERAPY FOR PSYCHOSIS

The evidence is that cognitive-behavioral therapy (CBT) approaches to medication-resistant, positive symptoms of psychosis such as delusions and hallucinations are moderately effective, particularly if continued for at least 6 months. This is now a recommended treatment in the United Kingdom, according to National Institute of Clinical Excellence (NICE) guidelines produced in 2003. Such treatments focus on engaging clients, discussing their view of events, and formulating a joint model of the interaction of certain life experiences (including negative schemas) with current concerns, emotional reactions, and their appraisal. The emphasis is primarily on increasing understanding, making sense of the experience, and reducing distress. There is evidence that this may also reduce the frequency of hallucinations and sometimes allow the level of conviction in distressing delusions to attenuate. The latter can be accomplished by helping people to increase their cognitive flexibility, to consider alterative views and their evidence, and to compensate for reasoning biases, such as jumping to premature conclusions.

It is not yet clear how far supportive relationships on their own can help with these processes. There is evidence that supportive counseling can reduce distress in psychosis, although effects do not appear to last beyond the end of the period in which it is provided, and they are weaker than those found with CBT.

INCREASING SOCIAL NETWORKS

There is also evidence that social isolation is associated with reduced insight and might plausibly contribute to the development of delusional ideas. We do know that the social networks of those with schizophrenia are typically extremely small (down from a norm of around 30 people to around three), and that formation of confiding relationships after episodes of psychosis is difficult. Although some attempts have been made to increase social networks, the evidence that this reduces symptoms is not conclusive. It seems likely that confiding relationships are most important, not just new people in a social network, and that the former are not so easy to provide outside of a therapeutic setting.

FAMILY INTERVENTION IN PSYCHOSIS

Given small social networks after the onset of psychosis, it is necessarily the case that family contacts, as there are in up to 50% of patients with longer term problems, may both be normalizing and provide confiding relationships. However, schizophrenia is a condition in which caring relationships can be put under immense strain, and family relationships can become conflictual. In these situations in particular, family intervention (FI) has been shown to be effective. The NICE guidelines on schizophrenia in the United Kingdom also recommend FI for patients with persistent symptoms and frequent relapses who are in contact with caregivers. Longer treatment (over 6 months), again, has been found to be more effective. The interventions that are useful focus on improving patients' communication and problem solving, increasing caregiver and client understanding and cognitive appraisal of difficulties, and emotional processing of the grief, loss, and anger that is commonly felt. We also know that psychoeducation on its own does not change outcomes. Although FI is effective, it has proved difficult to put into clinical practice, at least partly because it involves intensive use of staff time, and caregiver concerns are often not seen as primary by busy clinical teams. However, such interventions are indicated particularly for families where there are repeated relapses, and are likely to be cost-effective. Another recent approach is to offer FI help at an early stage of the illness, with the hope of preventing later difficulties. However, the evidence for this approach remains thin, mainly because many families do not wish to engage in discussion of possible long-term problems during early episodes.

Both CBT and FI can be seen as ways of managing emotional impact and social stress by aiding cognitive reappraisal. The evidence for the effectiveness of these interventions, in addition to medication, is at present moderate. Other psychological interventions, such as social skills training or cognitive remediation (which aims to improve more basic cognitions such as attribution and memory) have a less secure evidence base and are not recommended interventions in the United Kingdom at present. They are also not directly aimed at improving social reactivity. All of these interventions are discussed in much more detail in other chapters of this volume.

KEY POINTS

- Positive symptoms of schizophrenia seem to be related to emotional and social reactivity.
- There is good evidence that life events trigger episodes of schizophrenia, a link that is also seen in other disorders.
- Social networks are often restricted in schizophrenia; lacking a confidant seems particularly related to increased symptoms.
- Medication, the first line of treatment, is often not fully effective. Adjunctive psychological interventions such as CBT and FI have been shown to improve outcomes.
- Psychological interventions seem to work by improving both disturbed affect and cognitive appraisals.

REFERENCES AND RECOMMENDED READINGS

Bebbington, P., & Kuipers, L. (1994). The predictive utility of EE in schizophrenia: An aggregate analysis. *Psychological Medicine, 24,* 707–718.

Bebbington, P., & Kuipers, E. (2003). Schizophrenia and psychosocial stresses. In S. R. Hirsch & D. R. Weinberger (Eds.), *Schizophrenia* (2nd ed.). Malden, MA: Blackwell Scientific.

Bebbington, P. E., Bhugra, D., Brugha, T., Singleton, N., Farrell, M., Jenkins, et al. (2004). Psychosis, victimisation and childhood disadvantage: Evidence from the second British National Survey of Psychiatric Morbidity. *British Journal of Psychiatry, 185,* 220–226.

Birchwood, M., & Jackson, C. (2001). *Schizophrenia.* Sussex, UK: Psychology Press.

Broome, M. R., Wooley, J. B., Tabraham, P., Johns, L. C., Bramon, E., Murray, G. K., et al. (2005). What causes the onset of psychosis? *Schizophrenia Research, 79,* 23–34.

Brown, G. W., & Birley, J. L. T. (1968). Crises and life changes and the onset of schizophrenia. *Journal of Health and Social Behavior, 9,* 203–214.

Fowler, D., Garety, P., & Kuipers, E. (1995). *Cognitive behaviour therapy for people with psychosis.* East Sussex, UK: Wiley.

Freeman, D., & Garety, P. A. (2004). A cognitive model of persecutory delusions. In *Paranoia: The psychology of persecutory delusions* (Maudsley Monograph No. 45, pp. 115–135). Hove, UK: Psychology Press.

Garety, P. A., Kuipers, E. A., Fowler, D., Freeman, D., & Bebbington, P. (2001). A cognitive model of the positive symptoms of psychosis. *Psychological Medicine, 31,* 189–195.

Kapur, S. (2003). Psychosis as a state of aberrant salience: A framework linking biology, phenomenology, and pharmacology in schizophrenia. *American Journal of Psychiatry, 160*(1), 13–23.

Kuipers, E., Bebbington, P., Dunn, G., Fowler, D., Freeman, D., Watson, P., et al. (2006). Influence of carer expressed emotion and affect on relapse in non-affective psychosis. *British Journal of Psychiatry, 188,* 173–179.

Kuipers, E., Leff, J., & Lam, D. (2002). *Family work for schizophrenia: A practical guide* (2nd ed.). London: Gaskell Press.

Myin-Germeys, I., van Os, J., Schwartz, J., Stone, A., & Delespaul, P. (2001). Emotional reactivity in daily life stress in psychosis. *Archives of General Psychiatry, 58,* 1137–1144.

Steinberg, H. R., & Durell, J. (1968). A stressful situation as a precipitant of schizophrenic symptoms: An epidemiological study. *British Journal of Psychiatry, 114,* 1097–1105.

Wing, J. K., & Brown, G. W. (1970). *Institutionalism and schizophrenia: A comparative study of three mental hospitals 1960–68.* Cambridge, UK: Cambridge University Press.

CHAPTER 9

PSYCHOPATHOLOGY

IPSIT V. VAHIA
CARL I. COHEN

Over the course of the last century the conceptualization of schizophrenia has been subject to considerable debate. Unlike most disorders in medicine, no known pathophysiological mechanism can be linked to the symptoms of schizophrenia. This means that the diagnosis and symptoms of schizophrenia must be based on observations, verbal reports, and inferences, thereby making it more difficult to reach a consensus about how to conceptualize and define it. Thus, in this chapter, although we focus primarily on the symptoms of schizophrenia, we also illustrate how the cluster of symptoms thought to be associated with schizophrenia is dependent on how the disorder is conceptualized. These concepts remain in flux and have been influenced by historical, social, and cultural tendencies.

HISTORICAL BACKGROUND

Early Developments

Schizophrenia as a distinct clinical entity has existed for slightly over 100 years. Prior to that time, the existence of schizophrenia could only be inferred from case descriptions by 17th- and 18th-century physicians, such as those of Philippe Pinel and John Haslam. Émil Kraepelin (1856–1926) and Eugen Bleuler (1857–1939) have been recognized for establishing the modern foundation for the concept of schizophrenia. Their primary contribution was to bring unity to variety of overlapping symptom clusters by indicating which symptoms must be present to confirm the diagnosis. Although Karl Kahlbaum had proposed a longitudinal approach to schizophrenia prior to Kraepelin, it was Kraepelin's insight that a variety of psychotic entities could be combined into a single entity consisting of hebephrenia, paranoid deterioration, and catatonia subtypes. He used the term *dementia praecox* (translated from the term *demence precoce* coined by French psychiatrist Benedict Morel) to describe what he perceived as a deterioration process (dementia) with premature onset. Whatever the subtype, Kraepelin regarded the following symptoms as characteristic of dementia praecox: hallucinations, usually of an auditory or tactile form; decreased attention to the outside world; lack of curiosity; disorders of thought, especially of the *Zarfahrenheit* (scatter) type, with unusual and partly comprehensible associations; changes of speech resulting from the thought disorder, such as incoherence; lack of insight and judgment; delusions; emotional blunting; negativism; and stereotypy. These symptoms had to occur in the presence of a clear consciousness. Kraepelin's description is important because it has historically shaped the way schizophrenia is conceptualized. Many of his symptom descriptions and schizophrenia subtypes have served as a foundation for *Diagnostic and Statistical Manual of Mental Disorders* (DSM) and *International Classification of Diseases* (ICD) descriptors and classification. One of the essential elements of Kraepelin's nosology was the association between symptomatology and a poor prognosis, although it is often forgotten that he did recognize that recovery, albeit rare, could occur with the disorder.

In his original work, Eugen Bleuler used the phrase *group of schizophrenias* as synonymous with *dementia praecox*. One of Bleuler's aims was to apply Freud's ideas to reexamine the psychopathology in the disorder. Although the term *schizophrenia* did not carry the same negative prognosis as dementia praecox, Bleuler indicated that restitution of function did not occur. Bleuler viewed schizophrenia as a splitting of psychic functions. Thus, psychic complexes did not combine in a unified form, as in healthy persons. Rather, the personality seemed to lose its unity, so that different ideas and drives were split off. For example, processes of association became mere fragments of ideas and concepts, thinking stopped in the middle of a thought, and the intensity of emotional reactions was not consistent with the various events that caused the reaction (i.e., an excessive or inadequate response).

Bleuler's main contribution was his effort to separate the "primary" or core symptoms of schizophrenia (i.e., those related to the splitting) from "secondary" symptoms, which represented psychological reactions to the primary symptoms. The primary symptoms comprised disturbances in association, thought disorder, changes in affectivity, a tendency to prefer fantasy to reality and to seclude oneself from reality, and autism. Secondary symptoms included hallucinations, delusions, catatonic symptoms, and various behavioral abnormalities.

In response to those conceptions of schizophrenia that were etiologically driven, Kurt Schneider (1887–1967) proposed to define schizophrenia in purely symptomatic terms. Like Karl Jaspers (1883–1969), he championed diagnosis based on the form rather than the content of a sign or symptom. For example, he maintained that delusions should not be diagnosed by the content of the belief, but by the way in which a belief is held. He distinguished "first-rank" symptoms, which, rather than being conceived in any theoretical way, were seen as being primary or basic symptoms (i.e., of greatest diagnostic importance). His classification scheme played a strong role in the formation of DSM-III and ICD classifications. Schneider's first-rank symptoms may be summarized as follows:

- *Special auditory hallucinations.* This includes hearing one's own thoughts echoed by the voices, hearing two or more voices arguing or discussing a topic, or a voice commenting on the person's activities as they occur.
- *Special delusions.* This two-stage phenomenon comprises a normal perception followed by a delusional interpretation of it as having a special and highly personalized significance.
- *Passivity experiences.* These include somatic passivity or sensations imposed by an outside agency passivity of affect or emotions imposed by an external agency that are not the person's own, passivity of impulse or wishes that are not the person's own, and passivity of volition, in which a person's motor activity is controlled by an external agency.
- *Alienation of thought.* This includes thought withdrawal, thought insertion, and thought broadcasting.

The Influence of Psychoanalytic and Interpersonal Theories

The predominance of various psychoanalytic schools from the period 1930–1960 led to approaches that refocused symptoms within the intrapsychic and interpersonal arenas. Work by Heinz Hartmann and others highlighted disturbances in ego function and object relations. For example, Hartmann (1964) contended that schizophrenia was characterized by severe impairments in ego functioning. Hence, persons with schizophrenia could not deal easily with frustrations because of ego deficiencies in defensive mechanisms, a lack of stabilized object relations, and the ego's relation to reality. Harry Stack Sullivan (1953) conceptualized schizophrenia as arising from the organization of experience with significant people in early life (e.g., intense anxiety precipitated by an intense emotional response from the significant environment). This increased focus on impaired social interaction influenced Strauss and Carpenter (1974) in their pioneering study of outcome in schizophrenia to add problems of "rapport" to the classical schizophrenic dimensions of positive and negative symptoms.

The Influence of Socioenvironmental Theories

During the 1950s and 1960s, in tandem with the development of civil rights movements to address racial and gender inequalities, the rights of mental patients became more prominent. There was increased recognition that social and environmental factors played a role in the observed symptoms of schizophrenic persons. For example, several writers described "depersonalization syndromes" and "hospitalism" that developed in understimulated patients hospitalized long term. Such symptoms consisted of apathy and amotivation. Others noted how psychotic symptoms were exacerbated by overstimulation and conflicting messages from family or clinical staff. A number of models attempted to make schizophrenia symptoms more comprehensible in terms of the communication and alliances underlying family systems. Thus, psychotic symptoms might be symbolic expressions of persons who felt trapped or confused within a dysfunctional family system. For example, Laing and Esterson (1970) illustrated how a patient's ideas of reference could be explained by observing the family's interactions: "Her mother and father kept exchanging with each other a constant series of nods, winks, gestures, knowing smiles . . ." (p. 40), which they adamantly denied when commented on by the interviewer. Finally, labeling and postmodern theorists elucidated sociohistorical factors that influenced the construction of disease categories. Their work undermined the notion that symptoms were objectively conceived (i.e., "value-free").

The Era of DSM

Prior to DSM-III (American Psychiatric Association, 1980), the descriptive symptoms of schizophrenia were often interpreted in a broad sense, which led to inconsistencies in the diagnosis of schizophrenia. On the one hand, the World Health Organization landmark International Pilot Study of Schizophrenia (Hawk, Carpenter, & Strauss, 1975) in the 1960s demonstrated that schizophrenia was diagnosed far more commonly in the United States and the Soviet Union than in other countries. Although this was attributed to multiple factors, including culture, it also demonstrated a much broader interpretation of diagnostic criteria for schizophrenia in these two countries. On the other hand, the study found marked similarities in the key symptoms for rendering a diagnosis in all countries: delusions of control, thought broadcast, thought insertion, thought withdrawal, flattened affect, and auditory hallucinations of various kinds.

The first impetus in the United States for diagnostic clarity came from researchers who required standardization and uniformity in diagnosis. A group at the Washington University School of Medicine (1972) under the direction of John Feighner developed systematized inclusion and exclusion criteria for various psychiatric diagnoses. In a collaborative project between the National Institute of Mental Health (NIMH) and Robert Spitzer at Columbia, the "Feighner criteria" were modified and expanded to include more diagnostic categories. These new criteria, called the "Research Diagnostic Criteria," served as the basis for DSM-III, released in 1980 for general clinicians. Thus, DSM addressed the need for a more reliable diagnostic system based on formal operational criteria and observed manifestations. DSM-III authors noted that given a lack of proven theories about schizophrenia, the reliability of diagnosis depended on clinical observation. DSM-IV (American Psychiatric Association, 1994) served to distill this concept further and the organization of symptoms into categories and subtypes. At this point in time, psychopathology of schizophrenia is best understood as a combination of what is observed clinically and what patients themselves experience.

DSM-IV-TR DEFINITIONS OF SCHIZOPHRENIA AND ITS SYMPTOMS

According to the text revision of DSM-IV, "The essential features of Schizophrenia are a mixture of characteristic signs and symptoms (both positive and negative) that have been present for a significant portion of time during a 1-month period (or for a shorter time if successfully treated), with some signs of the disorder persisting for at least 6 months" (American Psychiatric Association, 2000, p. 298). It adds that the abnormality has to be associated with marked social or occupational dysfunction and not be better accounted for by an alternate diagnosis as defined by the manual. It further necessitates that the abnormality not result from the direct physiological effects of a substance or a general medical condition. It also distinguishes schizophrenia from autistic disorder (or another pervasive developmental disorder) by specifying that an additional diagnosis of schizophrenia in autistic persons can be made only if prominent delusions or hallucinations are present for at least a month. The characteristic symptoms of schizophrenia involve dysfunctions in multiple cognitive and functional spheres that include perception, inferential thinking, language and communication, behavioral monitoring, affect, fluency and productivity of thought and speech, capacity to experience pleasure, decision making, drive, and attention. Schizophrenia presents with a variety of symptoms and has no single pathognomonic symptom. The diagnosis involves identification of specific clusters of symptoms.

As described below, DSM-IV-TR describes the characteristic symptoms of schizophrenia as falling into two broad categories: positive and negative. The positive symptoms represent distortions or exaggerations of normal cognitive functions, whereas the negative symptoms represent a diminution or loss of normal functions. DSM-IV-TR specifies that the positive symptoms include distortions in thought content (delusions), perception (hallucinations), language and thought process (disorganized speech), and self-monitoring of behavior (grossly disorganized or catatonic behavior). It further divides positive symptoms into two "dimensions" that probably represent different underlying pathophysiological processes. The "psychotic dimension" includes delusions and hallucinations, whereas the "disorganization dimension" includes disorganized speech and behavior.

Positive Symptoms

Psychotic Dimension

DELUSIONS

Delusions are defined by DSM-IV-TR (American Psychiatric Association, 2000, p. 299) as "erroneous beliefs that usually involve a misinterpretation of perceptions or experiences." A delusional belief involves four features: It is objectively false, it is idiosyncratic, it is illogical, and it is stubbornly maintained. Although DSM-IV-TR classifies delusions based on their content (e.g., persecutory, grandiose, erotomanic, self-referential, grandiose, somatic, or nihilistic), recent research suggests that delusions can be clustered into three distinct entities: Delusions of influence (delusions of being controlled, thought insertion or withdrawal), self-significance delusions (grandeur, reference, guilt/sin), and delusions of persecution. It is hypothesized that each of these clusters may be linked to underlying neurobiological processes.

For the purpose of diagnosis, DSM-IV-TR acknowledges Schneider's description of "bizarre" delusions as being especially characteristic of schizophrenia. Delusions are deemed bizarre if they are clearly implausible and not understandable, and do not derive from ordinary life experiences or the person's cultural system. Delusions that express a loss of control over mind or body are generally acknowledged as bizarre; these include a person's belief that his or her thoughts have been taken away by some outside force ("thought withdrawal"), that alien thoughts have been put into his or her mind ("thought insertion"), or that his or her body or actions are being acted on or manipulated by some outside force ("delusions of control"). If the delusions are judged to be bizarre, this single symptom is considered as adequate evidence to make the diagnosis of schizophrenia.

HALLUCINATIONS

According to DSM-IV-TR, hallucinations may occur in any sensory modality (e.g., auditory, visual, olfactory, gustatory, and tactile), but auditory hallucinations are by far the most common. Auditory hallucinations are usually experienced as voices (though occasionally they may be limited to just sounds). Sometimes they are of the "command" type—a voice commanding the person to perform some action. The experience of hallucination is distinct from the person's own thoughts. DSM-IV-TR specifies that the hallucinations must be experienced in the context of a clear sensorium. It is important to keep in mind, however, that some hallucinations may fall within the context of normal experience (e.g., voices heard either at the time of falling asleep (hypnagogic) or waking up (hypnapompic), or an isolated experience of hearing one's name called out). They may also be considered normal in the context of certain religious rites and cultures.

The term "Schneiderian hallucinations" refers to a specific forms of auditory hallucinations (e.g., two voices having a dialogue independent of the person experiencing the hallucination, or hearing multiple voices commenting on the person's action). DSM-IV-TR identifies these as being sufficient by themselves to diagnose schizophrenia.

Disorganization Dimension

DISORGANIZATION OF THOUGHT

Disorganized thinking or *formal thought disorder* has been argued by some to be the single most important feature of schizophrenia. It refers to abnormalities in the form, structure, or processing of speech rather than its content. Because of the difficulty inherent in developing an objective definition of a thought disorder, and because in a clinical setting inferences about thought are based primarily on the individual's speech, the concept of disorganized speech has been emphasized in the definition for schizophrenia used in DSM-IV-TR. The speech of individuals with schizophrenia may be disorganized in a variety of ways. The person may "slip off the track" from one topic to another ("derailment" or "loose associations"); answers to questions may be obliquely related or completely un-related ("tangentiality"); and, rarely, speech may be so severely disorganized that it is nearly incomprehensible and resembles receptive aphasia in its linguistic disorganization ("incoherence" or "word salad"). Since mild disorganization of speech is common, the disorganization in schizophrenia should be sufficiently severe to impair meaningful com-munication.

DISORGANIZATION OF BEHAVIOR

According to DSM-IV-TR,

> Grossly disorganized behavior may manifest itself in a variety of ways, ranging from child-like silliness to unpredictable agitation. Problems may be noted in any form of goal-directed behavior, leading to difficulties in performing activities of daily living such as preparing a meal or maintaining hygiene. The person may appear markedly disheveled, may dress in an unusual manner (e.g., wearing multiple overcoats, scarves, and gloves on a hot day), or may display clearly inappropriate sexual behavior (e.g., public masturbation) or unpredictable and untriggered agitation (e.g., shouting or swearing). (American Psychiatric Association, 2000, p. 300)

The manual also stresses the importance of clinical discretion in determining this. Mild disorganization of behavior may be present in a variety of clinical disorders, and as in the case of thought disorganization, the importance of severity is emphasized.

CATATONIA AND MOTOR SYMPTOMS

According to DSM-IV-TR,

> Catatonic motor behaviors include a marked decrease in reactivity to the environment, sometimes reaching an extreme degree of complete unawareness (catatonic stupor), main-taining a rigid posture and resisting efforts to be moved (catatonic rigidity), active resis-tance to instructions or attempts to be moved (catatonic negativism), the assumption of inappropriate or bizarre postures (catatonic posturing), or purposeless and unstimulated excessive motor activity (catatonic excitement). (American Psychiatric Association, 2000, p. 300)

Abnormalities of psychomotor activity such as pacing, rocking, apathetic immobil-ity, or other stereotyped movements are also common in patients with schizophrenia. Gri-macing, posturing, and odd ritualistic movements are often noted. Motor abnormalities are associated with the catatonic subtype of schizophrenia.

Negative Symptoms

Three negative symptoms—*affective flattening*, *alogia*, and *avolition*—are included in the definition of schizophrenia in DSM-IV-TR.

- *Affective flattening*, described by DSM-IV-TR as being especially common, is characterized by facial immobility and unresponsiveness, with poor eye contact and re-duced body language. Although a person with affective flattening may smile and warm up occasionally, his or her range of emotional expressiveness is clearly diminished most of the time. DSM-IV-TR recommends observation of a person over a period of time, as well as in interactions outside those with the clinician, to determine presence of affective flattening. It is important to distinguish this from the affective blunting that may be seen in depressed patients.

- *Alogia* (poverty of speech) is manifested by brief, laconic, empty replies. There is an absence of ability to carry out engaging meaningful conversation. Alogia may reflect a more primary inability to form completely and then articulate thoughts, and must be differentiated from unwillingness to speak, which is often seen as part of a severe positive symptomatology.
- *Avolition* is characterized by an inability to initiate and persist in goal-directed activities. The person may sit for long periods of time and show little interest in participating in work or social activities.

Several additional negative symptoms have been identified. These include *anhedonia* (reduction in capacity to experience pleasure), *asociality* (reduction of interest in other people), and *inattentiveness* (difficulty in maintaining focused or engaged).

Although negative symptoms are common, they must be judiciously differentiated from a variety of other clinical features, including depressed mood, isolative behavior seen in paranoid individuals, or apathy, which is often seen in older persons with dementias, frontal lobe disorders, or parkinsonian features. In older persons who already carry a diagnosis of schizophrenia, this clinical distinction becomes critically important. Certain antipsychotic medications often produce extrapyramidal side effects, such as bradykinesia or akinesia, which may mimic affective flattening. The distinction between true negative symptoms and medication side effects often depends on clinical judgment and detailed evaluation by the clinician.

It is prudent to approach a clinical estimation of negative symptoms with discretion, and a person's overall functioning and broader clinical and social picture must be assessed as well. Ideally, negative symptoms are diagnosed only after observation over a prolonged period of time.

Other Associated Clinical Features

DSM-IV-TR lists multiple symptoms that are present in schizophrenia and that may be strongly associated with certain subtypes:

- Dysphoric mood may take the form of depression, anxiety, or anger. Sleep patterns are often disturbed.
- Various cognitive dysfunctions such as poor concentration, disorientation, or impaired memory may be present acutely, but some deficits may persist.
- Depersonalization, derealization, and somatic concerns may occur and sometimes reach delusional proportions.
- Suicide risk remains higher than that in the general population over the whole lifespan, and is often elevated immediately after an acute psychotic episode.
- Many studies have reported that subgroups of individuals diagnosed with schizophrenia have a higher incidence of assaultive and violent behavior.
- There are high rates of comorbidity with substance-related disorders and with anxiety disorders, such as obsessive–compulsive and panic disorders.

INTERNATIONAL CLASSIFICATION OF DISEASES

The first version of the ICD appeared in 1900, and was designed to establish comparable nomenclature among different countries. In 1946, it was entrusted to the newly established WHO. The authors of the ICD-10 (WHO, 2003) section on schizophrenia acknowledged that none of the symptoms categorized under schizophrenia could be considered pathognomic. However, they specified that there was a practical usefulness in dividing the symptoms into groups based on their importance to diagnosis and patterns of occurrence. These include the following symptoms:

1. Thought echo, thought insertion or withdrawal, and thought broadcasting.
2. Delusions of control, influence, or passivity, clearly referred to body or limb movements or specific thoughts, actions, or sensations; delusional perception.
3. Hallucinatory voices giving a running commentary on the patient's behavior, or discussing the patient among themselves, or other types of hallucinatory voices coming from some part of the body.
4. Persistent delusions of other kinds that are culturally inappropriate and completely impossible, such as religious or political identity, or superhuman powers and abilities (e.g., being able to control the weather, or being in communication with aliens from another world).
5. Persistent hallucinations in any modality, when accompanied by either fleeting or half-formed delusions without clear affective content or persistent overvalued ideas, or when occurring every day for weeks or months on end.
6. Breaks or insertions into the train of thought, resulting in incoherence or irrelevant speech, or neologisms.
7. Catatonic behavior, such as excitement, posturing, or waxy flexibility, negativism, mutism, and stupor.
8. "Negative" symptoms such as marked apathy, paucity of speech, and blunting or incongruity of emotional responses, usually resulting in social withdrawal and lowering of social performance; it must be clear that these are not due to depression or to neuroleptic medication.
9. A significant and consistent change in the overall quality of some aspects of personal behavior that manifests as loss of interest, aimlessness, idleness, a self-absorbed attitude, and social withdrawal.

DIFFERENCES BETWEEN DSM-IV-TR AND ICD-10

There are several differences between the latest versions of DSM and ICD diagnostic systems with respect to symptoms. DSM is more general, whereas ICD is more specific regarding the types of psychotic symptoms. ICD requires three symptoms, whereas DSM requires that two of five categories to be present (although if certain Schneiderian symptoms are present, only one category has to be met). ICD requires that symptoms be present for only 1 month, whereas DSM requires a duration of illness of 6 months.

FUTURE DIRECTIONS

With the increasing influence of the neuroscience in schizophrenia research, a new paradigm shift has occurred regarding the conceptualization of symptom domains in schizophrenia. Each symptom domain is thought to be associated with unique neurocircuitry regulated by distinct neurotransmitters, receptors, and genes. Neuroscience suggests that (1) positive symptoms are influenced by dopaminergic systems involving the striatum and the nucleus accumbens; (2) affective symptoms involve dopaminergic and serotonergic projections to the ventromedial cortex; and (3) cognitive symptoms involve dopaminergic projections to the dorsolateral prefrontal cortex. In this model, negative symptoms are viewed as being subsumed under affective or cognitive dysfunction.

KEY POINTS

- The definition of schizophrenia as a clinical entity has evolved over the last century and continues to be modified. It has been influenced by psychoanalytic, interpersonal, and socioenvironmental theories.
- The definition of schizophrenia used in current clinical practice is based on the DSM-IV-TR.
- DSM-IV-TR divides symptoms of schizophrenia into two broad categories: positive symptoms and negative symptoms, which it goes on to describe in greater detail.
- Positive symptoms are further divided into the psychotic dimension (which includes delusions and hallucinations) and the disorganization dimension (which includes disorganization of thoughts, disorganization of behavior, and catatonic symptoms).
- Negative symptoms are further divided into amotivation, alogia, and avolition.
- ICD-10, a classification system published by the WHO, is more general than the DSM-IV-TR and is used as a primary diagnostic manual in some parts of the world outside the United States.
- The DSM-IV-TR and ICD-10 both stress on the importance of clinical judgment in eliciting symptoms and making a diagnosis of schizophrenia.
- Current research revolves around identifying neurotransmitter and neurocircuitry that correlate with manifest symptoms of schizophrenia, and this may form the basis for redefining schizophrenia as a diagnostic entity in the future.

REFERENCES AND RECOMMENDED READINGS

American Psychiatric Association. (1994). *Diagnostic and statistical manual of mental disorders* (4th ed.). Washington, DC: Author.

American Psychiatric Association. (1980). *Diagnostic and statistical manual of mental disorders* (3rd ed.). Washington, DC: Author.

American Psychiatric Association. (2000). *Diagnostic and statistical manual of mental disorders* (4th ed., text rev.). Washington, DC: Authors.

Hartmann, H. (1964). *Essays on ego psychology: Selected problems in psychoanalytic theory.* Madison, CT: International Universities Press.

Hawk, A. B., Carpenter, W. T., Jr., & Strauss, J. S. (1975). Diagnostic criteria and five-year outcome in schizophrenia: A report from the International Pilot Study of Schizophrenia. *Archives of General Psychiatry, 32*(3), 343–347.

Jaspers, K. (1959). *General psychopathology* (1997 ed.). Baltimore: Johns Hopkins University Press.

Kimhy, D., Goetz, R., Yale, S., Corcoran, C., & Malaspina, D. (2005). Delusions in individuals with schizophrenia: Factor structure, clinical correlates, and putative neurobiology. *Psychopathology, 38*(6), 338–344.

Laing, R. D., & Esterson, A. (1970). *Sanity, madness, and the family: Families of schizophrenics.* Harmondsworth, UK: Penguin.

Nasrallah, H., & Smeltzer, D. (Eds.). (2002). *Contemporary diagnosis and management of the patient with schizophrenia.* Newtown, PA: Handbooks in Health Care.

Sadock, B. J., & Sadock, V. A. (Eds.). (2002). *Kaplan and Sadock's synopsis of psychiatry* (9th ed.). Philadelphia: Lippincott, Williams & Wilkins.

Siris, S. G. (2001). Suicide in schizophrenia. *Journal of Psychopharmacology, 2,* 127–135.

Strauss, J. S., & Carpenter, W. T., Jr. (1974). The prediction of outcome in schizophrenia, II: Relationship between predictor and outcome variables. *Archives of General Psychiatry, 31,* 37–42.

Sullivan, H. S. (1953). *Conceptions of modern psychiatry.* New York: Norton.

World Health Organization. (2003) *International statistical classification of diseases and related health problems* (10th rev. ed.). Geneva: Author.

CHAPTER 10

COGNITIVE FUNCTIONING IN SCHIZOPHRENIA

GAURI N. SAVLA
DAVID J. MOORE
BARTON W. PALMER

Cognitive functioning is an important, yet underappreciated, dimension of schizophrenia. Schizophrenia is typically characterized by the overt psychopathological symptoms (i.e., positive symptoms, such as hallucinations, and negative symptoms, such as blunted affect and anhedonia). The currently available pharmacological treatments for schizophrenia largely target these symptoms (particularly the positive symptoms, with less effect on negative symptoms). Recent empirical research has consistently demonstrated that although psychopathological symptoms disrupt patients' lives, deficits in cognitive functioning have the strongest influence on their overall level of independent functioning. Research on cognition in schizophrenia has also shown that there is considerable heterogeneity in the severity and pattern of cognitive deficits among people with the illness. Understanding this heterogeneity, and how different cognitive deficit profiles affect functioning, is important in the consideration of the long-term-care needs of patients with schizophrenia.

This chapter briefly reviews historical perspectives on cognition in schizophrenia, contemporary research findings and conceptualizations of cognitive deficits in schizophrenia, the long-term course of these deficits, effects of impaired cognition on daily functioning, and efforts to develop effective cognitive treatments, as well as clinical recommendations in light of these findings.

THE EVOLVING VIEW OF COGNITION IN SCHIZOPHRENIA

Although Émil Kraepelin and Eugen Bleuler presented their conceptualizations of *dementia praecox* or the *schizophrenias* approximately a century ago, several of their observations continue to be replicated and validated today. Many of Kraepelin's descriptions of *dementia praecox* are similar in content to current discussions of disruptions in executive functions (Zec, 1995). For instance, Kraepelin viewed problems in volition or will as central to this disorder. He also put substantial emphasis on the role of attentional deficits; for instance, he distinguished between "active attention" (*aufmerksamkeit*), which he asserted is impaired at all stages of the illness, and "passive attention" (*auffassung*), which he described as being mostly impacted in acute stages of the illness.

Despite the awareness of cognitive deficits in schizophrenia from its earliest conceptualization, some of the prominent theories of schizophrenia in the United States in the mid–20th century were strongly influenced by psychoanalytic and interpersonal theories about the etiology of the illness, the popular (although not universal) notion being that schizophrenia was a "functional" (as opposed to "organic" or neurological) condition. A particularly notorious theory that arose in the 1930s was that of the so-called schizophrenogenic mother. This concept had roots in the writings of several influential figures in the early to mid–20th century (reviewed in Hartwell, 1996). For instance, Sullivan posited that personality is shaped by early interpersonal relationships, especially with the mother, and that schizophrenia is a result of pathological early relationships. Similarly, Levy concluded that an "overprotective mother" played a major etiological role in her child's later development of schizophrenia. It is interesting to note that while American psychiatry was emphasizing psychodynamic and interpersonal models of schizophrenia around the 1930s, Freud began emphasizing the neurobiological underpinning of this condition, and noted that patients with schizophrenia appeared to have a hereditary predisposition to the illness.

It would be a mischaracterization to suggest that the biological basis of schizophrenia was not recognized in American psychiatry. Practices, such as fever or seizure induction, as well as brain surgery (e.g., frontal lobotomy) before the introduction of neuroleptic medications in the 1950s clearly speak to 20th-century recognition of the involvement of the brain in the manifestation of symptoms of schizophrenia. The introduction of neuroleptic medications in 1952, and their increased use thereafter, as well as the rise of the dopamine hypothesis, also fostered wider recognition of schizophrenia as something than a "functional" disorder. However, full appreciation of the importance and central role of cognitive deficits in schizophrenia has only emerged on a widespread basis within the last few decades, with exponential growth in neuropsychological research consistent with the wider recognition of the importance of cognitive deficits in schizophrenia. Indeed, harkening back to Kraepelin, some have suggested that schizophrenia, at its core, may be a neurocognitive disorder.

THE NATURE OF COGNITIVE DEFICITS IN SCHIZOPHRENIA

Patterns and Level of Cognitive Impairment

The substantial growth in the empirical literature of neuropsychological deficits in schizophrenia over the past two to three decades has shown that the majority of patients with schizophrenia have mild-to-moderate neuropsychological deficits. Heinrichs and Zakzanis (1998) conducted a meta-analysis of 204 studies of cognition in schizophrenia and concluded that 60–80% of patients with schizophrenia have at least mild neurocognitive deficits. That figure is consistent with findings from our research group, showing that about a quarter of patients with schizophrenia continue to function in the "normal" range of neurocognition (Palmer et al., 1997). No single pattern of deficits is unique or common to all patients with schizophrenia, but some of the most frequently impaired abilities include attention, working memory, visual and verbal learning, psychomotor speed, and executive functions.

The attentional deficits in schizophrenia can include inability to distinguish between relevant and irrelevant stimuli or information (selective attention or "gating"), inability to stay mentally "on track" (sustained attention), and lack of vigilance (such as waiting for a particular stimulus or event to occur over time). Working memory is a concept closely related to attention as well as to executive functioning, and involves the ability to hold and manipulate information in one's mind for short periods of time for further processing. Working memory is a resource-limited process, and requires active rehearsal and allocation of attentional resources for retention. Goldman-Rakic (1994) and others have suggested that deficits in working memory may underlie some of the other aspects of schizophrenia, including executive dysfunction and some aspects of thought disorder.

Episodic memory is often mentioned as one of the most frequently impaired abilities in schizophrenia. However, it is important to distinguish between difficulties with acquisition of new information and/or efficiency of its retrieval, and actual loss of the memory trace. As yet another example of his astute observational skills, in his 1919 textbook, Kraepelin accurately noted, "Memory is comparatively little disordered. The patients are able, when they like, to give a correct detailed account of their past life, and often know accurately to a day how long they have been in the institution" (pp. 18–19). Kraepelin's descriptions are consistent with contemporary neuropsychological research on memory functions in schizophrenia. In particular, most patients with schizophrenia have difficulties with initial acquisition of information (such as number of words recalled over a series of trials on a word list learning task) but are generally able to retain the information they actually learn. Some patients may have difficulty showing such retention under the demands of a free recall test, but they generally benefit from cued or multiple-choice testing, indicating that the information does in fact remain stored. This pattern contrasts sharply with that typically seen in cortical dementias, such as dementia due to Alzheimer's disease, wherein there is not only difficulty with acquisition but also "rapid forgetting" (loss of the memory trace) of the acquired information (Heaton et al., 1994). Whether the acquisition and retrieval deficits reflect memory processes per se, or are instead more accurately conceived of as secondary effects of deficits in attention and executive functioning, remains an open question. Another common misconception is that the memory deficits associated with schizophrenia are primarily deficits in acquisition of verbal information. Recent research suggests that both visual and verbal learning deficits are common among individuals with schizophrenia.

Psychomotor speed, as measured with common tasks, such as the Trail Making Test or Digit Symbol from the Wechsler Adult Intelligence Scale—Third Edition (WAIS-III), can be thought of as comprising two components: (1) mental processing speed and (2) efficiency of psychomotor integration. Both may be affected by schizophrenia and/or its treatment. The conventional neuroleptics were noted in particular for their tendency to elicit extrapyramidal symptoms, including psychomotor slowing, which can affect performance on tests designed to measure an array of other cognitive ability areas.

The cognitive dimension most widely studied in schizophrenia may be executive functions. As noted in Palmer and Heaton (2000), "A simple definition of the term executive skills remains elusive, but in general, this construct appears to involve those cognitive processes which permit an adaptive balance of initiation, maintenance, and shifting of responses to environmental demands permitting goal-directed behavior" (pp. 62–64). Some of the specific abilities that may fall under this rubric include abstraction, planning, mental flexibility, response inhibition, self-monitoring, evaluation, and decision making.

The Wisconsin Card Sorting Test (WCST), a measure sensitive to abstraction, problem solving, and mental flexibility, has been among the most widely used neuropsychological measures in the schizophrenia literature. For instance, a recent search of the

PsycINFO database [accessed December 13, 2007] for published articles with the words *schizophrenia* or *schizophrenic* in the title, and *WCST* or *Wisconsin Card* in the title or abstract resulted in 392 citations in peer-reviewed journals, the earliest being Elizabeth Fey's 1951 report demonstrating worse performance on the WCST among patients with schizophrenia relative to healthy controls. Two hundred and one such articles were published between January 1, 2001, and December 13, 2007. The sheer volume of ongoing schizophrenia research using the WCST speaks to the perceived importance of executive deficits in patients with schizophrenia.

At least when studied on a group level, the cognitive deficits in schizophrenia tend to be diffuse/nonfocal (across a number of ability areas). However, it is interesting to note that the findings in terms of executive dysfunction and initial acquisition of new information are consistent with Kraepelin's speculations regarding potential pathology in the frontal and temporal lobes in schizophrenia. Although there is no identified, specific neuropathological cause associated with this disorder, the temporal and frontal regions, including the frontal–subcortical circuits, remain areas of intense research focus.

Heterogeneity in virtually any conceivable dimension among patients with schizophrenia is probably the single, most consistent attribute one can apply to the findings from the larger schizophrenia literature in the past century. Attempts to divide schizophrenia into meaningful or homogenous subgroups date back to the earliest conceptualizations of this disorder. Indeed, Bleuler spoke of this disorder as the *schizophrenias*. Modern diagnostic systems such as the fourth, text revised edition of the *Diagnostic and Statistical Manual of Mental Disorders* (DSM-IV-TR; American Psychiatric Association, 2000) and the *International Classification of Diseases* (ICD-10; World Health Organization, 1990) continue this tradition; the schizophrenia subtypes in these contemporary diagnostic systems are largely based on patterns of psychopathological rather than cognitive or functional symptoms. Seaton, Goldstein, and Allen (2001) estimated that there are over 100 potential combinations of variables under three broad categories: causes of heterogeneity (age, education–socioeconomic status, comorbidity, etc.), heterogeneous characteristics (i.e., neurological, cognitive, and symptom profile), and course and outcome of illness (stability or decline in symptoms, age of onset, etc.). Their own proposed model of heterogeneity in schizophrenia focused on cognitive aspects and was based on a four-cluster solution: (1) uniform mild-to-moderate impairment across domains; (2) similar pattern as that in (1), but with intact psychomotor skills; (3) impairment in shifting between reasoning strategies, but intact abstraction skills; and (4) significantly impaired (dementia-like) performance. However, the authors listed numerous other cluster-analytic studies that yielded cognitive subtypes of schizophrenia, but with widely different solutions based on different patterns of cognitive performance. More recently, functional imaging techniques have also been applied to identification of homogenous subtypes. Unfortunately, consensus on the utility of any particular categorization scheme remains elusive.

Trajectory of Cognitive Impairment in Schizophrenia

Preonset Cognitive Functioning

The contemporary model of schizophrenia is that of a neurodevelopmental condition. This view is not completely new. Kraepelin noted that some cases of schizophrenia may be attributable to early brain insults. Barney Katz, in his 1939 doctoral dissertation from the University of Southern California, presented evidence that patients with psychosis experienced a higher incidence of obstetrical complications at the time of their birth.

More recent evidence for the neurodevelopmental nature of schizophrenia comes from an array of converging lines of evidence. A large literature suggests that certain forms of maternal influenza and/or malnutrition during key stages of pregnancy are associated with statistical increases in the risk of schizophrenia. Cannon, Jones, and Murray (2002) conducted a meta-analysis and found that complications during gestation (e.g., maternal bleeding or diabetes), abnormal prenatal growth and development (e.g., low birthweight, reduced head circumference), and complications during birth (e.g., asphyxia, emergency caesarean section delivery) were each significantly associated with psychosis in later life. There is also evidence of early abnormalities in motor development or functioning among at least some of those who later develop schizophrenia. In addition, patients with schizophrenia are more likely than the general population (and patients with some other forms of serious mental illness) to show an increased number of minor facial anomalies (which are thought to be correlated with neurodevelopmental aberrations during gestation). Also, those at genetic risk for schizophrenia (first- and second-degree relatives), show a higher risk of subtle deficits (which consistently remain stable over time) relative to the general population.

Given a neurodevelopmental model (i.e., with the possibility of abnormal neurodevelopment present even during gestation), why does schizophrenia typically manifest later in life (most typically, albeit not always, in adolescence or early adulthood)? A possible answer to this puzzle comes from a theory proposed by Feinberg (1982). Based on the empirical finding that an extensive reorganization of connections between cortical structures (synaptic "pruning") occurs during adolescence, Feinberg proposed that the onset of schizophrenia symptoms may be associated with deficits in this "pruning" process. Although this idea was viewed as somewhat speculative at the time, an increasing body of empirical research supports the notion of excessive "pruning" of certain cortical structures (particularly, the prefrontal cortex), and "underpruning" or complete failure of "pruning" of certain subcortical structures (e.g., the lenticular nuclei) among patients with schizophrenia. In this regard, many neuroscientists now view schizophrenia as a "disconnection" syndrome; that is, at least some aspects of schizophrenia may be characterized not only by abnormalities within specific brain regions but also in terms of disruptions in communication/interaction between different brain areas. This notion melds nicely with that of "adolescent pruning," in which the interconnections are "pruned" to permit more efficient communication/interaction.

Perionset Cognitive Functioning

In addition to any subtle premorbid neurocognitive deficits, there is also evidence that further decline in cognitive functioning (at a level equivalent to about 5–10 IQ points or one-third to two-thirds of a standard deviation) generally occurs during the perionset period. Bilder and colleagues (2006) demonstrated that objective tests scores obtained from academic records (achievement test scores, and Scholastic Aptitude Test scores) of children who developed schizophrenia in adolescence or adulthood were significantly lower than those of their healthy peers. Furthermore, they also demonstrated that the change in cognitive ability at first onset of schizophrenia approximated about 11.5 IQ-equivalent points.

Long-Term Course of Cognitive Functioning

As may be implied by his use of the term *dementia praecox*, Kraepelin's original view of schizophrenia was that the typical course was one of progressive decline in functioning. Although there were dissenters, this rather bleak prognostic view greatly influenced thinking about the common course of schizophrenia throughout much of the 20th century. However, recent longitudinal neuropsychological studies of schizophrenia suggest that, at least after the first few years from the time of symptom onset, the level of cognitive functioning in patients with schizophrenia (compared to the level expected among same-age people in the general population) remains stable. For instance, results a study from a large-scale longitudinal study by Heaton and colleagues (2001) found that the level of cognitive deficits remains stable regardless of the specific cognitive domain examined, current age, age of illness onset, or changes in severity of positive or negative symptoms. There is some evidence, however, such as that from Harvey (2001), that a proportion of "poor outcome" chronically institutionalized older adult patients with schizophrenia may be prone to show greater than age-normal declines in cognitive functioning. The specific factors responsible for decline in this subgroup remain an area of ongoing research.

FUNCTIONAL IMPACT OF COGNITIVE DEFICITS IN SCHIZOPHRENIA

There is strong evidence that neuropsychological impairment is related to deficits in everyday functioning abilities among persons with schizophrenia. As shown in the classic review of the functional outcome literature by Green (1996), level of cognitive impairment is a stronger predictor of patients' level of functional independence/disability than severity of psychopathology. Verbal, concentration, and executive functioning skills are consistently related to activities of daily living, social skills, and benefits derived from social skills training programs. Neuropsychological abilities have also been shown to be related to performance-based measures of everyday functioning and social skills among older patients with schizophrenia, as well as ability to manage their own medications and capacity to consent to treatment or research.

TREATMENT OF COGNITIVE DEFICITS

Pharmacological Treatments

Given the availability of pharmacotherapy for schizophrenia and its effectiveness for certain positive symptoms, most patients receive treatment when they first report psychotic symptoms. Since the introduction of clozapine in 1988, followed by other second-generation (or "atypical") antipsychotic agents such as risperidone, olanzapine, quetiapine, ziprasidone, and aripiprazole, there has been some suggestion that these second-generation medications may partially improve certain aspects of neurocognitive functioning in schizophrenia (Keefe, Silva, Perkins, & Lieberman, 1999). The question of functionally relevant degrees of cognitive benefit from second-generation antipsychotic medications remains at least partially open for debate (Gold, 2004). It is yet unclear whether these medications actually enhance underlying cognitive abilities or simply lack the harmful extrapyramidal side effects associated with conventional neuroleptics, as well as the potential adverse effects of the anticholinergic medications typically prescribed to manage such side effects.

Regardless of how the debate resolves, however, the possibility of such benefits, together with the growing literature showing the importance of cognitive deficits as predictors of functional living skills in schizophrenia (reviewed earlier), have catalyzed interest in developing new agents that directly target the cognitive symptoms of schizophrenia for intervention. For instance, Measurement and Treatment Research to Improve Cognition in Schizophrenia (MATRICS) and Treatment Units for Research on Neurocognition and Schizophrenia (TURNS) are ongoing NIMH-sponsored efforts that aim to foster the development of cognition-enhancing medications for schizophrenia (Buchanan et al., 2005).

Psychosocial Treatments

In recent years, there has been an increasing recognition of the need for psychosocial rehabilitative interventions for schizophrenia. Cognitive Training, originating in neurorehabilitation research in traumatic brain injury, targets neurocognitive abilities such as attention, learning and memory, and executive functioning. Cognitive Training is not a restorative intervention (i.e., it does not reverse lost functions); rather, it is compensatory in nature (i.e., it teaches patients, via strategy coaching and task practice, to use external aids or to modify their environments to make up for deficit areas).

CLINICAL IMPLICATIONS

Cognitive functioning is a core dimension of schizophrenia that has been traditionally ignored in treatment contexts. Given the considerable heterogeneity in the level of deficits among patients, the remarkable stability of these deficits within patients, and the strong relationship between such deficits and everyday functioning, clinical attention to the level and pattern of cognitive deficits in individual patients with schizophrenia is clearly warranted as part of treatment planning. In that regard, we offer the following recommendations.

Neuropsychological assessment is generally provided and interpreted by a licensed doctoral-level clinical psychologist with specific training in neuropsychological principles. The evaluation generally includes administration of a battery of standardized tests to measure a range of cognitive functions. However, neuropsychological assessment involves more than mere testing; it involves synthesizing the standardized test results with other information, including clinical history, behavioral observations, medical and neurological data, as well as information about the patient's premorbid and current psychosocial functioning. Because such an evaluation requires some cooperation on the part of the patient to attend to the neuropsychological tests, the actual evaluation may be most useful after the most acute symptoms have been stabilized, but briefer testing may be helpful in documenting what a patient is able to attend to and understand, even when in more acutely psychotic states. After stabilization, comprehensive assessment should be considered part of the overall treatment planning for patients with schizophrenia.

Neuropsychological evaluation can be helpful in the clinical care of patients with schizophrenia in a number of important ways. For instance, having schizophrenia does not make one immune to other neurological conditions. Neuropsychological assessment can be helpful in evaluating the possible presence of secondary neurological conditions. For instance, as noted earlier, patients with schizophrenia frequently have difficulty with initial acquisition of information but generally show adequate retention of information once learned (at least if evaluated through cued recall or recognition methods). Thus, presence of "rapid forgetting" in a patient with schizophrenia may be an indication of the presence of a secondary condition; therefore, such persons should receive further, more comprehensive cognitive evaluation.

Neuropsychological evaluation of patients with schizophrenia is generally more useful in determining not only areas and levels of cognitive limitations/deficits but also, importantly, the presence and degree of spared cognitive capacities that may be drawn upon in implementing rehabilitative interventions. With the emergence of newer treatments that have beneficial effects on cognitive deficits, repeated neuropsychological evaluation will also be important in tracking the effectiveness of such interventions for individual patients.

KEY POINTS

- Schizophrenia is commonly, although not always, associated with mild-to-moderate neuropsychological deficits.
- The pattern of deficits varies widely among patients, although some of the most commonly impaired areas include attention and working memory, episodic learning (but not retention), psychomotor speed, and executive functioning.
- The level of neuropsychological deficits varies widely between patients with schizophrenia and has a stronger influence on the level of independent functioning than do the primary psychopathological symptoms.
- Contrary to Kraepelin's notion of schizophrenia as a dementia praecox, the typical course of the cognitive deficits in this disorder is one of remarkable stability, even when psychopathological symptoms fluctuate.
- Standard pharmacological treatments for schizophrenia primarily help with the positive symptoms of this disorder. The influence of even second-generation antipsychotics in terms of yielding functionally relevant relief from neuropsychological deficits is unclear.
- Neuropsychological evaluation for schizophrenia is helpful not only to characterize the nature of cognitive deficits but also to identify abilities that are relative strengths in the development of plans for treatment and long-term care.

REFERENCES AND RECOMMENDED READINGS

American Psychiatric Association. (2000). *Diagnostic and statistical manual of mental disorders* (4th ed., text rev.). Washington, DC: Author.

Bilder, R. M., Reiter, G., Bates, J., Lencz, T., Szeszko, P., Goldman, R. S., et al. (2006). Cognitive development in schizophrenia: Follow-back from the first episode. *Journal of Clinical and Experimental Neuropsychology, 28,* 270–282.

Buchanan, R. W., Davis, M., Goff, D., Green, M. F., Keefe, R. S., Leon, A. C., et al. (2005). A summary of the FDA-NIMH-MATRICS workshop on clinical trial design for neurocognitive drugs for schizophrenia. *Schizophrenia Bulletin, 31,* 5–19.

Cannon, M., Jones, P. B., & Murray, R. M. (2002). Obstetric complications and schizophrenia: Historical and meta-analytic review. *American Journal of Psychiatry, 159,* 1080–1092.

Feinberg, I. (1982). Schizophrenia: Caused by a fault in programmed synaptic elimination during adolescence? *Journal of Psychiatric Research, 17,* 319–334.

Fey, E. T. (1951). The performance of young schizophrenics and young normals on the Wisconsin Card Sorting Test. *Journal of Consulting Psychology, 15*(4), 311–319.

Gold, J. M. (2004). Cognitive deficits as treatment targets in schizophrenia. *Schizophrenia Research, 72,* 21–28.

Goldman-Rakic, P.S. (1994). Working memory dysfunction in schizophrenia. *Journal of Neuropsychiatry and Clinical Neurosciences, 6,* 348–357.

Green, M. F. (1996). What are the functional consequences of neurocognitive deficits in schizophrenia? *American Journal of Psychiatry, 153,* 321–330.

Hartwell, C. E. (1996). The schizophrenogenic mother concept in American psychiatry. *Psychiatry, Interpersonal and Biological Processes, 59*(3), 274–297.

Harvey, P. D. (2001). Cognitive impairment in elderly patients with schizophrenia: Age-related changes. *International Journal of Geriatric Psychiatry, 16*(Suppl. 1), S78–S85.

Heaton, R., Paulsen, J. S., McAdams, L. A., Kuck, J., Zisook, S., Braff, D., et al. (1994). Neuropsychological deficits in schizophrenics: Relationship to age, chronicity, and dementia. *Archives of General Psychiatry, 51,* 469–476.

Heaton, R. K., Gladsjo, J. A., Palmer, B. W., Kuck, J., Marcotte, T. D., & Jeste, D. V. (2001). Stability and course of neuropsychological deficits in schizophrenia. *Archives of General Psychiatry, 58,* 24–32.

Heaton, R. K., & Marcotte, T. D. (2000). Clinical neuropsychological tests and assessment techniques. In F. Boller, J. Grafman, & G. Rizzolatti (Eds.), *Handbook of neuropsychology* (Vol. 1, 2nd ed., pp. 27–52). New York: Elsevier Science.

Heinrichs, R. W., & Zakzanis, K. K. (1998). Neurocognitive deficit in schizophrenia: A quantitative review of the evidence. *Neuropsychology, 12,* 426–445.

Keefe, R. S., Silva, S. G., Perkins, D. O., & Lieberman, J. A. (1999). The effects of atypical antipsychotic drugs on neurocognitive impairment in schizophrenia: A review and meta-analysis. *Schizophrenia Bulletin, 25,* 201–222.

Kraepelin, É. (1919). *Dementia praecox and paraphrenia.* Huntington, NY: Krieger.

Mednick, S. (1991). *Fetal neural development and adult schizophrenia.* Cambridge, UK: Cambridge University Press.

Palmer, B. W. (2004). The expanding role of neuropsychology in geriatric psychiatry. *American Journal of Geriatric Psychiatry, 12,* 338–341.

Palmer, B. W., & Heaton, R. K. (2000). Executive dysfunction in schizophrenia. In T. Sharma & P. D. Harvey (Eds.), *Cognition in schizophrenia: Impairments, importance and treatment strategies* (pp. 51–72). New York: Oxford University Press.

Palmer, B. W., Heaton, R. K., Paulsen, J. S., Kuck, J., Braff, D., Harris, M. J., et al. (1997). Is it possible to be schizophrenic yet neuropsychologically normal? *Neuropsychology, 11,* 437–446.

Seaton, B. E., Goldstein, G., & Allen, D. N. (2001). Sources of heterogeneity in schizophrenia: The role of neuropsychological functioning. *Neuropsychology Review, 11*(1), 45–67.

Twamley, E. W., Jeste, D. V., & Bellack, A. S. (2003). A review of cognitive training in schizophrenia. *Schizophrenia Bulletin, 29,* 359–382.

World Health Organization. (1990). *International classification of diseases* (10th ed.). Geneva: Author.

Zec, R. F. (1995). Neuropsychology of schizophrenia according to Kraepelin: Disorders of volition and executive functioning. *European Archives of Psychiatry and Clinical Neuroscience, 245*(4–5), 216–223.

CHAPTER 11

COURSE AND OUTCOME

HEINZ HÄFNER
WOLFRAM AN DER HEIDEN

Schizophrenia is a disorder that can be treated successfully. Ethical considerations prevent us from studying the untreated illness course. For this reason, our chapter focuses on the treated course as it presents itself under current conditions of care. This limitation does not apply to the untreated early course that precedes first contact.

TIME TRENDS

Since the beginning of the 20th century, lengths of stay of patients hospitalized for the first time with a diagnosis of schizophrenia have shortened dramatically. The reason lies in the change in strategy from long-term custodial care to a primarily open, therapeutically active system of community-based care. This fundamental change, however, does not permit us to infer that the natural course of the illness has also changed.

Comparisons of the illness course over long periods of time require homogenization of the study designs (diagnosis, representative study samples, appropriate assessments, etc.). In the largest meta-analysis so far, which covered 320 studies from a period of almost 100 years, the increase in global recovery rates that occurred with the advent of traditional antipsychotics (1895–1955: 35%; 1956–1985: 49%) disappeared unexpectedly in the subsequent period (1986–1992: 36%) of the new generation of antipsychotic medications (Hegarty, Baldessarini, Tohen, Waternaux, & Oepen, 1994). But a combination of factors underlies these figures. At any rate, it should be noted that the medications currently available reduce the intensity and frequency of psychotic episodes but have little impact on negative symptoms, and cognitive and functional impairment, which play the greatest role in global outcome. The only treatment-related improvement that has occurred is an enormous decrease in hospital stays and catastrophic outcomes such as life-threatening catatonia in countries with fully developed mental health care systems.

DIAGNOSIS AND ILLNESS COURSE

Given the ubiquitousness and cross-cultural robustness of the schizophrenic core syndrome, the disorder is broadly accepted as both common and consistent with the concept of a disease. The diagnosis of schizophrenia shows good reliability over long periods of time (e.g., from first admission to 10 years later). Furthermore, the negative symptoms of schizophrenia and characteristic cognitive impairment are even more stable.

The *International Classification of Diseases* (ICD) distinguishes diagnostic subtypes with different patterns of symptoms, onset, and course. The simple type—a rare diagnosis that does not involve psychotic symptoms—and the hebephrenic type show an insidious onset and a chronic, unfavorable course. The undifferentiated type contains a mixture of symptoms from the other types except for catatonia. The rare catatonic type usually shows an acute onset, a remitting course, and an outcome involving only a low degree of disability. The paranoid type, the most frequent subtype, is characterized by delusions, hallucinations, and, in many cases, also pronounced thought disorder. The early illness course of the paranoid type varies considerably from acute to insidious onsets.

Longitudinal studies have shown a considerable overlap in the symptoms of the most common types (i.e., paranoid and undifferentiated, or hebephrenic, schizophrenia). Hence, these subtypes are suboptimal constructs. The most simple categorization of the symptoms of schizophrenia, for which the terms negative versus positive, or psychotic, are used, goes back to Émil Kraepelin. Attempts to distinguish these two symptom dimensions as discrete etiological disease entities (type I: psychotic, attributed to dopaminergic dysfunction, type II: negative, with cognitive impairment attributed to early neurodevelopmental disorder) are not sufficiently supported by empirical data.

Efforts to identify core symptom dimensions of schizophrenia have been more successful. Factor analyses of schizophrenia have consistently yielded at least four symptom dimensions: positive symptoms (i.e., reality distortion), negative symptoms (e.g., psychomotor poverty, anhedonia), disorganization (e.g., inappropriate affect, thought disorder, disturbed speech, bizarre behavior), and depression. These factors constitute the main symptom dimensions of schizophrenia over the course of illness.

WHEN DOES SCHIZOPHRENIA START?

The neurodevelopmental hypothesis has made the question of the onset of schizophrenia a topical issue. The risk factors, which comprise pre- and perinatal complications, viral encephalitis and bacterial meningoencephalitis in infancy, early developmental delays and premorbid deficits in cognitive and social functioning, and morphological changes in the brain that persist during the illness course, suggest that the disorder starts during embryonic life or soon afterwards.

Critical views of the "simple neurodevelopmental model" argue that these risk factors are not specific to schizophrenia and account only for a small proportion of cases. Furthermore, schizophrenia also develops in old age. The occurrence of psychosis and the preceding onset of and increase in nonpsychotic symptoms should be regarded as representing a new disorder characterized by different types of symptoms and associated impairments. Anomalies of brain development *in utero* and in childhood are better seen as risk factors, and the concomitant dysfunctions, as precursors of the disorder. The actual course of schizophrenia begins with the onset and accumulation of prepsychotic prodromal and subsequent psychotic symptoms.

ONSET, PRODROMAL STAGE, AND FIRST PSYCHOTIC EPISODE

Kraepelin (1896) first described minor changes in mood, which may be recurrent or persist for weeks, months or even for years as the only premonitory signs of an imminent mental disorder. Subsequent research has supported his observation. In about 75% of cases, schizophrenia onset occurs with slowly mounting depressive and negative symptoms that involve increasing functional impairment and cognitive dysfunction. Less than 10% of cases start with positive symptoms only. Reports on the duration of the prepsychotic prodromal stage vary widely. Because of differences in study designs and nonrepresentative populations, mean values range from a few months to 9 years. In a population-based sample of 232 first-episode cases of schizophrenia assessed by the Interview for the Retrospective Assessment of the Onset and Course of Schizophrenia (IRAOS), 18% of patients had an acute type of onset (1 month from onset to first admission), 15% had a subacute onset (1 month to 1 year), and the majority, 68%, had a chronic early illness course of more than 1 year before first admission. The mean duration of the prepsychotic prodromal stage was 4.8 years, with a median of 2.3 years, indicating that shorter durations predominated (Häfner, Löffler, Maurer, Hambrecht, & an der Heiden, 1999).

The *onset of psychotic symptoms,* which marks the beginning of a psychotic episode, is easier to assess. The duration of untreated psychosis (DUP)—in most studies about 1 year—and the duration of untreated illness(DUI)—from first symptom to first contact—depend on help-seeking behavior and the availability of appropriate treatment. In Norway a program for promoting public awareness, including information toward the general public, health services, and schools, managed to reduce DUP from 2.5 to 0.5 years (Johannessen et al., 2001).

The illness course preceding first contact can be studied in a state uninfluenced by antipsychotic or antidepressive medications. Table 11.1 shows the period prevalence and ranks of the 10 most frequent symptoms of schizophrenia spectrum disorder and severe unipolar depression from onset to first admission in samples individually matched by age and sex, and in "healthy" controls from the population of the study area. The two disease groups differ significantly from healthy controls at this early stage.

Table 11.1 also shows a high degree of similarity at the prepsychotic stage between the symptoms of schizophrenia and severe depression. This suggests that the first episode in these disorders is frequently preceded by a common prodromal syndrome comprising depressive and negative symptoms, and increasing functional impairment. Only a small fraction of depressive and negative syndromes go on to develop psychotic symptoms or a full-blown psychosis.

PSYCHOTIC AND DEPRESSIVE SYMPTOMS AS RISK FACTORS AND SYMPTOM DIMENSIONS OF PSYCHOSIS

Children and adults with single psychotic symptoms without psychotic illness are at an increased risk for developing psychosis. An increase in depressive symptoms or anxiety in early adulthood also increases the risk for developing psychosis in the following years, whereas a decrease in anxiety and depression reduces that risk. Only a small proportion of patients with a schizophrenia spectrum disorder (e.g., 17% in the Age Beginning Course study; Häfner et al., 1999) do not experience any depressive episodes before first contact. Most of these patients have negative symptoms, particularly affective blunting. More depressive symptoms at the prodromal stage predict more psychotic relapses. The mean prevalence of depressive symptoms in a psychotic episode ranges from 60 to 80%.

TABLE 11.1. Comparison of the Period Prevalences of the 10 Most Frequent Symptoms in the Early Course of Schizophrenia and Depression and Among Normal Controls

Symptom	Schizophrenia		Depression		Normal Controls		Sz vs. Dep	Sz vs. NC	Dep vs. NC
	%	Rank	%	Rank	%	Rank			
Worrying	74.6	9	94.6	4	26.9	6.5	***	***	***
Headaches, other aches and pains	49.2	—	66.9	—	30.8	4	**	**	***
Nervousness, restlessness	88.3	3	81.5	10.5	27.7	5	n.s.	***	***
Anxiety	88.1	4	81.5	10.5	26.9	6.5	n.s.	***	***
Difficulties of thinking, concentration	93.8	1.5	96.9	3	20.8	—	n.s.	***	***
Depressed mood	84.9	5	100.0	1	46.9	1	***	***	***
Loss of self-confidence	68.3	10.5	89.2	7	35.7	3	***	***	***
Social withdrawal, suspiciousness	79.8	8	90.8	6	13.8	—	*	***	***
Disturbed appetite and/or sleep	93.8	1.5	98.5	2	43.4	2	n.s.	***	***
Loss of energy/ slowness	82.5	6	93.8	5	15.4	—	**	***	***
Irritability	65.4	—	68.5	—	26.2	8	n.s.	***	***
Delusional mood	68.3	10.5	4.6	—	0.0	—	***	***	*
Delusional misinterpretations, delusions of reference	80.3	7	6.2	—	0.0	—	***	***	**
Oversensitivity	22.3	—	52.3	—	25.4	9	***	n.s.	***
Dissocial behavior	15.3	—	14.6	—	22.3	10	n.s.	n.s.	n.s.
Reduced spare-time activities	63.5	—	89.1	8	15.5	—	***	***	***
Reduced interests/ citizen role	33.9	—	87.7	9	3.8	—	***	***	***

The symptoms—17 in total—were assessed, retrospectively, at age of first admission; symptoms with rank 1 to 10 in any of the three groups. Sz, schizophrenia; Dep, depression; NC, normal controls. McNemar test: n.s., not significant. Data from Häfner et al. (2005).
* $p < .05$; ** $p < .01$; *** $p < .001$.

A heuristic explanation of this finding is that processes of brain dysfunction may first result in the neuropathological pattern of depression, accompanied by some negative symptoms and functional impairment. These dysfunctional brain processes may or may not progress into more negative symptoms and psychosis (Häfner et al., 2005).

DUI AND DUP AS INDICATORS OF AN UNFAVORABLE ILLNESS COURSE

DUP and DUI have been found to predict an unfavorable course of the first episode of schizophrenia, including delayed or incomplete remission, reduced level of global functioning, longer duration of hospitalization, and higher treatment costs. In addition, over the long-term DUP and DUI tend to be associated with a higher risk and a greater severity of relapses, more days in the hospital, poorer global functioning, poorer quality of life, and a greater burden on the family. There is some evidence that DUP and DUI predict the course of different dimensions of the illness. Prolonged DUP (maximum of psychotic symptoms) has been found to predict psychotic symptoms but not negative symptoms. In contrast, prolonged DUI (maximum of negative symptoms) has been found to predict more negative symptoms, social impairment, and downward social drift. The finding that duration of each symptom dimension significantly predicts the severity of that same symptom dimension is in line with the relative independence of the positive and negative symptoms in the long-term course of schizophrenia.

After it became clear that functional impairment and the bulk of the social consequences frequently emerge before first therapeutic contact, interest grew in delaying psychosis onset or ameliorating the illness by early recognition and early intervention. There is evidence that cognitive-behavioral therapy in combination with low doses of antipsychotic medication significantly reduce transition to psychosis within 1 year in compliant, high-risk patients compared to controls. But it is not yet clear whether transitions to psychosis are merely postponed, or whether the effect is permanent that also leads to a better course and social outcome of schizophrenia in the long term.

An explanation of the association between DUP and an unfavorable illness course as a result of a neurotoxic effect of psychosis has to consider the possibility that the effect might be confounded by preceding disease-inherent factors. A highly acute onset without more severe negative symptoms is generally associated with a good functional and social prognosis, whereas an insidious, lengthy onset, with a high frequency of negative symptoms and severe cognitive impairment, predicts a poor outcome.

DESCRIPTIVE ASSESSMENT AND CLASSIFICATION OF TYPES OR TRAJECTORIES OF ILLNESS COURSE

Many studies of the course of schizophrenia before 1990 were based on patients whose histories of illness duration already differed considerably at the time of inclusion in the studies. As a result, unfavorable courses were overrepresented in these samples. Not until recently have a growing number of large-scale follow-up studies starting in the first psychotic episode been published.

Because representative population samples of first-episode probands are difficult to recruit, most follow-up studies proceed from first admissions to a particular service or hospital. Depending on the clients served by the particular services, this approach may lead to distorted samples. For example, due to an overrepresentation of young black males in public mental hospitals, most of the older follow-up studies in the United States arrived at higher incidence rates for young men and a less favorable course compared to women. Recent studies show that only young males fall ill with schizophrenia more frequently and more severely than do premenopausal women. Postmenopausal women show higher incidence rates and frequently more severe illness courses than their male counterparts. One possible reason is that women at this age lose the protective effect of estrogen.

Kraepelin attempted to reduce the multitude of trajectories representing descriptive types of illness course. All constructs proposed so far are unsatisfactory, as demonstrated by the comparison of proportions of cases and different types of course from five long-term studies of schizophrenia (Figure 11.1). This lack of concordance with hypothesized trajectory types reflects the high degree of interindividual variability in the course of schizophrenia.

The only sensible and practical solution at present is to distinguish a few typical trajectories on the basis of a limited number of parameters, as done by Shepherd, Watt, Falloon, and Smeeton (1989) in their four types based on two parameters (number of episodes with psychotic symptoms and amount of functional impairment) measured over time.

DOMAINS OF COURSE AND OUTCOME

Following Strauss and Carpenter's (1972) examination of single, not fully intercorrelated components of the disease process instead of global outcome, more recent longitudinal studies usually focus on symptom dimensions (positive, negative, depressive, etc.), functional indicators (cognitive and other neuropsychological test results, social and work performance), structural changes visible in sMRI scans and neurophysiological parameters (electroencephalogram [EEG], evoked potential [EVP]), as well as illness behavior and quality of life. Further characteristics of the course of schizophrenia are environmentally rooted parameters, such as social network and support, and the economic and social dimensions of quality of life. Cognitive impairment and negative symptoms correlate with poor functional capacity and poor social adaptation. Positive symptoms usually do not have a significant impact on overall functioning, even if clinical and demographic characteristics are controlled. Contributing to this difference are the different temporal dimensions of these symptom dimensions (e.g., persistent cognitive impairment and nega-

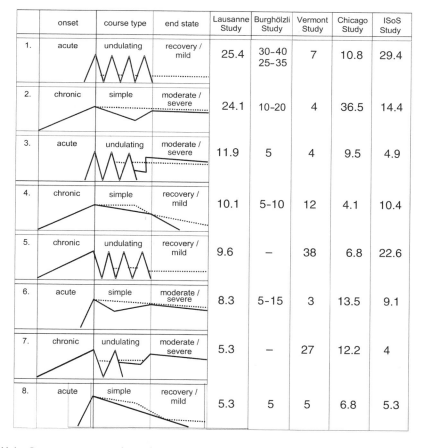

	onset	course type	end state	Lausanne Study	Burghölzli Study	Vermont Study	Chicago Study	ISoS Study
1.	acute	undulating	recovery / mild	25.4	30–40 25–35	7	10.8	29.4
2.	chronic	simple	moderate / severe	24.1	10–20	4	36.5	14.4
3.	acute	undulating	moderate / severe	11.9	5	4	9.5	4.9
4.	chronic	simple	recovery / mild	10.1	5–10	12	4.1	10.4
5.	chronic	undulating	recovery / mild	9.6	–	38	6.8	22.6
6.	acute	simple	moderate / severe	8.3	5–15	3	13.5	9.1
7.	chronic	undulating	moderate / severe	5.3	–	27	12.2	4
8.	acute	simple	recovery / mild	5.3	5	5	6.8	5.3

FIGURE 11.1. Course types in schizophrenia. Five studies are represented. The numbers indicate the percentage of patients, with the course type depicted on the left (e.g., 7% of the patients in the Vermont Study demonstrated an acute onset, an undulating course, and a recovered/mild end state (type I), in contrast to the ISoS study, where 29.4% of the patients belong to this course type. Data from Häfner and an der Heiden (2003).

tive symptoms vs. recurrent and disappearing psychotic episodes). Cognitive deficits are also more resistant than psychotic symptoms to environmental factors.

Social disability, characterized by deficits in social role performance, social functioning, and social handicap, is an interaction between disease-related factors, such as symptoms, and poor self-care. Thus, social disability is more dependent on environmental influences than on symptoms or impaired self-care. Social stigma unfavorably influences the social course of schizophrenia, especially the social and occupational reintegration of patients.

SHORT-TERM ILLNESS COURSE

Due to the remarkable decrease in long-term inpatient treatment over the past several decades, the frequency of readmissions and the number of hospital days per year are no longer reliable indicators of illness course. According to sound first-episode studies of ICD-9 or -10, or the fourth edition of the *Diagnostic and Statistical Manual of Mental Disorders* (DSM-IV; American Psychiatric Association, 1996) schizophrenia spectrum disorder, the proportion of patients who stay symptom-free in the following 5 years ranges from about 20% to over 30%.

Depressive symptoms are prevalent in the early course of schizophrenia. In the International Pilot Study of Schizophrenia (IPSS; Harrison et al., 2001), 17% of patients with schizophrenia also had a diagnosed episode of depression at 2-year follow-up, and 15% at 5-year follow-up. Depressive mood is the most frequent symptom at any stage in the course of schizophrenia and is present in about 80% of patients at first psychotic episode. With a modal rate of 35% over the entire illness course, depression constitutes a fairly stable dimension of schizophrenia (an der Heiden, Könnecke, Maurer, Ropeter, & Häfner, 2005).

Factors predicting an unfavorable short-term functional outcome (at 1–2 years) are poor premorbid functioning; more severe negative symptoms, which is the most stable determinant of poor social functioning; cognitive impairment; prolonged DUI and DUP; and male gender until about midlife (45 years). At postmenopausal age and thereafter, the sex ratio is reversed, with the female sex indicating poorer prognoses.

PRECIPITATION OF PSYCHOTIC RELAPSES

Irregularly recurring psychotic episodes may be triggered by stressful life events and by a high degree of tension in interpersonal relationships (expressed emotion [EE] paradigm). High EE in family members, including critical comments, hostility, and emotional overinvolvement (e.g., extreme self-sacrificing behavior, overprotectiveness) is associated with relapses in other mental disorders as well, and even in chronic somatic illness.

Apart from the precipitating factors, the main predictors of short- and medium-term risk for psychotic relapses, independent of therapy variables, are the number of previous psychotic episodes, severity of depressive symptoms, DUP and substance abuse (cannabis in particular), but not negative symptoms or cognitive impairment.

LONG-TERM ILLNESS COURSE

All studies of the long-term course of schizophrenia, whether retrospective or prospective, rely on data collected retrospectively. Follow-up studies that include a great number of cross-sectional assessments done at short intervals and/or that supplement the information given by the patients with interviews of key persons and study of case records, teachers' reports, and so forth, reduce the risk of error in retrospective assessments, but such studies are rare. Two examples are the Mannheim–World Health Organization (WHO) first-episode study, with 10 assessments conducted over 15.5 years (an der Heiden et al., 1995), and the Marengo, Harrow, Herbener, and Sands (2000) study, with five assessments conducted over 10 years. The few prospective first-episode follow-up studies covering at least 10 years and published between 1976 and 2000 included an average of three assessments (Häfner & an der Heiden, 2003).

Because medical interventions may modify the illness course, data on the type, dose, and time of intake of psychotropic medications would be of great interest. But all these parameters vary a great deal over the long-term course and are difficult to control. For this reason, very little is known about how pharmacotherapy influences risk of relapse and other domains of the long-term course of illness.

By the early 1990s, most of the studies recruited their samples retrospectively from among the patients of a single hospital and did only one follow-up to examine illness courses covering 20 years and more. This first generation of studies, all based on very broad diagnostic definitions (Bleuler's criteria, ICD-8 or -9, DSM-III), came to the conclusion that globally, on average, schizophrenia is not a progressive illness. This conclusion is to some extent supported by more sophisticated, modern follow-up studies. Specifically, the 12-, 15-, and 25-year follow-ups of the transnational samples of the WHO schizophrenia studies (IPSS sample: World Health Organization, 1973; International Study of Schizophrenia [ISoS]: Harrison et al., 2001) and 10- to 15-year follow-ups of samples from the WHO Determinants of Outcome of Severe Mental Disorders (DOSMD) study (Jablensky et al., 1992) fairly consistently show a high degree of heterogeneity in the course and outcome of schizophrenia, with no or only mild deterioration on average in the first years following first admission. Marked deterioration occurs only in a small proportion of cases in the long term.

Full remissions without subsequent relapses persist in about 20% of cases in the long-term. According to the WHO studies, the course of schizophrenia is more favorable in many, but not all, developing countries, in part because the samples included comparatively larger proportions of cases with acute transient psychoses even at later follow-ups.

Recovery or major sustained improvement occurs mostly in the first years following illness onset. Patients who do not improve in the first years, or who deteriorate slightly or markedly, tend to continue this trend in the long term, too. First-episode studies have failed to confirm consistently a period of stability after the first episode and a period of improvement in the long term.

Concerning the single domains of the course of schizophrenia, the highest degree of stability is shown by negative symptoms and cognitive impairment, and, consequently, by global and social functioning. Patients with pronounced cognitive impairment in the long-term course of schizophrenia show a considerable neuropsychological deficits already at first admission. These deficits usually develop premorbidly or at the prodromal stage.

Four studies examined the medium- or long-term course on the basis of Liddle's (1987) three-factor model of the symptoms of schizophrenia. One covered 2 years (Arndt et al., 1995), two covered 5 years (Salokangas, 1997; cf. Häfner & an der Heiden, 2003), and one covered 10 years (Marengo et al., 2000). In agreement with the long-term follow-up studies of global symptom measures, none showed a clear-cut trend for improvement or deterioration. As expected, the course of the negative factor was fairly independent of the two other factors and in all studies showed a high degree of stability over the illness course (Figure 11.2). The positive factor showed a lower degree of stability and was partly correlated with the disorganization factor.

Marengo and colleagues (2000) included the depression factor in addition to the three other factors and did follow-ups at 2.0, 4.5, 7.5, and 10.0 years after first admission. In agreement with more recent studies, the authors concluded that "depression constituted an independent and stable dimension of schizophrenia" (p. 61) over the entire course of the illness. These findings underscore the heterogeneity of the symptom dimensions subsumed under the disease concept of schizophrenia.

Because there is clear overlap between the clinically defined depressive and the negative syndrome, an der Heiden and colleagues (2005) studied a depressive core syndrome (depressive mood, lack of self-confidence, feelings of guilt, suicidal ideation) and a manic core syndrome (elated mood, reduced need for sleep, pressure of speech, hyperactivity, flight of ideas) over an illness course of 11.3 years in a sample of 107 patients with schizophrenia. They found a modal rate of 35% for the depressive core syndrome and of 6–7% for the manic syndrome, and a high degree of stability for both syndromes over the long-term. Figure 11.3, based on IRAOS data for 134 months, validated at seven cross sections with the Present State Examination (PSE) interview, illustrates the remarkable stability of—and the lack of a trend in—the prevalence rates for depression and the manic core syndrome. Months spent with depressive symptoms are the most frequent (47.1), compared to months of psychotic symptoms (13.7). Purely depressive relapse episodes occur at a frequency of about 1 to 5 compared with psychotic relapses. This means that depressive symptoms increase with the emerging disorder and occur as an integral part of psychotic episodes at all stages of the course of schizophrenia. So far depression has not been given the attention it deserves in the treatment of schizophrenia, despite its great importance for patients' subjective quality of life, coping, and increased risk for suicide.

The frequency of psychotic relapses is difficult estimate, because their number varies depending on the patients' living environments and can be triggered by stressful life events and stressful home environments, and because precise information on antipsychotic treatment is not available. In the population-based ABC Schizophrenia Study (an der Heiden et al., 2005) covering an 11.3-year illness course under treatment, the fre-

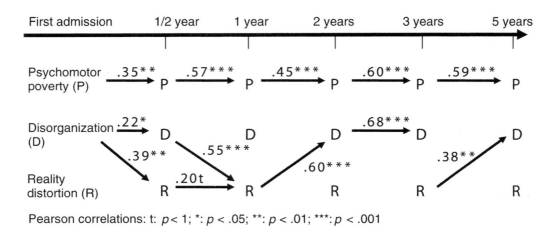

Pearson correlations: t: $p < 1$; *: $p < .05$; **: $p < .01$; ***: $p < .001$

FIGURE 11.2. Correlation within and between syndrome ratings at six points in time over 5 years. The factors were tested by explorative orthogonal factor analysis at each of the five follow-ups; ABC subsample of 115 first-illness episodes. Data from Löffler and Häfner (1999).

quency of relapses varied from zero to several per year, with an average of three and a maximum of 22 in 11.3 years.

SOCIAL COURSE

Schizophrenia is on average not a progressive illness characterized by deterioration and social decline after the first illness episode. Many patients already have considerable impairment and social disadvantage at the prodromal stage. Because of impaired social development in early-onset illness or social decline from a relatively high status in late-onset illness, this disadvantage often makes schizophrenia a permanently disabling disorder.

In the ABC Schizophrenia Study (an der Heiden et al., 2005) 31% of the first-episode sample had full-time jobs at first admission, and 32% at 11.3-year follow-up, compared with 70% for individually matched controls. Similar differences were found in the mean rates for patients living independently and for those divorced. Considerably more female than male patients had remarried. These results further corroborate the stable trend in the main domains of illness course in schizophrenia despite some changes that occur both for the better and for the worse (high divorce and remarriage rates, job loss, and reemployment).

The quality of life of patients with a long, chronic course of illness, when measured by objective criteria, is significantly reduced in several domains. But after a history of illness of several years, their subjective life satisfaction often does not differ significantly from that of healthy controls, because most patients manage to cope emotionally with the disorder and reduce their expectations. Factors detrimental to the subjective quality of

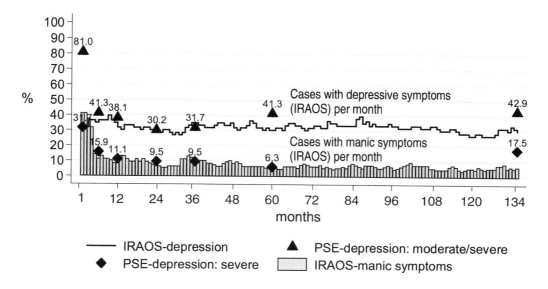

FIGURE 11.3. The prevalence of purely depressive and manic symptoms (no overlap with negative or positive symptoms) in the long-term course of schizophrenia. Depressive and manic symptoms ($n = 107$) were assessed retrospectively per month over 136 months with the IRAOS. Depressive symptoms were validated prospectively with the Present State Examination (PSE) at seven cross sections over that same period ($n = 13$).

life in the long term are male gender, the amount of anxiety and depression, insufficient social support, and social stigma.

PROGNOSTIC INDICATORS OF THE LONG-TERM COURSE

As stated earlier, prognostic indicators are not identical with etiological risk or protective factors whose existence or amount contributes to the risk of developing the disorder. Examples of such risk factors are a family history of schizophrenia or viral encephalitis infection in early childhood. Prognostic indicators are phenomena associated with the illness course that predict the further course of illness (e.g., cognitive impairment, negative symptoms). The most important predictors across both categories are family load of schizophrenia in first-degree relatives; several susceptibility genes (or loci; e.g., G30/72 on chromosome 13q); disturbed development of the brain *in utero* and peripartum (obstetric complications, hypoxia in particular), encephalitis or bacterial meningitis infection in early childhood; pronounced structural changes in the brain prior to illness onset; male sex, with onset before age 45 years; female sex, with onset after ages 45–50 years; and cannabis misuse before onset of the illness.

With regard to their relevance to a patient's life, the main domains are symptomatology (negative, positive, depressive), amount of cognitive, functional, and social impairment and disability, frequency of relapses, and quality of life. The best predictor of the social course is premorbid work and social performance. Because first contact in 75% of cases is preceded by a prodromal period of more than 1 year, during which the bulk of social consequences emerge, social performance prior to first contact is not clearly premorbid. The use of social functioning as a prognostic indicator of the future illness course requires prediction based on the past course of fairly stable factors, such as cognitive impairment. For this reason, psychological tests (e.g., cognitive testing, persistence, motivation, and stress tolerance), social functioning, and social and marital status measured at the end of the early illness course, which mostly coincides with first admission, are good prognostic indicators of the social course and outcome of schizophrenia.

A predictor directly associated with the disorder is an early age of onset, especially the rare onset in childhood and youth. It is usually associated with a high genetic load and particularly severe morphological changes on the one hand, and developmental delays and cognitive deficits on the other. Onset of illness later in life usually involves full-blown psychotic symptoms comprising fully elaborated delusions and hallucinations that are rarely accompanied by mental disorganization. In late-onset cases, particularly in men, clarity of the thought process is usually not affected. In addition, in old and very old adults, social status is fairly stable (retirement pension; a network of long-lasting, stable relationships; etc.) and more or less immune to the adverse effects of the disorder. For this reason schizophrenia in older adults is associated with a lower risk for social decline.

As mentioned earlier, male gender is an unfavorable predictor of early-onset illness, but a favorable predictor of illness developed later in life. In contrast, female gender is a favorable predictor of premenopausal illness, but an unfavorable predictor of peri- and postmenopausal illness. Not only a prolonged DUP, but also a prolonged DUI, as stated, does predict a more severe, extended first episode and an unfavorable illness course.

Severe negative symptoms and considerable cognitive impairment are predictors of the dimension "negative symptoms, cognitive and functional impairment" and, hence, of an unfavorable functional and social course. A high frequency of psychotic episodes and, to a smaller degree, depressive symptoms predict a greater frequency of psychotic relapses. All types of comorbidity with severe misuse of or dependence on psychoactive substances predict a poor social course, poor cognitive functioning, and more severe psychotic symptoms.

RISK OF SUICIDE IN THE COURSE OF SCHIZOPHRENIA

Patients with schizophrenia compared with the general population show elevated rates of unnatural causes of death, of which suicide is the most frequent. In recent studies the portion of suicides in total deaths (proportional mortality) of people with schizophrenia is estimated at about 30%. Exact estimates are hampered by transnational variability of the rates and by the fact that suicides are frequently masked (e.g., as car accidents). Although several reviews have reported that about 10% of people with schizophrenia commit suicide, single studies show a high degree of variance in the rates.

In a sophisticated meta-analysis of 29 studies published between 1966 and 2000, and based on a total of 22,600 patients with schizophrenia, Palmer, Pankratz, and Bostwick (2005) calculated a weighted lifetime incidence of 4.9% (95% confidence interval [CI]: 4.3–5.6%). Schizophrenia itself does not seem to be the only risk factor for suicide over the course of the disorder. Heilä and colleagues (1999) analyzed by means of psychological autopsy all suicides committed in a year in Finland. In 46% of people with schizophrenia, stressful life events had occurred in the 3 months preceding the suicide. Most of these events were beyond the influence of the persons in question, such as death or severe illness of a family member.

Risk for suicide in people with schizophrenia markedly decreases with age as opposed to that for most general populations, which increase with age. Severe depressive symptoms and comorbid alcohol and drug abuse are main risk factors both in people with schizophrenia and in the general population, whereas severe negative symptoms tend to be a protective factor, reducing the risk.

Apart from these mostly observable risk factors is consideration of individual psychological risk factors and coping abilities, which can only be assessed in a personal interview. For example, suicidal ideation has been found to be a better predictor of future suicidal behavior than depressed mood (Young et al., 1998).

In a small number of studies suicide rates are increased, particularly in the first years following illness onset. The somewhat lower rates reported by those studies for subsequent periods are probably accounted for by selective suicide mortality, resulting in a decline of high-risk cases. But the risk remains increased throughout the lifetime. According to a majority of studies, unlike in the general population, the risk does not differ essentially between males and females with schizophrenia.

KEY POINTS

- The main domains of schizophrenia spectrum disorders—symptom dimensions, frequency of relapses, cognitive impairment, and social disability—on average show a stable course, without a trend for either the better or the worse.
- The course of schizophrenia shows a high degree of interindividual variability, with about 20% of individuals with a first psychotic episode staying free of symptoms for 10 years.
- The traditional subtypes of schizophrenia are not stable over time (e.g., paranoid, undifferentiated).

- The disease construct of schizophrenia comprises several relatively independent symptom dimensions, with negative symptoms and cognitive impairment remaining relatively stable over the illness course, and psychotic symptoms occurring in most patients on an episodic basis.
- The onset of schizophrenia usually occurs with depressive and negative symptoms, and functional impairment during a prepsychotic prodromal phase that on average lasts for several years, followed by a *psychotic prephase,* defined as the period between the first positive symptom and the maximum of positive symptoms, lasting on average for 1 year.
- The power of prognostic indicators of illness course is limited to the domains to which they belong: symptom dimensions, psychotic relapses, social functioning, and so forth.
- A very early age of onset (under age 15), male gender and onset before middle age, female gender and onset after menopause, poor premorbid adjustment, an insidious onset, and a prolonged psychotic prephase with pronounced negative symptoms and cognitive impairment at first treatment contact are reliable predictors of a poor long-term social course of schizophrenia.
- Comorbidity of alcohol and cannabis abuse predicts more severe positive symptoms, more relapses, and a poor social course, whereas a short prodromal stage characterized by few or no negative symptoms, minor functional impairment, and an acute onset of psychosis predicts a favorable social course.
- Depressed mood is the most frequent symptom in schizophrenia throughout the entire illness course, including psychotic relapses.
- Risk of suicide is slightly elevated in schizophrenia (5–10% over the illness course), which is increased by depressive symptoms and decreased by severe negative symptoms, particularly affective flattening.

REFERENCES AND RECOMMENDED READINGS

American Psychiatric Association (1996). *Diagnostic and statistical manual of mental disorders* (4th ed.). Washington, DC: Author.

an der Heiden, W., Könnecke, R., Maurer, K., Ropeter, D., & Häfner, H. (2005). Depression in the long-term course of schizophrenia. *European Archives of Psychiatry and Clinical Neuroscience, 255,* 174–184.

an der Heiden, W., Krumm, B., Müller, S., Weber, I., Biehl, H., & Schäfer, M. (1995). Mannheimer Langzeitstudie der Schizophrenie (Mannheimer Long-Term Schizophrenia Project). *Nervenarzt, 66,* 820–827.

Arndt, S., Tyrrell, G., Flaum, M., & Andreasen, N. C. (1992). Comorbidity of substance abuse and schizophrenia: The role of pre-morbid adjustment. *Psychological Medicine, 22,* 379–388.

Bleuler, M. (1972). *Die schizophrenen Geistesstörungen im Lichte langjähriger Kranken- und Familiengeschichten* [The schizophrenic disorders in the light of long-term case and family histories]. Stuttgart, Germany: Thieme.

Bromet, E. J., Naz, B., Fochtmann, L. J., Carlson, G. A., & Tanenberg-Karant, M. (2005). Long-term diagnostic stability and outcome in recent first-episode cohort studies of schizophrenia. *Schizophrenia Bulletin, 31,* 639–649.

Ciompi, L., & Müller, C. (1976). *Lebensweg und Alter der Schizophrenen* [Life course and age of schizophrenic patients]. Berlin: Springer.

Häfner, H., & an der Heiden, W. (2003). Course and outcome of schizophrenia. In S. R. Hirsch & D. R. Weinberger (Eds.), *Schizophrenia* (2nd ed., pp. 101–141). Oxford, UK: Blackwell.

Häfner, H., Löffler, W., Maurer, K., Hambrecht, M., & an der Heiden, W. (1999). Depression, negative symptoms, social stagnation and social decline in the early course of schizophrenia. *Acta Psychiatrica Scandinavica, 100,* 105–118.

Häfner, H., Maurer, K., Trendler, G., an der Heiden, W., Schmidt, M., & Könnecke, R. (2005). Schizophrenia and depression. *Schizophrenia Reseach, 77,* 11–24.

Harding, C. M., Brooks, G. W., Ashikaga, T., Strauss, J. S., & Breier, A. (1987). The Vermont longitudinal study of persons with severe mental illness. II. Long-term outcome of subjects who retrospectively met DSM-III criteria for schizophrenia. *American Journal of Psychiatry, 144,* 727–735.

Harris, M. G., Henry, L. P., Harrigan, S. M., Purcell, R., Schwartz, O. S., Farrelly, S. E., et al. (2005). The relationship between duration of untreated psychosis and outcome: An eight-year prospective study. *Schizophrenia Research, 79,* 85–93.

Harrison, G., Hopper, K., Craig, T., Laska, E., Siegel, C., Wanderling, J., et al. (2001). Recovery from psychotic illness: A 15 and 25 year international follow-up study. *British Journal of Psychiatry, 178,* 506–517.

Hegarty, J. D., Baldessarini, R. J., Tohen, M., Waternaux, C., & Oepen, G. (1994). One hundred years of schizophrenia: A meta-analysis of the outcome literature. *American Journal of Psychiatry, 151,* 1409–1416.

Heilä, H., Heikkinen, M. E., Isometsä, E. T., Henriksson, M. M., Marttunen, M. J., & Lönnqvist, J. K. (1999). Life events and completed suicide in schizophrenia: A comparison of suicide victims with and without schizophrenia. *Schizophrenia Bulletin, 25,* 519–531.

Jablensky, A., Sartorius, N., Ernberg, G., Anker, M., Korten, A., & Cooper, J. E. (1992). Schizophrenia: Manifestations, incidence, and course in different cultures: A World Health Organization ten-country study. *Psychological Medicine, Monograph Supplement, 20,* 1–97.

Johannessen, J. O., McGlashan, T. H., Larsen, T. K., Horneland, M., Joa, I., Mardal, S., et. al. (2001). Early detection strategies for untreated first-episode psychosis. *Schizophrenia Research, 51,* 39–46.

Kraepelin, E. (1896). *Psychiatry. Ein Lehrbuch fuer Studierende und Aerzte* [Psychiatry: A textbook for students and physicians]. Leipzig, Germany: Barth.

Löffler, W., & Häfner, H. (1999). Dimensionen der schizophrenen Symptomatik [Dimensions of schizophrenic symptomatology]. *Nervenarzt, 70,* 416–429.

Liddle, P. F. (1987). The symptoms of chronic schizophrenia: A re-examination of the positive–negative dichotomy. *British Journal of Psychiatry, 151,* 145–151.

Marengo, J., Harrow, M., Herbener, E. S., & Sands, J. (2000). A prospective longitudinal 10-year study of schizophrenia's three major factors and depression. *Psychiatry Research, 97,* 61–77.

Marengo, J. T., Harrow, M., Sands, J., & Galloway, C. (1991). European versus U.S. data on the course of schizophrenia. *American Journal of Psychiatry, 148,* 606–611.

Marshall, M., Lewis, S., Lockwood, A., Drake, R., Jones, P., & Croudace, T. (2005). Association between duration of untreated psychosis and outcome in cohorts of first-episode patients. *Archives of General Psychiatry, 62,* 975–983.

Norman, R. M., & Malla, A. K. (2001). Duration of untreated psychosis: A critical examination of the concept and its importance. *Psychological Medicine, 31,* 381–400.

Olesen, A. V., & Mortensen, P. B. (2002). Readmission risk in schizophrenia: Selection explains previous findings of a progressive course of disorder. *Psychological Medicine, 32,* 1301–1307.

Opjordsmoen, S. (1991). Long-term clinical outcome of schizophrenia with special reference to gender differences. *Acta Psychiatrica Scandinavica, 83,* 307–313.

Palmer, B. A., Pankratz, V. S., & Bostwick, J. M. (2005). The lifetime risk of suicide in schizophrenia: A reexamination. *Archives of General Psychiatry, 62,* 247–253.

Salokangas, R. K. R. (1997). Structure of schizophrenic symptomatology and its changes over time: Prospective factor-analytical study. *Acta Psychiatrica Scandinavica, 95,* 32–39.

Shepherd, M., Watt, D., Falloon, I. R. H., & Smeeton, N. (1989). The natural history of schizophrenia: A five-year follow-up study of outcome and prediction in a representative sample of schizophrenics. *Psychological Medicine, Monograph Supplement, 15,* 1–46.

Strauss, J. S., & Carpenter, W. T. J. (1972). The prediction of outcome in schizophrenia: I. Characteristics of outcome. *Archives of General Psychiatry, 27,* 739–746.

Wiersma, D., Wanderling, J., Dragomirecka, E., Ganev, K., Harrison, G., an der Heiden, et al. (2000). Social disability in schizophrenia: Its development and prediction over 15 years in incidence cohorts in six European centres. *Psychological Medicine, 30,* 1155–1167.

World Health Organization. (1973). *The International Pilot Study of Schizophrenia* (Vol. 1). Geneva: Author.

Young, A. S., Nuechterlein, K. H., Mintz, J., Ventura, J., Gitlin, M., & Liberman, R. P. (1998). Suicidal ideation and suicide attempts in recent-onset schizophrenia. *Schizophrenia Bulletin, 24,* 629–634.

PART II

ASSESSMENT AND DIAGNOSIS

CHAPTER 12

DIAGNOSTIC INTERVIEWING

ABRAHAM RUDNICK
DAVID ROE

Schizophrenia, which is considered the most severe psychiatric disorder, is characterized by many impairments, such as psychosis and apathy, cognitive deficits and comorbid symptoms, as well as disrupted functioning and behavioral problems. Diagnostic interviewing is the "gold standard" for establishing a psychiatric diagnosis. In this chapter, we review diagnostic interviewing strategies for what are currently considered to be the characteristic symptoms of schizophrenia, recognizing that diagnostic criteria may change (as they have in the past).

Current classifications—hence, diagnostic criteria—of schizophrenia are based primarily on the work of Kraepelin, who focused on the deteriorating course of the illness (which he termed *dementia praecox*), and Bleuler, who emphasized the core symptoms of the disorder as difficulties in thinking consistently and concisely (loose associations); restriction in range of emotional expression, and emotional expression that is incongruent with the content of speech or thought (flat and inappropriate affect, respectively); loss of goal-directed behavior (ambivalence); and retreat into an inner world (autism). The two current major classification systems in psychiatry, the *Diagnostic and Statistical Manual of Mental Disorders* (DSM; American Psychiatric Association, 2000) and the *International Classification of Diseases* (ICD; World Health Organization, 1992) both specify that the diagnosis of schizophrenia is based on the presence of characteristic symptoms, the absence of others, and psychosocial difficulties that persist over a significant period of time. Symptoms must be present in the absence of general medical or so-called "organic" conditions (e.g., substance abuse, neurological disorders such as Huntington's disease, and more) that could lead to a similar clinical presentation.

The characteristic symptoms of schizophrenia are divided into positive and negative symptoms, although cognitive impairments and perhaps some comorbid symptoms may be core deficits of schizophrenia as well (American Psychiatric Association, 2000).

Positive symptoms refer to the *presence* of perceptual experiences, thoughts, and behaviors that are ordinarily absent in individuals without a psychiatric illness. The typical positive symptoms are hallucinations (primarily hearing, but also tactile feelings, seeing, tasting, or smelling in the absence of environmental stimuli), delusions (false or patently absurd beliefs that are not shared by others in the person's environment), and disorganization of thought and behavior (disconnected thoughts and strange or apparently purposeless behavior). Some positive symptoms are considered highly specific, such as first-rank symptoms (e.g., delusions of thought insertion and auditory hallucinations with a running commentary), and perhaps even pathognomonic (i.e., inappropriate affect). For many people with schizophrenia, positive symptoms fluctuate in their intensity over time and are episodic in nature, with approximately 20–40% experiencing persistent positive symptoms (Curson, Patel, Liddle, & Barnes, 1988). Of note is that the term *psychosis* usually addresses delusions and hallucinations (Rudnick, 1997).

Negative symptoms are the opposite of positive symptoms, in that they are defined by the *absence* of behaviors, cognitions, and emotions ordinarily present in persons without psychiatric disorders. Common examples of negative symptoms include flat affect, avolition (lack of motivation to perform tasks), and alogia (diminished amount or content of speech). All of these negative symptoms are relatively common in schizophrenia, and they tend to be stable over time. Furthermore, negative symptoms have a particularly disruptive impact on the ability of people with schizophrenia to engage and to function socially, and to sustain independent living.

The diagnosis of schizophrenia, according to DSM-IV-TR (American Psychiatric Association, 2000), which is the most current diagnostic system in psychiatry, requires the following criteria: (a) two or more characteristic symptoms, each present for a significant portion of time during a 1-month period (or less if successfully treated); (b) social/occupational dysfunction; (c) persistence of the disturbance for at least 6 months, of which at least 1 month must fully meet criterion a (active-phase symptoms). The other criteria exclude other psychiatric disorders, particularly schizoaffective disorder, mood disorders, substance use disorders, general medical condition, and pervasive developmental disorders (unless delusions and hallucinations exist, in which case schizophrenia can be diagnosed in conjunction with pervasive developmental disorders). There are various subtypes of schizophrenia (i.e., paranoid, disorganized, catatonic, undifferentiated, and residual [American Psychiatric Association, 2000]), but their validity is not well established, and a patient can present with more than one of them over time.

INTERVIEWING STRATEGIES

The current most widely accepted approach for diagnostic interviewing in psychiatric assessment is the use of structured interviews. The main advantage of structured interviews is that they provide a standardized approach for gathering information, which increases the (interrater) reliability of the assessment. Another advantage is that they provide guidelines for determining whether a specific symptom exists or not. On the downside, to benefit fully from the advantages of structured interviews, a fair amount of training, as well as ongoing fidelity evaluation, is required. A comprehensive assessment interview should commence with evaluation of basic characteristics of the disorder, followed by frequently associated features and common comorbid diagnoses. In the following section we focus on interviewing strategies for assessing characteristic symptoms of schizophrenia, recognizing that various assessment instruments can support a given interviewing strategy.

A wide range of assessment instruments, divided primarily into self-report and interview-based instruments, have been developed to evaluate the existence and severity of psychiatric symptoms. The Structured Clinical Interview for DSM-IV (SCID; First, Spitzer, Gibbon, & Williams, 1995) is the most widely used diagnostic assessment instrument in the United States for research studies with persons who have psychiatric disabilities. Psychiatric rating scales based on semistructured interviews have also been developed to provide a useful, reliable measure of the wide range of psychiatric symptoms commonly present in people with psychiatric disorders. These scales typically contain from 1–50 or so specifically defined items, each rated on a 5- to 7-point severity scale. Some interview-based scales have been developed to measure the full range of psychiatric symptoms, such as the Brief Psychiatric Rating Scale (BPRS; Overall & Gorham, 1962) and the Positive and Negative Syndrome Scale (PANSS; Kay, Opler, & Fiszbein, 1987), whereas other interview-based scales have been designed to tap specific dimensions, such as the Scale for the Assessment of Negative Symptoms (SANS; Andreasen, 1982). The same classification holds true for self-report scales.

Interview-based psychiatric rating scales typically assess a combination of symptoms elicited through direct questioning and symptoms or signs observed in the course of the interview, as well as symptoms elicited by collateral history taking (from caregivers and clinical documentation). For example, in the BPRS, depression is rated by asking questions such as "What has your mood been lately?" and "Have you been feeling down?". Ratings of mannerisms and posturing, on the other hand, are based on the behavioral observations of the interviewer. Psychiatric symptom scores can either be added up for an overall index of symptom severity, or summarized in subscale scores corresponding to symptom dimensions, such as negative, positive, and comorbid (affective and other) symptoms.

INTERVIEWING GUIDELINES

Psychiatric diagnosis involves use of generic clinical assessment skills, such as combining open-ended and close-ended questions, as well as specialized skills needed to address challenges associated with psychiatric impairments. In this section we discuss guidelines for interviewing people with schizophrenia, focusing on particular challenges to interviewing, and highlighting clinical communication skills in particular.

Guideline 1: Preinterview "Baggage"

Some challenges to interviewing may begin even before the interviewee has actually attended the interview or met the interviewers. These may be related to the interviewees' feelings, expectations, and concerns generated perhaps by past experience. For instance, even before coming to the interview, the interviewee may feel threatened, expect to be harshly judged and criticized, and be concerned about the possible consequences of the interview. Such preinterview feelings may manifest themselves in a range of different ways. For example, an interviewee who is feeling threatened may be very guarded or may be aggressive as a response to his or her perceived threat. Similarly, an interviewee who expects to be harshly judged may be hesitant and reluctant to interact or even hostile and antagonistic toward the interviewer. Finally, an interviewee who is concerned with the consequences of the interview might be busy trying to guess how he or she might "best" respond to questions asked by the interviewer, which would seriously threaten the validity of the information elicited.

Because the effectiveness and quality of all interviews depend on rapport, a starting point for the interviewer meeting an interviewee with features described earlier would be to develop empathy and understanding of the potential origins of the interviewee's "baggage." This may include recognizing that the interviewee may have been in several clinical settings and situations in the past that he or she perceived as threatening (e.g., being interviewed at a teaching hospital in front of trainees who were all strangers), that he or she was indeed judged harshly (e.g., for discontinuing medication against medical advice or using substances), or suffered from perceived consequences of previous interviews (e.g., forced interventions or involuntarily hospitalization). In addition, the interviewer may use his or her clinical skills to help the interviewee feel more comfortable and at ease by expressing concern and empathy, and reacting to the interviewee and his or her story in a nonjudgmental manner. It is often useful in such cases not to ignore the "elephant in the room" but rather to focus first on the interviewee's immediate feelings and address the discomfort that he or she might be feeling ("I have a sense that you are not feeling very comfortable. I was wondering if you might be willing to share how you are feeling right now"). In addition to addressing the interpersonal context, there are several practical ways in which the interviewer might be able to help the interviewee feel more at ease. Examples include introducing him- or herself, describing what to expect in terms of the format of the interview (its nature, rationale, and length) and what will follow. The interviewer should offer the interviewee the option to ask questions and to have his or her concerns addressed before proceeding. Forming a collaborative atmosphere in which the interviewee is viewed as an active participant rather than a passive subject of an interview is important. In addition, respecting the interviewee's style and pacing oneself to better match his or her tempo gradually increase the interviewee's trust and participation. Finally, when the interviewee is uncomfortable, it is particularly useful to start the actual interview with a "warm-up" phase that includes easy-to-answer, factual questions to help the interviewee gradually become more at ease. As the interviewee feels more comfortable, follow-up questions can be particularly helpful in gathering more information about particular areas of significance.

Guideline 2: Lack of Insight into Illness

Because the interview usually takes place in a clinical setting (outpatient clinic or hospital), a typical early question is "What brought you here?" or "How did you come to be in the hospital?". These questions are meant to provide a neutral stimulus to encourage the interviewee to reveal the sequence of events that preceded the current situation. One potential challenge is that the interviewee may lack insight into his or her behaviors, experiences or beliefs that impacted the events preceding the interview. The interviewee may deny having a problem ("I do not know. Everything was just fine") or believe that what led to being treated is not his or her problem ("They [family] wanted me taken away, because they needed the room in the house"), or that he or she has a problem but not a mental problem ("I was feeling weak, but they wanted me to go to the psychiatrist"). These various degrees and styles reflecting a lack of insight are common among people with schizophrenia and present a potential obstacle for the interviewer seeking to obtain an overview of the current episode and psychiatric history.

Although it may be frustrating for the interviewer, it is not useful to be confrontational or to repeat the question with the hope that the interviewee will eventually "gain insight." It is important instead to acknowledge the potential value in the information collected rather than to get angry or anxious about failing to elicit the "required" information. There are a number of reasons why information collected "even" with an interviewee who seems to have limited insight into his or her condition may be of value: First, discrepancies between the perceptions of interviewees and mental health providers may not always indicate lack of insight (Roe, Leriya, & Fennig, 2001). Second, even if the interviewee clearly lacks insight, it is clinically useful to explore and to understand how he or she perceives and experiences different events (Roe & Kravetz, 2003). In addition, lack of insight may in some cases serve as a defense against the threat to self posed by the illness, and its social and personal meaning (Roe & Davidson, 2005). Thus, acknowledging the clinical value of the interviewee's report, even if it is not concurrent with one's own, may help the interviewer to convey genuine respect for the interviewee's views rather than to become impatient, angry, or confrontational regarding the interviewee's "lack of insight."

Guideline 3: Challenges of the Extremes: The Guarded and the Suggestible Interviewee

The validity of the information collected may be seriously compromised in the extreme case of a particularly guarded or suggestible interviewee. At one extreme, the guarded interviewee may not reveal much information, particularly in relation to symptoms. Because clinical assessment in psychiatry is dependent to a great degree on self-report, interviews with guarded interviewees may create the false impression that they experience fewer symptoms than they actually do. At the other extreme are the suggestible interviewees, who are easily influenced by the interviewer's questions and "convinced" that they have experienced symptoms they may never have had, and may therefore be assessed as more symptomatic than they are in actuality. Regardless of which extreme a person represents, the information collected through the interview may not reflect his or her condition in a valid manner.

There are a number of possible solutions to these issues. First, the interviewer can be explicit about the value of eliciting the most valid information and its importance in helping to generate the most beneficial and tailored treatment plan. Second, he or she can gently explore whether the interviewee has understood the questions. Third, once the interviewer identifies such a tendency, he or she should be particularly careful about asking leading questions that imply to the interviewee that there is a "right" answer (which would motivate the guarded interviewee to deny having the symptom, and the suggestible interviewee to become convinced that he or she has it). Finally, it is important that the interviewer use his or her judgment and clinical skills to evaluate whether other sources (including observations within the interview) are in concurrence with the interviewee's self-report.

Guideline 4: Assessing Symptoms

Many of the reviewed challenges in collecting reliable information during an interview are intensified when an interviewer tries to elicit information about symptoms. These challenges make it particularly difficult to achieve the primary goal of a diagnostic interview—to assess the interviewee's symptoms in a reliable manner. In the absence of laboratory test markers and indicators, psychiatric diagnosis depends heavily on self-report, which is subject to many distortions (although it may provide valuable information on subjective experience).

Fortunately, the interview's inherent limitations are also its strength: The complex process and data gathering that get in the way of generating a diagnostic hypothesis may also facilitate it. For instance, by evaluating the content and logical flow of the interviewee's verbalization, the interviewer may be able to learn about the presence of symptoms such as hallucinations and thought disorganization (e.g., loose associations, circumstantiality, and thought blocking). Although delusions may at times be readily assessed because of the interviewee's preoccupation with the theme or idea, at other times engagement in lengthier discussions is required before the interviewee begins to reveal much about his or her delusional ideas. In addition, observing the interviewee's behavior and affective expressivity during the interview can help the interviewer detect symptoms such as constricted or inappropriate affect. Finally, the interviewer may ask him- or herself whether he or she is losing track of the point the interviewee is trying to make, which can serve as a useful cue to consideration of different symptoms, such as tangential speech or derailing.

Guideline 5: Symptoms Getting in the Way

During some interviews, the characteristic symptoms of schizophrenia make it difficult to secure sufficient and sound information, for example, when the interviewee is actively hallucinating or delusional; displaying disorganized thought or behavior; and presenting severe negative symptoms, cognitive impairments, or comorbid symptoms such as anxiety. Common effects of these symptoms and impairments are distractions that disrupt the flow of the interview and hinder collaboration.

There are various ways to address such disruptions. One way is to break up the interview into smaller parts to accommodate the person's short attention span. This can involve taking more frequent rest breaks or conducting the interview over a few days. This approach can also be used within the interview by breaking questions down into smaller ones, so that the person can more easily retain and process them. Finally, it is also often useful to explain the benefits of the interview and provide token rewards, so that the person participates as fully as possible in the interview.

Guideline 6: Beyond Isolated Symptoms: The Importance of the Context

Another challenge may be a lack of sufficient information on the personal or cultural context within which the diagnostic information may be meaningfully understood. This may occur in transcultural situations, in which the interviewer is not versed in the interviewee's language and culture. Because the interviewer functions as a yardstick to some degree to evaluate the interviewee's beliefs, it is imperative that he or she be familiar with, or at least be sure to assess, the interviewee's general and health beliefs in relation to those of the culture to which the person belongs.

To understand the personal context it is useful to explore how symptoms relate to various domains of a person's life. To gather such information, it is important that the interviewer ask about a range of other contexts, including work, living, leisure, and social relationships, to try to identify the often complex mutual influences between these contexts and symptoms. Another important aspect of the context is its longitudinal course (e.g., time of onset of the first psychotic episode), which may have an impact on the developmental abilities of the interviewee (e.g., educational level and interpersonal experiences). The interviewer should also be sensitive to paranoia or to a traumatic history on the part of the interviewee that may disrupt the interview, and use appropriate communication skills to build trust. For instance, the interviewer should fully disclose the possible risks and expected benefits of the interview, give the interviewee as much control as possible over the interview (e.g., by asking open-ended questions and inviting the person to tell his or her life story), use empathic verbalizations, and more. Last but not least, the interviewer should be sensitive to the interviewee's cultural (and spiritual) context by using an interpreter when needed, recognizing that the interviewee's health beliefs and health-related behaviors may be very different from those of the interviewer.

Guideline 7: Differential Diagnosis

The symptoms of schizophrenia often overlap with those of many other psychiatric disorders; thus, the presence of other syndromes should be assessed and ruled out before the diagnosis of schizophrenia can be made. Schizoaffective and mood disorders are commonly confused with schizophrenia, because they are mistakenly thought to simply include both psychotic and affective symptoms (i.e., in bipolar disorder and major depressive disorder with psychotic features). But it is not the predominance of the psychotic versus the affective component that determines the diagnosis; rather, it is the timing of psychotic and affective symptoms. If psychotic symptoms and affective symptoms always overlap, the person is diagnosed with an affective disorder, whereas if psychotic symptoms are present some of the time, in the absence of an affective syndrome, the person meets criteria for either schizoaffective disorder or schizophrenia (the former, if the mood symptoms are prolonged).

Recent research has revealed high rates of exposure to trauma and posttraumatic stress disorder (PTSD) comorbidity among people with a severe mental illness such as schizophrenia (Switzer et al., 1999). These findings, and the overlap in symptom presentation, make PTSD a highly relevant disorder when assessing schizophrenia. Dissociative or intrusive (reexperiencing) symptoms, such as trauma-related auditory phenomena and flashbacks, may be mistakenly interpreted as schizophrenia, so special attention is required to rule them out.

Substance use disorders such as alcohol dependence or drug abuse can either be a differential diagnosis or a comorbid disorder of schizophrenia. With respect to differential diagnosis, substance use disorders can interfere with a clinician's ability to diagnose schizophrenia, and if the substance use is covert, lead to misdiagnosis (Kranzler et al., 1995). Psychoactive substances, such as alcohol, marijuana, cocaine, and amphetamines, can produce symptoms and dysfunction that mimic those found in schizophrenia, such as hallucinations, delusions, and social withdrawal (Schuckit, 1989). The most critical recommendations for diagnosing substance abuse in schizophrenia include (1) maintain a high index of suspicion of substance abuse, especially if an interviewee has a past history of substance abuse; (2) use multiple assessment techniques, including self-report instruments, interviews with interviewees, clinician reports, reports of significant others, and biological assays; and (3) be alert to signs that may be subtle indicators of the presence of a substance use disorder, such as unexplained symptom relapses, increased familial conflict, money management problems, and depression or suicidality.

Many general medical disorders, such as hyperthyroidism, and cognitive disorders, such as dementia of various types, can present with schizophrenia-like symptoms. In many of these disorders the cognitive impairments are similar (e.g., in some cases of head injury). Hence, the differential diagnosis of schizophrenia in relation to these disorders may be difficult, particularly when past history is not conclusive (e.g., when a first psychotic episode started after a head injury). Moreover, the impact of comorbidity, such as whether a head injury that occurred after the onset of schizophrenia is contributing to symptom severity and cognitive impairment, may be very difficult to determine, because the natural course of schizophrenia in itself is not a uniform one. Still, a thorough medical and psychiatric history is helpful in this respect, as are laboratory tests—blood tests for hormones and many other factors, brain imaging such as computed tomography and magnetic resonance imaging, and other tests—to rule out or to confirm general medical and cognitive disorders.

KEY POINTS

- Schizophrenia is a severe and complex psychiatric disorder; characteristic—positive and negative—symptoms, as well as other impairments, commonly accompany the disorder.
- Diagnostic interviewing for schizophrenia is facilitated by structured assessment tools.
- There are various challenges in diagnostic interviewing of people with schizophrenia, for which guidelines can be helpful.
- Many of the guidelines for diagnostic interviews of people with schizophrenia address clinical communication skills.
- Differential diagnosis should be given special attention in diagnostic interviews of people with schizophrenia.

REFERENCES AND RECOMMENDED READINGS

American Psychiatric Association. (2000). *Diagnostic and statistical manual of mental disorders* (4th ed., text rev.). Washington, DC: Author.

Andreasen, N. C. (1982). Negative symptoms in schizophrenia: Definition and reliability. *Archives of General Psychiatry, 39,* 784–788.

Curson, D. A., Patel, M., Liddle, P. F., & Barnes, T. R. E. (1988). Psychiatric morbidity of a long-stay hospital population with chronic schizophrenia and implications for future community care. *British Medical Journal, 297,* 819–822.

First, M. B., Spitzer, R. L., Gibbon, M., & Williams, J. B. W. (1995). *Structured Clinical Interview for DSM-IV Axis I Disorders—Patient Edition (SCID-I/P, Version 2.0).* New York: Biometrics Research Department, New York State Psychiatric Institute.

Kay, S. R., Opler, L. A., & Fiszbein, A. (1987). The Positive and Negative Syndrome Scale (PANSS) for schizophrenia. *Schizophrenia Bulletin, 13,* 261–276.

Kranzler, H. R., Kadden, R. M., Burleson, J. A., Babor, T. F., Apter, A., & Rounsaville, B. J. (1995). Validity of psychiatric diagnoses in patients with substance use disorders: Is the interview more important than the interviewer? *Comprehensive Psychiatry, 36,* 278–288.

Overall, G., & Gorham, D. (1962). The Brief Psychiatric Rating Scale. *Psychological Reports, 10,* 799—812.

Roe, D., & Davidson, L. (2005). Self and narrative in schizophrenia: Time to author a new story. *Journal of Medical Humanities, 31,* 89–94.

Roe, D., & Kravetz, S. (2003). Different ways of being aware of and acknowledging a psychiatric disability: A multifunctional narrative approach to insight into mental disorder. *Journal of Nervous and Mental Disease, 191,* 417–424.

Roe, D., Lereya, J., & Fennig, S. (2001). Comparing patients and staff member's attitudes: Does patient's competence to disagree mean they are not competent? *Journal of Nervous and Mental Disease, 189,* 307—310.

Rudnick, A. (1997). On the notion of psychosis: The DSM-IV in perspective. *Psychopathology, 30,* 298–302.

Schuckit, M. A. (1989). *Drug and alcohol abuse: A clinical guide to diagnosis and treatment, third edition.* New York: Plenum Press.

Switzer, G. E., Dew, M. A., Thompson, K., Goycoolea, J. M., Derricott, T., & Mullins, S. D. (1999). Posttraumatic stress disorder and service utilization among urban mental health center clients. *Journal of Traumatic Stress, 12,* 25–39.

World Health Organization. (1992). *International classification of diseases (ICD-10)* (10th ed.). Geneva: Author.

CHAPTER 13

ASSESSMENT OF CO-OCCURRING DISORDERS

KAREN WOHLHEITER
LISA DIXON

This chapter covers the assessment of a range of disorders that commonly co-occur with schizophrenia. These include use and abuse of different substances, such as alcohol, other drugs, and nicotine. The increased recognition of the important role that mental health professionals assume in the diagnosis and management of co-occurring somatic disorders has required that mental health practitioners perform routine monitoring and assessment of such disorders. Assessment of co-occurring addiction and somatic disorders often requires two types of approaches. The first approach involves asking the patient a series of questions. The second approach includes a variety of biophysical tests. Both are covered in this chapter.

SUBSTANCE ABUSE DISORDERS

Approximately 50% of persons with schizophrenia have a lifetime rates of co-occurring substance abuse, with rates approaching 70–80% in more acutely ill samples. Substance abuse is associated with a number of adverse clinical, social, and behavioral outcomes. Thus, assessment is critical, so that appropriate treatment can be initiated. Integrated, stage-specific treatments have been found to be effective for patients with co-occurring substance use disorders. Once patients are diagnosed with a substance abuse disorder, it is important to assess regularly for drug and alcohol abuse, using a multifaceted approach throughout treatment.

Studies report a number of methods for assessing substance use. Self-report is often a common technique; however, due to frequent underreporting by patients, this technique may best be utilized as a collateral data point with biochemical tests, such as urine toxicology or breath analysis and clinician ratings. Typically data are collected from multiple sources, and patients are assessed for substance use over a period of time.

Assessments

Clinician Rating Scales

The 5-point Clinician Rating Scale (CRS) is used to rate the extent of alcohol, cannabis, and cocaine abuse over the preceding 6 months. Patients are placed in one of five categories: abstinence, use without impairment, abuse, dependence, or dependence without institutionalization. The clinician is instructed to rate patients based on self-report, behavioral observation, and collateral reports. The CRS has been used frequently in a number of studies and has been found to have good reliability and validity.

Drug Abuse Screening Test

The Drug Abuse Screening Test (DAST) is used to identify drug-use-related problems in the past year. The DAST has been found to be internally stable and to discriminate between patients with and without current drug dependence. This scale asks patients to answer 10 yes–no questions on drug use. Patients are categorized as having no problems if they answer all questions "no" versus "low," "moderate," or "substantial" levels based on responses.

Michigan Alcoholism Screening Test

The Michigan Alcoholism Screening Test (MAST) is a simple, self-scoring scale that asks patients about alcohol use and related problems. It is frequently used in both clinical and research settings.

CAGE

This is a brief scale that mental health providers can use to assess alcohol use. The questions are as follows:

> C—Has anyone ever felt you should *Cut* down on your drinking?
> A—Have people *Annoyed* you by criticizing your drinking?
> G—Have you ever felt *Guilty* about your drinking?
> E—Have you ever had a drink first thing in the morning (*Eye-opener*) to steady your nerves or to get rid of a hangover?

One positive response suggests a drinking problem; two or more positive responses indicate a problem with approximately 90% reliability in most research studies.

DALI

The Dartmouth Assessment of Lifestyle Instrument (DALI), an 18-item questionnaire, is a useful screen for both current alcohol and drug (i.e., marijuana and cocaine) use disorders in people with severe mental illness.

Addiction Severity Index

The Addiction Severity Index (ASI) is one of the most widely used standardized instruments for assessing substance use. It can be used for multiple purposes, such as to assess severity of substance use or to assess periodic changes in patients' substance use prior to, during, and after treatment.

Time-Line Follow-Back

The Time-Line Follow-Back (TLFB) utilizes a calendar and tools to aid patient recall of substance use over varying lengths of time. Studies have found the TLFB useful in detected underreported use of alcohol.

Breathalyzer

Alcohol use can be measured within 40–70 minutes after consumption of any alcoholic drink. The amount of alcohol in the blood reaches its highest level about an hour after drinking. The rest of it is passed out of the body in urine and exhaled breath. A Breathalyzer can measure blood alcohol concentration (BAC) from a puff of air. According to the American Medical Association, impairment can occur at levels of 0.05; however, most states report legal limits of 0.08. Breathalyzer results cannot be used to indicate levels of use over time. The reading only provides for clinicians a current BAC level.

Toxicology Screening (Urine and Blood)

A toxicology test can be used to monitor specific drug use. A wide variety of substances, including cocaine, marijuana, alcohol, and amphetiamines, may be monitored. Though tests of urine and blood are available, urine tests are easier to do, and a wider number of drugs can be detected in the urine. Also, a drug (or its metabolized form) may be detectable for a longer period of time in urine than in blood. Clinicians should have access to a list of current medications (prescription and nonprescription), herbal supplements, vitamins, and other substances that the patient has taken in the prior 4 days, because they may interfere with testing. Most toxicology tests determine only the presence of drugs in the body, not the specific level or quantity. Follow-up testing is often required to determine the exact level of a certain drug in the body and confirm the results of the initial test. Results that indicate drug use or abuse should be confirmed by at least two different test methods because of the possibility of false-positive results. For suspected drug abuse, a trained person may need to witness the urine or blood collection.

Hair Analysis

Although hair analysis is being done more frequently to test for illegal drug use (e.g., cocaine or marijuana use), it is not always widely available. Hair samples are taken from a specific part of the body, such as from the back of the scalp by the neck or from the pubic area. Hair close to the skin or scalp includes the most recent growth, which provides the most accurate information about recent use. Hair samples do not indicate recent changes in the body, such as drug use within the past few days, or the amount of substance that was used.

NICOTINE DEPENDENCE

Persons with schizophrenia are more likely to be smokers than are people in the general population. Approximately 70–90% of people with schizophrenia smoke compared to about 25% of the general population. People with schizophrenia are more likely to be daily smokers compared to people in the general population. Daily smoking is usually considered a sign of nicotine addiction. Smoking in this population is associated with the same risks seen in the general population, such as higher rates of cardiovascular disease and higher rates of chronic obstructive pulmonary disease.

Assessment of cigarette dependence requires asking patients at each visit if they smoke, and determining the frequency and amount of smoking. An abstinence period is typically defined by no more than five cigarettes from the start of the abstinence period. A standard abstinence question is "Have you smoked at all since (date of abstinence)?", with the following possible responses: (1) No, not a puff; (2) one to five cigarettes; or (3) more than five cigarettes. For responses 1 and 2, a biochemical test is usually helpful to confirm a classification of abstinence.

A standardized questionnaire such as the Fagerstrom Test of Nicotine Dependence (FTND) can also be used to assess nicotine dependences. This scale is a six-item measure of behaviors related to dependence on nicotine. Items ask about time elapsed before smoking the first cigarette of the day, difficulty refraining from smoking, increased smoking in the morning, and the most difficult cigarette of the day to give up. The FTND shows good internal consistency and construct validity. Scores range from 0 to 10, with scores greater than 3 indicating dependence.

A Smokerlyzer may be used with patients to assess the level of carbon monoxide in expired air. Carbon monoxide (CO) measures of less than 9 parts per million (ppm) can be used to confirm abstinence. Alternative biochemical measures, such as cotinine concentration levels (saliva, urine, plasma), may be used. The cutoff for urine is 50 ng/ml, and 15 ng/ml for saliva. Cotinine levels do not discriminate between nicotine ingested by cigarettes and that derived from replacement products. It is therefore important to inquire about use of these products prior to testing nicotine levels. Although testing for the presence of cotinine is the preferred biochemical method to determine abstinence, CO verification can also determine use. This method only detects recent smoking. However, most smokers return to daily smoking if they relapse, and CO levels can be used for confirmation of cigarette use.

INFECTIOUS DISEASES: HIV AND HEPATITIS C

Individuals with schizophrenia are at increased risk of HIV infection compared to the general population. Current prevalence rates for persons with schizophrenia range between 2 and 5%, with rates of 2% in nonmetropolitan areas and 5% in observed urban areas. This prevalence is around eight times the overall estimate for the U.S. population. Women with schizophrenia are at even greater increased risk for HIV; the male-to-female ratio is 4:3, compared to 5:1 in the general population. A number of factors, such as increased injection drug use and unsafe sexual practices, may contribute to increased HIV rates in this population. Studies have also shown that persons with severe mental illnesses are more likely to engage in high-risk behaviors and less likely to modify their behaviors.

Patients with a dual diagnosis of schizophrenia and substance use disorder have a 22% greater chance of having HIV than patients without a mental illness. However, those without a substance abuse disorder are 50% less likely than people without a mental illness to contract HIV. This may be due to less socialization because of negative symptoms such as withdrawal and apathy (Himelhoch et al., 2007).

In addition to increased risk for HIV, high-risk behaviors and injection drug use contribute to higher rates of hepatitis C virus (HCV) in persons with schizophrenia. Rates of HCV in this population range from 9 to 20%, at a rate 11 times greater than that in the general population. Among those infected with HCV, 90% will develop chronic infections, and 20% will progress to hepatic cirrhosis.

Testing and Risk Assessment for Infectious Diseases: Screening for Risk Behaviors

The most common risks for persons with severe mental illness are drug use behaviors (e.g., sharing paraphernalia) and sexual behaviors related to drug use (e.g., unprotected sex with high-risk partners, exchanging sex for money). The use of crack cocaine and intravenous drugs are associated with the highest level of risk. Screening for these risk behaviors in people with severe mental illness can be accomplished in a clinical setting by face-to-face interviewing.

The AIDS Risk Inventory (ARI) and the DALI are both useful tools in screening for behaviors that may lead to increased risk for blood-borne infectious disease. The ARI is a structured interview used to assess knowledge, attitudes, and risk behaviors associated with acquiring and transmitting blood-borne infections. Studies that have used this scale with severely mentally ill participants have found that it is reliable and valid. The DALI is an 18-item questionnaire that contains two screening scales: one for current alcohol use disorders, and another for drug (i.e., marijuana and cocaine) use disorders in people with severe mental illness.

Those who report risk behaviors for HIV or hepatitis should be tested for infection. Recommended tests include HIV-1 enzyme immunoassay (EIA) antibody; HCV antibody, confirmed with polymerase chain reaction (PCR) viral load; hepatitis B surface antigen; and immunoglobulin M core antibody. These can be obtained in a single blood draw. Testing also should involve providing pre- and posttest counseling regarding test procedures and the implications of test results.

Laboratory Tests

HIV: HIV Enzyme-Linked Immunosorbent Assay and, If Positive, Western Blot

Tests for detecting antibodies to HIV proteins include enzyme-linked immunosorbent assay (ELISA), which is both highly sensitive and specific, but some false-positive ELISA tests occur. When reactive, ELISA should be repeated on the same sample. If it is positive a second time, a more specific test should be performed (e.g., the Western blot assay, which is an immunoelectrophoretic procedure for identifying antibodies to specific viral proteins separated by their molecular weight).

ELISAs that directly measure viral antigens rather than antiviral antibodies are relatively insensitive. Tests of antigen levels have been supplanted by more sensitive measurements of plasma ribonucleic acid (RNA).

Several sensitive assays of plasma RNA, such as reverse-transcription PCR (RT-PCR) that amplifies viral nucleic acids, or branched DNA (bDNA) that amplifies signal, are sensitive and accurate over a wide range of viral concentrations (up to 1,000,000 copies/ml of plasma). The lower limits of detection are about 50 copies/ml for both RT-PCR and bDNA. Other methods for nucleic acid amplification, such as nucleic acid sequence-based amplification (NASBA) and transcription-mediated amplification (TMA), are under development.

Whereas ELISA measures antibody to whole virus concentration and gives a "positive," "negative," or indeterminate test result, Western blotting is a more specific test. It allows one to visualize antibodies directed against specific viral proteins. For this reason, it is a confirmatory test for a positive HIV ELISA. In an HIV Western blotting, proteins are electrophoresed into a gel. As they migrate through the gel, the proteins are separated based upon size and charge. Characteristically, smaller proteins migrate through the gel faster than larger proteins.

HCV: Anti-HCV Screening Assays

Anti-HCV screening test kits licensed or approved by the U.S. Food and Drug Administration comprise three immunoassays: two EIAs (Abbott HCV EIA 2.0, Abbott Laboratories, Abbott Park, IL, and ORTHO® HCV Version 3.0 ELISA, Ortho-Clinical Diagnostics, Raritan, NJ) and one enhanced chemiluminescence immunoassay (CIA; VITROS® Anti-HCV Assay, Ortho-Clinical Diagnostics, Raritan, NJ). All of these immunoassays use HCV-encoded recombinant antigens.

Confirmatory Testing: Recombinant Immunoblot Assay and PCR

The Centers for Disease Control and Prevention have recommended that a person be considered to have serological evidence of HCV infection only after an anti-HCV screening-test-positive result has been verified by a more specific serological test (e.g., the recombinant immunoblot assay [RIBA®; Chiron Corporation, Emeryville, CA]) or a nucleic acid test (NAT). This recommendation is consistent with testing practices for hepatitis B surface antigen and antibody to HIV, for which laboratories routinely conduct more specific reflex testing before reporting a result as positive.

Treatment of HIV infection is recommended for almost all infected persons, preferably prior to the onset of significant immune deficiency. Treatment of HCV with antiviral medication may be recommended for persons with moderately severe liver disease, which is assessed by symptoms, physical examination, laboratory tests, and, in some cases, liver biopsy. Infected persons should be referred to a medical specialist for treatment.

METABOLIC CONDITIONS

Diabetes Mellitus

There is about an 8% prevalence rate of diabetes in the general population of North America. Rates among people with schizophrenia are much higher, with reported rates ranging from 16 to 25%. Second-generation antipsychotics, obesity, and lifestyle factors can all contribute to the increase in prevalence. Patients at high risk for developing diabetes should be assessed. Risk factors include obesity; age greater than 45 years; family history of diabetes; being African American, Native American, Asian American, Pacific Islander, or Hispanic American; and blood pressure greater than 140/90 or history of high blood pressure, high cholesterol, or inactive lifestyle. If a patient is 45 years or older and overweight, testing is recommended. If the patient is younger than age 45, overweight, and has at least one of the aforementioned risk factors, testing is recommended. Testing is able to indicate whether blood glucose is normal, prediabetic, or diabetic. If a patient is diagnosed with prediabetes, testing is indicated at least every 1–2 years. People diagnosed with prediabetes often develop diabetes within 10 years. Regular testing for diabetes is now generally recommended for patients who receive antipsychotic medications.

Testing Methods

Fasting plasma glucose measures blood glucose after the patient has fasted for at least 8 hours. A level of 99 or less is normal, and a level of 126 or above is consistent with diabetes. An oral glucose tolerance test measures blood glucose after the patient has fasted for at least 8 hours and 2 hours after drinking a glucose-containing beverage. A level of 139 or less is normal, and a level of 200 or above is consistent with diabetes. Levels in between are considered impaired fasting glucose, or prediabetic. A random plasma glucose test checks blood glucose without regard to eating. This test can be used with an assessment of symptoms to diagnosis diabetes, but not prediabetes. Positive test results should be confirmed by repeating the fasting plasma glucose test or the oral glucose tolerance test on a different day.

Obesity/Overweight

Patients with schizophrenia are at a greater risk for weight gain and obesity due to use of psychotropic agents and lifestyle factors. Obesity has been linked to stroke, coronary heart disease, type II diabetes, hypertension, and arthritis. Weight gain and obesity should be monitored closely at patient visits. Height and weight can be assessed to calculate body mass index (BMI). Typically a BMI of 25 or greater is considered overweight, with a body mass ≥30 indicating obesity. Waist circumference is also useful to define weight problems, because excess abdominal fat is associated with glucose intolerance, dyslipidemia, and hypertension. Waist circumferences should not exceed 40 inches in men and 35 inches in women.

Weight should be assessed frequently throughout treatment to assess any increases or decreases that may occur. This is especially important after introducing new antipsychotic medications. Though no specific guidelines are widely accepted, it is not unreasonable to obtain weights at each appointment.

Exercise and Diet

There are relatively few instruments available for assessing the eating and exercise habits of people with schizophrenia. The International Physical Activity Questionnaire (IPAQ) has been used with this population; it is simply worded and easily understood by a wide variety of populations. The IPAQ has brief and extended versions. Both versions include items about exercise habits; however, the extended version includes questions on inactivity that are often informative. The Self-Efficacy and Exercise Habits Survey, developed by Sallis, Pinski, Grossman, Patterson, and Nader (1998), measures exercise-related self-efficacy and has been shown be both valid and reliable.

Pedometers are also a simple, inexpensive, objective measure of activity. Step monitors are now being used successfully to estimate levels of movement expressed as "steps taken throughout the day" to document activity. Patients can be given log sheets to complete to indicate activity during the week or month to help clinicians understand their activity levels. Pedometers may also be used to help patients monitor exercise and fitness goals.

Eating habits are often to difficult to track. A simple food diary or log may be the easiest way to indicate eating habits. Logs can be filled out by patients on a daily basis and reviewed by health care providers at appointments. The Diet History Questionnaire (DHQ), a relatively easy to use food frequency instrument developed by the National Cancer Institute, has good validity for tracking eating habits. Food questionnaires are problematic because patients often over- or underestimate their food intake during the time period. This is often why daily food logs may be a more accurate way for clinicians to assess eating habits.

Metabolic Syndrome

This syndrome is closely associated with a generalized metabolic disorder called insulin resistance, in which the body cannot use insulin efficiently. The underlying causes of the syndrome are physical inactivity, genetic factors, and overweight/obesity. Patients who have the metabolic syndrome are at an increased risk for stroke, type 2 diabetes, and coronary heart disease.

There are no universally accepted criteria for diagnosing the metabolic syndrome. The criteria proposed by the third report of the National Cholesterol Education Program (NCEP) Expert Panel on Detection, Evaluation, and Treatment of High Blood Cholesterol in Adults (Adult Treatment Panel [ATP] III) are the most current and widely used. According to the ATP III criteria, the metabolic syndrome is identified by the presence of three or more of the following components: (1) central obesity, as measured by waist circumference: men > 40 inches, women > 35 inches; (2) fasting blood triglycerides greater than or equal to 150 mg/dl; (3) blood high-density lipoprotein (HDL) cholesterol: men < 40 mg/dl, women < 50 mg/dl; (4) blood pressure greater than or equal to 130/85 mm Hg; and (5) fasting glucose greater than or equal to 110 mg/dl.

CARDIOVASCULAR DISORDERS

Hypertension

Similar to diabetes due to obesity and lifestyle factors, persons with schizophrenia are at increase risk for high blood pressure. Blood pressure monitoring at patient visits can assess whether treatment is needed for hypertension. *Hypertension,* or *high blood pressure,* is often defined as mean systolic blood pressure (SBP) ≥140 mm Hg, mean diastolic blood pressure (DBP) ≥90 mm Hg.

Lipid Disorders

Persons with schizophrenia are also at increased risk for developing high cholesterol due to lifestyle factors such as poor diet, lack of exercise, and obesity. In addition, some studies have linked the use of clozapine and olanzapine to hypertriglyceridemia. Patients should have their lipid levels check on an annual basis, since high total cholesterol and low-density lipoprotein (LDL) cholesterol levels are strong, independent risk factors for coronary heart disease.

A lipid profile should be done after the patient has fasted for 9–12 hours. According to the NCEP, the following levels indicate borderline high to very high levels:

Total cholesterol levels
   200–239 mg/dl: Borderline high
   240 mg/dl or higher: High
Triglycerides
   150–199 mg/dl: Borderline high
   200–499 mg/dl: High
   500 mg/dl or higher: Very high
LDL
   130–159 mg/dl: Borderline high
   160–189 mg/dl: High
   190 mg/dl or higher: Very high

POLYDIPSIA

Polydipsia is the intake of greater than 3 liters of fluid per day. It can be primary or secondary to medical conditions or medication side effects. This excessive intake of fluids can increase symptoms of disorientation and confusion. In some extreme cases, polydipsia can lead to hyponatremia and seizures.

An interdisciplinary team approach can be very useful in helping assess and treat polydipsia. The initial goal in diagnosing this disorder is to gather baseline data and try to confirm or rule out presence of the problem. Prior to confirming or assigning a diagnosis of polydipsia, other causes such as diabetes mellitus, diabetes insipidus, chronic renal failure, malignancy, pulmonary disease, and hypocalcemia should be excluded. In many cases, this information is contained in medical records from the patient's primary care providers.

Multiple methods may be used to assess whether a patient has polydipsia. Observable symptoms may include mood swings, confusion, inability to follow commands, disorientation, and rambling speech. If a patient is in an observable setting, such as an inpatient unit, clinical staff may notice an increase in water or fluid consumption. In addition, some antipsychotic medications can increase a patient's risk for developing polydipsia. Therefore, an initial review of patient records and a medical evaluation can help confirm a diagnosis. Diagnostic lab work using urinalysis can also be used to determine whether polydipsia is present. Finally, weight monitoring can be used. If excessive fluid intake is suspected, patients should have their weight monitored. Such monitoring should be done closely, when possible, such as in an inpatient setting. Patients should be weighed at least twice a day, and not after eating a large meal. If patients' morning and evening weights differ by greater than 5%, they should be closely monitored for possible seizures due to a change in electrolytes. In addition, it is helpful to monitor the intake of water or fluids. Two simple techniques that can be used are intake logs or a bottle that contains the recommended amount daily of fluids.

KEY POINTS

- Assessment for drug and alcohol use optimally involves multiple sources of information.
- Assessment should be continuous throughout treatment, because substance use disorders tend to be relapsing and remitting.
- Objective measures of substance use include Breathalyzer tests and toxicology screening of urine, blood, and hair.
- Cigarette smoking, the most common addiction in schizophrenia, can be monitored with self-reported use and biological measures that test expired air and saliva or urine.
- The dangerous physical consequences of infectious diseases that can cause severe medical disability and even death require monitoring of both high-risk behaviors and exposure to hepatitis (both B and C) and HIV.
- Even patients who are currently abstinent may have infectious diseases of which they are unaware; thus, understanding patients' past use and behavior is important.
- Rates of obesity, diabetes, and metabolic syndrome are elevated among persons with schizophrenia and require close monitoring and coordination with primary care.
- Weight and blood pressure can be assessed regularly in psychiatric clinics and should become a part of routine monitoring and patient education.
- Fasting blood tests for lipids and glucose are critical for identifying and tracking metabolic problems.
- Although exercise and diet are difficult to track systematically, simple logs developed for individual patient monitoring can be helpful.

REFERENCES AND RECOMMENDED READINGS

Booth, M. L. (2000). Assessment of physical activity: An international perspective. *Research Quarterly for Exercise and Sport, 71*(2), 114–120.

Cancer Prevention Research Center. (2007). *Stages of change algorithm for the weight: Stages of Change—Short Form.* Available online at *www.uri.edu/research/cprc/masures/weight01.htm*

Carey, K. B., Carey, M. P., Maisto, S. A., & Henson, J. M. (2004). Temporal stability of the timeline followback interview for alcohol and drug use with psychiatric outpatients. *Journal of Studies of Alcohol, 65*(6), 774–781.

Carey, K., Cocco, K., & Simons, J. (1996). Concurrent validity of clinicians' ratings of substance abuse among psychiatric outpatients *Psychiatric Services, 47,* 842–847.

Chawarski, M., & Baird, J. (1998, June–July). *Comparison of two instruments for assessing HIV risk in drug abusers in social and behavioral science: Proceedings of the 12th World AIDS Conference.* Bologna, Italy, Monduzzi Editore.

Chawarski, M. C., Pakes, J., & Schottenfeld, R. S. (1998). Assessment of HIV risk. *Journal of Addictive Diseases, 17*(4), 49–59.

Craig, C. L., Marshall, A. L., Sjostrom, M., Bauman, A. E., Booth, M. L., Ainsworth, B. E., et al. (2003). The International Physical Activity Questionnaire (IPAQ): A comprehensive reliability and validity study in twelve countries. *Medicine and Science in Sports and Exercise, 35*(8), 1381–1395.

Drake, R. E., Osher, F. C., Noordsy, D. L., Hurlbut, S. C., Teague, G. B., & Beaudett, M. S. (1990). Diagnosis of alcohol use disorders in schizophrenia. *Schizophrenia Bulletin, 16,* 57–67.

Ewing, J. A. (1984). Detecting alcoholism: The CAGE questionnaire. *Journal of the American Medical Association, 252*(14), 1905–1907.

Heatherton, T. F., Kozlowski, L. T., Frecker, R. C., & Fagerstrom, K. O. (1991). The Fagerstrom Test for Nicotine Dependence: A revision of the Fagerstrom Tolerance Questionnaire. *Journal of Addictions, 86,* 1119–1127.

Himelhoch, S., McCarthy, J., Ganoczy, D., Medoff, D., Dixon, L., & Blow, F. (2007). Understanding associations between serious mental illness and HIV among patients in the VA health system. *Psychiatric Services, 58*(9), 1165–1172.

Irvin, E., Flannery, R., Penk, W., & Hanson, M. (1995). The Alcohol Use Scale: Concurrent validity data. *Journal of Social Behavior and Personality, 10,* 899–905.

Jarvis, M. J., Russell, M. A. H., & Soloojee, Y. (1980). Expired air carbon monoxide: A simple breath test of tobacco smoke intake. *British Medical Journal, 281,* 484–485.

Marcus, B. H., Selfby, V. C., Niaura, R. S., & Rossi, J. S. (1992). Self-efficacy and the stages of exercise behavior change. *Research Quarterly for Exercise and Sport, 63,* 60–66.

McHugo, G. J., Drake, R. E., Burton, H. L., & Ackerson, T. H. (1995). A scale for assessing the stage of substance abuse treatment in persons with severe mental illness. *Journal of Nervous and Mental Disease, 183,* 762–767.

McClellan, A., Kushner, H., & Metzger, D. (1992). The fifth edition of the Addiction Severity Index. *Journal of Substance Abuse Treatment, 9*(3), 199–213.

Rosenberg, S. D., Drake, R. E., Wolford, G. L., Mueser, K. T., Oxman, T. E., Vidaver, R. M., et al. (1998). Dartmouth Assessment of Lifestyle Instrument (DALI): A substance use disorder screen for people with severe mental illness. *American Journal of Psychiatry, 155,* 232–238.

Rosenberg, S. D., Swanson, J. W., Wolford, G. L., Osher, F. C., Swartz, M. S., Essock, S. M., et al. (2003). The five-site health and risk study of blood-borne infections among persons with severe mental illness. *Psychiatric Services, 54,* 827–835.

Sallis, J. F., Pinski, R. B., Grossman, R. M., Patterson, T. L., & Nader, P. R. (1998). The development of self-efficacy scales for health-related diet and exercise behaviors. *Health Education Research, 3,* 283–292.

Selzer, M. L. (1971). The Michigan Alcoholism Screening Test: The quest for a new diagnostic instrument. *American Journal of Psychiatry, 127,* 1653–1658.

Selzer, M. L., Vinokur, A., & Rooijen, L. (1975). A self-administered Short Michigan Alcoholism Screening Test (SMAST). *Journal of Studies on Alcohol, 36,* 117–126.

Skinner, H. A. (1982). The Drug Abuse Screening Test. *Addictive Behaviors, 7*(4), 363–371.

Steinberg, M., Williams, J., Steinberg, H., Krejci, J., & Ziedonis, D. (2005). Applicability of the Fagerstrom Test for Nicotine Dependence in smokers with schizophrenia. *Addictive Behaviors, 30,* 49–59.

Subar, A. F., Thompson, F. E., Kpnis, V., Midthune, D., Hurwitz, P., McNutt, S., et al. (2001). Comparative validation of the Block, Willett, and National Cancer Institute food frequency questionnaires: The Eating at America's Table Study. *American Journal of Epidemiology, 154*(12), 1089–1099.

CHAPTER 14

ASSESSMENT OF PSYCHOSOCIAL FUNCTIONING

TANIA LECOMTE
MARC CORBIÈRE
CATHERINE BRIAND

Psychosocial functioning assessments for individuals with severe mental illness have greatly evolved over the past two decades. Initially, their sole purpose was to determine an individual's readiness to return to the community after years of institutionalization, and the level of assistance needed to stay there. Assessments were later used by mental health professionals to determine whether their clients needed rehabilitation and how they fared in different treatment programs. With psychiatric rehabilitation moving toward the recovery model—which focuses on clients' strengths, self-determination, growth potential, and personal choices, and promotes full partnership with clinicians regarding services offered—psychosocial functioning assessments have become more a collaborative process between mental health professionals and clients. As such, social functioning measures are used by clients to self-monitor their progress, and by mental health professionals to guide them toward the appropriate programs or interventions. Large-scale psychosocial functioning assessments may also be conducted by health management organizations or other external funding agencies to determine the overall effectiveness of specific rehabilitation programs. Psychosocial functioning assessments are, of course, also used in the context of efficacy and effectiveness studies of specific rehabilitation treatments or programs. No longer considered the domain of psychometricians or psychologists, psychosocial functioning assessments are now an integral part of clinical practice in psychiatric rehabilitation.

Psychosocial functioning has been defined in different ways and may cover a large array of behaviors. Typically, *psychosocial functioning* includes everything needed to live successfully in today's society, namely, having the necessary independent living skills (cooking, cleaning, hygiene, etc.), engaging in positive relationships (social skills), studying or having a job, taking care of one's health and mental health, as well as avoiding problematic community behaviors (violence, substance abuse, etc.). For people with children, being a good parent and caregiver is also an important aspect of social functioning.

Other linked concepts that may be found in assessments are one's role in the community, social skills and social competence, family relations, as well as personal and professional goals. Although self-esteem, social support, expectations, and motivation are important for psychosocial functioning, they are not measures of functioning itself, because they do not relate to specific community behaviors, attitudes, feelings, and perceptions. Some authors argue that subjective quality of life should be considered as part of any social functioning assessment. Though determining satisfaction levels regarding different aspects of one's life, or treatment, can be quite relevant because dissatisfaction can at times precede motivation for change, quality-of-life measures can be misleading. In fact, it has often been observed that as individuals progress in their recovery and realize they have more options and goals than they originally believed, their satisfaction levels decrease.

A wide range of different measures exist for assessing psychosocial functioning. These measures vary in terms of who they were designed for (hospitalized clients, outpatients, first episodes), their purpose (e.g., guide policymakers, assess impact of treatment, obtain broad information on large samples, help consumers self-monitor their progress), the type of assessment (i.e. structured interview, self-rating scale, other-rating scale, behavioral task), their psychometric properties (reliability, validity), and the length of time needed to complete the assessment. The choice of the optimal scale to measure psychosocial functioning depends on a number of considerations:

- In what context is this assessment taking place (e.g., clinical intervention, research, mental health clinic external review)?
- What specific question(s) do I hope this assessment will help answer?
- If I'm following a specific theoretical model in my work with consumers, is the assessment still appropriate?
- Do I need specific training to use this assessment?
- Do I need to pay the copyright fees for each use of this assessment?
- Will I be able to interpret the results easily?
- Has this assessment ever been validated with the type of clients with whom I work?
- Does this assessment exist in other languages, if needed?

When answering all of these questions, it is preferable also to consider specific client preferences. For instance, some clients get really anxious if the assessment resembles a test too much, but they do really well in role-play situations. Others prefer self-rating questionnaires to semistructured interviews, and still others enjoy receiving a lot of assistance and very clear, multiple-choice answers. Some clinicians might feel that they know their clients well enough and prefer using clinician-rated scales. Though other-rated scales can be very useful in specific cases (e.g., research or cost-effectiveness evaluation), they actually have less therapeutic value than scales with more than one perspective, including the client's and the clinician's answers, and perhaps even information from family members. Not only is the client's evaluation often more comprehensive than that of the clinician but also the process of answering the questions or thinking about one's social functioning can by itself produce change or bring about new rehabilitation goals. Furthermore, when the assessment is used in the context of a working relationship between the clinician and client (and sometimes with the family as well), discrepancies in perceptions and questions regarding the performance, or absence of performance, of certain social behaviors can be discussed.

In our choice of instruments, we have focused on measures that we believe cover essential aspects of psychosocial functioning, namely, behaviors or difficulties in performing behaviors in the following domains: *independent living skills* (or community adjustment), *social competence* (including social skills, problem-solving skills, and interpersonal relations), and *vocational functioning* (overcoming barriers to employment, work behaviors). *Independent living skills* are an essential part of community functioning and include basic skills in terms of hygiene (personal hygiene, as well as taking care of one's living space), cooking and nutrition, managing money, using some mean of transportation, and taking care of one's physical and mental health (e.g., taking meds, making doctor's appointments, if needed). The presence and/or absence of these skills can guide clinicians and clients in determining the most appropriate housing option, as well as planning specific courses or training sessions. *Social competence* is perhaps the most important aspect of social functioning. Many individuals with schizophrenia live in isolation and have great difficulties in engaging in meaningful relationships, yet when asked, a vast majority mention wishing they had a significant other and close friends. Many rehabilitation programs are geared toward improving social competence; a careful assessment can therefore be extremely valuable. As such, it is important not only to ask how many friends a client has but who those friends are (e.g., does the client consider the clerk at the coffee shop who does not know his or her name a friend?), how many contacts the client has, and so forth. Social skills are included within social competence and imply abilities such as being able to engage in a conversation; to keep good eye contact, voice tone, body posture, and so on, as well as to know how to create friendships. It also means being able to recognize verbal and nonverbal cues from the person with whom one is trying to converse. One important aspect of social skills training is social problem solving, which should also be assessed. Because problems with landlords, employers, family members, or roommates are likely to occur, it is important to determine whether your clients know how to deal effectively with these situations. Given the motivation that most individuals with severe mental illness have to obtain and maintain a job, *vocational functioning* is an important aspect of social functioning to assess. Clients' abilities to overcome potential barriers to employment, as well as work behaviors, should be assessed to help clients improve their chances to obtain and maintain their jobs. Similar concepts should also be assessed for those who prefer to study or go back to school. However, other than looking at grades and teachers' comments, the dearth of instruments currently described in the literature regarding school functioning have led us to not present any here.

The following measures all tap into one or all three of the social functioning domains mentioned (i.e., independent living skills, social competence, and professional or vocational integration) and sometimes also assess other concepts, such as symptoms, health, goals, or roles. They are presented in three categories: (1) global measures: offer a global score or general scales that together measure several aspects of social functioning, as well as other clinical domains; (2) comprehensive measures: assess multiple specific aspects of social functioning; and (3) specific measures: address only one domain or aspect of social functioning in a detailed manner.

As mentioned previously, many psychosocial functioning measures exist, and others are still being developed. Following a thorough review, we propose a few measures that are either widely used or are so useful and well designed that we expect they will be adopted by many clinicians in the near future. To facilitate the reader's understanding, we have categorized the scales as global measures, comprehensive measures, or measures of a specific domain of social functioning. We also offer a brief description of each assessment and have grouped the following information in Table 14.1: the type of assessment (i.e. self-rated, other-rated, interview, role play), the length of administration, the type of clients with whom the assessment was validated, whether there is a need for training, the languages in which the measure is available, and where to get more information about obtaining or using the assessment.

GLOBAL MEASURES OF PSYCHOSOCIAL FUNCTIONING

Global Assessment of Functioning

The Global Assessment of Functioning (GAF; American Psychiatric Association, 1994; Hall, 1995) gives one global score of overall functioning based on the client's clinical, social, and professional state. The score is based on a continuum of functioning ranging from 1 to 100. The GAF gives one score that is compared to the highest score in the past year. It is a quick and global way of assessing clinical change and is often used by psychiatrists. The measure typically does not include questions, so the clinician must generate questions to obtain the needed information. However, there is a more comprehensive version with detailed anchor points, as well as a self-rated version, though these are not as widely used. The score obtained is in fact highly correlated to clinical symptoms. It does not allow assessment of details or variations in specific domains of functioning and only provides (in its most frequent use) the clinician's perspective. The scale is divided into nine intervals: 1–10, 11–20, 21–30, up to 91–100. The scale is not meant for people who function at a high level.

Behavior and Symptom Identification Scale

The Behavior and Symptom Identification Scale (BASIS-32; Eisen, Dill, & Grob, 1994) measures symptoms and social functioning with 32 items divided into five subscales: Psychosis, Impulsivity, Anxiety/Depression, Interpersonal Relations, and Living Skills. The scale measures the degree of difficulty the person has experienced in the last 7 days for each item. The BASIS-32 is quick and easy to administer, and offers the client's perspective. Since it only assesses the past week, it can also be used at regular intervals to assess change over time. The five subscales were statistically derived, meaning that they were determined by statistical analyses and not theoretically conceived; therefore, they may be difficult to interpret in a clinical context. The BASIS-32 is more often used for assessing large groups of clients and determining their clinical and social functioning than for specific treatment purposes.

Short Form 36-Item General Health Survey

The Short Form 36-Item General Health Survey (SF-36; Ware & Sherbourne, 1992) assesses eight areas of health, including physical functioning, physical limitation in role functioning, pain, general health, vitality, social functioning, emotional limitations in functioning, and general mental health. The SF-36 is quick to administer and is mostly useful for determining multiple aspects of health—not specifically psychosocial functioning only. It is widely used by health management authorities and is often reported in really large-scale studies. Because it is available in many languages and validated with so many samples, it is easy to compare the results from one clinical site with others. It is, however, of limited clinical relevance in terms of a detailed assessment of social functioning, because only a small number of items cover that domain.

COMPREHENSIVE MEASURES OF PSYCHOSOCIAL FUNCTIONING

Multnomah Community Ability Scale

The Multnomah Community Ability Scale (MCAS; Barker & Barron, 1997) offers scores on four subscales (Obstacles to Functioning, Adaptation to Daily Life, Social Competence, and Behavioral Problems) of the client's community functioning in the past 3–6 months.

TABLE 14.1. Measures of Psychosocial Functioning

	Psychosocial functioning domain	Type of measure	Length of administration	Validated	Need for training	Available languages	For more information
GAF (American Psychiatric Association, 1994; Hall, 1995)	Global measure	Clinician-rated	10–20 minutes	Validated with large range of clients	Clinical skills are needed.	Exists in as many languages as DSM-IV	Scale available in DSM-IV
BASIS-32 (Eisen et al., 1994)	Global measure	Self-rated	15–30 minutes	Multiple large-scale studies	No training is necessary.	English, Cambodian, Chinese, French, Finnish, German, Italian, Japanese, Korean, Portuguese, Tagalog and Vietnamese	*www.basissurvey.org/*
SF-36 (Ware & Sherbourne, 1992)	Global measure	Self-rated	15–30 minutes	Large-scale health surveys; not specific to serious mental illness	No training is necessary.	Available in more than 20 languages, including cultural variations (e.g., 11 different Spanish versions according to country)	*www.sf-36.org/*
MCAS (Barker & Barron, 1997)	Comprehensive measure	Clinician-rated	20–30 minutes	Validated with clients living in the community	Training is necessary; typically one day suffices.	English and French	Contact *sela@nbhc.org*
CASIG (Wallace et al., 2001)	Comprehensive measure	Self-Report (CASIG-SR) and Informant (CASIG-I) versions	60 minutes for the CASIG-SR and 45 minutes for the CASIG-I	Validated with clients living in the community	No training necessary; for administration; minimal training needed to convert collaborative scores into a well-designed treatment plan.	English and French; Spanish version to come	*www.psychrehab.com*
CAN (Phelan et al., 1995)	Comprehensive measure	Self-rated and clinician-rated	15–60 minutes	Multiple European studies with clients living in the community	Simple to use; training available.	Danish, English, French, German, Italian, Spanish, and Swedish	*www.rcpsych.ac.uk/ publications/gaskell/ 25_0.htm*

(continued)

TABLE 14.1. *Continued*

	Psychosocial functioning domain	Type of measure	Length of administration	Validated	Need for training	Available languages	For more information
ILSS (Wallace et al., 2000)	Independent living skills	Self-rated and informant-rated	30–60 minutes	Multiple studies; both a hospital and a community version exist	No training necessary.	English, French, Spanish and Portuguese (Brazilian)	*www.psychrehab.com*
AMPS (Fisher, 1993)	Independent living skills	Observational task	30–40 minutes	Validated in many countries, not just for people with severe mental illness (e.g., head injury, dementia, and intellectual deficiency)	Training is necessary; typically takes 5 days; designed to be administered by occupational therapists.	Dutch, Danish, English, French, Finnish, Slovenian, and Swedish	*www.ampsintl.com/*
SFS (Birchwood et al., 1990)	Social competence	Semistructured interview, and version for family members	20–30 minutes for each version	Validated with clients living in the community and their family members	No training is necessary to conduct the interview though some might be needed to score the results; a detailed scoring manual is provided.	English Spanish, German, Italian, and Chinese (also perhaps Japanese)	Contact *m,j,birchwood.20@ bham.ac.uk*
AIPSS (Donahoe et al., 1990)	Social competence	Role-play and video assessment	Average of 90 minutes	Validated with people with severe mental illness in various studies. Inpatients and outpatients.	Some training is needed to score the client's performance.	Has been used in multiple countries; only the English version is available by the author	Contact *Clyde.Donahoe@med.va. gov*
BECES (Corbière et al., 2004)	Vocational functioning	Self-rated or interview	15–30 minutes	Validated with clients registered in vocational programs.	No need for training.	English and French	Contact *marc.corbiere @usherbrooke.ca*
WBI (Bryson et al., 1997)	Vocational functioning	Observational measure that includes employer/ supervisor interview	15-minute behavioral observation plus a brief interview with employer or supervisor	Validated with working clients.	Some training (brief) is needed. Comes with a manual.	English	Contact *gary.bryson@med.va.gov*

140

The instrument has 17 items. The measure was developed by mental health professionals to assess individuals with severe and persistent mental illness. The higher the score, the more autonomous the person is considered. The MCAS allows us to assess different functioning domains over time and is fairly brief to fill out, but it only considers the clinician's input. Therefore, it can be useful for research, management, or program evaluations, but it is less useful clinically than measures that include more than one perspective, including the client's.

Client Assessment of Strengths, Interests, and Goals

The Client Assessment of Strengths, Interests, and Goals—Self-Report and Informant Versions (CASIG-SR and CASIG-I; Wallace, Lecomte, Wilde, & Liberman, 2001) is a comprehensive assessment of functioning that addresses most psychiatric rehabilitation treatment domains, namely, community living skills, cognitive skills, medication practices (compliance and side effects), quality of life and treatment, symptoms, consumer rights, and unacceptable community behaviors. Each scale ends with a goal question pertaining to that domain. The assessment also elicits goals in five broad areas (Residence, Financial, Relationships, Religion/Spirituality, and Physical and Mental Health) with open-ended questions. The CASIG assesses multiple outcomes relevant to clients and clinicians that focus on strengths and skills. It is capable of assessing changes over time (can be re-administered every 3 months) and includes multiple perspectives of family members, clinicians, and clients. The CASIG is ideal for treatment planning and assessing change over time in goals and skills. It is, however, considered time-consuming to administer.

Camberwell Assessment of Need

The Camberwell Assessment of Need (CAN; Phelan et al., 1995) measures level of difficulty and level of assistance needed in 22 areas of functioning, including housing, food, cleaning, hygiene, daily activities, physical health, psychotic symptoms, treatment or illness information, psychological distress, personal security, social security, security of others, alcohol, drugs, social relationships, emotional relationships, sexual life, care of children, education, financial tasks use of the telephone, and use of public transportation. The client and his or her clinician independently rate both the client's difficulty in functioning and the assistance provided to the respondent in each of the 22 areas (essentially one question per area). These two ratings are combined to yield one of three possible responses per area; (1) no difficulties, (2) no important difficulties, thanks to someone's intervention, or (3) important difficulties. This questionnaire covers many basic functioning areas in a general way (problem or no problem), rather than in depth. It does, however, cover more domains than most instruments, offers the advantage of two versions (clinician and client), and can be used at multiple time points.

DOMAIN-SPECIFIC ASSESSMENTS
OF PSYCHOSOCIAL FUNCTIONING

Independent Living Skills

Independent Living Skills Survey

The Independent Living Skills Survey (ILSS; Wallace, Liberman, Tauber, & Wallace, 2000) measures basic functional living skills in the past 30 days in the following areas: appearance/

clothing, personal hygiene, care of personal possessions, food preparation/storage, health maintenance, money management, transportation, leisure and community, job seeking, job maintenance, eating, and social relations. It is very useful for a thorough assessment of independent living skills. Most of the scales are also present in the CASIG, though the CASIG takes longer to administer, because it covers goals and other domains as well.

Assessment of Motor and Process Skills

The Assessment of Motor and Process Skills (AMPS; Fisher, 1993) is an observational assessment used to measure the quality of a person's activities of daily living (ADL) according to 16 motor and 20 process skills rated on effort, efficiency, safety, and independence. It involves having the person evaluated perform two or three personal or domestic tasks that he or she has had prior experience performing (e.g., pouring a glass of juice, making a bed, preparing eggs) from among a subset of culturally relevant and appropriately challenging tasks. The person chooses which tasks to perform. The AMPS is useful for clients who are more difficult to assess verbally. The tasks are designed to assess daily living skills, as well as motor skills, and some cognitive deficits. The AMPS is mostly recommended for settings that offer individually tailored occupational therapy treatments.

Social Competence

Social Functioning Scale

The Social Functioning Scale (SFS; Birchwood, Smith, Cochrane, Wetton, & Copestake, 1990) assesses social competence with seven subscales: Withdrawal/Social Engagement, Interpersonal Communication, Independence–Performance, Independence–Competence, Recreation, Prosocial, and Employment/Occupation. A scoring scale is provided for each subscale and allows identification of problem areas. Each scale is rated in various ways (Likert scales, ratings from 0 to 100, yes–no answers, straight answers (e.g., number of friends?). It covers in detail many aspects of social competence and is designed to assess change over time, particularly following clinical interventions, such as family therapy. The SFS offers the advantage of choice between two versions. The anchor points and scales might seem to some a bit confusing or questionable.

Assessment of Interpersonal Problem Solving Skills

The Assessment of Interpersonal Problem Solving Skills (AIPSS; Donahoe et al., 1990) assesses interpersonal problem solving in a behavioral manner through role playing. Videotaped vignettes describe 10 problematic situations and three neutral ones. The client must correctly solve the problem (when applicable) and is rated according to six aspects: (1) identifying whether there is a problem; (2) defining the problem; (3) processing the information to generate a solution; (4) verbal content of the client's response; (5) performance level of the role play according to verbal and nonverbal cues; and (6) overall quality of the role play. It is particularly useful for determining the need for or effects of a skills training intervention. The *in vivo* aspect of this assessment enables the clinician to observe the behaviors directly rather than simply relying on self-report.

Vocational Functioning

Most vocational outcomes can be assessed without using specific questionnaires. The most common vocational outcomes are whether or not the person is employed, whether or not employment is competitive, number of hours worked per week, wages earned, number of weeks the person has had the job, and whether the job provides benefits, such as medical insurance.

Barriers to Employment and Coping Efficacy Scale

The Barriers to Employment and Coping Efficacy Scale (BECES; Corbière, Mercier, & Lesage, 2004) assesses 43 potential barriers to work integration mentioned by people with mental illness seeking a job, along with perceived self-efficacy in overcoming the barriers. For each barrier, participants are first asked to what extent "in their current situation, could this item represent a barrier to employment?" Participants are also asked to evaluate the extent to which they feel able to overcome this barrier. People can perceive barriers to employment, yet feel able to overcome them. When clients encounter difficulties in overcoming barriers, their job coach or counselor can intervene by guiding them toward solutions or strategies.

Work Behavior Inventory

The Work Behavior Inventory (WBI; Bryson, Bell, Lysaker, & Zito, 1997) is a 36-item assessment that measures work performance with the following five subscales: Work Habits, Work Quality, Personal Presentation, Cooperativeness, and Social Skills. The WBI is very useful for job coaches or vocational rehabilitation specialists who wish to offer precise and useful support to their clients who are working. This measure is not appropriate for settings in which the clients do not wish to disclose to their employer that they have a severe mental illness diagnosis, because the assessment needs to be completed by the employer.

KEY POINTS

- Psychosocial functioning assessments are an important aspect of treatment planning and outcomes evaluation.
- When choosing the right measure, clinicians should consider multiple factors, including the purpose of the assessment, its psychometric properties, with whom it was validated, and the length of administration.
- Psychosocial functioning assessments can be grouped into three larger categories: global measures, comprehensive measures, and domain-specific measures.
- Global measures of psychosocial functioning often give one general score, include symptoms as well as functioning, and are mostly for large-scale health services or administrative studies rather than for specific clinical use.
- Comprehensive measures of psychosocial functioning assess multiple aspects of psychosocial functioning in a more detailed manner and are quite relevant clinically.
- Domain-specific assessments cover in depth a single aspect of psychosocial functioning, such as independent living skills, social competence, or vocational functioning, and can be very useful clinically for those with specific goals or needs in those domains.

REFERENCES AND RECOMMENDED READINGS

American Psychiatric Association. (1994). *Diagnostic and statistical manual of mental disorders* (4th ed.). Washington, DC: Author.

Barker, S., & Barron, N. (1997). *Multnomah Community Ability Scale: User's manual.* Portland, OR: Network Behavioral Health Care.

Birchwood, M., Smith, J., Cochrane, R., Wetton, S., & Copestake, S. (1990). The Social Functioning Scale: The development and validation of a new scale of social adjustment for use in family intervention programmes with schizophrenic patients. *British Journal of Psychiatry, 157,* 853–859.

Bryson, G., Bell, M. D., Lysaker, P., & Zito, W. (1997). The Work Behavior Inventory: A scale for the assessment of work behavior for people with severe mental illness. *Psychiatric Rehabilitation Journal, 20*(4), 47–55.

Corbière, M., Mercier, C., & Lesage, A. D. (2004). Perceptions of barriers to employment, coping efficacy, and career search efficacy in people with mental health problems. *Journal of Career Assessment, 12*(4), 460–478.

Donahoe, C. P., Carer, M. J., Bloem, W. D., Leff, G. L., Laasi, N., & Wallace, C. J. (1990). Assessment of Interpersonal Problem Solving Skills. *Psychiatry, 53,* 329–339.

Fisher, A. G. (1993). The assessment of IADL motor skills: An application of many-faceted Rasch analysis. *American Journal of Occupational Therapy, 47,* 319–329.

Eisen, S. V., Dill, D. L., & Grob, M. C. (1994). Reliability and validity of a brief patient-report instrument for psychiatric outcome evaluation. *Hospital and Community Psychiatry, 45,* 242–247.

Hall, R. C. W. (1995). Global Assessment of Functioning: A modified scale. *Psychosomatics, 36,* 267–275.

Phelan, M., Slade, M., Thornicroft, G., Dunn, G., Holloway, F., Wykes, T., et al. (1995). The Camberwell Assessment of Need: The validity and reliability of an instrument to assess the needs of people with severe mental illness. *British Journal of Psychiatry, 167*(5), 589–595.

Wallace, C. J., Lecomte, T., Wilde, J., & Liberman, R. P. (2001). CASIG: A consumer-centered assessment for planning individualized treatment and evaluating program outcomes. *Schizophrenia Research, 50,* 105–109.

Wallace, C. J., Liberman, R. P., Tauber, R., & Wallace, J. (2000). The Independent Living Skills Survey: A comprehensive measure of the community functioning of severely and persistently mentally ill individuals. *Schizophrenia Bulletin, 26*(3), 631–658.

Ware, J. E., Jr., & Sherbourne, C. D. (1992). The MOS 36-Item Short-Form Health Survey (SF-36): I. Conceptual framework and item selection. *Medical Care, 30*(6), 473–483.

CHAPTER 15

TREATMENT PLANNING

ALEXANDER L. MILLER
DAWN I. VELLIGAN

Much of this chapter is devoted to discussion of specifics of treatment planning. By way of introduction, however, we pose a series of questions that consider the rationale for and elements of treatment planning.

WHAT IS A TREATMENT PLAN?

A treatment plan is a document that relates treatments to desired outcomes (goals). To be operationally useful, the plan should specify how progress toward goals will be measured. For example, the goal of competitive employment might have days worked per quarter as a measure of progress. The treatment plan needs to cover all the areas that treatments are intended to affect. Goals should be specific and, where necessary, sequentially staged.

WHY HAVE A TREATMENT PLAN?

Schizophrenia is a chronic, multifaceted illness. Treatment responsibilities are typically divided among multiple providers, and priorities shift according to phase of illness. Treatments interact with one another and with life events (e.g., loss of stable housing likely impacts medication adherence). Providers come and go. Patients change treatment locations. Without a written record that pulls together the totality of treatments, their purposes, and their results, each provider tends to operate in a silo, attending to only one aspect of the illness, unaware of how that aspect fits and interacts with the rest of the picture. Thus, a dynamic treatment plan should be a mechanism for providing integrated, coordinated treatment over time.

145

WHO CREATES THE TREATMENT PLAN?

The treatment plan is a synthetic document that incorporates the goals of the treatment team and of the patient. Substantial research has shown that patient participation in treatment planning and decision making improves outcomes. It is essential that the treatment plan capture the goals and aspirations of the patient, as well as those of his or her treatment team. Patient goals are typically not framed in medical terms, such as absence of psychotic symptoms, but are expressed as desired functional outcomes ("working," "married," etc.). A critical aspect of creating and reshaping the treatment plan is to bring patient and treatment team goals into alignment with one another. When patients see a relationship between, for example, reducing symptoms by taking medication regularly and achieving their own goals in life, they are more likely to adopt the treatment team goals relative to medication adherence.

HOW ARE TREATMENT PLAN ELEMENTS PRIORITIZED?

One can think of treatment plan goals along different dimensions, such as urgency, criticality, and feasibility. Urgent goals typically deal with acute problems, such as decompensation or living situation difficulties, and take precedence over long-term goals, because progress on long-term goals does not occur until the urgent problems are resolved. Critical goals are those that form the building blocks for achievement of other goals. Earning a general equivalency degree (GED), for example, may be a critical goal en route to a particular employment goal. Whereas urgent goals usually deal with critical issues, critical goals are not necessarily urgent. Much of the work of formulating the long-term treatment plan goes into achieving treatment team and patient consensus about critical steps on the paths toward long-term goals. Criticality changes both with illness stage (stable vs. unstable) and with progress along goal paths, requiring ongoing reassessment. Feasibility (achievability) of treatment plan goals must also be factored into decisions about how to prioritize use of time and resources. There is nothing wrong with having lofty aims, but a compilation of unattainable goals is an invitation to discouragement with and abandonment of the treatment planning process. When goals are very remote in time or seemingly beyond the patient's present capabilities, it is important to establish intermediate goals—logical steps along the way that are within reach. Ultimately, decisions about prioritization of treatment plan elements need to be made by a team leader who knows the plan and the patient well, and who has decision-making authority.

WHEN SHOULD THE TREATMENT PLAN BE CHANGED?

Treatment plan changes are prompted by one of two events: (1) change in patient status, or (2) availability of relevant new treatments or knowledge about existing treatments. Treatment plan changes most often occur at team meetings, with provider and patient input. If the document and plan are to be dynamic, however, they should reflect current realities rather than catching up with them weeks or months later. This means that it should be the task of one treatment team member to update the treatment plan in real time. Electronic medical records on computer networks greatly simplify the logistics of changing the treatment plan and communicating it to other treatment team members.

WHAT DOES A TREATMENT PLAN LOOK LIKE?

There is no standard treatment plan format, but if a treatment plan is to be a useful tool for communication, then it should contain key elements of information in visually accessible form. Table 15.1 presents a suggested template with two examples of problems and interventions. Even in systems without electronic medical records, we suggest creating and storing the treatment plan electronically and designating one person to be responsible for keeping it current and putting the latest version in the medical record.

TREATMENT PLAN DEVELOPMENT

Appropriate use of evidence-based and promising practices is at the core of treatment planning. That is to say, practices supported by good scientific evidence are key tools of treatment plan implementation. The potential value of each practice for an individual patient tends to change over time, with the exception of antipsychotic medication, which should be consistently maintained as treatment for chronic schizophrenia. A list of practices with one or more controlled trials is in Table 15.2. Evidence-based practices are those for which two or more independent randomized controlled trials have shown evidence of efficacy. Other practices that show promise have not yet attained this level of evidence. Other chapters in this book review the evidence for many of these practices. Cognitive adaptation training (CAT) is a relatively new treatment that promotes desired behaviors by restructuring the patient's living environment and by providing external prompts and cues (e.g., to take medication).

It is useful to characterize treatment goals in terms of the applicable practices. Table 15.3 lists problem areas frequently encountered in schizophrenia treatment and practices that have evidence for effectiveness in each area. *Proven* efficacy means that there is at least one randomized controlled trial and that results are unambiguous. In a couple of instances, ineffective treatments are listed because they have historically been widely used, but controlled trials have shown them to not be useful compared to the effective treatments listed.

The choice of which practice to use, when there is more than one choice, is determined by the patient's condition and local availability of the intervention. Not every patient care setting is able to make all these practices available to all patients for whom they are suitable. Under these circumstances we suggest that it is preferable to include the practice in the treatment plan and document its lack of availability. This illustrates aware-

TABLE 15.1. Treatment Plan Example

Problem	Intervention(s)	Measure	Goal	Start date	Expected goal achievement date	Responsible person	Contact information
Psychosis	Drug A	Brief Positive Symptom Scale	Reduction to no more than mild symptoms	2-14-07	5-10-07	Dr. Jones	555-5555
Repeated hospitalizations	Assertive community treatment	Days in hospital per year	Reduction of > 50% compared to prior year	1-15-07	4-14-07	Ms. Smith	123-4567

TABLE 15.2. Evidence-Based and Promising Practices for Treatment of Schizophrenia

1. Medications
2. Psychosocial approaches
   a. Cognitive-behavioral therapy (CBT)
   b. Compliance therapy/motivational interviewing/shared decision making
   c. Cognitive remediation
   d. Social skills training
   e. Assertive community treatment (ACT)
   f. Cognitive adaptation training (CAT)
   g. Supported employment
   h. Family therapies
   i Integrated dual-diagnosis treatment
   j. Supported housing

ness of the potential value of the practice for the patient and, cumulatively, is a basis for estimating the need for the practice, if resources can be channeled into providing it.

MEDICATION TREATMENT PLANNING

There is general agreement that antipsychotics are mainstays in the treatment of chronic schizophrenia, and that psychotic symptoms are their primary target. Often, however, treatment plans do not specify how symptoms will be measured, or which side effects will be assessed and how often. In addition, explication of the rationale for choosing a particular antipsychotic and discussion of possible alternatives in the event of poor responses occur infrequently. The value of including these items is that they help lay out a road map for treatment to guide other prescribers who see the patient in other settings, or when the primary prescriber is absent, or if the primary prescriber ceases seeing the patient for whatever reason. It is a common and frustrating experience to see a patient on a complex medication regimen for the first time and not be able to discern why the regimen is being used and whether it is producing better results than prior, simpler treatment programs.

Many persons with schizophrenia have coexisting conditions and symptoms that warrant treatment with other medications, such as antidepressants, antianxiety agents, and sedative–hypnotics. Use of these medications for appropriate indications is completely warranted and desirable. It is, however, a common observation that, once started, these adjunctive medications are continued indefinitely. A key part of medication treatment planning is ongoing review of the entire medication regimen, with the goal of discontinuing medications that are no longer needed. Simplification of the medication regimen enhances adherence, decreases the likelihood of undesirable side effects and drug–drug interactions, and reduces costs.

Many practitioners and organizations choose to follow a recent medication guideline or algorithm for schizophrenia. This approach takes advantage of the expert knowledge and opinions that have gone into construction of the algorithm or guideline and helps define the sequence of medications to be used in the event of inadequate response. Moreover, when followed by a clinic or group of providers, it brings desirable consistency to medication management across time and patients. Some recent guidelines and algorithms are listed in Table 15.4, with comments about their content and utility.

Implementation of a guideline or algorithm requires that there be enough specificity in the recommendations that a prescriber can apply them to specific patient care circum-

TABLE 15.3. Matching Practices with Problem Areas in Treating Schizophrenia

Problem area	Proven efficacy	Possible efficacy	Not efficacious
Positive symptoms	Antipsychotic, CBT (added)		Individual psychodynamic psychotherapy
Negative symptoms		Antipsychotic, social skills training	
Cognitive deficits		Cognitive remediation, antipsychotic	
Social/family	Family therapies, social skills training		
Occupational/school	Supported employment		Sheltered workshops
Activities of daily living (ADLs)	CAT, independent living skills training		
Housing	Supported housing		
Substance abuse	Integrated dual diagnosis treatment, medications specific to category of abused substance (e.g., methadone)		
Depression	Antidepressants, CBT		
Anxiety	Antianxiety medications	Antipsychotic	
Medication adherence	Behavioral tailoring	CAT, compliance therapy/ motivational interviewing/ shared decision making/ regimen simplification	
Relapses/ rehospitalizations	ACT, CAT, family therapies, antipsychotic	Relapse prevention training	

stances. Documentation needs to be detailed enough that a reviewer can determine whether the recommendations are being followed. Documentation in over half of medical records that are not structured to capture the elements being rated has repeatedly been found to be inadequate to rate prescriber adherence to medication guidelines. Thus, guideline implementation includes restructuring medical records to prompt recording of the necessary information to judge whether the guideline is being used. Examples of documentation geared to implementation of a specific guideline or algorithm can be found in the appendices at *www.dshs.state.tx.us/mhprograms/timasczman.pdf.*

Medication algorithms and guidelines should not be confused with standards of care. They are recommendations for typical patients. Individual patient characteristics and clinical judgment ultimately determine whether it is appropriate to apply the algorithm or guideline in individual situations.

PLANNING PSYCHOSOCIAL INTERVENTIONS

Consumer-Centered Plan

One of the most important aspects of planning successful psychosocial treatment is to ensure that the goals and objectives of the consumer lie at the center of the plan. Each spe-

TABLE 15.4. Recent Medication Algorithms/Guidelines for Schizophrenia

Algorithm/guideline	Content	Utility
Practice Guideline for the Treatment of Patients with Schizophrenia (American Psychiatric Association, 2004)	Comprehensive literature review, some sequence recommendations.	Not manualized. No specific measures of or criteria for "response."
Expert Consensus Guidelines (McEvoy, Scheifler, & Frances, 1999)	Based on expert consensus around case examples. Defined sequence of antipsychotic choices, up to clozapine.	Not manualized. No specific measures of or criteria for "response."
International Psychopharmacology Algorithm Project (IPAP) (*www.ipap.org*)	Expert consensus. Defined sequence of antipsychotic choices, up to clozapine. Links to specific recommendations based on individual side effects and associated symptoms.	Interactive website. Discussions with references go with each problem area and recommendation. No specific measures of or criteria for "response."
Patient Outcomes Research Team (PORT) (Lehman et al., 2004)	Set of recommendations based solely on results of randomized controlled trials (RCTs).	Not manualized. Limited in scope to questions addressed by RCTs. Good basis for quality control measures.
Texas Medication Algorithm Project (TMAP) (Moore et al., 2007)	Expert consensus. Defined sequence of antipsychotic choices, including clozapine failures/refusals.	Manual on website. Specific symptom rating scales and criteria for "response." Forms for documentation.

cific goal of the plan should link back to one of the consumer's stated goals. Goals often expressed by consumers include a desire to obtain work or return to school, to find a girl-friend, or to get along better with family members. Although some goals are not immediately attainable for a specific client (e.g., returning to work), each goal included in the treatment plan may be viewed as a stepping-stone toward the individual's ultimate ambition. All too often, treatment goals (e.g., medication adherence, grooming) are imposed because members of the treatment team are convinced that such goals are in the best interests of the client. Although the treatment team's view may be accurate, clients must endorse treatment plan goals as their own. If the treatment team's goal can be tightly linked with what the client wants, progress toward the goal is more likely.

Assessment of Psychosocial Issues

The development of a good treatment plan for psychosocial functioning requires a detailed assessment of the client's residual symptomatology, medication adherence, and social and environmental context. In addition, the consumer's ability to perform ADLs, to interact socially, and to work need to be examined to identify appropriate targets for intervention.

Targets of the Psychosocial Treatment Plan and Potential Treatments

Medication Adherence

Many aspects of the patient's functioning can be targeted by psychosocial treatment. Given the vast array of potential treatment targets, it is important to prioritize goals.

Poor adherence to oral antipsychotic medication leads to relapses, derails the process of recovery, and contributes to the high cost of treating schizophrenia. With this in mind, it is important to ensure good adherence to medication. Medication adherence is important in determining whether the selected treatment is effective, whether there should be dosage adjustments, and whether concomitant medications should be added. Because prescribers typically are not able to identify accurately how much of the prescribed medication an individual is taking, decisions about medication changes are often made with little or no accurate data. To optimize treatment, adherence is extremely important. However, medication adherence is infrequently a client-stated goal. Linking medication adherence to staying out of the hospital, getting along better with family, and other client-identified goals is essential in making adherence an objective of the treatment plan. The use of motivational interviewing can be helpful in raising the client's awareness of the need for medication, and in dealing with his or her ambivalence regarding taking medication. However, the intention to take medication is not the same as adherence. Forgetting, failure to establish routines consistent with taking medication, and chaotic environments contribute to problem adherence even when the consumer is very willing to take medication. Environmental adaptations such as signs, alarms, and pill containers may be used to prompt and to cue the client to take medications as prescribed. A thorough assessment of how the client remembers to take medication, where medication is kept, and an understanding of when missed doses occur can assist in planning strategies to enhance adherence. In-home interventions to promote medication adherence are part of the CAT intervention.

Positive Symptoms

Antipsychotic medications may reduce but not eliminate the positive symptoms of schizophrenia. Hallucinations and delusions often continue and may cause a substantial amount of distress to clients. Cognitive-behavioral approaches are designed to address these enduring psychotic symptoms by helping clients to examine evidence for their perceived power and origins ("What is the evidence that the voice is that of the Devil?"), and to alter cognitive attributions associated with these symptoms, so that the symptoms, although present, create less distress. CBT can be a helpful adjunct to medication treatment.

Negative Symptoms

Negative symptoms such as amotivation, asociality, and poverty of speech and movement are predictive of poor community outcomes for patients with schizophrenia. Targeting negative symptoms is important in improving outcomes for these individuals. There are no available psychosocial treatments designed specifically with negative symptoms as the primary target. However, a variety of treatments may lead to decreases in negative symptoms on standard assessments. Interventions that engage individuals' participation and increase functioning, ADLs, or leisure and recreational skills may lead to decreased negative symptom scores.

Cognitive Functioning

Deficits in psychomotor speed, attention, memory, and planning characterize individuals with schizophrenia. Evidence suggests that these cognitive impairments may underlie deficits in social and role functioning. Cognitive remediation (CR) techniques seek to improve cognitive functions directly, utilizing a variety of pen-and-paper or computerized tests requiring attention, planning, problem-solving, and memory skills. Several models of remediation are currently being studied. Some CR interventions provide individual treatment, whereas others are conducted in small group settings. There is emerging evidence that CR may improve cognitive functioning, and that these improvements may generalize to broader outcomes, such as improvements in social functioning and work-related performance.

Social Functioning/Family Interaction

Many patients complain about difficulty in making friends, initiating conversations, following complex social interactions, and solving interpersonal problems with friends or family members. Social skills can be improved by formal social skills training. Training focuses on helping the patient to maintain appropriate nonverbal behavior (e.g., eye contact, voice volume), to learn standard techniques to initiate and maintain conversations, and strategies to solve interpersonal problems. Although social skills may improve with social skills training, additional work may need to address the client's often limited opportunity to use newly developed skills in the home environment.

Family Interventions

Families may not know where to turn or what to do when a relative is diagnosed with schizophrenia. Family psychoeducation helps family members to learn about the diagnosis, symptoms, warning signs of relapse, and the purpose and side effects of medication. Key information for family members includes understanding the need for continued medication even when their relative's symptoms have been minimized. Psychoeducation can be helpful in decreasing the risk for relapse or rehospitalization. Other family programs, such as behavioral family management, train family members to communicate better, to solve problems with their ill relative, and to decrease stresses that may lead to relapse. Finally, many family members become expert at how to help their relative to manage schizophrenia. Their expertise is often shared in self-help groups, such as those run by the National Alliance on Mental Illness (NAMI). Relatives often have sound advice regarding symptom control, medication, and providers. Many NAMI organizations provide psychoeducation and host workshops conducted by experts on various topics related to mental health. These resources can help the family to help the patient.

Activities of Daily Living

Individuals with schizophrenia are impaired relative to age-matched control subjects on a variety of independent living skills. Problems with grooming and hygiene, care of living quarters, and shopping and budgeting are important targets for intervention. When these important aspects of everyday functioning are not attended to, problems can magnify. For example, poor money management may lead to problems paying for needed medication. Improving specific ADLs may be required before work or social function can be improved. For example, it is very difficult for someone with poor grooming and hygiene to get a job or a girlfriend. Independent living skills can be taught in groups or in one-on-one sessions. Teaching these skills in the consumer's home environment is preferable to teaching that occurs in a clinic setting, because generalization of skills from clinic to home environments may not occur without direct training in the home. An in-home intervention such as CAT uses environmental supports (signs, alarms, pill containers, hygiene supplies, and organization of belongings) in the patient's home to improve everyday functioning. These supports cue and sequence appropriate behaviors (e.g., bathing) and discourage inappropriate behavior (e.g., taking extra medication).

Occupational/School Functioning

Despite the fact that only 10–20% of individuals with schizophrenia hold jobs in the competitive marketplace, many consumers have a desire to work. Obstacles to work, including disincentives based on the fear of losing disability benefits, can be formidable. For some consumers, rather than competitive employment, the goal is volunteer work for a few hours weekly, whereas for others it is part- or full-time employment in the competitive marketplace. Supported employment programs emphasize rapid job search for consumers with a stated preference to work. Although supported employment is very successful at getting consumers working, job tenure typically lasts only a few months on average, with as many as 50% of patients who attain work having unsatisfactory job terminations. Using job coaches and environmental supports such as tape-recorded instructions, checklists, and alarms may help improve consumers' job performance and tenure.

For consumers who may be reluctant to try or who cannot access supported employment programs, it may be best to include small steps toward increased community involvement in the treatment plan to build their confidence. This might begin with following an agreed-upon schedule (waking at a specific time, showering, etc.). It may be helpful to aid the consumer to engage in volunteer work for a few hours weekly and gradually increase the number of hours, until volunteer work is at least part time. These steps can help the person to develop the necessary skills, discipline, and self-confidence to enter supported employment and to work successfully in the competitive marketplace.

Housing

As many as 15% of patients with schizophrenia are homeless. Without stable and safe housing it is difficult for these individuals to keep track of medications and appointments, to perform behaviors that require a routine, and to feel comfortable in their surroundings. In addition, homelessness is associated with higher use of psychiatric inpatient care and emergency room services. In some communities, programs provide for temporary housing until individuals obtain the benefits that pay for a stable living environment.

Living environments for individuals with schizophrenia vary in terms of the structure they provide. In some residential facilities, complete care is provided, such that consumers are responsible only for keeping up their area of a shared bedroom. Medication is provided, all meals are prepared, and cleaning and laundry are done by staff in these locations. Other residential facilities may require that residents share duties for cooking and cleaning. Some facilities do not provide transportation to medication appointments. It is important for the treatment team to be aware of these differences. Some consumers elect to live on their own in apartments, where family members may assist them, or where they are responsible for managing all tasks on their own. The level of structure in the living situation ideally should match the consumer's abilities. Because abilities may change over time or illness phase, reassessment at specific intervals should be considered. Group homes following the Fairweather Lodge Program that combine a shared living environment and a work program have been successful in helping consumers reach their potential for independent living.

Substance Abuse

Between 20 and 65% of individuals with schizophrenia have comorbid substance abuse disorders. Comorbid substance abuse increases the likelihood of poor adherence to medication and is associated with more severe symptoms, more frequent hospitalizations, and poorer prognosis. Although traditional 12-step programs such as Alcoholics Anonymous or Narcotic Anonymous may be helpful for some patients, available data suggest that outcomes are better for patients in programs that integrate mental health and substance abuse treatments. Successful treatments address motivational issues and teach individuals how to develop skills for recovery. A relatively new treatment that has shown promise for this group of patients, called behavioral treatment for substance abuse in schizophrenia, involves motivational interviewing to develop treatment goals; urinalysis contingency, in which social and small monetary reinforcement are provided for "clean" urine; social skills training aimed at providing patients the skills necessary to refuse drugs when offered and to develop friendships with those who do not use drugs; education about medications for psychiatric illness and how drugs affect the brain; and learning to cope with high-risk situations. This treatment has been found to decrease patients' substance use and increase the frequency of "clean" urine drug screens.

Additional common problems for individuals with schizophrenia include comorbid depression, anxiety, posttraumatic stress and obsessive–compulsive symptoms. Cognitive-behavioral approaches have been found to be effective with each of these syndromes in persons without schizophrenia. While it seems reasonable to extrapolate from these studies that this approach is efficacious in schizophrenia, studies to demonstrate this are lacking. Evidence is mixed for the usefulness of CBT for the treatment of depression associated with psychotic symptoms.

KEY POINTS

- Treatment plans should match specific treatments with individual needs and goals.
- Treatments are more successful when the individual participates in developing his or her treatment plan.
- Treatment plans should prioritize based on the urgency, criticality, and feasibility of specific treatment goals.
- Documentation of interventions and of their effects is critical to making rational changes in the treatment plan.
- The range of evidence-based practices and promising new treatments permits the creation of treatment plans that comprehensively address symptoms *and* problems in daily functioning in schizophrenia.

REFERENCES AND RECOMMENDED READINGS

American Psychiatric Association. (2004). *Practice guideline for the treatment of patients with schizophrenia* (2nd ed.). Washington, DC: Author.

Bond, G. R. (2004). Supported employment: Evidence for an evidence-based practice. *Psychiatric Rehabilitation Journal, 27,* 345–359.

Bell, M., Bryson, G., Greig, T., Corcoran, C., & Wexler, B. E. (2001). Neurocognitive enhancement therapy with work therapy: Effects on neuropsychological test performance. *Archives of General Psychiatry, 58*(8), 763–768.

Bellack, A. S. (2004). Skills training for people with severe mental illness. *Psychiatric Rehabilitation Journal, 27*(4), 375–391.

Bennett, M. E., Bellack, A. S., & Gearon, J. S. (2001). Treating substance abuse in schizophrenia: An initial report. *Journal of Substance Abuse Treatment, 20*(2), 163–175.

Dolder, C. R., Lacro, J. P., Leckband, S., & Jeste, D. V. (2003). Interventions to improve antipsychotic medication adherence: Review of recent literature. *Journal of Clinical Psychopharmacology, 23*(4), 389–399.

Drake, R., & Mueser, K. T. (2000). Psychosocial approaches to dual diagnosis. *Schizophrenia Bulletin, 26,* 105–118.

Drake, R. E., Becker, D. R., & Bond, G. R. (2003). Recent research on vocational rehabilitation for persons with severe mental illness. *Current Opinion in Psychiatry, 16*(4), 451–455.

Drake, R. E., Mueser, K. T., Brunette, M. F., & McHugo, G. J. (2004). A review of treatments for clients with severe mental illness and co-occurring substance use disorder. *Psychiatric Rehabilitation Journal, 27,* 360–374.

Folsom, D. P., Hawthorne, W., Lindamer, L., Gilmer, T., Bailey, A., Golshan, S., et al. (2005). Prevalence and risk factors for homelessness and utilization of mental health services among 10,340 patients with serious mental illness in a large public mental health system. *American Journal of Psychiatry, 162*(2), 370–376.

Keith, S. J., Matthews, S. M., & Schooler, N. R. (1991). A review of psychoeducational family approaches. In C. A. S. Tamminga & S. Charles (Eds.), *Schizophrenia research* (pp. 247–254). New York: Raven Press.

Lehman, A. F., Kreyenbuhl, J., Buchanan, R. W., Dickerson, F. B., Dixon, L. B., Goldberg, R., et al. (2004). The Schizophrenia Patient Outcomes Research Team (PORT): Updated treatment recommendations 2003. *Schizophrenia Bulletin, 30,* 193–217.

Lehman, A. F., Lieberman, J., Dixon, L. B., McGlashan, T. H., Miller, A., Perkins, D., et al. (2004). Practice guideline for the treatment of patients with schizophrenia, second edition. *American Journal of Psychiatry, 161*(Suppl. 2), 1–56.

McEvoy, J. P., Scheifler, P. L., & Frances, A. (Eds.). (1999). The Expert Consensus Guidelines: Treatment of schizophrenia, *Journal of Clinical Psychiatry, 60*(Suppl. 11).

Miller, A., Chiles, J. A., Chiles, J. K., Crismon, M. D., Shon, S. P., & Rush, A. J. (1999). The TMAP Schizophrenia Algorithms. *Journal of Clinical Psychiatry, 60*(10), 649–657.

Moore, T. A., Buchanan, R. W., Buckley, P. F., Chiles, J. A., Conley, R. R., Crismon, M. L., et al. (2007). The Texas Medication Algorithm Project antipsychotic algorithm for schizophrenia: 2006 update. *Journal of Clinical Psychiatry, 68,* 1751–1762.

Mueser, K. T., Corrigan, P. W., Hilton, D., Tanzman, B., Schaub, A., Gingerich, S., et al. (2002). Illness management and recovery for severe mental illness: A review of the research. *Psychiatric Services, 53,* 1272–1284.

O'Donnell, C., Donohoe, G., Sharkey, L., Owens, N., Migone, M., Harries, R., et al. (2003). Compliance therapy: A randomised controlled trial in schizophrenia. *British Medical Journal, 327,* 1–4.

Phillips, S. D., Burns, B. J., Edgar, E. R., Mueser, K. T., Linkins, K. W., Rosenheck, R. A., et al. (2001). Moving assertive community treatment into standard practice. *Psychiatric Services, 52,* 771–779.

Tarrier, N., & Wykes, T. (2004). Is there evidence that cognitive behaviour therapy is an effective treatment for schizophrenia?: A cautious or cautionary tale? *Behaviour Research and Therapy, 42*(12), 1377–1401.

Velligan, D. I., Bow-Thomas, C. C., Huntzinger, C. D., Ritch, J., Ledbetter, N., Prihoda, T. J., et al. (2000). Randomized controlled trial of the use of compensatory strategies to enhance adaptive functioning in outpatients with schizophrenia. *American Journal of Psychiatry, 157*(8), 1317–1323.

Velligan, D. I., Lam, F., Ereshefsky, L., & Miller, A. L. (2003). Psychopharmacology: Perspectives on medication adherence and atypical antipsychotic medications. *Psychiatric Services, 54*(5), 665–667.

PART III

SOMATIC TREATMENT

CHAPTER 16

ANTIPSYCHOTICS

ERIC C. KUTSCHER

The treatment of schizophrenia has significantly evolved since the early 20th century. The discovery of chlorpromazine in 1954 helped shape the current pharmacological options in the treatment of schizophrenia. Although many medications target various subtypes of receptors, their general mechanisms of action are similar in that they decrease dopamine activity to some degree. Various treatment algorithms and guidelines exist to help direct practice by individualizing therapy, and utilization of these resources improves patient outcomes drastically.

This chapter is organized into various sections based on the classification of antipsychotic medications. Additionally, current treatment guideline recommendations for various aspects of the illness are discussed to provide a concise, evidence-based approach to decision making.

PHARMACOLOGICAL TREATMENT GOALS

Acute Illness

Oftentimes patients with schizophrenia are first seen in the acute hospitalization setting. Many patients present with thoughts of self-harm and agitation. During the initial states of the acute stabilization, many treatment goals should be achieved:

1. Reduce the potential for harm.
2. Decrease agitation and uncooperativeness.
3. Reduce the severity of the patient's positive symptoms.
4. Improve sleep and self-care issues.

During the first few days of acute stabilization, clinicians may administer many as-needed medications to control the patient's symptoms, realizing that improvement in the core features of schizophrenia will take 4–6 weeks (Table 16.1). However, this does not preclude the use of medications to control the acute symptoms. Patients should be encouraged to take oral medications prior to the administration of injectable medications. Treatment guidelines suggest that benzodiazepines and/or antipsychotic medications

TABLE 16.1. Time Course of Symptom Improvement in Response to Antipsychotic Treatment

First 5 days	Weeks 1–2	Weeks 3–6	Week 6 and beyond
• Agitation • Hostility • Aggression • Anxiety • Sleep • Eating patterns	• Socialization • Self-care/activities of daily living • Mood symptoms • Delusions and hallucinations become less bothersome	• Decreases in delusions and hallucinations • Improved interpersonal skills	• Minimal improvement in insight and judgment • Some delusions/hallucinations remain fixed

should be used in this phase. The recognized standard of care for acute psychosis with agitation is 5 mg of haloperidol and 2 mg of lorazepam, otherwise known by nursing staff as the "B-52 Bomber." This combination has been shown to be synergistic, and is preferable administration of the individual medications. Many of the second-generation antipsychotics, and one third-generation antipsychotic, that are available may provide adequate treatment of acute symptoms, including olanzapine, risperidone, quetiapine, ziprasidone, and aripiprazole, with less of a risk of adverse effects; these medications are discussed later in this chapter.

Stabilization

Once treatment goals for the acute phase have been achieved, the patient then progresses into the stabilization phase, which is the transition phase from hospitalization to the outpatient setting. The treatment goals of this phase are as follows:

1. Optimization of medications (decrease dosing frequency; stop as-needed medications; reduce medications, if needed, to reduce adverse effects).
2. Medication adherence education: Taking medications for 6 months after discharge can reduce the risk of relapse by 30% compared to not taking the medications as prescribed.
3. Insight therapy to help patients understand their illness and the necessity for medications.

This is the most important phase of treatment, because it directs the patients' care into the maintenance, or outpatient, phase. Medications should be optimized and patients should be educated about all of their medications to decrease the risk of nonadherence. Additionally, all adverse effects must be addressed; otherwise, patients are very unlikely to continue the medication after discharge from the hospital.

Maintenance

This phase of treatment is generally completed on an outpatient basis and is a continual process. Treatment goals should strive to improve patients' quality of life and social functioning, reduce adverse medication effects, improve medication adherence, and address all residual symptoms not addressed during hospitalization. It is important to remember that most medications take 4–6 weeks to achieve their full benefit. Relapse on average is 20% per year when patients are adherent with their medications; 5–15% of patients never have complete resolution of their symptoms with medications (Table 16.2). Guidelines suggest treatment with medications for at least 1–2 years after the first episode and for at least 5 years after subsequent episodes. Any patient who poses a danger to self or others should be treated indefinitely after the first episode.

MEDICATION DECISION MAKING

Various methods help to direct decisions about the utilization of antipsychotic medications. Some of the basic standards are as follows:

1. Utilize treatment guidelines (see References and Recommended Readings).
2. Utilize family history. If a family member has responded to a medication, then this may predict response in the patient.
3. Always involve the patient; informed patients are more adherent with prescribed medications.
4. Utilize the STEPS decision model, which looks at a multitude of factors to help decide on medications for specific patients. The following sequence helps the clinician choose medications for specific patients:

S: Safety. How safe are the medication choices for this patient?

T: Tolerability. What are the side effects, and how do they compare to side effects of other medications for this patient?

E: Efficacy. Are there efficacy differences between the medications that may suggest response in the patient?

P: Price. How much does this medication cost compared to alternative treatments, and can the patient afford these medications?

S: Simplicity. How complex is the regimen (multiple dosages per day may reduce medication adherence rates)?

ANTIPSYCHOTIC MEDICATIONS

Medications used to treat schizophrenia have been classified into many different categories. Two primary classes referred to in the literature are the typical and atypical antipsychotics. The typical antipsychotics include medications such as phenothiazines, butyrophenones, thioxanthenes, dihydroindolines, and dibenzoxazepines. The atypical

TABLE 16.2. Degree of Symptom Improvement with Antipsychotic Treatment

Symptoms	Percentage of patients that show improvement
Insight	10–15
Judgment	20–25
Sociability/interpersonal skills	40–45
Delusions	45–50
Appetite	50–55
Sleep	55–60
Negativism	55–60
Hallucinations	55–60
Tension/hostility	65–75
Combativeness	75–80

antipsychotics include clozapine, risperidone, olanzapine, quetiapine, ziprasidone, and aripiprazole. The term *atypical* originated from the idea that these medications reduce the risk of extrapyramidal side effects (EPS).

Most recently the classification of these medications has been changed based on pharmacology. The terms *first-generation antipsychotics* (FGAs), *second-generation antipsychotics* (SGAs), and *third-generation antipsychotics* (TGAs) have replaced *typical* and *atypical*. This newer classification is used in this chapter.

It is important to note that all antipsychotic medications have equal efficacy in the treatment of positive symptoms of schizophrenia when equally dosed, although responses of individual patients may vary. Dosing until side effects emerge without efficacy is not standard of practice. Subsets of research suggest that the utilization of clozapine provides better efficacy than all other antipsychotic medications in the treatment of refractory patients.

First-Generation Antipsychotics

These medications are oftentimes referred to as *typical* antipsychotic medications. They can be subclassified into low-potency, high-potency, and very-high-potency agents. This classification also helps clinicians understand the adverse effect profiles of these medications, which are discussed by Dolder in Chapter 17, this volume. All of these medications have a similar mechanism of action by antagonizing dopamine receptors in the mesolimbic pathway, subsequently decreasing positive symptoms. Additionally, various actions may cause bothersome adverse events. Potency levels provide a simplified explanation of the medications. The high-potency medications are for the most part pure dopamine receptor antagonists and have little to no other mechanisms. Whereas the low-potency medications are pure dopamine receptor antagonists, they also have other mechanisms to various degrees, including anticholinergic, calcium channel–blocking, alpha-blocking, and antihistamine properties.

Dosing of these medications should be conservative and take place once (preferred) to twice daily to avoid unwanted side effects. It is recommended that clinicians start at the lowest available dosage strength and increase the dosage as needed during the acute phase of the illness. Dosage minimization should be attempted once the patient has reached the stabilization phase of the illness. Equivalent dosing of FGA medications is provided in Table 16.3.

For patients with poor compliance two first-generation medications are available in a long-acting, intramuscular, injectable form. Haloperidol and fluphenazine are available as decanoate injections utilized every 4 weeks and every 1–3 weeks, respectively. Z-track intramuscular administration is required for both medications. Dosing of these medications is recommended only after the patient has been stabilized on oral medications to provide an adequate conversion to the long-acting formulation. Conversion from oral to decanoate therapy is recommended as follows.

Haloperidol Decanoate

Various strategies exist for dosing haloperidol decanoate. Loading dose and dose conversion strategies have been utilized. The first dose (load dose) starts at 20 times the oral dose, then 15 times for the second dose, and then 10 times for the third dose (dosing once a month). It is recommended, if the first dose is over 100 mg, to utilize two injections: always giving a test dose for the first injection, followed by a second injection 3–5 days later. Steady states of haloperidol decanoate are not reached for about 3 months, so a cross-taper from the oral medication is suggested, especially if the loading dose is not used.

TABLE 16.3. Dosing of the First-Generation Antipsychotics

	Dose range	Equivalent dosages (oral)	Half-life (hours)	Intramuscular dosing (short acting)
Low-potency agents				
Chlorpromazine (Thorazine)	200–2,000 mg	100 mg	3–40	25–50 mg
Thioridazine (Mellaril)	200–800 mg	100 mg	10–30	N/A
High-potency agents				
Loxapine (Loxitane)	10–250 mg	2 mg	6–8	N/A
Molindone (Moban)	10–225 mg	10 mg	2–6	N/A
Very-high-potency agents				
Haloperidol (Haldol)	5–40 mg	2 mg	15–30 (decanoate = 21 days)	2–10 mg
Fluphenazine (Prolixin)	5–60 mg	2 mg	8–32 (decanoate = 1–3 days)	2.5–10 mg
Perphenazine (Trilafon)	8–64 mg	10 mg	10–20	N/A
Thiothixine (Navane)	10–80 mg	2–5 mg	34	N/A
Trifluoperazine (Stelazine)	5–60 mg	5 mg	3–40	N/A

Note. Trade names are in parentheses.

Fluphenazine Decanoate

Conversion to the long-acting formulation is not well established due to variability of metabolism. There is a suggestion to take the total daily dose and multiply by 1.5 for the every 2-week injection amount, although there is no consensus on conversion from oral to deacanoate dosing established in the literature.

Second-Generation Antipsychotics

These medications, often referred to as *atypical* antipsychotics, have a similar mechanism of action in the treatment of schizophrenia. These agents functionally antagonize dopamine (D_2) receptors in the mesolimbic pathway and antagonize serotonin (5-HT_{2A}) receptors in the mesocortical pathway. The difference between these and the FGA medications is the specificity of the dopamine antagonism at recommended dosages and the serotonin activity. The serotonin antagonist activity is thought to increase dopamine activity in the frontal cortex, which potentially alleviates the negative symptoms of schizophrenia. These medications have various other minimal mechanisms, the most common of which is histamine antagonism.

Dosing of SGA medications should be conservative, but for many patients the target dose can be achieved in a few days. Additionally, these medications can be dosed once daily, with the exception of ziprasidone, which requires twice-daily dosing with food for increased absorption. Without food absorption, dosing is limited to 30–35% of the dose; with food, the patient will absorb upwards of 70% of the dose. Dose minimization should be attempted once the person has reached the stabilization phase of his or her illness. Equivalent dosing of second- and third-generation medications is provided in Table 16.4.

Clozapine is considered a medication for refractory illness, due to its side effect profile and monitoring parameters. Weekly white blood cell (WBC) counts are required for the first 6 months of treatment, then changed to every other week. If the patient has not had any significant WBC changes after 1 year, that person is eligible for every 4-week monitoring.

Clozapine utilization guidelines
(See guidelines provided with each specific clozapine product.)

- Failure of at least three antipsychotics, of which two must be second-generation agents.
- WBC $\geq$ 3,500/mm^3 required to start therapy; a very slow dose titration is required to avoid medication side effects.
- Any WBC changes by 3,000/mm^3 within a 3-week period must be evaluated.
- Any WBC below 2,000/mm^3 or an absolute neutrophil count below 1,000/mm^3 requires stopping clozapine.
- After discontinuation of clozapine, WBC should be monitored for 4 weeks.
- Therapeutic blood level is > 500 ng/dl and may take up to 6 months to achieve a full response.

For patients with poor compliance one second-generation medication is available in long-acting, intramuscular injectable form. Risperdal (risperidone) Consta is available and is dosed every 2 weeks. Z-track intramuscular administration is not required, but injections should rotate between alternating buttocks. Dosing of these medications is recommended only after the patient has been stabilized on oral medications to provide an adequate conversion to the long-acting formulation. Dosing guidelines suggest that oral risperidone should be continued for 3 weeks after the long-acting agent is started. This provides adequate blood level coverage until the injection starts to release from the injection site. Risperdal Consta uses a unique delivery system called Medisorb. This system encapsulates active medication into polymer-based microspheres that gradually release the drug at a controlled rate due to hydrolysis. Doses cannot be subdivided due to the formulation of this product. Steady state levels of the long-acting risperidone formulation are not achieved until about 8 weeks after the first injection. For conversion from oral risperidone to Risperdal Consta the following is recommended:

- 0–2 mg daily: 25 mg every 2 weeks intramuscularly.
- 2–4 mg daily: 50 mg every 2 weeks intramuscularly.
- Maximum recommended dosage of 50 mg every 2 weeks.

Third-Generation Antipsychotics

Aripiprazole is oftentimes referred to as an atypical antipsychotic, but current classification suggests this agent has a distinct mechanism and should be classified separately. Aripiprazole is unique in it mechanism of action compared to all other D_2 antipsychotic medications. This medication is a partial agonist at dopamine D_2 receptors in the mesolimbic pathway. This mechanism is believed to provide a constant dopamine signal of about 35%. This essentially correlates to either a reduction of dopamine transmission or an increase, depending on the occupancy of the receptor prior to aripiprazole therapy. Many clinicians refer to the medication as a "thermostat" for the D2 receptor. This medication also antagonizes 5-HT$_{2A}$ receptors in the mesocortical pathway, which is thought to increase dopamine activity in the frontal cortex and potentially alleviate the negative symptoms of schizophrenia. One additional mechanism is the partial antagonist activity at 5-HT$_{1A}$ receptors, which is similar to that of buspirone and may provide benefit for patients with anxiety symptoms. Dose minimization should be attempted once the person has reached the stabilization phase of the illness. Current research suggests that aripiprazole may be as effective as other antipsychotic medications, but conclusive data are not available at the current time. Equivalent dosing of this medication with SGA medications is provided in Table 16.4.

Basic Pharmacological Parameters of Antipsychotic Medications

The pharmacokinetics of all antipsychotics are summarized in the following general statements (differences may occur with specific medications and patients):

- All medications are highly lipophilic, which helps with fast central nervous system penetration.
- All medications are highly protein bound, which may limit central nervous system penetration.
- The majority of medications have long half-lives that allow once-daily dosing (see Tables 16.3 and 16.4).
- Most medications do not have established therapeutic blood concentrations.
- In patients with renal or hepatic disease the dose should be started at 50% usual daily dose.
- Improvements are gradual with time; maximal improvement can be observed at 4–6 months (Table 16.1).

Antipsychotic Drug Interactions

There is a large potential for drug–drug interactions with the antipsychotic medications. Although many of these are not clinically important, some common interactions must be

TABLE 16.4. Dosing of the Second- and Third-Generation Antipsychotics

	Dose range	Approximate equivalent dosages (oral)	Half life (hours)	Intramuscular dosing (short acting)
Clozapine	300–450 mg	400 mg	12–66	N/A
Olanzapine	5–20 mg	15 mg	20–50	5–10 mg every 2–4 hours, maximum daily dose of 30 mg
Risperidone	0.5–6 mg	4 mg	20 (3–6 days with long-acting injection)	N/A (25–50 mg long-acting injection)
Ziprasidone	40–160 mg (divided twice daily with food); twice the increased bioavailability with food	120 mg	7	10 mg every 2 hours or 20 mg every 4 hours, maximum daily dose of 40 mg (20 mg intramuscular = 120 mg oral)
Quetiapine	200–800 mg	600 mg	6	N/A
Aripiprazole	5–30 mg	15 mg	75–96	9.75 mg every 2 hours, maximum daily dose of 30 mg
Paliperidone	6–12 mg	6 mg[a]	23	N/A

[a]Dosing equivalence for paliperidone, the active metabolite of risperidone, has not been established in comparison to other second-generation antipsychotics.

recognized. Table 16.5 describes how the most commonly prescribed antipsychotics are metabolized. The following is a selection of common interactions with the antipsychotic medications.

• Smoking induces cytochrome P450 1A2 enzyme (CYP450 1A2) production. Smokers may need higher doses of clozapine, olanzapine, and possibly haloperidol or even ziprasidone, and monitoring for increased antipsychotic adverse effects during and after smoking cessation. This is important even if nicotine replacement is utilized, because the aromatic hydrocarbons in smoke may be largely responsible for the induction.

• Atypical antipsychotic concentrations may be affected by many CYP450-inhibiting drugs, such as paroxetine, fluoxetine, and others. But the atypical antipsychotics are unlikely to alter the metabolism of drugs metabolized by CYP450.

• Haloperidol may affect the metabolism of various opiates and other drugs through CYP450 2D6 inhibition.

TREATMENT RECOMMENDATIONS

Various treatment guidelines direct selection of antipsychotic medication and duration of therapy. Overall, treatment guidelines suggest initiating the SGA or TGA medications as first-line therapy. There are a variety of reasons for these recommendations: They are more tolerated compared to FGA medications, they have less side effects, and they have been shown to reduce hospitalization, improve compliance and patients' reported feelings of wellness. Selection of these medications has been described previously in this chapter. All the guidelines have recommendations on when to choose clozapine therapy or a long-acting antipsychotic medication. Additionally, switching from one agent to another should be done with a cross-taper and titration of the new agent. Please refer to the recommended readings for the specific guidelines.

KEY POINTS

• Second- and third-generation antipsychotics are considered the first line in the treatment of schizophrenia.
• Patients must have completed blood work before clozapine prescriptions may be written.

TABLE 16.5. Antipsychotic Medication Metabolism

Drug	How metabolized	Induces	Inhibits
Aripiprazole	**2D6**, 3A4	None	None
Clozapine	**1A2**, 2C19, 2D6, 3A4	None	None
Haloperidol	1A2, **2D6**, **3A4**	None	2D6
Olanzapine	**1A2**, 2D6	None	None
Quetiapine	3A4	None	None
Risperidone	**2D6**, 3A4	None	Mild 2D6
Ziprasidone	1A2, **3A4 (primarily via aldehyde oxidase)**	None	None

Note. Bold type indicates the primary metabolic pathway.

- Therapeutic dosages of antipsychotics can take 4–6 weeks to provide clinical improvements; time must be given for a medication to be effective.
- Antipsychotic polypharmacy is not considered standard practice unless a patient cannot utilize clozapine or has failed clozapine therapy.
- Complete resolution of the symptoms of schizophrenia with antipsychotics is uncommon; oftentimes the symptoms are reduced to tolerable levels.
- Single daily dosages of antipsychotics should be used, if possible, to improve medication adherence.
- Drug interactions are possible with all antipsychotics and must be monitored.
- Following published treatment guidelines and using the STEPS process of medication selection helps to improve patient outcomes.

REFERENCES AND RECOMMENDED READINGS

Alam, D. A., & Janicak, P. G. (2005). The role of psychopharmacotherapy in improving the long-term outcome of schizophrenia. *Essential Psychopharmacology, 6*(3), 127–140.

American Psychiatric Association. (2004). American Psychiatric Association Practice Guidelines for the Treatment of Psychiatric Disorders Compendium 2004. *American Journal of Psychiatry, 161*(Suppl. 2), 1–56.

Davis, J. M., & Chen, N. (2005). Old versus new: Weighing the evidence between the first- and second-generation antipsychotics. *European Psychiatry, 20*(1), 7–14.

Davis, J. M., Chen, N., & Glick, I. D. (2003). A meta-analysis of the efficacy of second-generation antipsychotics. *Archives of General Psychiatry, 60*(6), 553–564.

Dolder, C. R., Lacro, J. P., Leckband, S., & Jeste, D. V. (2003). Interventions to improve antipsychotic medication adherence: Review of recent literature. *Journal of Clinical Psychopharmacology, 23*(4), 389–399.

Janssen Pharmaceutica. (2007). *Product Information for Invega™*. Mountain View, CA: Author.

Lehman, A. F., Kreyenbuhl, J., Buchanan, R. W.. Dickerson, F., Dixon, L. B., Goldberg, R., et al. (2004). The Schizophrenia Patient Outcomes Research Team (PORT): Updated treatment recommendations 2003. *Schizophrenia Bulletin, 30*(2), 193–217.

Leucht, S. L., Barnes, T. R., Kissling, W., Engel, R. R., Correll, C., & Kane, J. M. (2003). Relapse prevention in schizophrenia with new-generation antipsychotics: A systematic review and exploratory meta-analysis of randomized, controlled trials. *American Journal of Psychiatry, 160,* 1209–1222.

Leucht, S., Wahlbeck, K., Hamann, J., & Kissling, W. (2003) New generation antipsychotics versus low-potency conventional antipsychotics: A systematic review and meta-analysis. *Lancet, 361,* 1581–1589.

Lieberman, J. A., Tollefson, G., Tohen, M., Green, A. I., Gur, R. E., Kahn, R., et al. (2003). Comparative efficacy and safety of atypical and conventional antipsychotic drugs in first-episode psychosis: A randomized, double-blind trial of olanzapine versus haloperidol. *American Journal of Psychiatry, 160*(8), 1396–1404.

Miller, A. L., Chiles, J. A., Chiles, J. K., Crismon, M. D., Shon, S. P., & Rush, A. J. (1999). The TMAP schizophrenia algorithms. *Journal of Clinical Psychiatry, 60,* 649–657. (Electronic updates available at *www.dshs.state.tx.us/mhprograms/tmaptoc.shtm.*)

Moncrieff, J. (2003). Clozapine v. conventional antipsychotic drugs for treatment-resistant schizophrenia: A re-examination. *British Journal of Psychiatry, 183,* 161–166.

Perry, P. J. (2007). *Psychotropic drug handbook* (8th ed.). Philadelphia: Lippincott Williams & Wilkins.

Rummel, C., Hamann, J., Kissling, W., Leucht, S., et al. (2003). New generation antipsychotics for first episode schizophrenia. *Cochrane Database of Systematic Reviews, 4,* CD004410.

Stahl, S. M. (2005). *Essential psychopharmacology: Neuroscientific basis and practical applications* (2nd ed.). Cambridge, UK: Cambridge University Press.

CHAPTER 17

SIDE EFFECTS
OF ANTIPSYCHOTICS

CHRISTIAN R. DOLDER

The modern era of antipsychotic pharmacotherapy began in the 1950s with the introduction of chlorpromazine. This agent, along with other conventional antipsychotics such as haloperidol, fluphenazine, and thioridazine, enabled health care providers to improve significantly the positive symptoms of schizophrenia (e.g., delusions, hallucinations). Unfortunately, the gains in symptom improvement seen with conventional antipsychotics were often offset by substantial toxicity, especially neurological side effects. The limitations associated with these agents spurred the development of atypical antipsychotics such as clozapine, risperidone, and olanzapine. As a class, the atypical antipsychotics were developed to be at least as efficacious as conventional agents, but with significantly reduced neurological side effects. The ability of the atypical antipsychotics to do just this have propelled them as the antipsychotics of choice for the treatment of schizophrenia and related psychotic disorders. Despite the advantages of atypical antipsychotics over conventional agents, atypical antipsychotics are not without side effects. This chapter reviews the most common side effects of antipsychotics (see Table 17.1), focusing on atypical agents, and discusses options to treat and to minimize antipsychotic-induced side effects.

Recent results from the Clinical Antipsychotic Trials of Intervention Effectiveness (CATIE) schizophrenia study highlight the negative impact side effects have on antipsychotic therapy. Findings from this National Institute of Mental Health–sponsored trial that involved nearly 1,500 patients also questions whether the efficacy and safety benefits associated with the atypical antipsychotics are really as large as some investigators and clinicians have thought. Over the course of the trial, 74% of participants discontinued the study before 18 months. The time to the treatment discontinuation for any cause among risperidone, olanzapine, quetiapine, ziprasidone, and perphenazine groups was found to be significantly longer only in the olanzapine-treated group when compared to the quetiapine or risperidone groups. The rates of medication discontinuation due to intolerable side effects ranged from 10 to 19% of patients, but the times to discontinuation were similar among groups. Olanzapine was associated with higher rates of discontinua-

TABLE 17.1. Antipsychotic-Induced Side Effect Potential

	EPS	TD	Prolactin elevation	Weight gain	Dyslipidemia	Glucose intolerance	Anticholinergic effect
High-potency conventional antipsychotics	+++	+++	+++	+	+	+	++
Low-potency conventional antipsychotic	++	++	++	++	+	+	+++
Clozapine	+/–	+/–	+	+++	++	++	++
Risperidone	++	+	++	+	+	+	+
Olanzapine	+	+	+	+++	++	++	++
Quetiapine	+	+	+	+	+	+	+
Ziprasidone	+	+	+	+/–	+/–	+/–	+/–
Aripiprazole	+	+	+	+/–	+/–	+/–	+/–

Note EPS, extrapyramidal symptoms; TD, tardive dyskinesia; +/–, minimal potential and/or insufficient data; +, mild potential; ++, moderate potential; +++, substantial potential.

tion for metabolic side effects, and perphenazine was associated with higher rates of discontinuation for extrapyramidal side effects (Lieberman et al., 2005).

NEUROLOGICAL SIDE EFFECTS

Extrapyramidal side effects (EPS; i.e., acute dystonia, Parkinsonism, akathisia) have long been known to be an adverse result related to the use of antipsychotics, especially high-potency conventional antipsychotics. The bothersome and often distressing results of EPS have been shown to inhibit significantly patients' desire to take antipsychotics. The pervasive and bothersome nature of these side effects was one of the major driving forces prompting the development of the atypical antipsychotics. With the exception of high-dose risperidone, all of the atypical antipsychotics have been reported in a variety of study designs to be associated with a significantly reduced risk of EPS compared to conventional antipsychotics. Despite the lower incidence of EPS with the atypical antipsychotics, the widespread use of these agents makes it necessary for clinicians to remain aware of the clinical presentation and treatment of EPS.

Acute dystonia often occurs within the first week of initiating antipsychotic therapy and is associated with muscular rigidity and cramping that usually involves muscles of the face, tongue, and neck. A subset of patients may experience prodromal tongue thickness or swallowing difficulty up to 6 hours prior to full-blown acute dystonia. An episode of acute dystonia is generally treated with anticholinergic medications such as benztropine (1–2 mg) or diphenhydramine (25–50 mg) administered intramuscularly or intravenously. A repeat injection is possible if symptoms remain 20–30 minutes following the first dose of the anticholinergic agent. Unresponsive dystonia can also be addressed with a low-dose benzodiazepine. Resolution of the acute dystonia should be followed by a 1- to 2-week course of an anticholinergic medication, and the use of antipsychotic therapy should be limited to an atypical antipsychotic with low propensity to cause EPS.

Antipsychotic-induced Parkinsonism often occurs after several weeks of antipsychotic therapy, is more common in the elderly, and usually presents with the classic symptoms of rigidity, tremor, and bradykinesia. The presence of antipsychotic-induced

Parkinsonism is addressed by one of two methods: (1) switching to an atypical antipsychotic with a low propensity to induce Parkinsonism or (2) adding an anticholinergic medication such as benztropine, trihexyphenidyl, or diphenhydramine. In general, switching to an atypical antipsychotic is preferred over adding a medication that may cause its own side effects in an attempt to treat or prevent an antipsychotic-induced side effect.

Akathisia is experienced subjectively as an unpleasant sensation of restlessness and observed objectively as restlessness, anxiety, and agitation. Akathisia can be very frightening and distressful to patients, and is a known risk factor for antipsychotic nonadherence. Similar to antipsychotic-induced Parkinsonism, akathisia is most commonly associated with the use of high-potency conventional antipsychotics and is unlikely with low-dose risperidone, uncommon with olanzapine and quetiapine, and extremely unlikely with clozapine. Although akathisia is unlikely to be caused by ziprasidone and aripiprazole, both agents can produce anxiety and agitation as side effects that may resemble akathisia. Antipsychotic-induced akathisia can be treated by switching to an atypical antipsychotic with a low risk of akathisia, or by adding one of several medications: (1) a low-dose beta-blocker (e.g., propanolol, 10–20 mg three times daily); (2) an anticholinergic (e.g., benztropine, 1–2 mg twice daily; or (3) benzodiazepine (e.g., lorazepam, 1 mg three times daily).

Tardive Dyskinesia

Tardive dyskinesia (TD) is a syndrome of chronic or permanent abnormal, involuntary movements that presents usually with athetoid movements of the tongue, facial, and neck muscles, extremities, or trunk usually after at least 3–6 months of antipsychotic treatment in younger adults and 1 month of treatment in older adults. This often irreversible side effect is a well-known consequence of typical antipsychotics, with long-term studies reporting incidence rates of 5% per year in adults, and rates 5–6 times that in older adults. Although the mechanism of antipsychotic-induced TD remains unclear, it is clear that the use of conventional antipsychotics and age (i.e., patients 50 years of age and older) are associated with an increased risk of developing TD. Other clinical correlates of TD in schizophrenia, confirmed in the results from the CATIE schizophrenia study, include duration of antipsychotic use, presence of EPS, treatment with anticholinergics, and substance abuse (Miller et al., 2005). Atypical antipsychotics have been shown to involve a substantially lower risk of EPS compared to conventional antipsychotics, and researchers have hoped that this would also translate into less TD—a hope that has been confirmed in a number of studies. A scholarly review of all long-term trials (i.e., at least 1 year) involving both typical and atypical antipsychotics that reported newly identified cases of TD was conducted. Eleven such studies involving over 2,700 patients were identified. The investigators reported that the weighted mean annual incidence of TD related to atypical antipsychotic use was 0.8% in adults, 6.8% in mixed adult and older adult patients, and 5.3% in patients 54 years of age and older. In contrast, adults treated with haloperidol were found to have a weighted mean annual incidence of 5.4% (Correll, Leucht, & Kane, 2004). Thus, these findings support the idea that long-term use of atypical antipsychotics is associated with a lower incidence of TD, but that important consideration must be given to patients prescribed any antipsychotic on a long-term basis.

Because there is no reliable treatment for TD, prevention is crucial. The risk of TD can be minimized by prescribing antipsychotics only when there is a clear indication and by avoiding conventional antipsychotics. Prior to initiating any antipsychotic therapy, clinicians should establish baseline motor functioning with a standardized scale such as the

Abnormal Involuntary Movements Scale (AIMS; Simpson, Lee, Zoubok, & Gardos, 1979). An AIMS examination should be repeated at least every 6 months during the use of antipsychotics. Should a patient develop problematic TD while being prescribed an antipsychotic, the clinician should consider stopping antipsychotic treatment if possible, switching the patient to an atypical antipsychotic (a different atypical antipsychotic, if one is currently prescribed), or switching to clozapine. A number of studies have shown symptomatic benefit when switching patients who developed TD during treatment with a conventional antipsychotic or an atypical antipsychotic to a different atypical antipsychotic (especially clozapine). For example, in an open-label study involving seven patients with schizophrenia and severe TD, the effects of clozapine treatment (mean dose, 428 mg/day) were evaluated over 5 years. Symptom scores decreased 83% from baseline after 3 years and 88% from baseline after 5 years. The effects of risperidone (mean dose, 3.6 mg/day) on preexisting severe TD were examined over 48 weeks in 40 patients with schizophrenia. At the end of the trial, mean AIMS scores had decreased significantly from baseline (from 15.7 to 10.6). Significant improvement was noted after 8 weeks of risperidone treatment and maintained throughout the study period. Individually, total AIMS scores decreased from baseline in 35 of the 40 patients treated, and increased in 5 of the patients (Bai et al., 2005).

A variety of adjunctive treatments for TD, including lithium, physostigmine, melatonin, and benzodiazepines, have been tried but without consistent benefit. Beneficial use of antioxidants such as vitamin E to prevent TD also has not been convincingly proven.

Neuroleptic Malignant Syndrome

Neuroleptic malignant syndrome (NMS) is a serious and potentially life-threatening idiosyncratic reaction to antipsychotics. Although the risk of developing NMS appears to be greater with the use of high-dose, high-potency conventional antipsychotics, reports of NMS linked to atypical antipsychotics exist. The most common symptoms of NMS, often with an onset of hours to days, are (lead pipe) rigidity, fever, autonomic instability, and delirium. Renal failure, cardiac arrhythmias, seizures, and coma may also occur. Treatment of NMS includes prompt removal of the offending antipsychotic and aggressive supportive care. Use of the muscle relaxant dantrolene (1–3 mg/kg per day in divided doses) to decrease rigidity and secondary hyperthermia, with or without bromocriptine (2.5–10 mg, three times daily) to potentially speed recovery has been advocated. Prudent selection of antipsychotics is necessary when restarting therapy in patients with schizophrenia. Atypical antipsychotics with a low likelihood of EPS and NMS, such as quetiapine and clozapine, should be considered.

HYPOTHALAMIC- AND PITUITARY-RELATED SIDE EFFECTS

Hyperprolactinemia, resulting from dopaminergic receptor (D_2) blockade on lactotroph cells, occurs frequently in patients prescribed high-potency conventional antipsychotics and high-dose risperidone but is uncommon with other atypical antipsychotics. For example, in a study involving approximately 400 inpatients prescribed a conventional antipsychotic or risperidone for at least 3 months, prolactin levels above the upper range of normal occurred in 60% of women and 40% of men. Prolactin levels usually returned to normal within 2–4 days of antipsychotic discontinuation. Symptoms of hyperprolactinemia can be problematic and include gynecomastia, galactorrhea, sexual dysfunction, and amenorrhea. Methodologically sound studies of women treated with conventional antipsychotics have reported prevalence rates of approximately 45% for oligomenorrhea/amenorrhea and 19% for galactorrhea. Furthermore, high prolactin levels inhibit the hypothalamic–pituitary–gonadal axis, resulting not only in high circulating prolactin levels but also reduced gonadal hormone levels. Long-term consequences of antipsychotic-related hypogonadism include premature bone loss and osteoporosis. Clozapine and quetiapine do not produce sustained elevations of plasma prolactin across their dosage range. Olanzapine has been shown to produce little effect on prolactin levels, although hyperprolactinemia can occur at higher doses. Ziprasidone and aripiprazole, based on limited data, appear to be prolactin-sparing agents. The development of symptomatic hyperprolactinemia during antipsychotic therapy should prompt clinicians to switch to a more prolactin-sparing agent.

METABOLIC SIDE EFFECTS

The association between metabolic side effects and antipsychotics, especially atypical antipsychotics, is well publicized. Hypertension, hyperlipidemia, obesity, and hyperglycemia, when examined individually or together (as part of the metabolic syndrome), represent a tremendous source of cardiovascular risk. Patients with schizophrenia have high rates of these metabolic disorders. For example, analysis of baseline data from the CATIE schizophrenia study revealed that approximately 40% of patients met criteria for metabolic syndrome.

Weight Gain

The prevalence of obesity in the U.S. general population has been estimated to be 20–30%. In contrast, the prevalence of obesity in the U.S. schizophrenia population (medicated) has been estimated to be between 40 and 60%. Although patients with schizophrenia may be overweight for a variety of reasons, both conventional and atypical antipsychotics have been shown to cause weight gain in some patients. This is far more than a cosmetic issue. A link between antipsychotic nonadherence and antipsychotic-induced weight gain has been demonstrated. In addition, obese patients have an increased risk of heart disease, hypertension, and diabetes. An increased risk of these medical disorders is important to consider, because a diagnosis of schizophrenia carries with it a relative risk of mortality that is 1.6–2.6 times greater than that of the general population. Furthermore, the life expectancy of an individual with schizophrenia is 20% less than that of the general population. Cardiovascular disease is the number one cause of death in patients with schizophrenia.

Important differences exist among the antipsychotics in terms of weight gain potential. Low-potency conventional antipsychotics have been implicated in weight gain for years. Data from randomized, controlled trials of atypical antipsychotics in adults demonstrate that weight gain cannot be considered a class effect. Clozapine and olanzapine are associated with the greatest likelihood of clinically significant weight gain. In a meta-analysis that examined mean weight change at 10 weeks at standard dosages of antipsychotic medications, clozapine and olanzapine were associated with the greatest weight gain (4.0–4.5 kg). Studies have reported that risperidone and quetiapine are associated with moderate weight gain. Ziprasidone and aripiprazole are associated with the least likelihood of weight gain and have been described as weight neutral. Although ziprasidone and aripiprazole are associated with substantially less weight gain potential, significant weight gain (i.e., at least 7% of initial body weight) was experienced by 9%

and 8%, respectively, of patients enrolled in clinical trials. In contrast, some studies have reported that up to 40% of patients prescribed olanzapine will experience significant weight gain. The actual magnitude of antipsychotic-associated weight gain may be minimized by weight gain results reported from clinical trials that are usually of short duration. Long-term studies of antipsychotic use have reported that weight gain tends to continue beyond the common 8- to 12-week duration of clinical trials.

A variety of hypotheses exist regarding how antipsychotics produce weight gain. One of the most common relates to the fact that many antipsychotics bind to histamine receptors. The affinity for histamine receptor subtypes has been reported to correlate with weight gain. For example, olanzapine has the highest affinity of all the atypical antipsychotics for the histamine type 1 receptor. Conversely, aripiprazole and ziprasidone exhibit some of the lowest affinities for similar histamine receptor subtypes. Many atypical antipsychotics exhibit activity at several serotonin receptor subtypes, including the 5-HT_{2C} subtype. Weight gain associated with antipsychotics may also be a consequence of such serotonergic activity.

There is currently no accurate method to predict which patients will experience substantial antipsychotic-induced weight gain. Thus, patients must be informed of the risk, and behavioral interventions such as diet and exercise counseling should be offered. In patients who are already overweight, or who have a predisposition to become overweight, selecting an antipsychotic with a reduced potential to cause weight gain is warranted. Behavioral and lifestyle modifications that include both reduced-calorie diets and increased physical activity have been reported to help prevent and treat antipsychotic-induced weight gain. In patients who become overweight as a result of an antipsychotic despite nonpharmacological treatment, switching to an antipsychotic that is weight neutral is also warranted. The use of medications with weight-lowering potential (e.g., sympathomimetic agents, orlistat, metformin, topiramate, and amantadine) have been examined in a limited amount of trials and have been shown generally to have limited efficacy on their own.

Dyslipidemia

A variety of studies (retrospective database analyses, controlled trials, observational investigations) have reported that individual atypical antipsychotics have differing effects on dyslipidemia. In general, clozapine and olanzapine are the largest potential offenders in terms of worsening a patient's lipid profile, although increases in weight associated with these medications likely play an important role. Results of clinical trials, chart reviews, and health care database analyses suggest that clozapine and olanzapine therapy are associated with increases in triglyceride levels. In a Medi-Cal database that included over 4,000 cases of schizophrenia and 8,000 matched controls, the risk of hyperlipidemia was increased with the use of both clozapine and olanzapine, but not risperidone or quetiapine. Additionally, a U.K. database study that included over 18,000 patients with schizophrenia and 7,000 case controls compared rates of hyperlipidemia among antipsychotics. No significant increase in the risk of hyperlipidemia was noted with risperidone or conventional antipsychotics, but patients treated with olanzapine therapy had a significantly higher risk of developing hyperlipidemia compared to controls (odds ratio = 4.65, 95% confidence interval = 2.44–8.85). In a retrospective chart review that examined cholesterol levels following initiation of antipsychotics, patients in the olanzapine group experienced significant increases from baseline in fasting triglycerides (88.2 mg/dl) and fasting total cholesterol (23.6 mg/dl). These changes were significantly greater than those found with risperidone-treated patients.

Reports of hyperlipidemia with risperidone and quetiapine are limited, but the likelihood of these agents causing adverse changes in lipid levels appears lower than that of clozapine or olanzapine. Similarly, data are too limited to determine definitively the potential impact of ziprasidone and the risk of developing dyslipidemia. Nonetheless, a handful of investigations have reported that ziprasidone does not have an adverse effect on lipid levels and may even lead to beneficial changes in some lipid parameters. Data currently available suggest that aripiprazole has a desirable lipid profile. A 26-week trial of 310 patients with chronic schizophrenia investigated the effects of aripiprazole versus placebo on cholesterol levels. The investigators reported similar changes compared to placebo in total cholesterol, high-density lipoprotein (HDL) cholesterol, low-density lipoprotein (LDL) cholesterol, and triglycerides. In other studies of aripiprazole in patients with lipid elevations due to prior antipsychotic treatment, lipid levels often decreased to patients' baseline levels with the switch to aripiprazole.

In summary, some atypical antipsychotics have the ability to increase cholesterol levels, namely, triglyceride levels. The selection of an antipsychotic with a decreased likelihood of worsening existing dyslipidemia may be an important consideration. Patients whose cholesterol levels substantially worsen while they receive atypical antipsychotic treatment may need to be switched to an agent with a lower likelihood of elevating cholesterol. In addition, the ability of antipsychotics to produce metabolic side effects such as dyslipidemia necessitates monitoring (see Table 17.2).

Diabetes/Glucose Intolerance

The last several years have seen considerable attention focused on the potential of atypical antipsychotics to cause new cases of diabetes or to worsen existing diabetes. It is difficult to clearly separate the apparent increase in diabetes risk and use of antipsychotics in patients with schizophrenia. For instance, the prevalence of diabetes and obesity among individuals with schizophrenia appears to be up to two times higher than that of the general population. Additionally, individuals with psychiatric illness may also have a higher prevalence of impaired glucose tolerance. Cigarette smoking, an extremely common habit in patients with schizophrenia, can exacerbate insulin resistance despite possible reductions in body weight. Increased visceral adiposity, a risk factor for diabetes, also appears to be greater in patients with schizophrenia compared to the general public.

Numerous case reports and review articles have documented both the onset of new cases of diabetes and worsening of existing diabetes following initiation of treatment with atypical antipsychotics. Retrospective cohort studies have consistently reported that patients prescribed clozapine and olanzapine are at increased risk of developing diabetes compared to individuals prescribed conventional antipsychotics. The risk associated with risperidone and quetiapine varies among studies, and limited data for both ziprasidone and aripiprazole suggest a very limited risk for diabetes. In a group of patients prescribed

TABLE 17.2. Monitoring Recommendations for Atypical Antipsychotics

	Baseline	4 weeks	8 weeks	12 weeks	Quarterly	Annually
Weight and BMI	×	×	×	×	×	
Waist circumference	×					×
Blood pressure	×			×		×
Fasting plasma glucose	×			×		×
Fasting lipid profile	×			×		×

Note. BMI, body mass index.

a variety of antipsychotics, an oral glucose tolerance test revealed that fasting glucose and insulin levels were higher with olanzapine, risperidone, and clozapine compared to levels in psychiatric patients taking typical antipsychotics and normal volunteers. These results suggest a link between insulin resistance and several atypical antipsychotics. The incidence of newly diagnosed diabetes was retrospectively assessed over a 2-year period in more than 56,000 veterans with schizophrenia who were consistently prescribed clozapine, risperidone, olanzapine, quetiapine, or a conventional antipsychotic. Overall, 4.4% of patients were diagnosed with diabetes annually, and the attributable risk of developing diabetes was low but varied among medications: clozapine, 2.0%; quetiapine, 0.8%; olanzapine, 0.6%; and risperidone, 0.1% (Leslie & Rosenheck, 2004).

Although the risk of developing diabetes or exacerbating existing diabetes cases as a result of atypical antipsychotic therapy appears small, the seriousness of diabetes necessitates that clinicians obtain baseline parameters (height, weight, waist circumference, body mass index, and fasting blood sugar; see Table 17.2), then monitor such parameters throughout treatment (American Diabetes Association, 2004). Patients should be encouraged to monitor their own weight as well. Clinicians should consider switching patients whose glycemic control worsens to an antipsychotic with a low propensity to cause or worsen diabetes. The development of severe hyperglycemia, with or without symptoms, should prompt immediate medical care.

CARDIAC SIDE EFFECTS

There has been a concern that atypical antipsychotics may slow cardiac conduction, producing QT interval prolongation and predisposing patients to arrhythmias. In general, atypical antipsychotics have only modest and usually clinically unimportant effects on the QT interval. Among the atypical antipsychotics, ziprasidone has the greatest potential to prolong a patient's QT interval, although published data generally do not report significant electrocardiographic (ECG) abnormalities. In patients with preexisting QT prolongation, the use of ziprasidone may not be warranted. In general, patients older than age 45 and individuals with preexisting cardiac conduction abnormalities should have a baseline EKG performed prior to initiating any antipsychotic therapy and periodically thereafter (see Table 17.2).

Of all the atypical antipsychotics, clozapine has been singled out because of its potential cardiac toxicity. Recently, investigators reviewed the published literature to examine the risk of myocarditis, pericarditis, and cardiomyopathy in patients treated with clozapine. The authors found 65 cases of myocarditis, 6 cases of pericarditis, and 52 cases of cardiomyopathy in patients treated with clozapine. Although the incidence rate of clozapine-associated cardiac side effects is undetermined, there clearly is a relationship between clozapine and myocarditis and cardiomyopathy. It is important to note that these side effects are uncommon yet serious. Some authors have suggested that patients prescribed clozapine should be assessed for myocarditis in the first month of treatment and assessed regularly for cardiomyopathy. Most importantly, health care professionals should remain vigilant if any cardiac symptoms develop in patients prescribed clozapine.

Orthostatic Hypotension

Orthostasis has been reported to occur most commonly with the use of low-potency conventional antipsychotics, especially chlorpromazine and thioridazine. Postural hypotension is also relatively common with the atypical antipsychotic clozapine. Other atypical antipsychotics also occasionally lead to orthostasis, especially risperidone and quetiapine. The potential for quetiapine to cause orthostasis, particularly in older adults, is one of the reasons that it is commonly titrated up to a target dose. Because of the risk of falls related to postural hypotension in susceptible patients, and the rare possibility of severe postural hypotension leading to syncope, patients should be warned to get up from a seated or prone position slowly. If symptomatic orthostasis persists, switching to a different atypical antipsychotic should be considered. In general, the ability of an antipsychotic to produce orthostasis can be predicted by its level of alpha-1 receptor blockade. The above-mentioned agents (i.e., clozapine, chlorpromazine, and thioridazine) have significant alpha-1 blocking activity.

HEMATOLOGICAL SIDE EFFECTS

The only antipsychotic associated with clinically significant hematological toxicity is clozapine. Although relatively uncommon (1% of treated patients), the ability of clozapine to cause agranuloctyosis necessitates regular monitoring and prompt action in response to substantial reductions in white blood cell counts. The appropriate use of clozapine is discussed in detail by Sajatovic, Madhusoodanan, and Fuller (Chapter 18, this volume).

OVERDOSAGE

Antipsychotics, in general, have a low potential for causing death when taken by themselves in overdose situations. Although there is substantially less experience with atypical antipsychotics compared to conventional antipsychotics in overdose situations, the atypical antipsychotics appear safer, although isolated published reports of death exist. Generally, the most serious results of an antipsychotic overdose are coma and hypotension. Cardiac arrhythmias and seizures have also been reported. Central nervous system depression and excitation have both been reported in patients who overdose on antipsychotics.

KEY POINTS

- Atypical antipsychotics represent the treatment of choice for patients with schizophrenia when clinicians consider efficacy and safety.
- Atypical antipsychotics, compared to conventional agents, are associated with a decreased risk of EPS and TD but still have a substantial side effect potential.
- The risk of metabolic side effects associated with atypical antipsychotics necessitates baseline and follow-up monitoring of patients.
- Clozapine and olanzapine have the greatest potential to cause weight gain, dyslipidemia, and impaired glucose control.
- Selection of an antipsychotic should be made on a patient-by-patient basis to minimize the potential for antipsychotic-related side effects.

REFERENCES AND RECOMMENDED READINGS

American Diabetes Association, American Psychiatric Association, American Association of Clinical Endocrinologists, & North American Association for the Study of Obesity. (2004). Consensus development conference on antipsychotic drugs and obesity and diabetes. *Diabetes Care, 27,* 596–601.

Ananth, J., Venkatesh, R., Burgoyne, K., Gadasalli, R., Binford, R., & Gunatilake, S. (2004). Atypical antipsychotic induced weight gain: Pathophysiology and management. *Annals of Clinical Psychiatry, 16,* 75–85.

Bai, Y. M., Yu, S. C., Chen, J. Y., Lin, C. Y., Chou, P., & Lin, C. C. (2005). Risperidone for pre-existing severe tardive dyskinesia: A 48-week prospective follow-up study. *International Clinical Psychopharmacology, 20,* 79–85.

Bergman, R. N., & Ader, M. (2005). Atypical antipsychotics and glucose homeostasis. *Journal of Clinical Psychiatry, 66,* 504–514.

Correll, C. U., Leucht, S., & Kane, J. M. (2004). Lower risk for tardive dyskinesia associated with second-generation antipsychotics: A systematic review of 1-year studies. *American Journal of Psychiatry,161,* 414–425.

Leslie, D. L., & Rosenheck, R. A. (2004). Incidence of newly diagnosed diabetes attributable to atypical antipsychotic medications. *American Journal of Psychiatry,161,* 1709–1711.

Lieberman, J. A., Stroup, T. S., McEvoy, J. P., Swartz, M. S., Rosenheck, R. A., Perkins, D. O., et al. (2005). Effectiveness of antipsychotic drugs in patients with chronic schizophrenia. *New England Journal of Medicine, 353,* 1209–1223.

Lindenmayer, J. P., Czobor, P., Volavka, J., Citrome, L., Sheitman, B., McEvoy, J. P., et al. (2003). Changes in glucose and cholesterol levels in patients with schizophrenia treated with typical or atypical antipsychotics. *American Journal of Psychiatry, 160,* 290–296.

Miller, D. D., McEvoy, J. P., Davis, S. P., Caroff, N., Saltz, B. L., Chakos, M. H., et al. (2005). Clinical correlates of tardive dyskinesia in schizophrenia: Baseline data from the CATIE schizophrenia trial. *Schizophrenia Research, 80,* 33–43.

Rosenbaum, J. F., Arana, G. W., Hyman, S. E., Labbate, L. A., & Fava, M. (Eds.) (2005). *Handbook of psychiatric drug therapy* (5th ed.). Philadelphia: Lippincott Williams & Wilkins.

Simpson, G. M., Lee, J. H., Zoubok, B., & Gardos, G. (1979). A rating scale for tardive dyskinesia. *Psychopharmacology, 64,* 171–179.

Wirshing, D.A. (2004). Schizophrenia and obesity: Impact of antipsychotic medications. *Journal of Clinical Psychiatry, 65*(Suppl. 18), 13–26.

CHAPTER 18

CLOZAPINE

MARTHA SAJATOVIC
SUBRAMONIAM MADHUSOODANAN
MATTHEW A. FULLER

Clozapine is the prototype drug from the antipsychotic class often referred to as *atypical*. Subsequent to the approval of clozapine by the U.S. Food and Drug Administration (FDA), additional atypical antipsychotic agents received FDA approval, including (in chronological order) risperidone, olanzapine, quetiapine, ziprasidone, aripiprazole, and paliperidone. With the introduction of newer antipsychotic agents over the last decade, atypical agent use has vastly increased, and the atypical compounds are now the dominant therapeutic agents in the management of patients with schizophrenia.

A European review (Seshamani, 2002) on clozapine therapy cost-effectiveness and impact on patient quality of life suggested improvement on multiple levels: (1) Treatment with clozapine significantly improves patient symptoms and quality of life; (2) patients who receive clozapine experience a reduction in the number of hospitalizations, which can lead to a decrease in hospital costs; (3) treating patients with clozapine shifts the cost structure from inpatient care to outpatient care and drug therapies; and (4) patients who receive clozapine can experience reduction in overall treatment costs.

In spite of these advantages, clozapine use is limited by its adverse effect profile and need for regular laboratory monitoring. Thus, clozapine use represents only a small proportion of patients treated in most clinical settings (5% or less) and current use is generally reserved for only the most severe forms of schizophrenia.

PHARMACOKINETICS AND PHARMACODYNAMICS OF CLOZAPINE

Clozapine binds to multiple receptors, particularly to dopaminergic $(D_1–D_5)$ serotoninergic $(5\text{-}HT_{2A}, 5\text{-}HT_{2C}, 5\text{-}HT_6)$, adrenergic (alpha$_1$), cholinergic (M_1, M_2, M_4) and histaminergic (H_1) receptors.

The absorption of orally administered clozapine is 90–95%. However, clozapine is subject to first-pass metabolism, resulting in an absolute bioavilability of 50–60%. Food does not affect the systemic bioavailablity of clozapine. Therefore, it may be administered with or without food.

Plasma concentrations show large interindividual variation, with average steady-state peak plasma concentrations occurring at approximately 2.5 hours (range: 1–6 hours) after dosing. Clozapine is 95–97% bound to plasma proteins. The elimination of clozapine is biphasic, with a mean elimination half-life of 8 hours (range: 4–12 hours) after a single 75 mg dose and 12 hours (range: 4–66 hours) after reaching steady state with 100 mg twice-daily dosing. This suggests the possibility of concentration-dependent pharmacokinetics. However, at steady state, the area under the curve (AUC) and peak and trough plasma concentrations increase linearly in a dose-related fashion.

Clozapine is almost completely metabolized prior to excretion, and only trace amounts of unchanged drug are detected in the urine and feces. Approximately 50% of the administered dose is excreted in the urine, and 30% in the feces. The desmethyl metabolite has only limited activity while the hydroxylated and N-oxide derivatives are inactive. The metabolism of clozapine occurs via multiple cytochrome P450 (CYP450) enzymes. However, clozapine is primarily a substrate for CYP450 1A2.

A correlation between clozapine plasma levels and clinical response has been suggested. Optimal response appears to be reached in individuals whose clozapine plasma level is at least 350 ng/ml.

TREATMENT STUDIES IN SCHIZOPHRENIA

Approximately 30% of patients with schizophrenia do not respond to conventional antipsychotic agents and are labeled as treatment resistant. Clozapine is considered the treatment of choice for this refractory patient population. Clozapine has been compared to conventional antipsychotics in patients with schizophrenia in over 30 studies involving more than 2,500 patients. These studies have largely been of short duration (< 13 weeks) and have included mostly young (mean age, 38 years) men. Although there were no differences in mortality, ability to work, or suitability for discharge at the end of the studies, clinical improvement was seen more frequently in those taking clozapine both in the short and long term. In the short-term trials, patients on clozapine had fewer relapses. Symptom assessment scales showed a greater reduction of symptoms in clozapine-treated patients. Patients were more satisfied with clozapine, and it was more acceptable in the long-term treatment compared to conventional antipsychotic agents. However, clozapine was associated with more hypersalivation, temperature increase, and drowsiness, but fewer motor side effects and dry mouth. The clinical efficacy in terms of clinical improvement and symptom reduction was most prominent in those patients who were resistant to conventional antipsychotics. Approximately one-third of patients with treatment-resistant illness improved with clozapine treatment. More recently, a multicenter, randomized, international study compared the risk for suicidal behavior in patients treated with clozapine versus olanzapine in 980 patients with schizophrenia/schizoaffective disorder (Meltzer et al., 2003). The major finding from this randomized study was that clozapine therapy demonstrated superiority to olanzapine in reducing key measures of suicidality in patients with schizophrenia/schizoaffective disorder, who are at high risk for suicide.

IDENTIFICATION OF THE INDIVIDUAL WHO IS A GOOD CANDIDATE FOR CLOZAPINE THERAPY

The FDA-approved indications for use of clozapine include (1) treatment of severely ill patients with schizophrenia who fail to show an acceptable response to adequate course of standard antipsychotic drug treatment and, (2) for reduction of the risk of recurrent suicidal behavior in patients with schizophrenia or schizoaffective disorder who are judged to be at risk of reexperiencing suicidal behavior. One generally accepted norm to establish treatment resistance is failure in at least two trials of antipsychotic drugs for at least 6 weeks each at doses equal to 10–20 mg of haloperidol per day, or its equivalent. Treatment-resistant patients often have at least moderate positive, negative, or disorganization (incoherence, loose association, inappropriate affect, and poverty of thought content) symptoms and impaired social functioning despite at least two adequate trials of antipsychotic drugs chosen from two or more different classes of these agents. Off-label uses of clozapine sometimes seen in clinical settings include use for patients with unmanageable extrapyramidal symptoms (EPS), tardive dyskinesia (TD), refractory bipolar disorder, refractory obsessive–compulsive disorder (OCD), and Parkinson's disease.

CLOZAPINE THERAPY INITIATION AND ISSUES RELATED TO EARLY STAGES OF TREATMENT

Medical Assessments

The patient should have a thorough history and physical examination (Table 18.1). The history should include information regarding any history of blood dyscrasias, seizure disorder, cardiovascular disease, hepatic and renal disease, as well as any immunosuppressive diseases such as HIV. Laboratory testing should include a complete baseline blood count with white blood cell (WBC) count and absolute neutrophil count (ANC), complete metabolic assay including serum electrolytes and renal function tests, and an electrocardiogram (ECG) with QTc interval. Clozapine dosing and titration may require modification in individuals with any of the aforementioned preexisting conditions.

Patient and Family Education

Risks, benefits, and treatment alternatives should be discussed with the patient and family, and documented in the treatment record (Table 18.1). The hematological and cardiovascular risks must be discussed in detail. The specific monitoring protocol regarding blood draws should be discussed with patients and families, and agreed upon in advance. In some treatment settings, home visits for blood drawing may be arranged to facilitate adherence with monitoring.

Dosing and Titration

The starting dose of clozapine is 12.5 mg once or twice daily (Table 18.1). The small starting dose helps to assess for early hypotensive reactions. Patient should be observed for sedation and changes in blood pressure and pulse. The dose can be increased by 25–50 mg daily up to a target dose of 300–450 mg/day by the end of 2 weeks for young, medically healthy individuals. Subsequent dosage increments may be made once or twice weekly in increments not to exceed 100 mg. Twice-daily dosage is recommended in view of the half-life of clozapine. The dose generally need not exceed 450–600 mg/day in most adults < 60 years old in the initial phase of treatment. The maximum recommended dose is 900 mg/day, if response is unsatisfactory at 600 mg/day. The dosage of clozapine in older adults is usually 100–300 mg/day. A quick-dissolving formulation of clozapine is now available for individuals who have difficulty swallow-

TABLE 18.1. Clinical tips for clozapine initiation and management

Clinical point/adverse effect	Management tips
Medical assessment prior to clozapine initiation	• History and physical. • Screen for blood dyscrasia, seizure disorder, cardiovascular disorder, immunosuppressive disease. • Labs: complete blood count with differential, metabolic assay. • ECG
Patient and family education	• Discussion of hematological and cardiovascular risk. • Agreed upon (in advance) monitoring schedule, arrange in-home blood draws if possible.
Initial dosing and titration	• Healthy adults: 12.5mg once or twice daily, increased as tolerated in increments of 25–50 mg/day to a target dose of 300–450 mg/day. May require doses of 600–900 mg/day for treatment of schizophrenia. • Median dose to reduce suicidal behavior on the order of 300 mg/day.
Hematological effects	• Weekly WBC/ANC for first 6 months. • Every-other-week WBC/ANC for Months 6–12 if no complications. • Monthly WBC/ANC after 12 months and beyond, if no complications.
Sedation	• Most pronounced in first month; minimize with slow titration and lowest effective dose.
Seizure risk	• Most pronounced with high overall dosage and fast titration. Minimize with slow titration. Use valproate if anticonvulsant is needed.
Cardiovascular risks (hypotension, myocarditis, etc.)	• Low starting dose, slow titration. • ECG follow-up, especially in those with past cardiac history. • Increase fluid intake, potential use of fludrocortisone for hypotension.
Long-term weight gain	• Follow ADA guidelines for monitoring parameters. • Education, diet control, and behavioral measures (involve family, case managers). • Potential benefit with sibutamine.
Continued refractory symptoms	• Add on high-potency conventional antipsychotic (haloperidol). • Add on risperidone. • Add on anticonvulsant (valproate or lamotrigine).

ing pills. Patients who respond to clozapine should be continued on the lowest dose required to maintain remission.

Management of Potential Early Side Effects

Hematological Effects

Agranulocytosis (granulocyte count < 500/mm^3) and granulocytopenia (granulocyte count < 1,500/mm^3) are rare (less than 1%), but serious potential side effects of clozapine therapy. Agranulocytosis and granulocytopenia, if they occur, usually develop in the first 2–6 months of therapy. The risk is higher in older adults, women, and in patients of Ashkenazi Jewish descent with the human leukocyte antigen HLA-B38 phenotype. Mortality is higher in African American populations who develop agranulocytosis. Coadministration of drugs such as carbamazepine, which have bone marrow–suppressing effects, can potentially increase the risk for agranulocytosis. It is necessary to monitor hematological status (white blood cell count [WBC] and absolute neutrophil count [ANC]) on a weekly basis for the first 6 months of clozapine therapy (Table 18.1). Patients should be instructed to report onset of fever, sore throat, weakness, or other signs of infection promptly. If the total WBC falls below 3,000 or if the ANC falls below 1,500, medical or hematological consultation should be obtained. Agranulocytosis is a medical emergency and is managed by reverse isolation and prophylactic broad-spectrum antibiotics. Treatment with granulocyte colony-stimulating factor (G-CSF) and granulocyte–macrophage colony-stimulating factor (GM-CSF) have been reported to decrease morbidity and to shorten the duration of illness secondary to agranulocytosis. Other hematological side effects associated with clozapine therapy include benign leukocytosis (0.6%), leukopenia (3%), eosinophilia (10%), and elevated erythrocyte sedimentation rate.

Neurological/Mental Status Effects

Sedation, occurring in 10–58% of clozapine-treated individuals, is perhaps the most common and immediately troubling neurological side effect. Fortunately, some sedation is likely to resolve gradually after early phases of titration. Additionally, effects of daytime sedation can be minimized by giving most of the clozapine dose at night.

Clozapine reduces seizure threshold and the occurrence of seizures is dose related— 0.7% per 100 mg dose. Valproate is preferred by many clinicians as the safest and best-tolerated anticonvulsant in clozapine-treated patients experiencing seizures.

During the first few months of clozapine treatment some patients develop benign fevers (100–103°F). This is usually self-limiting, and can be managed with antipyretics. However, the more serious condition of neuroleptic malignant syndrome (NMS) also is more common in the first 14 days of clozapine treatment. Concurrent treatment with lithium is a risk factor for NMS. Management of NMS includes discontinuation of antipsychotic and supportive measures to reduce the body temperature, including use of a hypothermia blanket and hydration. Drugs such as amantadine, benzodiazepines, dantrolene, and bromocriptine can be effective. Electroconvulsive therapy (ECT) also has been used in refractory cases.

Finally, approximately 10% of clozapine-treated patients experience obsessive–compulsive symptoms such as repeated handwashing. Decreasing clozapine dose or addition of a serotonin selective reuptake inhibitor (SSRI) may help to alleviate these symptoms.

Cardiovascular and Other Side Effects

Cardiovascular side effects that may be associated with clozapine therapy include tachycardia, orthostatic hypotension, prolongation of QTc interval, deep vein thrombosis, myocarditis, and cardiomyopathy. Clozapine should be discontinued in patients who develop myocarditis or cardiomyopathy. Tachycardia is due to vagal inhibition and can be treated with beta-adrenergic antagonists such as atenolol; however, this may also potentiate the hypotensive effects of clozapine. Low starting dose and gradual titration can reduce the hypotensive side effects. Additional treatment measures include fluid intake of at least 2 liters/day, support stockings, increased sodium intake, and fludrocortisone treatment.

Sialorrhea (hypersalivation) occurs in 31–54% of individuals on clozapine therapy. Sialorrhea may respond to clonidine patches (0.1 mg weekly). Anticholinergic agents may be helpful for some patients but should be approached cautiously because of additive effects and the possibility of anticholinergic delirium. Clozapine itself has strong anticholinergic effects that can lead to urinary retention, constipation, and gastrointestinal (GI) obstruction. It has been postulated (McGurk et al., 2005), that anticholinergic effects may be responsible for worsening of spatial working memory in individuals with schizophrenia. Slow titration of clozapine and use of lowest effective dose minimize anticholinergic effects.

Enuresis/urinary incontinence (0.23%) is a potential additional embarrassing side effects of clozapine. Avoiding fluids in the evening, voiding before going to bed, scheduling middle-of-the-night awakening to empty the bladder, and using enuresis alarms can be of help. Ephedrine, intranasal desmopressin (DDAVP), and oxybutynin have been reported to be beneficial in the management of clozapine-induced enuresis.

MAINTENANCE CLOZAPINE THERAPY IN CLINICAL SETTINGS

Once clozapine has been initiated and a stable, maintenance dose achieved, tasks for the clinician include (1) ongoing hematological monitoring, (2) monitoring for long-term, adverse medication effects and physical health monitoring, and (3) ongoing symptom assessment and functional outcome evaluation (Table 18.1).

Hematological Monitoring

Fortunately, recommendations for regular serum monitoring with respect to hematological effects were modified in 2005. Current monitoring frequency suggests weekly WBC counts and ANC monitoring for the first 6 months of therapy, then every 2 weeks (if no complications) for months 6–12 of treatment, and after 12 months of therapy (if no complications) every 4 weeks ad infinitum. If therapy is discontinued, monitoring should continue for an additional 4 weeks from time of discontinuation.

Long-Term Health Monitoring

Monitoring for long-term adverse medication effects with clozapine is largely centered on evaluation of weight gain and development of metabolic abnormalities such as development of type 2 diabetes. Many studies overwhelmingly confirm that atypical antipsychotic medications produce substantially more weight gain compared to conventional antipsychotic agents, and clozapine is generally agreed to have significant weight gain potential. Additional related consequence of the atypical antipsychotics are their effect on serum lipids. Clozapine, which often produces substantial weight gain, may also be associated with increases in total cholesterol, low-density lipoprotein (LDL) cholesterol, and triglycerides, and with decreased high-density lipoprotein (HDL) cholesterol. The American Diabetes Association (ADA) and the American Psychiatric Association (APA) have recommended that individuals maintained on atypical antipsychotic medications (including clozapine) should have baseline assessment of personal and family history of obesity–diabetes–cardiovascular risk factors, weight and height, waist circumference, blood pressure, and fasting plasma glucose and lipid profiles. Weight should be measured at weeks 4 and 8 of treatment, week 12 of treatment, and quarterly thereafter. Additional monitoring recommendations are personal history reassessment annually, waist circumference annually, blood pressure and fasting plasma glucose at 12 weeks, then annually thereafter, and fasting lipid profile at 12 weeks, then every 5 years thereafter. Hypertension may be associated with weight gain and lipid abnormalities in some clozapine-treated patients. Education, diet control, and behavioral measures may prevent excessive weight gain. In those with weight gain, medication treatment can be attempted (e.g., sibutamine), with careful monitoring of side effects. Additional adverse effects that may be associated with long-term treatment include somnolence, sialorrhea, and urinary incontinence (all of which may be dose dependent to some degree). Myocarditis may occur with patients maintained on clozapine therapy. In rare cases, agranulocytosis may occur even after years of uncomplicated treatment, and isolated cases of apparent movement disorders or TD have been reported.

It is known that schizophrenia is associated with several chronic physical illnesses and a shorter life expectancy compared with that in the general population. A recent expert consensus panel has recommended that mental health care providers perform appropriate physical health monitoring that typically occurs in primary care settings for their patients with schizophrenia who do not receive such monitoring. Patients with severe, treatment-refractory illness are likely to belong to this group of disadvantaged individuals who often have difficulty accessing care in standard primary settings. Physical health consensus recommendations overlap somewhat with ADA–APA guidelines (body mass index, plasma glucose levels, lipid profiles). Additional parameters of physical health monitoring include monitoring for signs of myocarditis, sexual dysfunction, and EPS–TD in patients on clozapine (particularly individuals age 50 and older).

Ongoing Symptom Evaluation and Functional Outcome Assessment

Cognitive functioning and quality of life may improve in those who have good response to clozapine therapy. Additionally, potential reduction in suicidality maintains safety and allows patients to engage in recovery interventions. There is also fairly consistent evidence that clozapine therapy may reduce aggressive behavior and allow some individuals with previously extremely severe illness to transition to more independent, less restrictive residential settings. Maximization of clozapine dosage on the order of 600–900 mg/day should be attempted in patients who tolerate the drug but appear to be refractory (checking serum levels may be somewhat useful, although there are no clear, standardized target levels). The median dose to reduce risk of suicidal behavior in clinical trials was approximately 300 mg/day (range: 12.5–900 mg/day).

Treatment adherence should remain an ongoing concern, although, perhaps because of the need for ongoing serum monitoring, a number of reports suggest that treatment adherence is actually better for clozapine compared to other antipsychotic compounds. For individuals who are refractory with optimized clozapine dosing there have been reports that adjunctive treatment with other antipsychotics (high-potency conventional agents such as haloperidol, or atypical agents such as risperidone), or anticonvulsant compounds, such as lamotrigine, may be of benefit for some patients.

KEY POINTS

- Clozapine is the prototype drug from the antipsychotic class often referred to as *atypical* antipsychotics.
- Clozapine use is generally reserved for the most severe forms of schizophrenia and is the treatment of choice for refractory patients.
- In addition to its efficacy in severely ill/refractory patients with schizophrenia, clozapine has been demonstrated to reduce the risk of recurrent suicidal behavior.
- Clozapine therapy may reduce aggressive behavior and allow some individuals with previously severe illness to transition to more independent, less restrictive residential settings.

- Common side effects of clozapine therapy include sedation, tachycardia, orthostasis, sialorrhea, and weight gain/metabolic abnormalities (e.g., elevated serum glucose and development of diabetes).
- Due to the potential for rare but serious hematological effects (agranulocytosis or granulocytopenia) it is necessary to monitor hematological status continuously for as long as individuals are maintained on clozapine therapy.
- Because risk of clozapine-related hematological effects are greatest in the first 6 months of therapy, the need for frequent serum monitoring decreases over time and is only necessary on a monthly basis after 12 months of therapy without complications.

REFERENCES AND RECOMMENDED READINGS

American Diabetes Association, American Psychiatric Association, American Association of Clinical Endocrinologists, & North American Association for the Study of Obesity. (2004). Consensus development conference on antipsychotic drugs and obesity and diabetes. *Diabetes Care, 27*(2), 596–601.

Kane, J., Honigfeld, G., Singer, J., Meltzer, H. Y., & the Clozapine Collaborative Study Group. (1988). Clozapine for the treatment-resistant schizophrenia: A double blind comparison with chlorpromazine. *Archives of General Psychiatry, 45,* 789–796.

Marder, S. R., Essock, S. M., Miller, A. L., Buchanan, R. W., Casey, D. E., Davis, J. M., et al. (2004). Physical health monitoring of patients with schizophrenia. *American Journal of Psychiatry, 161*(8), 1334–1349.

McGurk, S. R., Carter, C., Goldman, R., Green, M. F., Marder, S. R., Hie, H., et al. (2005). The effects of clozapine and risperidone on spatial working memory in schizophrenia. *American Journal of Psychiatry, 162*(5), 1013–1016.

Meltzer, H. Y., Alphs, L., Green, A. I., Altamura, A. C., Anand, R., Bertoldi, A., et al. (2003). Clozapine treatment for suicidality in schizophrenia: International Suicide Prevention Trial. *Archives of General Psychiatry, 60*(1), 82–91.

Meltzer, H. Y., Burnett, S., Bastani, B., & Ramirez, L. F. (1990). Effect of six months of clozapine treatment on the quality of life of chronic schizophrenic patients. *Hospital and Community Psychiatry, 41,* 892–897.

National Alliance on Mental Illness. Available online at *www.nami.org.*

Physicians' Desk Reference (59th ed.). (2005). Montvale, NJ: Thompson.

Seshamani, M. (2002). Is clozapine cost-effective?: Unanswered issues. *European Journal of Health Economics, 3*(Suppl. 2), S104–S113.

U.S. Food and Drug Administration. Available online at *www.fda.gov.*

Wahlbeck, K., Cheine M., & Essali, M. A. (2000). Clozapine versus typical neuroleptic medication for schizophrenia. *Cochrane Database of Systematic Reviews, 2,* CD000059.

CHAPTER 19

OTHER MEDICATIONS

BRITTON ASHLEY AREY
STEPHEN R. MARDER

Although antipsychotics are the first-line agents for the treatment of schizophrenia, large areas of need are still unmet. First, many patients with schizophrenia demonstrate only partial responses to antipsychotics. Second, as the Clinical Antipsychotic Trials of Intervention Effectiveness (CATIE) revealed, a large proportion of patients discontinue their antipsychotic due to lack of efficacy or tolerability issues. Last, neither the first- nor second-generation antipsychotics adequately address symptom domains such as cognition and negative symptoms. Both of these domains have been shown to have significant impact on functional outcomes in schizophrenia.

In this chapter, we discuss alternative and adjunctive medication strategies for the treatment of schizophrenia, including mood stabilizers, benzodiazepines, and antidepressants. Furthermore, we present the evidence supporting treatments for co-occurring disorders such as depression, mania, anxiety, and obsessive–compulsive disorder. Finally, we mention new medications and mechanisms in development for the treatment of schizophrenia. We do not discuss treatment strategies for the side effects of antipsychotics, such as extrapyramidal symptoms, tardive dyskinesia, weight gain, or metabolic issues (for a discussion of these side effects, see Dolder, Chapter 17, this volume).

MOOD STABILIZERS

Mood stabilizers or antiepileptic agents have been widely used in the treatment of schizophrenia. Citrome, Jaffe, Levine, and Allingham (2002) showed that the use of mood stabilizers in the New York State mental health system nearly doubled from 1994 to 2001, with 47.1% of inpatients diagnosed as having schizophrenia in 2001 receiving a mood stabilizer.

We discuss the evidence for the use of mood stabilizers as monotherapy and as augmentation agents to address the core symptoms of schizophrenia. We also discuss data that support using these medications as adjunctive treatment for affective symptoms and agitation in schizophrenia. Finally, we make recommendations for the use of mood stabilizers in schizophrenia based on the evidence presented.

Lithium

There is little evidence that lithium has any inherent antipsychotic properties; indeed, studies to date show that as a sole agent, lithium is ineffective in the treatment of schizophrenia.

There is some support for increasing response rates in schizophrenia by augmenting antipsychotics with lithium. However, in a meta-analysis, Leucht, Kissling, and McGrath (2004) showed that the advantage of lithium augmentation was not significant when patients with affective symptoms were excluded from the studies. Additionally, more patients taking lithium discontinued the studies, suggesting a lower tolerability of lithium augmentation. Thus, despite some evidence in favor of lithium augmentation, the overall results are inconclusive and suggest that it may only be effective for patients with affective symptoms.

A limited body of evidence indicates that lithium, as augmentation to antipsychotics, helps atypical mania, schizoaffective disorder, or schizophreniform disorder, both as an acute treatment and to prevent recurrence. Indeed, some literature suggests that it may be useful to subtype schizoaffective disorders into primarily affective versus schizophrenia types, and to treat them accordingly. To this end, adding mood stabilizers such as lithium to the treatment of patients with predominant affective or manic symptoms appears to be effective. Further support for this strategy comes from a literature review by Keck, McElroy, Strakowski, and West (1994), which demonstrated that the combination of lithium and antipsychotics is superior to antipsychotics alone for schizoaffective, bipolar-type patients. Last, some literature suggests that concomitant administration of lithium alongside an antipsychotic may be useful in certain patients with aggression, agitation, or psychomotor excitement.

At present, however, available data do not support the use of lithium montherapy or adjunctive therapy in the treatment of the core symptoms of schizophrenia. On the other hand, lithium does appear to be a useful comedication when added to an antipsychotic for patients with either concomitant affective symptoms or agitation and aggression.

Valproate

Valproate is currently one of the most frequently prescribed drugs in treatment of schizophrenia spectrum disorders. A study by Citrome et al. (2002) showed that in the New York State mental health system between 1994 and 2001, adjunctive use of valproate nearly tripled among patients with a diagnosis of schizophrenia, and was ultimately prescribed for 35% of patients with schizophrenia, making it the most commonly prescribed mood stabilizer for that population.

A Cochrane Database review by Basan and Leucht (2004) showed that studies evaluating valproate as monotherapy to treat schizophrenia are extremely limited and show no benefit. Furthermore, this review concluded that the effectiveness of adjunctive valproate on overall outcomes in schizophrenia remains unclear.

A more promising strategy involves the use of valproate to augment antipsychotics in the short-term treatment of patients who demonstrate agitation or excitement. In a study of 249 patients hospitalized with acute exacerbation of schizophrenia, with a moderate degree of uncooperativeness and hostility or excitement and tension, Citrome and colleagues (2004) showed that adding valproate to either risperidone or olanzapine was well tolerated, produced a faster onset of action in the combination group, and indicated reduced hostility and core psychotic symptoms. This advantage for valproate augmentation was not sustained, however, beyond the first week of treatment.

Based on the randomized trial–derived evidence currently available, therefore, no data support or refute the use of valproate as an adjunctive agent in the long-term treatment of schizophrenia. However, it may be reasonable to consider valproate for acutely ill inpatients with agitation in the first weeks of treatment and when more rapid improvement is important. We also support the use of valproate in patients with unstable moods when an antipsychotic alone fails to lead to mood stability.

Carbamazepine

A review of the available literature by Leucht et al. (2002) determined that carbamazepine monotherapy has not been shown to be effective in the treatment of schizophrenia when compared to placebo or antipsychotic. Some studies have shown a trend indicating a benefit from carbamazepine as an adjunct to antipsychotics in the treatment of schizophrenia, but the trials have had small numbers of subjects, and a review of the available data has indicated inconsistent and inconclusive results.

Some preliminary data show that carbamazepine may be useful in treating affective symptoms of schizophrenia, and may decrease violent behavior in psychotic patients. However, the studies are extremely limited, and further research is warranted on the use of carbamazepine in patients with excitement, aggression, mania with psychosis, and bipolar-type schizoaffective disorder.

Furthermore, it is important to note that because carbamazepine induces metabolic activity and can therefore lower the dose of certain antipsychotics (e.g., haloperidol, thiothixene) when administered adjunctively, when it is withdrawn, a corresponding increase of the antipsychotic may occur. Indeed, studies of patients on haloperidol demonstrated that the adjunctive use of carbamazepine was associated with a dramatic fall in haloperidol plasma levels and a worse clinical outcome compared to the monotherapy group.

Thus, at present, neither carbamazepine monotherapy nor augmentation can be recommended on the basis of the available evidence for routine use in the treatment of schizophrenia.

Lamotrigine

Several lines of evidence suggest that glutamate may be involved in schizophrenia pathophysiology. Postmortem studies have revealed a lower density of glutamatergic receptors in patients with schizophrenia; and lower levels of cerebrospinal fluid (CSF) glutamate have been found in patients with schizophrenia compared to normal controls. The most compelling evidence is provided by the psychomimetic effects of the N-methyl-d-aspartic acid (NMDA) antagonists phencyclidine and ketamine. When administered to normal controls, both agents can induce positive, negative, and cognitive symptoms similar to those observed in patients with schizophrenia. Hence, there has been much interest and speculation about the role of lamotrigine, which acts on the glumatate system, in the treatment of schizophrenia.

Despite this, there are few studies in the literature about the effects of lamotrigine in the treatment of schizophrenia. There are no reported randomized, controlled clinical trials of lamotrigine monotherapy in schizophrenia, and few trials of adjunctive treatment.

Small, open-label trials of clozapine-treated patients with treatment-resistant schizophrenia have shown that the addition of lamotrigine to clozapine resulted in significant improvement in Brief Psychiatric Rating Scale (BPRS) total scores. These results are further supported by one randomized controlled trial of lamotrigine added to clozapine, in which both positive and general psychopathological symptoms improved with lamotrigine augmentation.

However, data for lamotrigine augmentation with other antipsychotics are less clear. Indeed, there have been mixed results when lamotrigine was used as an adjuvant to antipsychotics other than clozapine. Kremer and colleagues (2004), in a double-blind, placebo-controlled study of 38 patients with treatment-resistant schizophrenia, found that the addition of lamotrigine to either first- or second-generation antipsychotics resulted in improvement in positive symptoms and general psychopathology in patients who completed the study, regardless of whether they were on a typical or atypical antipsychotics. In contrast, in a small, naturalistic outcome study of 17 patients with treatment-resistant schizophrenia, Dursun and Deakin (2001) showed that only when lamotrigine was added to clozapine did patients experience a reduction in psychotic symptoms; there was no significant improvement when lamotrigine was added to risperidone, haloperidol, olanzapine, or fluphenthixol.

Therefore, although the addition of lamotrigine may be useful for some patients with treatment-resistant schizophrenia who are currently being treated with clozapine, further use of lamotrigine in schizophrenia treatment is not supported by the available literature.

Summary

As monotherapy for schizophrenia, mood stabilizing drugs have no documented beneficial effect. However, when these drugs are used as adjunctive therapies to antipsychotics, some positive effects have been demonstrated. Lithium has demonstrated effects on affective symptoms associated with schizophrenia and schizophrenia-related illnesses. Evidence for antiaggressive effects exists for several of the mood stabilizers, but it is perhaps best validated for the use of adjunctive valproate in acutely ill inpatients to hasten recovery and reduce agitation in the first week of treatment, although there is no evidence supporting the long-term use of adjunctive valproate for the treatment of aggression in schizophrenia at this time. Finally, preliminary evidence suggests that the addition of lamotrigine to clozapine may be beneficial in treatment-resistant schizophrenia, but more studies are needed to substantiate this effect, and to validate the same findings with other antipsychotics.

BENZODIAZEPINES

Medications that affect gamma-aminobutyric acid (GABA), such as benzodiazepines, may have a potential role in the treatment of schizophrenia. This is supported by data indicating that schizophrenia may be associated with a down-regulation in cortical GABAergic function. Because GABA can reduce dopaminergic activity, increasing GABA function with certain benzodiazepines could be effective in treating positive and negative symptoms of schizophrenia.

To date, the literature contains no consistent evidence that benzodiazepines in monotherapy effectively treat the core symptoms of schizophrenia. A review of the data reveals that the majority of available studies indicate some positive benzodiazepine effects in reducing agitation, anxiety, or global impairment. However, only slightly more than half of the double-blind, controlled trials published on benzodiazepines as monotherapy demonstrated specific effects of benzodiazepines on psychotic symptoms; the other half fared no better than placebo.

Although monotherapy with benzodiazepines in schizophrenia cannot be recommended on the basis of the available literature, benzodiazepines are commonly used along with antipsychotics in the management of acutely agitated patients with psychosis. In a review of randomized, double-blind studies using benzodiazepines as adjunctive therapy, Wolkowitz and Pickar (1991) concluded that benzodiazepines may have some positive effects in improving the response to antipsychotic medications; however, other literature suggests that this response may not be maintained beyond the acute phase of the illness. Nevertheless, it is our opinion that short-term use of oral or intramuscular benzodiazepines is often a safer alternative for treatment of agitation in acute schizophrenia than increasing the dose of antipsychotic.

One area in which the data appear to be more consistent concerns the use of benzodiazepines in catatonia. A review of the international literature by Pommepuy and Januel (2002) concluded that lorazepam is safe and 80% effective in the treatment of catatonia. The *APA Guidelines for the Treatment of Schizophrenia* (*www.psych.org*) report that most studies use lorazepam at doses of 1–2 mg intravenously or 2–4 mg by mouth, repeated as needed over 48–72 hours, after which treatment can progressively be reduced. Clonazepam, oxazepam, and diazepam have also been used successfully in the treatment of catatonia.

Finally, although benzodiazepines are frequently used in the treatment of anxiety disorders that co-occur with schizophrenia, there are only case reports and case series reporting the use of benzodiazepines (e.g., alprazolam and diazepam) in panic disorder and other anxiety states in schizophrenia. There are no randomized, placebo-controlled studies; thus, no evidence-based rationale supports or refutes their use in anxiety disorders and schizophrenia.

Although benzodiazepines may produce some beneficial effects in the acute phase of schizophrenia, both in helping to control agitation and in treating catatonia, they may not be ideal drugs in the long-term treatment of this illness because of their significant side effect profile. Benzodiazepines contribute to sedation and to the development of tolerance after even a brief period of treatment. Ataxia, sedation, dysarthria, nausea, vomiting, confusion, excitation, disinhibition, and/or assaultiveness have all been reported. Furthermore, withdrawal from benzodiazepines may include psychosis and seizures. Thus, although benzodiazepines may benefit some patients, they may be counterproductive in others.

Summary

In summarizing these results, there appears to be no evidence-based rationale for the use of benzodiazepine monotherapy in the treatment of schizophrenia. The adjunctive use of benzodiazepines with antipsychotics is often helpful for the short-term treatment of agitation and anxiety during the acute phase of the illness. Benzodiazepine augmentation may be particularly useful when patients are receiving antipsychotics that do not have intrinsic sedating properties, such as risperidone, ziprasidone, or aripiprazole. Moreover, these agents should be withdrawn as agitation diminishes. Although no data compare the different benzodiazepines to one another, we recommend use of the high-potency benzodiazepines, such as lorazepam and clonazepam. Benzodiazepines such as lorazepam do have a role in the treatment of catatonia, in which they may produce rapid, dramatic, and sustained improvement. However, the adverse effects of benzodiazepines, such as sedation, tolerance, and potential withdrawal effects, limit their utility in the long-term treatment of schizophrenia.

ANTIDEPRESSANTS

In a 2002 Cochrane Database review, Leucht and colleagues reported that true depressive symptoms are found in 50% of patients with newly diagnosed schizophrenia, and 33% of people with chronic schizophrenia who have relapsed. Depression is common in schizophrenia and is associated with disability, reduction of motivation to accomplish tasks and the activities of daily living, increased duration of illness, more frequent relapses, and increased risk of suicide. Diagnosing schizophrenia with depression requires a careful separation of confounding factors, such as negative symptoms, side effects of medications, substance abuse, and other possible contributing factors.

Antidepressants, especially tricyclics, have been studied in patients with schizophrenia and comorbid depression. However, studies of antidepressants in the treatment of schizophrenia are generally small and of poor quality, and provide weak evidence for the effectiveness of antidepressants in persons with schizophrenia. The Schizophrenia Patient Outcomes Research Team (PORT; Lehman et al., 2004) study also acknowledged the existence of several single-blind, randomized controlled trials of antidepressants in patients with schizophrenia, and similarly concluded that the results were mixed.

The evidence regarding whether antidepressants worsen the course of schizophrenia during the actively psychotic phase is also conflicting. A study by Kramer and colleagues (1989) showed that combining antidepressant medications and antipsychotics for the treatment of actively psychotic patients with both schizophrenia and depression did not alleviate the depression and actually exacerbated some of the positive symptoms of schizophrenia. However, a study by Müller-Siecheneder and colleagues (1998) demonstrated that amitriptyline added to haloperidol improved both psychotic and depressive symptoms among persons with schizophrenia who had both disorders. Similarly, in a small trial of patients with schizophrenia and depression, the addition of fluoxetine, 20 mg per day, produced an improvement in dysphoria and sleep problems and reduced suicidality, without exacerbation of psychosis.

A review of the literature on controlled studies of antidepressants in schizophrenia indicates that the therapeutic efficacy of these agents is primarily a function of the phase in the disorder during which they are administered. Indeed, evidence-based medicine largely supports the value of adjunctive antidepressant medication for patients with schizophrenia who experience a full depressive syndrome after their psychosis has remitted. In patients with schizophrenia or schizoaffective disorder, antidepressants are likely to be most effective in patients whose acute psychotic episode has been adequately treated with an antipsychotic medication, but who subsequently develop a depressive syndrome that meets criteria for major depressive disorder. Further evidence of this comes from Siris, Morgan, Fagerstrom, Rifkin, and Cooper (1987), whose randomized, double-blind, controlled studies showed that treatment of postpsychotic depression in patients with schizophrenia with the first-generation antipsychotic imipramine was significantly more efficacious than placebo in relieving depression and in preventing relapse of depression. Furthermore, the addition of imipramine to an antipsychotic had a significant effect in preventing relapse of psychosis after 12 months among these patients.

On the basis of the available evidence, the 2004 PORT recommends that persons with schizophrenia who experience an episode of depression, despite an adequate reduction in positive psychotic symptoms with antipsychotic therapy, should receive a trial of an antidepressant. Although data are currently most conclusive for the tricyclics, such as imipramine and clompiramine, there is some evidence that selective serotonin reuptake inhibitors (SSRIs), such as fluoxetine, sertraline, and citalopram, may be equally effective in this regard.

Although the majority of the literature on the use of antidepressants in schizophrenia involves tricyclics and SSRIs, several studies reported on the use of bupropion in schizophrenia. In a double-blind, randomized, placebo-controlled study (Evins et al., 2005) on the use of bupropion for smoking cessation in patients with schizophrenia, subjects in the bupropion group had no worsening of clinical symptoms and had a trend toward improvement in depressive and negative symptoms, as well as increased rates of smoking cessation. Other placebo-controlled trials of bupropion for smoking cessation in schizophrenia have found that the addition of bupropion does not worsen positive symptoms, significantly reduces negative symptoms, and greatly enhances smoking abstinence rates compared to placebo. Despite the studies showing that the use of bupropion in patients with schizophrenia does not exacerbate psychotic symptoms, is effective for smoking cessation, and may improve depression, there is not enough evidence-based literature as yet to warrant its use for depression in this population.

OBSESSIVE–COMPULSIVE DISORDER AND ANXIETY DISORDERS

Obsessive–compulsive symptoms (OCSs) and obsessive–compulsive disorder (OCD) frequently occur in schizophrenia and appear to worsen long-term outcomes. Data suggest that patients with schizophrenia and OCSs benefit from treatment with both an antipsychotic and an antidepressant medication. In support of this, two controlled trials exist in the literature involving OCS treatment in schizophrenia: one with clomipramine, and the other with fluvoxamine. Both have shown positive results, but both were small, limited studies.

Except for the two pharmacological studies in OCD, there are no double-blind randomized controlled trials on the treatment of anxiety in schizophrenia. A review of the literature by Braga, Petrides, and Figueira (2004) indicates that anxiety disorders such as OCD, panic disorder, social phobia, and posttraumatic stress disorder (PTSD) are prevalent in schizophrenia, and treatment for anxiety can help alleviate symptoms in those patients. Most of the literature on anxiety disorders in schizophrenia comprise case reports and open-label trials using antidepressants such as imipramine and fluoxetine with some degree of success. However, more studies are needed that further define evidence-based treatment for anxiety disorders in schizophrenia.

Important Considerations

Care must be taken to monitor plasma levels of antipsychotics, which may rise when combined with SSRIs or other, related antidepressants, due to their ability to inhibit various cytochrome P450 isoenzymes. This is especially important when antidepressants are coadministered with clozapine, because increasing levels of clozapine can lead to risk of seizures. Since bupropion itself lowers the seizure threshold, the combination of clozapine and bupropion should be avoided.

Summary

Although the literature is inconsistent regarding the use of antidepressants in acutely psychotic patients with depression, evidence-based data robustly support the use of these medications in postpsychotic patients who have been adequately treated with an antipsychotic medication and still display depressive symptomatology. At present, data supports the use of tricyclic medications, as well as several of the SSRIs in the treatment of depression in schizophrenia. Bupropion has been shown to be effective in smoking cessation in patients with schizophrenia and does not seem to exacerbate positive psychotic symptoms; however, robust data on the clinical efficacy of bupropion in depression are lacking. A sparse literature supports the use of antidepressant medication in obsessional states in schizophrenia, but further studies on the treatment of other anxiety states in schizophrenia are warranted. Finally, clinicians must be careful about drug interactions when prescribing antidepressant medications alongside antipsychotics.

CO-MEDICATIONS FOR NEGATIVE SYMPTOMS AND COGNITIVE IMPAIRMENTS

Patients with schizophrenia who have been stabilized on an antipsychotic commonly have persistent negative symptoms (including restricted affect, alogia, apathy, asociality, and anhedonia), as well as cognitive impairments (including impairments in memory, attention, and executive function). These symptom domains are important, because their severity is related to the severity of the social and vocational impairments associated with schizophrenia. When the second-generation antipsychotics were first introduced, reports suggested that these agents were more effective than first-generation agents for both of these symptoms domains. More recent data indicate that these advantages may have been exaggerated by early trial designs, and that when found these advantages are relatively small. As a result, both domains are seen as important targets for drug development. Although it would be simpler if broadly effective drugs for treating psychosis were also effective for one or both of these domains, it is also conceivable that the most effective strategy may be to supplement an antipsychotic with a co-medication to enhance cognition or to improve negative symptoms.

Translating discoveries from basic neuroscience into new drugs is receiving considerable attention, including a National Institute of Mental Health (NIMH) program whose goal is to facilitate drug development for cognition enhancement in schizophrenia. The program, titled MATRICS (Measurement and Treatment Research to Improve Cognition in Schizophrenia; *www.matrics.ucla.edu*), has already developed methods to measure outcome in clinical trials, proposed trial designs in collaboration with the U.S. Food and Drug Administration (FDA), and developed a consensus on promising molecular targets for drug development. A parallel process has been initiated for negative symptoms.

NOVEL MECHANISMS

As illustrated earlier, the second-generation antipsychotics have limitations in treating the wide variety of symptoms that may be present in schizophrenia, including mood symptoms, agitation, and cognitive difficulties. However, as mentioned earlier, a significant number of patients' core symptoms only partially respond to antipsychotic medications. As a result, novel mechanisms are being investigated as both monotherapy and adjunctive therapy to improve efficacy in treating positive and negative symptoms of this disease, including substance P inhibitors, glutameric drugs, glycine transporter inhibitors, and other agents.

Although most of these new agents are still in the preliminary phases of discovery, one mechanism that has received quite a bit of clinical and scientific interest of late is that of the omega-3 polyunsaturated fatty acids. The hypothesis for the efficacy of fatty acids is based on the premise that phospholipids are a significant component of neuronal membranes, and that abnormalities of phospholipid metabolism may be present in patients with schizophrenia. This has given rise to the theory that omega-3 polyunsaturated fatty acids, and eicosapentanoic acid (EPA) in particular, may have a role in treating this illness.

However, clinical data thus far in support of the role of fatty acids in treating schizophrenia are far from definitive. In a 2005 review, Peet and Stokes concluded that five of six double-blind, placebo-controlled trials on the effect of fatty acids in schizophrenia reported therapeutic benefit from omega-3 fatty acids in either the primary or secondary statistical analysis, particularly when EPA was added to existing psychotropic medication. However, in a Cochrane Database review of five short studies using EPA, Joy, Mumby-Croft, and Joy (2003) found evidence that EPA may have some antipsychotic properties when compared to placebo, but many of the studies were too small to be conclusive and ultimately demonstrated mixed results and no evidence of clear dose–response relationship to omega-3 fatty acids. Finally, Emsley, Oosthuizen, and van Rensburg (2003) summarized four randomized, controlled trials of EPA versus placebo as supplemental medication, and concluded that two of these trials showed the significant benefit of EPA on the positive and negative symptom scale total scores, whereas the other two did not show any effects on this primary efficacy measure.

Therefore, although some preliminary evidence may suggest that EPA might be an effective adjunct to antipsychotics, the data are far from conclusive. Large, randomized, controlled studies are needed to validate further the role of omega-3 fatty acids in the treatment of schizophrenia.

KEY POINTS

- A significant number of patients only partially respond to current antipsychotic medications.
- Second-generation antipsychotics do not adequately address negative symptoms or cognitive deficits in schizophrenia.
- Adjunctive medications are commonly used to potentiate efficacy of antipsychotics, address agitation and aggression, and treat affective symptoms in schizophrenia.
- Mood stabilizers such as lithium, carbamazepine, and valproate may play a key role in treating mania, as well as aggression, associated with schizophrenia. In particular, valproate has shown utility in reducing aggression in acutely agitation inpatients during the first week of hospitalization.
- Antidepressants have a significant, well-validated role in treating depression associated with schizophrenia, after the patient has been optimized on antipsychotic therapy. A limited amount of data also validate their use in treating anxiety disorders associated with schizophrenia.
- Benzodiazepines are commonly used to treat acute agitation associated with schizophrenia in the short term, and have a well-defined role in the treatment of catatonia.
- The treatment of negative symptoms and cognitive deficits in schizophrenia will likely require the use of adjunctive medications alongside antipsychotics, and ongoing research is examining medications that can address these symptom domains.
- Finally, novel mechanisms are being explored in the treatment of schizophrenia, and may offer promise to the significant number of patients who do not fully respond to conventional antipsychotic medications.

REFERENCES AND RECOMMENDED READINGS

Basan, A., & Leucht, S. (2004). Valproate for schizophrenia. *Cochrane Database of Systematic Reviews, 1,* CD004028.

Braga, R. J., Petrides, G., & Figueira, I. (2004). Anxiety disorders in schizophrenia. *Comprehensive Psychiatry, 45,* 460–468.

Citrome, L., Casey, D. E., Daniel, D. G., Wozniak, P., Kochan, L. D., & Tracy, K. A. (2004). Adjunctive divalproex and hostility among patients with schizophrenia receiving olanzapine or risperidone. *Psychiatric Services, 55*(3), 290–294.

Citrome, L., Jaffe, A., Levine, J., & Allingham, B. (2002). Use of mood stabilizers among patients with schizophrenia, 1994–2001. *Psychiatric Services, 53*(10), 1212.

Dursun, S. M., & Deakin, J. F. (2001). Augmenting antipsychotic treatment with lamotrigine or topiramate in patients with treatment-resistant schizophrenia: A naturalistic case-series outcome study. *Journal of Psychopharmacology, 15*(4), 297–301.

Emsley, R., Oosthuizen, P., & van Rensburg, S. J. (2003). Clinical potential of omega-3 fatty acids in the treatment of schizophrenia. *CNS Drugs, 17*(15), 1081–1091.

Evins, A. E., Cather, C., Deckersbach, T., Freudenreich, O., Culhane, M. A., Olm-Shipman, C. M., et al. (2005). A double-blind placebo-controlled trial of bupropion sustained-release for smoking cessation in schizophrenia. *Journal of Clinical Psychopharmacology, 25*(3), 218–225.

Joy, C. B., Mumby-Croft, R., & Joy, L. A. (2003). Polyunsaturated fatty acid supplementation for schizophrenia. *Cochrane Database Systematic Reviews, 2*, CD001257.

Keck, P. E., Jr., McElroy, S. L., Strakowski, S. M., & West, S. A. (1994). Pharmacologic treatment of schizoaffective disorder. *Psychopharmacology, 114*(4), 529–538.

Kramer, M. S., Vogel, W. H., DiJohnson, C., Dewey, D. A., Sheves, P., Cavicchia, S., et al. (1989). Antidepressants in "depressed" schizophrenic inpatients: A controlled trial. *Archives of General Psychiatry, 46*, 922–928.

Kremer, I., Vass, A., Gorelik, I., Bar, G., Blanaru, M., Javitt, D. C., et al. (2004). Placebo-controlled trial of lamotrigine added to conventional and atypical antipsychotics in schizophrenia. *Biological Psychiatry, 56*(6), 441–446.

Lehman, A. F., Kreyenbuhl, J., Buchanan, R. W., Dickerson, F. B., Dixon, L. B., Goldberg, R., et al. (2004). The Schizophrenia Patient Outcomes Research Team (PORT): Updated treatment recommendations 2003. *Schizophrenia Bulletin, 30*(2), 193–217.

Leucht, S., Kissling, W., & McGrath, J. (2004). Lithium for schizophrenia revisited: A systemic review and meta-analysis of randomized controlled trials. *Journal of Clinicial Psychiatry, 65*, 177–186.

Leucht, S., McGrath, J., White, P., & Kissling, W. (2002). Carbamazepine for schizophrenia and schizoaffective psychoses. *Cochrane Database Systematic Reviews, 3*, CD001258.

Lieberman, J. A., Stroup, T. S., McEvoy, J. P., Swartz, M. S., Rosenheck, R. A., Perkins, D. O., et al. (2005). Clinical Antipsychotic Trials of Intervention Effectiveness (CATIE) Investigators: Effectiveness of antipsychotic drugs in patients with chronic schizophrenia. *New England Journal of Medicine, 353*(12), 1209–1223.

Müller-Siecheneder, F., Müller, M. J., Hillert, A., Sgegedi, A., Wetzel, H., & Benkert, O. (1998). Risperidone versus haloperidol and amitriptyline in the treatment of patients with a combined psychotic and depressive syndrome. *Journal of Clinical Psychopharmacology, 18*, 111–120.

Peet, M., & Stokes, C. (2005). Omega-3 fatty acids in the treatment of psychiatric disorders. *Drugs, 65*(8), 1051–1059.

Pommepuy, N., & Januel, D. (2002) Catatonia: Resurgence of a concept: A review of the international literature. *Encephale, 28*(6), 481–492.

Siris, S. G., Morgan, V., Fagerstrom, R., Rifkin, A., & Cooper, T. B. (1987). Adjunctive imipramine in the treatment of postpsychotic depression. *Archives of General Psychiatry, 44*, 533–539.

Wolkowitz, O. M., & Pickar, D. (1991). Benzodiazepines in the treatment of schizophrenia: A review and reappraisal. *American Journal of Psychiatry, 148*, 714–726.

CHAPTER 20

ELECTROCONVULSIVE THERAPY

SHAWN M. McCLINTOCK
NAJEEB RANGINWALA
MUSTAFA M. HUSAIN

Convulsive therapy was introduced by Meduna in the early 1930s as a treatment for severe catatonia in dementia praecox by use of camphor oil injections. Refinement of convulsive therapy with electricity in the late 1930s by Cerletti and Bini in Rome was the precursor of modern electroconvulsive therapy (ECT). Resulting from the broad application, and misapplication, to other psychiatric conditions in the 1940s, the criticism ECT received both inside and outside the psychiatric community resulted in a limitation in its beneficial, therapeutic use. Also, the discovery of neuroleptic pharmacotherapy further decreased the use of ECT as a treatment modality in patients with schizophrenia. However, because a significant number of patients have medication resistance and adverse effects from prolonged neuroleptic treatment, ECT continues to be effective in alleviating psychotic symptoms in patients with chronic schizophrenia.

The use of ECT to treat patients with schizophrenia varies by country. Although its use is substantially greater in European countries, it remains limited in the United States for patients with schizophrenia. For example, approximately 2.9–36.0% of patients receiving ECT in other countries have a primary diagnosis of schizophrenia compared to 1% of such patients receiving ECT in the United States. This is a relatively small number given that after depression, schizophrenia is the next most common diagnostic category for which ECT is recommended. Presently, ECT is recommended for patients with schizophrenia who are diagnosed with medication resistance, catatonia, unmanageable aggressive behavior, first-break psychosis in young adulthood, or acute schizophrenic exacerbations (see Table 20.1).

In 2004, the American Psychiatric Association (APA) recommended ECT for use in patients diagnosed with schizophrenia and/or schizoaffective disorder who have persistent severe psychosis and/or suicidal ideation, prominent catatonic features, and comorbid depression. The APA also suggested that ECT be used in severe cases in which patients have not responded to pharmacotherapy and in those that require a rapid response to treatment.

TABLE 20.1. Symptoms of Acute Exacerbation and Catatonia for Which ECT Is Recommended

Acute exacerbation symptoms	Catatonia symptoms
Delusions	Mutism
Hallucinations	Stupor
Disorganized thoughts	Waxy flexibility
Disorganized behavior	Posturing
Excitement and	Stereotypies
Overactivity	Rigidity

Note. From Keuneman, Weerasundera, and Castle (2002). Copyright 2002 by Blackwell Publishing. Adapted by permission.

ECT is generally a safe procedure, with a documented mortality rate of 0.002% (i.e., similar to patients receiving brief anesthesia). Two broad side effect categories for ECT include medical sequelae and cognitive impairments. Common medical side effects include hyper- or hypotension, tachy- or bradycardia, headache, muscle ache, and nausea (usually related to anesthesia). Less common side effects include myocardial infarction and prolonged seizure activity (status epilepticus). The major cognitive impairments resulting from ECT include anterograde and retrograde amnesia. For many patients these cognitive impairments are mild and transient; however, for some, the side effects may be long term.

TREATMENT

Indications for ECT

Major Depressive Disorder

ECT is indicated for major depressive disorder that is severe, chronic, and debilitating. The presence of psychotic or melancholic features is predictive of positive treatment outcome. ECT is also indicated when the depression is considered to be treatment resistant.

Bipolar Disorder

ECT is indicated for the treatment of severe, acute mania, as well as the depressive episode in the context of bipolar disorder. ECT is also indicated when the bipolar depression is determined to be treatment resistant.

Schizophrenia

ECT is indicated for schizophrenia that has an acute onset and presence of hallucinations or delusions, and that has been found to be nonresponsive to psychotropic medications.

Schizoaffective Disorder

ECT is indicated for schizoaffective disorder that has an acute onset, presence of hallucinations or delusions, and acute and severe mania, and that has been found to be nonresponsive to psychotropic medications.

Catatonia

ECT is indicated for catatonia secondary to any etiopathology that is unresponsive to treatment with medication.

Pretreatment Evaluation

A comprehensive evaluation for patients undergoing ECT should include a complete psychiatric history, mental status examination, and medical/surgical history. The patient's right- or left-handedness should be assessed to recognize the pattern of cerebral hemispheric dominance. A physical examination should be performed, and laboratory tests, including electrolytes, hemogram, electrocardiogram (ECG), computed tomography (CT) or magnetic resonance imaging (MRI) of the head, and a chest X-ray, should be obtained.

The patient's current and prior pharmacotherapy should be reviewed because of possible interactions between medications, anesthetic medications, and ECT. For example, lithium taken during ECT treatment may increase post-ECT incidence of delirium or confusion. Benzodiazepine use can reduce the seizure duration and should be tapered or discontinued. Prior to beginning a course of acute ECT, monoamine oxidase inhibitors (MAOIs) have been found to result in drug–drug interactions with anesthetic agents and should be discontinued. Antipsychotic medications have a synergistic effect with ECT, except reserpine, which can lead to sudden death in certain cases. Anticonvulsant medications interfere with the induction of seizure activity and should be tapered or discontinued. Tricyclic antidepressants (TCAs) and selective serotonin reuptake inhibitors (SSRIs) are usually safe to use with ECT. The patient should not take anything by mouth for 8 hours before the ECT treatment.

ECT Procedure

The patient is closely monitored (i.e., vital signs, ECG recording, pulse oximetry) during the ECT procedure. A short-acting barbiturate, such as methohexital, is administered intravenously (IV) at a dose of 1 mg/kg body weight, followed by succinylcholine IV at the dose of 0.75–1.5 mg/kg body weight. Methohexital is typically preferred over other anesthetics such as etomidate and alfentanil which can increase—or thiopental, propofol, thiamylal, midazolam, and lorazepam, which can decrease—the duration of ECT-induced seizure activity (relative to methohexital or saline, respectively) (Zhengnian & White, 2002). The patient is ventilated with 100% oxygen during the procedure.

After the scalp is properly prepared by cleaning the skin, the electrodes are placed. For safety, a bite block is placed in the patient's mouth to avoid tongue bite. Seizure activity is monitored by electroencephalography (EEG), and motor movements are observed on the isolated arm or foot. Upon completion of the ECT treatment, the patient is transported to the recovery room, where he or she is continuously monitored until he or she attains complete recovery. The ECT procedure takes approximately 15 minutes and is followed by a recovery time of 20–30 minutes. The patient is generally allowed to eat within an hour of recovery.

Electrode Placement

The three different methods of electrode placement in ECT include bitemporal placement, bifrontal placement, and right unilateral placement (see Figure 20.1).

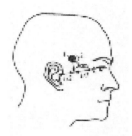 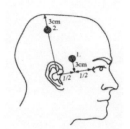 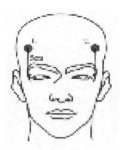

FIGURE 20.1. Diagram of electrode placement sites. *Left:* Bitemporal electrode placement—The center of the stimulus electrode is applied 2–3 cm above the midpoint of the line connecting the outer canthus of the eye and the external auditory meatus on each side of the patient's head. *Middle:* Unilateral electrode placement—One electrode is positioned as in bitemporal electrode placement on the right side. The center of the other electrode is placed 2–3 cm to the right of the vertex of the skull. *Right:* Bifrontal electrode placement—The center of each electrode is placed 4–5 cm above the outer canthus of the eye along a vertical line perpendicular to a line connecting the pupils. From Letemendia et al. (1993). Copyright 1993 by Cambridge University Press. Adapted by permission.

For bitemporal (BT) electrode placement, an electrode is placed on each temple, with the midpoint of each electrode 1 inch above the midpoint of the canthomeatus line.

For right unilateral (RUL) electrode placement, one electrode is placed on the right temple 1 inch above the midpoint of the canthomeatus line, and the other is placed 1 inch to the right side of the vertex of the skull.

For bifrontal (BF) electrode placement, each electrode is place 2.5 inches above the outer external canthus of the eye.

The general long-standing consensus is that BT electrode placement produces cognitive side effects with high efficacy. Relative to BT electrode placement, RUL electrode placement at low dose may be less effective and slower in relieving depressive symptoms. At high-stimulus doses of greater than 378 mC for RUL, the difference between electrode placements in terms of outcome decreases (McCall, Dunn, Rosenquist, & Hughes, 2002). Patients with schizophrenia may be treated with RUL, BT, or BF electrode placement, and electrode placement may be adjusted based on treatment outcome and side effects.

Stimulus Dosing

Stimulus dosing can be influenced by many variables. For example, age and stimulus dosing are positively correlated; that is, the greater the age, the greater the stimulus dosage to elicit seizure activity. Moreover, the placement of the electrodes can influence stimulus dosage. For initial and subsequent treatments, BT electrode placement dosing is the same and generally should be performed at moderately suprathreshold stimulation, defined as 150% above the seizure threshold (1.5 times above seizure threshold). RUL ECT placement should be performed at moderately to markedly suprathreshold stimulation, which is 250–600% above the seizure threshold (2.5 to 6.0 times above seizure threshold).

The empirical titration procedure (ETP), a commonly used method to ascertain and quantify the seizure threshold, is conducted by administering an initial dose of subconvulsive stimulus that is followed by restimulation with increased intensity after an interval of 20 seconds until motoric or EEG manifestation of a seizure is observed. The ETP is used to provide an amount of stimulus dosage with a high efficacy:low side effects ratio.

Seizure Monitoring

Seizures are monitored during ECT based on EEG, motor convulsion, tachycardia, and blood pressure. Tachycardia signals the ECT-induced cerebral seizure. The motor convulsions are observed in the isolated limb. It is recommended that both the motor seizure and the EEG be observed.

The EEG monitoring of ECT treatments shows characteristic patterns of the tonic and clonic phases of seizure activity (see Figure 20.2). The sites for EEG recording are frontal–mastoid and frontal–frontal montage. The frontal–mastoid montage is preferred because it maximizes the EEG seizure expression. During the tonic phase, hypersynchronous polyspike complexes are followed by polyspike and slow wave complexes. The clonus phase of the seizure is evidenced by sudden or gradual suppression of the polyspike and slow wave complexes. Most ECT-induced seizures last less than 90 seconds. For a seizure to have therapeutic benefit, it must be adequate, which means the motoric seizure activity should last for a minimum of 20 seconds; the EEG seizure activity should last a minimum of 30 seconds, and it should also show bilateral generalization (i.e., grand mal seizure). Regarding motoric manifestation, if there is an adequate seizure without motor activity, it may be possible that the cuff was inflated late or an increase in ictal blood pressure exceeded the restriction in circulation.

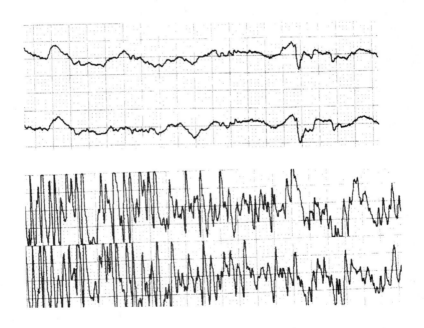

FIGURE 20.2. EEG recording. The top image is a normal EEG. The bottom EEG was created during a seizure (notice the sharp peaks and valleys).

Missed Seizures

If no seizure occurs after electrical stimulation, the patient is restimulated after an interval of 20 seconds at a higher energy level. Generally, the maximum number of restimulations permitted during the session is three or four.

Abortive or Brief Seizures

If the seizure duration is less than 15 seconds on both the motoric and EEG reading, the cause may be excessive anesthetic dosages, anticonvulsive medications, poor electrode contact, or device malfunction. The patient can be restimulated at a higher energy after a time interval of about 30–60 seconds.

Prolonged Seizures

A seizure is considered prolonged if it lasts more than 180 seconds (status epilepticus) by motoric or EEG manifestation. Should a prolonged seizure occur, the first step is to rule out any artifact in the reading. If no artifact is found, the seizure should be immediately terminated with an IV anesthetic agent. Continue oxygenation and close monitoring after a prolong seizure is stopped. A medical consultation should be considered if there is difficulty in termination of a prolonged seizure or if a spontaneous seizure occurs.

Inadequate Seizure Activity

If the patient experiences inadequate seizure activity with maximal electric stimulus, then etomidate can be used for induction of anesthesia. Alternatively, methohexital dosage can be reduced, and a combination of alfentanil or remifentanil can be added to extend the duration of seizure.

Frequency and Total Number of Treatments

In the acute treatment course, ECT is usually performed three times a week, regardless of electrode placement. The maximum number of acute treatments ranges from 12 to 20 treatments. If the patient responds to the acute course, then maintenance treatment is administered, with gradual interval increases between each treatment. ECT can be terminated if remission is achieved, or if the patient has severe side effects. Patients with acute onset of schizophrenic symptoms are more likely to benefit from ECT treatment. Combination treatment with antipsychotic medications and ECT have been found to be more effective than either treatment alone. For example, the relapse rate has been found to be less when the two treatments are combined rather than used separately.

ADVERSE EFFECTS

Postictal Delirium

Acute confusion can occur during the immediate postictal phase. Patients may present with restless agitation, disorientation, and repetitive, stereotyped limb and body movements. Also, patients may become uncooperative and show impaired comprehension. A quiet, relaxing environment post-ECT usually results in a smooth recovery. Postictal delirium can be treated with benzodiazepine IV or barbiturate medication. Alternately, increasing or decreasing the dose of succinylcholine and adding a small dose of methohexital at the end of the seizure may decrease the incidence of postictal delirium.

ECT-Induced Myalgias and Headaches

Myalgias and headaches are two common side effects following ECT treatment. To decrease and prevent ECT-induced myalgias and headaches, the patient can be premedicated with enteric-coated aspirin (650 mg) or acetaminophen (650 mg). In severe cases, ketorolac (30 mg IV) can be administered before the induction of anesthesia. Also, intranasal administration of sumatriptan may be beneficial if the patient develops post-ECT-induced headache despite ketorolac prophylaxis.

ECT-Associated Cognitive Side Effects

Anterograde and retrograde amnesia are common cognitive side effects following ECT treatment. Therefore, memory should be assessed before, during, and after the course of ECT treatment. Treatment should be adjusted according to the severity of the cognitive side effects. These modifications include changing the electrode placement (i.e., from BT to RUL), modifying the intensity of electrical stimulation from sinus wave to brief pulse stimulus, increasing the time interval between successive treatments, and altering the dose of the anesthetic medications. Typically, following the termination of ECT, cognitive difficulties resolves.

EVIDENCE SUPPORTING INTERVENTION

Research supporting the use of ECT in schizophrenia treatment has predominantly focused on its use as an adjunctive treatment to pharmacotherapy. ECT has been shown to increase the speed of response and efficacy, and ultimately leads to a decrease in both positive and negative symptoms. However, ECT may only improve positive symptoms and may in some cases have a minimal effect on negative symptoms.

Prior research has indicated that up to 25% of patients with schizophrenia do not adequately benefit from pharmacotherapy alone; thus, ECT is recommended as a treatment option. Predictors of response and benefit of ECT in patients with schizophrenia include an acute onset of schizophrenia, short duration of schizophrenia episode and presence of mood symptoms, delusions or hallucinations, and catatonic features. Negative indicators of response include long length of episode, older age during illness, previously failed neuroleptic pharmacotherapy, paranoid features, and high prevalence of negative symptoms.

As is the case with affective disorders, ECT is limited in treating schizophrenia due to high relapse rates and cognitive side effects. It is uncertain why the relapse rate is high; however, ECT is recommended in combination with pharmacotherapy as a maintenance and continuation therapy after acute treatment. There is limited research on optimizing ECT for schizophrenia, including dosing requirements and electrode placement site. For example, one study examined the effects of stimulus intensity during bilateral ECT placement using one, two, and four times the seizure threshold. The investigators concluded that clinical response time was positively related to the degree of stimulus dosing

(Chanpattana, Chakrabhand, Buppanharun, & Sackeim, 2000). Thus, a trend in research will be to find both the optimal ECT dosing strategy and electrode placement site to increase efficacy and minimize adverse cognitive effects.

TREATMENT GUIDELINES

The following treatment guidelines are adapted from the APA's *The Practice of Electroconvulsive Therapy* (see References and Recommend Readings) and the second edition of *APA Practice Guidelines for the Treatment of Patients with Schizophrenia* (2004, *www.psych.org*).

1. ECT should be considered in patients with persistent and severe psychosis, suicidal ideation, and or behaviors for which prior treatments failed.
2. ECT should be considered in patients whose catatonic features have not responded to acute pharmacotherapy.
3. ECT should be considered in patients with schizophrenia and comorbid depressive symptomatology with treatment resistance.
4. The number of ECT treatments to administer varies between a minimum of 12 and a maximum of 20 treatments. If more than 20 treatments are to be administered, a new consent should be obtained from the patient.
5. The comparative efficacies of unilateral and bilateral ECT have not been established in patients with schizophrenia; thus, either lead placement can be used.

KEY POINTS

- ECT is generally a safe and effective procedure in patients with schizophrenia. Immediate medical side effects include headache and muscle ache, and occasionally temporary or long-standing cognitive side effects.
- Initial indications for ECT were catatonia and dementia praecox. Presently, the main psychiatric indications for ECT are affective disorders, including unipolar and bipolar disorder that are severe, debilitating, and treatment resistant.
- Before ECT is initiated, a comprehensive evaluation should include a patient's medical and psychiatric history, laboratory exams, as well previous and current treatment history. It is important that certain medications, such as anticonvulsants, not be used due to interference with seizure activity.
- Safety and efficacy of the ECT procedure are increased by preparing the patient to receive ECT, using anesthesia, and monitoring body functions such as EEG, blood pressure, and motoric movement.
- The three main types of electrode placement include BT, which has the highest efficacy rate and the highest cognitive side effect profile; BF, which has a high efficacy rate and a mild-to-moderate cognitive side effect profile; and RUL, which, depending on the stimulus dosage, has a low-to-high efficacy rate and a mild-to-moderate cognitive side effect profile.
- Predictors of a positive response to ECT in patients with schizophrenia include acute schizophrenia onset, short duration of schizophrenia episode, and presence of delusions, hallucinations, or catatonic features.
- Predictors of a negative response to ECT in patients with schizophrenia include long length of schizophrenic episode, prior treatment failure with neuroleptic pharmacotherapy, paranoid features, and high negative symptom severity.

- The efficacy of acute ECT is high, with response rates that range from 70% to as high as 80%.
- The relapse rate within 6 months after acute ECT can range between 50 and 60%. For continuation treatment, ECT may be enhanced by the addition of pharmacotherapy.

REFERENCES AND RECOMMENDED READINGS

American Psychiatric Association. (2001). *The practice of electroconvulsive therapy: Recommendations for treatment, training, and privileging: A Task Force Report of the American Psychiatric Association.* Washington, DC: Author.

American Psychiatric Association. (2004). *Practice guideline for the treatment of patients with schizophrenia* (2nd ed.). Arlington, VA: Author.

Chanpattana, W., & Andrade, C. (2006). ECT for treatment-resistant schizophrenia: A response from the Far East to the UK NICE report. *Journal of ECT, 22*(1), 4–12.

Chanpattana, W., Chakrabhand, M. L. S., Buppanharun, W., & Sackeim, H. A. (2000). Effects of stimulus intensity of the efficacy of bilateral ECT in schizophrenia: A preliminary study. *Biological Psychiatry, 48*(3), 222–228.

Coffey, C. E. (1993). *Clinical science of electroconvulsive therapy.* Washington, DC: American Psychiatric Publishing.

Dodwell, D., & Goldberg, D. (1989). A study of factors associated with response to electroconvulsive therapy in patients with schizophrenic symptoms. *British Journal of Psychiatry, 154,* 635–639.

Fink, M., & Sackeim, H. A. (1996). Convulsive therapy in schizophrenia. *Schizophrenia Bulletin, 22*(1), 27–39.

Hoenig, J., & Chaulk, R. (1977). Delirium associated with lithium therapy and electroconvulsive therapy. *Canadian Medical Association Journal, 116,* 837–838.

Keuneman, R., Weerasundera, R., & Castle, D. J. (2002). The role of ECT in schizophrenia. *Australian Psychiatry, 10*(4), 385–388.

Letemendia, F. J., Delva, N. J., Rodenburg, M., Lawson, J. S., Inglis, J., Waldron, J. J., et al. (1993). Therapeutic advantage of bifrontal electrode placement in ECT. *Psychological Medicine, 23,* 349–360.

Lisanby, S. H. (2007). Electroconvulsive therapy for depression. *New England Journal of Medicine, 357,* 1939–1945.

McCall, V. W., Dunn, A., Rosenquist, P. B., & Hughes, D. (2002). Markedly suprathreshold right unilateral ECT verse minimally suprathreshold bilateral ECT. *Journal of ECT, 18,* 126–129.

Ottosson, J. O., & Fink, M. (2004). *Ethics in electroconvulsive therapy.* New York: Taylor & Francis.

Zhengnian, D., & White, P. F. (2002). Anesthesia for electroconvulsive therapy. *Anesthesia and Analgesia, 94,* 1351–1364.

PART IV

PSYCHOSOCIAL TREATMENT

CHAPTER 21

ENVIRONMENTAL SUPPORTS

DAWN I. VELLIGAN
ALEXANDER L. MILLER

Wykes (Chapter 25, this volume) describes cognitive rehabilitation (or cognitive remediation), a treatment designed to improve cognition and functional outcomes for patients with schizophrenia. Whereas cognitive rehabilitation utilizes computerized or pen-and-paper tests designed to improve attention, memory, and problem solving, environmental supports focus on structuring the environment to compensate for or work around impairments in these cognitive functions. Therapies that mainly work through the systematic use of environmental compensatory strategies and supports are relatively uncommon for schizophrenia but have a growing evidence base.

Compensatory strategies and environmental supports attempt to bypass cognitive deficits, negative symptoms, and disorganization by establishing supports in the environment that specifically cue and sequence adaptive behavior, and discourage maladaptive behavior. For example, pill containers with alarms can cue an individual to take medication on time. Daily-use pill containers can be used to discourage an individual from taking multiple doses of medication. Checklists can be used to prompt specific behaviors that are necessary to live more independently (e.g., cleaning the kitchen). These techniques have been utilized for years in the rehabilitation of individuals with head injuries and with mental retardation. More recently, these supportive strategies have been extended to treatment of schizophrenia in an intervention known as cognitive adaptation training (CAT) with very encouraging results.

COGNITIVE ADAPTATION TRAINING

CAT is a series of manual-driven compensatory strategies and environmental supports (signs, checklists, electronic cueing devices) based on a comprehensive assessment of the individual's neurocognitive function and behavior. We know that impairments in executive functions (the abilities needed to plan and carry out goal-directed behavior) can lead to one of several types of behavior when performing daily living skills; (1) apathy; (2)

disinhibition; (3) a combination of these. *Apathy* is characterized by poverty of speech and movement, and the inability to initiate and follow through on behavioral sequences. Someone with apathetic behavior is likely to have difficulty initiating each step in a multistep task. Obviously, for such a person, a task with many steps is unlikely to be initiated or, if initiated, will not likely be completed. *Disinhibition* is characterized by distractibility and behavior that is highly driven by cues in the environment. An individual with disinhibited behavior may start a task but become easily distracted and not complete it. A person with mixed behavior will have trouble both in initiating tasks and in not becoming distracted during the performance of tasks once they have been initiated.

Prior to participating in CAT, patients receive a comprehensive assessment of cognitive functioning, including tests of psychomotor speed, attention, memory, and problem solving. Behavior is rated with the Frontal Systems Behavior Scale (Grace & Malloy, 2002), an instrument that assesses apathy and disinhibition as observed during the performance of everyday tasks. In addition, the person's ability to perform basic and higher level daily activities is measured with a variety of performance-based assessments and behavioral observation. Finally, there is an assessment of the patient's environment, which examines whether the individual has items that are necessary to perform everyday tasks (soap, toothpaste, bug spray), where those items are placed (e.g., a toothbrush in a bottom dresser drawer is not likely to be used), and whether there are any safety hazards that need immediate attention (exposed electrical wires). Moreover, the assessment examines the availability of public transportation and whether supportive family members or friends are available for assistance.

Interventions in CAT are based on two dimensions: (1) level of impairment in executive functions (as determined by scores on a set of cognitive tests) and (2) whether the overt behavior of the individual is characterized more by apathy, disinhibition, or a combination of these styles. The poorer a person's executive functioning, the greater the need for high levels of structure and more obviously placed environmental cues. Those with somewhat better executive functioning need less structure and more subtle cues. Behaviors characterized by apathy can be altered by providing prompts and cues to initiate each step in a sequenced task. Examples of environmental alterations for apathetic behavior include utilizing checklists for tasks that involve complex behavioral sequencing, placing signs and equipment for daily activities directly in front of the patient (e.g., placing toothbrush and toothpaste in a basket directly attached to bathroom mirror), and utilizing labels and electronic devices (tape recorders) to cue and sequence behavior. Individuals with disinhibited behavior respond well to the removal of distracting stimuli and to redirection. For disinhibited behavior, supplies are organized to minimize inappropriate use. For example, outfits with one shirt, one pair of pants, and so forth, are placed in individual boxes in the closet to prevent the patient from putting on multiple layers of clothing. Differently colored bins for sorting laundry can prevent patients from mixing clean and soiled clothing. Individuals with mixed behavior (apathy and disinhibition) are offered a combination of these strategies.

Assessment results yield one of six CAT classifications for which interventions can be targeted. CAT classifications are presented in Table 21.1, along with problems that may be observed and possible interventions for impairments in dressing. Figure 21.1 illustrates three approaches for problems in dressing, one for each behavioral type, for individuals with poorer executive functioning.

Once an individual's CAT classification has been determined, strategies for specific functional problems (dental hygiene, laundry, leisure activity) are chosen from a series of tables. These basic strategies are then altered for strengths or weaknesses (relative to other outpatients with schizophrenia) in the areas of attention, memory, and fine motor

TABLE 21.1. Example Interventions by CAT Classification for Problems with Dressing

CAT classification	Example problem observed	Possible intervention
Apathetic—poorer executive function	Stays in bed clothes all day.	Place a clothing rack at the foot of the bed to prompt dressing. Each hanger should contain a complete set of clothing (i.e., shirt, pants, underwear, socks, and shoes) so that little initiation is required to complete the process (i.e., the person does not have to go to the dresser and then to the closet, etc.) (Figure 21.1A).
Apathetic—better executive function	May stay in bedclothes. Does not complete steps in dressing adequately due to poor initiation and inability to follow through on behavioral sequences (e.g., shirt is not tucked in, fly is not zipped, does not notice stains on clothing, puts on dirty clothing).	Use a customized recording alarm clock that prompts, "It's time to get dressed." Place a full-length mirror in the place the patient dresses (e.g., on the closet door). Tape a checklist to the mirror to prompt patient to check the specific problem areas (e.g., Tuck in your shirt, check for stains . . .)
Disinhibited—poorer executive function	Wears three shirts because they are hanging in the closet. Does not finish dressing due to distraction by irrelevant environmental stimuli.	Place complete outfits (shirt, pants, underwear, and socks) in separate plastic containers labeled with the day of the week. No clothes are hanging in the closet so there is no cue to put on additional clothing. Caretaker can start an audiotape that asks the patient a series of questions while dressing to keep him or her on task: for example, "Is your shirt on yet? Have you put on socks?" (Figure 21.1B).
Disinhibited—better executive function	Skips important steps in dressing due to distractibility by irrelevant stimuli (e.g., neglects to wear socks) or selects inappropriate items (e.g., heavy shirt in 100-degree heat, nonmatching clothes).	Remove distractions from dressing area. Remove items that are too small or inappropriate for current temperature. Place a sign on the closet door (e.g., "Don't forget your socks"). Color-code clothing that matches.
Mixed—poorer executive function	Does not initiate dressing and, once initiated, chooses inappropriate items.	Place a clothing rack at the foot of the bed to prompt dressing. To minimize distraction, enclose complete outfits, each in a plastic bag, and label for the day of the week (Figure 21.1C).
Mixed—better executive function	Slow to initiate dressing and, once initiated, may select inappropriate items.	Use a customized alarm to prompt dressing at a specified time. Remove all distractions from dressing area and clothing items that are too small or inappropriate for the current temperature. Color-code clothing that matches.

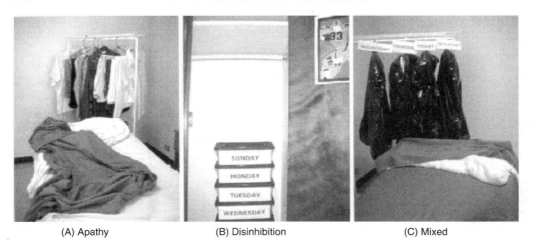

(A) Apathy   (B) Disinhibition   (C) Mixed

FIGURE 21.1. Examples of three CAT interventions, one for each behavioral type—apathetic (A), disinhibited (B), and mixed (C)—for someone with poorer executive functioning.

skills. For example, for someone with poor attention, the color of signs can be changed regularly or fluorescent colors can be used to capture attention. For someone with memory problems (particularly those with good auditory attention) audiotapes can be used to sequence behavior.

CAT interventions are established and maintained in the home by weekly visits from a CAT therapist/trainer. Individuals with bachelor's and master's degrees have been trained to do CAT. Fidelity to the model has been high. Intervention in studies published to date has lasted for 9 months. Studies of the effect of fading visits from weekly to monthly following 9 months are currently under way. During fading, we work to train the individual to set up the supports on his or her own (e.g., filling his or her own pill container weekly) and provide a month's worth of supports where possible (e.g., checklists that cover 5 weeks). Treatment typically begins by targeting client-identified goals, safety issues, and medication adherence. Over time, treatment targets a broad range of functional behaviors that include finding employment and engaging in leisure activities.

Patients who participated in a 9-month CAT treatment program were found to have lower levels of symptomatology and fewer relapses than those in standard treatment and control conditions. In addition, CAT has been found to improve adaptive functioning and community adjustment compared to standard and control treatments. Moreover, CAT has been found to improve adherence to medication regimens, as assessed by unannounced in-home pill counts. In summary, CAT strategies can improve a broad range of outcomes for individuals with schizophrenia.

OTHER WAYS TO USE ENVIRONMENTAL SUPPORTS

Generic Environmental Supports

Full CAT treatment is somewhat labor intensive and requires individualized treatment plans and home visits. As an alternative to CAT, it might be possible to provide important environmental supports, such as medication containers, calendars, watches, reminder signs, and hygiene checklists and supplies to patients when they come in for routine medication visits. When intensive treatments such as CAT or assertive community treatment are shown to be effective in randomized controlled trials, they are often scaled down for delivery in overburdened health care systems. A generic or scaled-down version of CAT has recently been systematically studied. Preliminary data suggest that individuals who use the supports provided improve on specific target behaviors. However, generic supports provided in a clinic setting, and expected to be set up by the client, are not as likely to be used as CAT supports, which are more individually tailored and established in the client's home by the CAT therapist and client working together.

Specific Supports for Specific Problems

Using environmental supports to cue and to reinforce taking medication has been found to be among the most effective strategies for individuals with physical illnesses. Environmental supports include advances in technology, such as the development of highly sophisticated pill containers. A recent invention known as the Med-eMonitor™ (see Figure 21.2) is capable of storing a month's supply of up to five different medications. The device prompts the patient when to take medication, reminds him or her of the goal of taking each medication, alerts the patient who is taking the wrong medication or taking it at the wrong time, records when containers are opened, and automatically downloads data to a secure website when placed into a cradle connected to a telephone line. The monitor can also ask a number of questions about side effects or symptoms on a regular basis. Based upon the patient's answers, a branching logic capability can provide further instructions or ask for more detailed information. Moreover, if problem adherence is identified after checking the website, treatment providers can contact the patient to identify barriers to adherence (e.g., "I left my medication at my sister's house"), to apply problem-solving techniques, and to remind the patient of important personal goals enhanced by taking medication as prescribed. In a recent *New England Journal of Medicine* review, Osterberg and Blaschke (2005) identified the following key factors for promoting adherence: identifying the problem; providing simple, clear instructions; reinforcing desired behavior; customizing treatment to the patient's schedule; and using supportive devices. Each of these features is incorporated into the design and function of smart pill containers such as the Med-eMonitor. In a recent pilot study at our site, the device significantly improved adherence to oral medication regimens in a sample of 15 subjects with

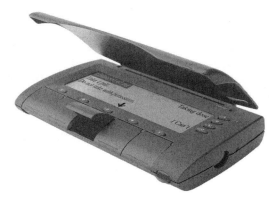

FIGURE 21.2. Med-eMonitor device. Photo courtesy of InforMedix, Inc.

schizophrenia, who went from a mean oral medication adherence rate of 52.11% (SD = 34.46) to a mean of 94.57% (SD = 7.33) over a 2-month period (p < .002).

Smart Homes

Smart homes have been suggested as supportive environments that may facilitate community adaptation for patients with schizophrenia. Smart homes have embedded technology designed to provide support, to prevent dangers, and to cue specific behaviors. This technology, used to compensate for cognitive deficits, is similar to the environmental supports provided in CAT. Smart homes have the capacity for remote data collection, interaction with the resident, and intervention. For example, a smart home may be able to transmit data about water faucets or ovens left on, to communicate with the resident about taking medication or other behaviors, or to shut off equipment automatically from a remote location. Whether such engineered living environments are economically feasible and can be developed and used in a way to promote the dignity and privacy of individuals with schizophrenia are open questions.

SUMMARY

Environmental supports have been found to improve functional outcomes for patients with schizophrenia. Given the advances in the development of new technologies, it is likely that the use of electronic environmental supports will continue to increase in the treatment of multiple medical conditions.

KEY POINTS

- Cognitive deficits, negative symptoms, and disorganized behavior lead to impairments in functional outcomes of individuals with schizophrenia.
- Environmental supports, such as signs, calendars, checklists, and medication containers with alarms, can bypass these problems, and cue and sequence adaptive behavior.
- Supports can be customized for level of impairment in executive functions and whether the person's behavior is characterized more by apathy (difficulty initiating every step of a multistep task) or disinhibition (being highly distracted by inappropriate cues in the environment).
- Individuals with apathy need supports to prompt and cue each step of a sequenced task.
- Individuals with disinhibition respond well to the reorganization of belongings and the removal of distracting stimuli.
- Environmental supports have been found to effectively improve adaptive functioning and decrease rates of relapse and symptom exacerbation in individuals with schizophrenia.
- As technology continues to advance, a wider range of supports may become available to address specific problems and difficulties.

REFERENCES AND RECOMMENDED READINGS

Bendle, S., Velligan, D. I., Mueller, J. L., Davis, B. V., Ritch, J. L., & Miller, A. L. (2005). The Med-eMonitor™ for improving adherence to oral medication in schizophrenia. *Schizophrenia Bulletin, 31,* 519.

Epstein, L. H., & Cluss, P. A. (1982). A behavioral medicine perspective on adherence to long-term medical regimens. *Journal of Consulting and Clinical Psychology, 50,* 950–971.

Frith, C. D. (1992). *The cognitive neuropsychology of schizophrenia*. East Sussex, UK: Erlbaum/Taylor & Francis.

Grace, J., & Malloy, P. F. (2002). *Frontal Systems Behavior Scale™*. Providence, RI: Brown University.

Osterberg, L., & Blaschke, T. (2005). Adherence to medication. *New England Journal of Medicine, 353*, 487–497.

Ruskin, P. E., Van Der Wende, J., Clark, C. R., Fenton, J., Deveau, J., & Thapar, R., (2003). Feasibility of using the Med-eMonitor system in the treatment of schizophrenia: A pilot study. *Drug Information Journal, 37*, 1–8.

Stip, E., & Rialle, V. (2005). Environmental cognitive remediation in schizophrenia: Ethical implications of "smart home" technology. *Canadian Journal of Psychiatry, 50*, 281–291.

Velligan, D. I., & Bow-Thomas, C. C. (2000). Two case studies of cognitive adaptation training for outpatients with schizophrenia. *Psychiatric Services, 51*, 25–29.

Velligan, D. I., Bow-Thomas, C. C., Huntzinger, C., Ritch, J., Ledbetter, N., Prihoda, T. J., et al. (2000). Randomized controlled trial of the use of compensatory strategies to enhance adaptive functioning in outpatients with schizophrenia. *American Journal of Psychiatry, 157*(8), 1317–1323.

Velligan, D. I., Mahurin, R. K., Diamond, P. L., Hazelton, B. D., Eckert, S. L., & Miller, A. L. (1997). The functional significance of symptomatology and cognitive function in schizophrenia. *Schizophrenia Research, 25*, 21–31.

Velligan, D. I., Prihoda, T. J., Ritch, J. L., Maples, N., Bow-Thomas, C. C., & Dassori, A. (2002). A randomized single-blind pilot study of compensatory strategies in schizophrenia outpatients. *Schizophrenia Bulletin, 28*(2), 283–292.

Zygmunt, A., Olfson, M., Boyer, C. A., & Mechanic, D. (2002). Interventions to improve medication adherence in schizophrenia. *American Journal of Psychiatry, 159*, 1653–1664.

CHAPTER 22

FAMILY INTERVENTION

CHRISTINE BARROWCLOUGH
FIONA LOBBAN

Families play an essential role in supporting people with long-term mental illness in the community and are focal in the social networks of people with a schizophrenia diagnosis. Over 60% of persons with a first episode of a major mental illness return to live with relatives, and this percentage is reduced only by 10–20% when those with subsequent admissions are included. Living with a close relative who experiences psychosis can present many challenges and may be associated with considerable personal costs. In schizophrenia, estimates from different studies suggest that up to two-thirds of family members experience significant stress and subjective burden as a consequence of their caregiver role. Such stress is not only likely to affect the well-being of the relatives and compromise their long-term ability to support the patient, but it may also have an impact on the course of the illness itself and on outcomes for the client. Hence, one of the most important advances in the treatment of schizophrenia in the last two decades has been the development of family-based intervention programs. The efficacy of this form of treatment is now well established, with many randomized controlled trials having demonstrated the superiority of family intervention over routine care in terms of patient relapse and hospitalization outcomes. This chapter outlines the background to this area of work, describes intervention approaches, summarizes the research findings to date, draws attention to important areas for future development, and provides treatment guidelines based on current knowledge.

BACKGROUND

The development of multifactorial models of the processes determining risk and relapse in schizophrenia provided the general rationale for the development of family interventions. These "stress–vulnerability" models emphasized the contribution of psychological and socioenvironmental stressors to the illness course, thereby opening up the way to psychological interventions. In particular family interventions found much of their initial impetus in the research on expressed emotion (EE). High EE is assessed on the basis of a critical, hostile or overinvolved attitude toward the patient on the part of a relative living in the same household. Early studies found that when patients were discharged to go home after being hospitalized for a schizophrenic relapse, their risk of subsequent relapse in the short term was greatly increased if one or more family members was assessed to be "high EE." These results have been replicated many times, and a meta-analysis of 27 studies (Butzlaff & Hooley, 1998) confirmed the elevated risk of relapse for patients in high-EE households. Within the context of stress–vulnerability models, an individual's home may be viewed as an environment capable of influencing the illness for better or worse. If attributes of certain households are responsible for precipitating relapse, then they might be identified and modified, with a resulting reduction in relapse rates. A series of studies testing this theory throughout the last two decades is described below.

DESCRIPTION OF FAMILY INTERVENTION APPROACHES

In the past two decades many studies have evaluated the impact of family interventions on schizophrenia. Typically, the controlled trials recruited families at the point of patient hospitalization for an acute episode of schizophrenia and commenced the family intervention when the patient was discharged back to the home. At the end of the intervention period lasting from 6 to 12 months, relapse rates of patients who received the family intervention as an adjunct to routine care were compared with those of patients who received routine care only. Routine care included the use of prophylactic medication. Table 22.1 presents a summary of studies that have compared family intervention with routine or standard care for patients with a schizophrenia diagnosis. Although we selected only studies in which the intervention lasted for at least 10 sessions it is apparent that there has been considerable variation in the programs of family interventions. Interventions developed by the various research groups differed on some important dimensions, including the location of the family sessions (home- vs. hospital-based); the number of sessions offered and the time period of delivery; the extent of the patient's involvement; and, last but not least, the precise content of the sessions and the mode of delivery. Because the researchers did not have a clear understanding of the mechanisms of patient relapse in the home environment, or why some relatives appeared to fare better in their approach than others, determining session content involved making certain assumptions about the kinds of problems associated with high-EE or stressed families, then deciding what issues needed to be targeted. In practice, all the studies assumed that families had inadequate knowledge or misunderstandings regarding the illness to the extent that some reviewers subsumed all family intervention under the category "psychoeducation," emphasizing that educating relatives about schizophrenia was an essential session component. The other commonly targeted area was helping the family members cope with symptom-related difficulties either by a specific problem-solving approach (Falloon, Laporta, Fadden, & Graham-Hole, 1993) or through assessment of individual problems and application of appropriate cognitive-behavioral techniques applied to a family context (Barrowclough & Tarrier, 1992). Despite differences in approaches, Mari and Streiner (1994) provided a useful summary of the common "ingredients" or "overall principles" of the treatments: to build up an alliance with relatives who care for the family member with schizophrenia; to reduce the adverse family atmosphere; to enhance the problem-solving capacity of relatives; to decrease expressions of anger and guilt; to maintain reasonable expectations of patient performance; to set limits safeguarding relatives' own well-being; and to achieve changes in relatives' behavior and beliefs. Clearly, to encompass all of these goals requires

TABLE 22.1. Controlled Studies Comparing Family Intervention with Standard Treatment for Patients with Schizophrenia

Study	Treatment conditions	N	Type of family intervention	Frequency and duration of treatment	Relapse
Kottgen et al. (1984)	Family intervention, high expressed emotion. Customary care, high expressed emotion. Customary care, low expressed emotion.	49	Psychodynamic: separate groups for patients and relatives	Weekly or monthly up to 2 years	2 years: family intervention equal to customary care for families with either high or low expressed emotion
Falloon et al. (1982, 1985)	Behavioral family therapy. Individual management.	36	Home-based behavioral family	Weekly for 3 months Biweekly for 6 months Monthly for 15 months	2 years: behavioral family therapy better than individual management
Leff et al. (1982, 1985)	Family intervention. Customary care.	24	Psychoeducation to help relatives with high expressed emotion model coping of low expressed emotion relatives	Biweekly for relatives groups for 9 months	2 years: family intervention better than customary care
Tarrier et al. (1988, 1989, 1994)	Behavioral family therapy enactive. Behavioral family therapy symbolic. Education only. Customary care.	77	Behavioral family therapy comprising stress management and training in goal setting	Three stress management and eight goal-setting sessions over 9 months	2 years: behavioral family therapy better than education or customary care; education and customary care equal
Vaughan et al. (1992)	Single-family psychoeducation and support. Customary care.	36	Psychoeducation	Ten weekly sessions	9 months: single-family education and support equal to customary care
Randolph et al. (1994)	Behavioral family therapy. Customary care	39	Clinic-based behavioral family therapy	Weekly for 3 months Biweekly for 3 months Biweekly for 6 months	2 years: behavioral family therapy better than customary care
Xiong et al. (1994)	Behavioral family therapy. Customary care.	63	Clinic-based psychoeducation, skills training, medication/symptom management	Bimonthly for 3 months Family sessions for 2 years (plus individual sessions with family members and patients): maintenance sessions every 2–3 months.	18 months: behavioral family therapy better than customary care

(continued)

TABLE 22.1. (*continued*)

Study	Treatment conditions	N	Type of family intervention	Frequency and duration of treatment	Relapse
Zhang et al. (1994)	Multiple- and single-family psychoeducation and support. Customary care.	78	Multiple-family clinic-based psycho-education counseling, medication/symptom management.	Individual and group counseling sessions every 1–3 months for 18 months.	18 months: family education and support better than customary care
Buchremer et al. (1997)	Relatives group. Customary care.	68	"Therapeutic" relatives groups and initiated relatives.	Every 2 weeks for 2 years	No differences between groups at 1 year or 2 years.
Telles et al. (1995)	Behavioral family management. Individual case management.	— —	Clinic-based behavioral family management	Weekly for 6 months, every 2 weeks for 3 months, monthly for 3 months	12 months: for total group conditions equal; for "poorly acculturated" patients, individual management better for "highly acculturated" patients, conditions equal
Leff et al. (1990)	Multiple-family psychoeducation and support. Single-family psychoeducation and support.	23	Multiple-family groups in the clinic; single family sessions at home	Biweekly for 9 months, varying amounts afterward	2 years: conditions equal
Zastowny et al. (1992)	Behavioral family therapy. Single-family psychoeducation and support.	30	Hospital-based behavioral family therapy; hospital based single-family psychoeducation and advice on handling common problems	Weekly for 4 months, monthly for 12 months	16 months: conditions equal
McFarlane et al. (1995)	Multiple-family psychoeducation and support. Single-family psychoeducation and support.	83 89	Multiple-family groups or single-family sessions in the clinic	Biweekly sessions for 2 years	2 years: multiple-family conditions better than single-family condition
Schooler et al. (1997)	Applied family management. Supportive family management.	157 156	Applied management comprising home-based behavioral family therapy sessions plus supportive family management; supportive family management comprising clinic-based multiple-family groups	Applied family management: behavioral family therapy weekly for 3 months, biweekly for 6 months, and monthly for 3–6 months plus concurrent monthly supportive family management for 24–28 months; supportive family management monthly for 24–28 months.	2 years: conditions equal

commitment over a considerable time period, and there have been large variations in the intensity of the interventions.

The content and format of family interventions have also been modified to address the differing needs of particular families.

First-Episode Psychosis

Relatives of individuals experiencing their first episode of psychosis report a higher risk of distress compared to family members of individuals who have a more chronic course of illness. Family members have numerous concerns at this time and are likely to have less knowledge and understanding of psychosis on which to draw. This may be an opportune time to engage family members, because they are likely to be searching for support and information (Addington & Burnett, 2004). Families need to be offered support to manage crises and an initial explanatory model of psychosis that they can use to understand their experiences. This can then be built on gradually, along with other aspects of family interventions, including problem-solving skills, communication training, cognitive reappraisal, and working with relapse prevention plans.

Substance Use and Psychosis

It is widely recognized that many people with psychosis misuse street drugs or alcohol, and that this "dual diagnosis" is associated with many complex problems for families. Specialist approaches to working with these difficulties have been described by Barrowclough (2003), who described an intervention that sought to promote a family response to match the patient's stage of change regarding substance use. This family intervention was conducted alongside individual work with the patient to address substance use. This randomized controlled trial combining family and individual treatment demonstrated good outcomes for patients.

Group Family Work

Working with groups of families who share similar problems has a number of advantages: Participants can be encouraged to share experiences and coping strategies that have worked for them. Many variations on the group format have been used; some have included patients, and others have been largely restricted to relatives, so that they can talk openly without fear of upsetting the patient. Evaluation studies of multiple-family intervention formats have shown inconsistent results, and in a meta-analysis, Pilling and colleagues (2002) found that, compared to single-family treatments, group treatments had a poorer outcome.

RESULTS FROM THE STUDIES AND DISCUSSION OF EVIDENCE BASE FOR FAMILY INTERVENTIONS

A number of meta-analytic reviews (Mari & Streiner, 1994; Pharoah, Mari, & Streiner, 1999; Pilling et al., 2002; Pitschel-Walz, Leucht, Bauml, Kissling, & Engel, 2001) of the family intervention have been published, including studies in which patients had a diagnosis of schizophrenia or schizoaffective disorder; in which there was some form of control or comparison group against which to evaluate any benefits from the experimental treatment; and in which patient relapse or hospitalization was examined as the main outcome. The Pharoah and colleagues (1999) analysis adopted more stringent inclusion criteria (excluding studies with nonrandom assignment, those restricted to an inpatient intervention, those not restricted to schizophrenia, and those in which intervention was less than five sessions) and included 13 studies. The review confirmed the findings of earlier, descriptive accounts of the studies. It concluded that family intervention as an adjunct to routine care decreases the frequency of relapse and hospitalization, and that these findings hold across the wide age ranges, sex differences, and variability in the length of illness in the different studies. Moreover, the analysis suggested that these results generalize across care cultures in which health systems are very different: Trials from the United Kingdom, Australia, Europe, the People's Republic of China, and the United States were included. However, more recent reviews have been less conclusive and have highlighted the large degree of heterogeneity in findings.

Pitschel-Walz and colleagues (2001) examined 25 studies spanning 20 years (1977–1997). Table 22.1 contains a subgroup of these studies, selecting those that had a treatment duration of at least 10 sessions. Their meta-analysis confirmed the superiority of family treatment over control groups relative to patient relapse rates, with a relapse rate decrease of 20% in patients whose families received an intervention. Although this treatment effect may seem relatively low, one must bear in mind that this analysis included studies in which the intervention was extremely brief, with little resemblance to the intensive programs in the original studies. For example, as shown in Table 22.1, the studies of Falloon and colleagues (1982), Leff, Kuipers, Berkowitz, Eberlein-Fries, and Sturgeon (1982), and Tarrier and colleagues (1988) demonstrated decreased relapse rates of approximately 40% in patients whose families received treatment. Unfortunately, the absence of treatment fidelity measures makes it very difficult to judge quality control within or between studies. Further comparison analyses within the Pitschel-Walz and colleagues review drew attention to some of the wide variations in the content and duration of programs in recent years. It seems that there was considerable dilution of the potency of the family interventions in the large meta-analyses in which there was no quality control. Categorizing studies into those lasting more or less than 10 weeks, they found that long-term interventions were more successful than short-term interventions, and that more intensive family treatments were superior to a more limited approach (e.g., in which relatives were offered little more than brief education sessions about schizophrenia). For families provided with a longer and more intense intervention, the Pitschel-Walz and colleagues review suggested some evidence of the long-lasting effects from family treatment. However, it must be emphasized that all the studies indicated that relapses increased with the number of years from termination of the intervention.

The more recent meta-analysis by Pilling and colleagues (2002) included 18 studies, and its conclusions were in line with previous reviews in confirming the efficacy of family intervention for reducing patient relapse. In a comparison of single-family and group family treatments, group treatments had poorer outcomes in terms of the reemergence of patients' psychotic symptoms or readmission to hospital. Pilling and colleagues agreed with previous reviewers (Mari & Streiner, 1994) that the effects from family interventions have decreased over the years, and suggested that this might in part be explained by the increased use of family group approaches. However, they added that this might not be due to the group format per se, but rather to other factors: the variable content of the group treatments; the fact that group treatments may have benefits not measured by the studies (e.g., on caregiver burden); or the fact that group treatments may have particular benefit for subpopulations.

One of the criticisms of family intervention studies has been their narrow focus on the end results of reductions in patient relapse and hospitalizations. The inclusion of other outcome measures has been variable; consequently, there are usually inadequate systematic data subjected to meta-analytic review. The Pitschel-Walz and colleagues (2001) review is more optimistic than that of Pilling and colleagues (2002) in the conclusions drawn about wider patient and family outcomes. With regard to patient outcomes, both reviews agree that there is some evidence of better medication compliance. Pitschel-Walz and colleagues also assert that there are indications of improved quality of life and better patient social adjustment in patients whose families were treated. Several studies have demonstrated that these improved outcomes are achieved with reduced costs to society.

As noted by Pilling and colleagues (2002), the potential benefit of the interventions for family members themselves has received relatively little attention. We must remember that although the trials sought to reduce stress in families, improvement in patient outcomes, and not family outcomes, was the prime target. When family burden was assessed as a secondary outcome, the results appear to be inconsistent. Szmukler and colleagues (2003) identified three randomized controlled trials aimed specifically at caregivers, although with very brief interventions. Although these studies showed some advantages, in terms of outcomes the advantages were only indirectly related to distress and burden (e.g., knowledge and attitudes). The use of different measures makes comparisons between studies assessing caregiver outcomes problematic. A recent trial with a longer duration of intervention, which did focus primarily on improving caregiver outcomes, did not produce encouraging results (Szmuckler et al., 2003). A two-phase intervention with six single-family sessions, followed by 12 group family sessions, was compared with standard care. Engagement in the trial was poor, and the authors reported that the caregiver program did not offer any significant advantage on any of the outcome measures: psychological morbidity, negative appraisal, coping, or support. Szmuckler and colleagues concluded that there is still uncertainty about the most effective interventions for caregivers of patients with psychotic disorders.

DISSEMINATION OF FAMILY INTERVENTIONS

In recent years there have been attempts to disseminate the benefits of family intervention in schizophrenia into routine service delivery. This has been largely through training programs designed to provide clinicians, mainly community psychiatric nurses, with the knowledge and skills required to implement the family work (see Tarrier, Barrowclough, Haddock, & McGovern [1999] for a review of dissemination programs). Despite the solid evidence base for the efficacy of family-based psychological treatment programs in schizophrenia, and the efforts of the training programs, the implementation of family work in routine mental health services has at best been patchy. The consensus view in the literature is that family intervention implementation faces complex organizational and attitudinal difficulties (e.g., McFarlane, Dixon, Lukens, & Luckstead, 2003), and insufficient attention has been paid to these problems in dissemination programs. In discussing the factors that might make the transference from research to practice difficult, Mari and Streiner (1994) suggested that the requirements of durable service-oriented interventions may differ from those based on time-limited research models. In an attempt to demonstrate the effectiveness of family interventions in standard psychiatric settings that accounted for these differences, a randomized controlled pragmatic trial was carried out by Barrowclough and colleagues (1999). The family intervention was based on the formal assessment of caregiver needs, and the program was carried out by a clinical psychologist in conjunction with the patient's social worker; thus, training was *in situ*. The fact that the intervention was found to effectively reduce caregiver needs and patient relapse at 12-month posttreatment suggests that there are advantages in developing dissemination models based within services. The need for changing the clinical practice of the whole service rather than training individuals is demonstrated in the work of Corrigan and colleagues (1997). However, difficulties arise not only with staff but also with caregiver reluctance to engage in family work. Several studies of community samples have shown that caregiver participation in family intervention is relatively low, with only 50% or so of caregivers taking up the offer of either a support service or family intervention (Barrowclough et al., 1999), with possibly higher rates when help is offered at a time of crisis or at first episode. It has been suggested that the professional-led, time-intensive model on which family interventions are based may not be the most optimal approach, and that multiple family psychoeducation groups led by trained caregivers, as described by Dixon and colleagues (2004), may offer a more acceptable alternative. Further evaluation of the impact of such interventions on both patient and caregiver outcomes is required.

RESEARCH INTO PSYCHOLOGICAL PROCESSES INFLUENCING FAMILY RESPONSES TO PSYCHOSIS AND IMPLICATIONS FOR INTERVENTIONS

A number of studies have now demonstrated that relatives' appraisals of the illness are important mediators of the relationship between illness factors and caregiver responses. Most work in this area has focused on one type of appraisal—the kind of explanations or causal attributions that relatives make about problematic behaviors associated with schizophrenia (see Barrowclough & Hooley [2003] for a review). Attributions of relatives who are high EE by virtue of being critical or hostile are different than those of low-EE relatives. More specifically, because high-EE relatives are critical, they consistently attribute more control to patients for their symptoms and problems than do relatives low in criticism; that is, they are more likely to hold patients responsible for their difficulties. Relatives rated as high EE because they are more hostile also attribute control to the patient, but they are even more likely to attribute problems to factors internal to the patients (i.e., seeing negative events as caused solely by the patients, to the exclusion of other potential contributory factors). In contrast, relatives rated as high EE because of emotional overinvolvement, tend to make sense of the illness in terms of factors outside the patients' control, and see the patient as an unfortunate victim of a severe illness.

Appraisals linked to EE have focused almost exclusively on an attributional framework of causal explanations. There may be some merit in increasing the scope of the study of relatives' cognitions about mental illness as a means of understanding variability in how people respond to close relatives with a severe mental illness. In the area of physical health, it is widely accepted that cognitive processes mediate people's adaptation to their own health problems, and the most notable theoretical framework adopted in this work is the self-regulation model of Leventhal, Diefenbach, and Leventhal (1992) and Leventhal, Nerenz, and Steele (1984). It has been demonstrated that patients' illness representations, or models of illness, are based on distinct components—identity, cause, time line, and illness consequences, as well as controllability. These representations have been shown to carry emotional, behavioral, and coping implications, and are related to health outcomes. It has been suggested that illness representations may also have important implications for people's responses to ill individuals, particularly in mental illness (Lobban, Barrowclough, & Jones, 2003). A preliminary study by Barrowclough, Lobban, Hatton, and Quinn (2001) supported the utility of this model in the context of relatives of patients with schizophrenia by using the Illness Perception Questionnaire. As with previous studies, there was little association between the measures of caregiver functioning (using measures of distress and burden) and patient functioning. However, when relatives perceived greater negative consequences for the patient because of the illness, they showed greater distress and subjective burden.

FUTURE DIRECTIONS

In summary, a number of important conclusions can be drawn from recent analyses of family intervention studies. First, although there is robust evidence for the efficacy of family interventions in schizophrenia, it is also clear that short family education or counseling programs do not affect relapse rates: "[receiving] a few lessons on schizophrenia . . . was simply not sufficient to substantially influence the relapse rate" (Pitschel-Walz et al., 2001, p. 84). The quality of interventions needs to be enhanced and monitored to ensure that families are offered the intensity of help likely to provide substantial benefits. Successful family interventions require considerable investment in time, skills, and commitment; and because for many patients the effect is to delay rather than to prevent relapse, many patients and families need long-term, continuing intervention. Work with relatives of recently diagnosed patients with schizophrenia indicates that this help needs to begin from the first onset of the psychosis. Second, we need to concentrate more research effort on developing interventions that are beneficial to the relatives' own well-being. Third, we need to continue to address dissemination and engagement issues. Although many patients and families benefit greatly from the intervention programs, a substantial number of families are difficult to engage, and the implementation of family programs within services presents many challenges. Finally, further work needs to identify optimum techniques for changing family attitudes when problems are particularly complex, for example, in schizophrenia and comorbid substance misuse.

TREATMENT RECOMMENDATIONS

1. Family interventions should be offered as part of a cohesive treatment package, tailored to meet the individual needs of each family. A systematic nonblaming rationale should be made clear to emphasize that although family members are not seen as responsible for causing the mental health problems, they may be able to play an important role in recovery.

2. Repeated attempts may be necessary to engage the family. Offering support and information at key times of distress, such as the first schizophrenia episode, relapse, or crisis, may be a useful way to begin to involve the family in a more structured intervention.

3. A long-term commitment to offer a minimum of 10 sessions over a period of about 6 months may be necessary to achieve an effective outcome. Short-term, limited interventions appear to be less effective.

4. The exact mechanism of change in successful family interventions remains unclear. Therefore, it is impossible to identify precisely what the key components of any intervention should be, and it is likely that these components may vary depending on the specific needs of the family. However, interventions should include the following components:

• Providing practical and emotional support to family members

- Providing information about the illness, mental health services, and other available support systems
- Helping the family to develop a working explanatory model of the illness
- Modifying beliefs about the illness that are unhelpful or inaccurate
- Increasing perceived coping for all family members
- Enhancing problem-solving skills
- Enhancing positive communication within the family
- Involving family members in an ongoing relapse prevention plan

5. Family interventions should aim to improve outcome for both patients and caregivers. The focus should be on recovery in terms of social relationships, employment, housing, dating and marriage, quality of life, and so forth, for both the patient and relatives, rather than exclusively on symptom reduction.

6. Despite the many barriers to offering family interventions, an attempt should always be made to work in collaboration with relatives who support people with mental health problems, and to do the best we can to support their efforts.

KEY POINTS

- Families play an essential role in supporting people with long-term mental health problems.
- Family intervention for schizophrenia reduces patient relapses and hospitalizations.
- Special programs have been developed for working with relatives of patients with a first episode and families of patients with co-occurring substance misuse.
- There is a lot of variation in approaches, but longer term, more intensive approaches seem to be more successful.
- More research effort is required for developing interventions that benefit relatives' well-being.
- Engagement of families can sometimes be problematic.
- More effort to disseminate family interventions into services is required.

REFERENCES AND RECOMMENDED READINGS

Addington, J., & Burnett, P. (2004). Working with families in the early stages of psychosis. In J. Gleeson & P. McGorry (Eds.), *Psychological interventions in early psychosis: A treatment handbook*. New York: Wiley.

Barrowclough, C. (2003). Family intervention for substance use in psychosis. In H. L. Graham, A. Copello, M. Birchwood, & K. T. Mueser (Eds.), *Substance misuse in psychosis: Approaches to treatment and service delivery*. Chichester, UK: Wiley.

Barrowclough, C., & Hooley, J. M. (2003). Attributions and expressed emotion: A review. *Clinical Psychology Review, 23*, 849–880.

Barrowclough, C., Lobban, F., Hatton, C., & Quinn, J. (2001). An investigation of models of illness in carers of schizophrenic patients using the Illness Perception Questionnaire. *British Journal of Clinical Psychology, 40*, 371–385.

Barrowclough, C., & Tarrier, N. (1992). *Families of schizophrenic patients: Cognitive behavioural intervention*. London: Chapman & Hall.

Barrowclough, C., Tarrier, N., Lewis, S., Sellwood, W., Mainwaring, J., Quinn, J., et al. (1999). Randomised controlled effectiveness trial of a needs-based psychosocial intervention service for carers of people with schizophrenia. *British Journal of Psychiatry, 174*, 505–511.

Buchremer, G., Klinberg, S., Holle, R., Schulze-Monking, H., & Hornung, P. (1997). Psychoeducational psychotherapy for schizophrenic patients and their key relatives: Results of a two year follow up. *Acta Psychiatrica Scandinavia, 96*, 483–491.

Butzlaff, R. L., & Hooley, J. M. (1998). Expressed emotion and psychiatric relapse: A meta-analysis. *Archives of General Psychiatry, 55,* 547–552.

Corrigan, V. A., McCracken, S. G., Edwards, M., Brunner, J., Garman, A., Nelson, D., et al. (1997). Collegial support and barriers to behavioural programs for severely mentally ill. *Journal of Behavior Therapy and Experimental Psychiatry, 28,*193–202.

Dixon, L., Luckstead, A., Stewart, B., Burland, J., Brown, C. H., Postrado, L., et al. (2004). Outcomes of the peer taught 12-week family-to-family education program for severe mental illness. *Acta Psychiatrica Scandinavica, 109,* 207–215.

Falloon, I. R. H., Boyd, J. L., McGill, C. W., Razini, J., Moss, H. B., & Gilderman, A. M. (1982). Family management in the prevention of exacerbrations of schizophrenia. *New England Journal of Medicine, 306,* 1437–1440.

Falloon, I. R. H., Boyd, J. L., McGill, C. W., Williamson, M., Razini, J., Moss, H. B., et al. (1985). Family management in the prevention of morbidity in schizophrenia: Clinical outcome of a 2 year longitudinal study. *Archives of General Psychiatry, 42,* 887–896.

Falloon, I. R. H., Laporta, M., Fadden, G., & Graham-Hole, V. (1993). *Managing stress in families: Cognitive and behavioural strategies for enhancing coping skills.* London: Routledge.

Jones, S., & Hayward, P. (2004). Coping with schizophrenia: A guide for patients, families and caregivers. Oxford, UK: Oneworld.

Kottgen, C., Soinnichesen, I., Mollenhauer, K., & Jurth, R. (1984). Results of the Hamburg Camberwell Family Interview study, I–III. *International Journal of Family Psychiatry, 5,* 61–94.

Leff, J. P., Berkowitz, R., Shavit, A., Strachan, A., Glass, I., & Vaughn, C. E. (1990). A trial of family therapy versus relatives' groups for schizophrenia. *British Journal of Psychiatry, 157,* 571–577.

Leff, J. P., Kuipers, L., Berkowitz, R., Eberlein-Fries, R., & Sturgeon, D. (1982) A controlled trial of intervention with families of schizophrenic patients. *British Journal of Psychiatry, 141,* 121–134.

Leff, J. P., Kuipers, L., & Sturgeon, D. (1985). A controlled trial of social intervention in the families of schizophrenic patients. *British Journal of Psychiatry, 146,* 594–600.

Leventhal, H., Diefenbach, M., & Leventhal, E. A. (1992). Illness cognition: Using common sense to understand treatment adherence and affect cognition interactions. *Cognitive Therapy and Research, 16*(2), 143–163.

Leventhal, H., Nerenz, D. R., & Steele, D. F. (1984). Illness representations and coping with health threats. In A. Baum & J. Singer (Eds.), *Handbook of psychology and health* (pp. 219–252). Hillsdale, NJ: Erlbaum.

Lobban, F., Barrowclough, C., & Jones, S. (2003). A review of models of illness for severe mental illness. *Clinical Psychology Review, 23,* 171–196.

Mari, J. J., & Streiner, D. L. (1994). An overview of family interventions and relapse in schizophrenia: Meta-analysis of research findings. *Psychological Medicine, 24,* 565–578.

Mari, J. J., & Streiner, D. L. (1996). Family intervention for people with schizophrenia (Cochrane Review). *The Cochrane Library,* Issue 1. Oxford, UK: Update Software.

McFarlane, W. R., Dixon, L., Lukens, E., & Luckstead, A. (2003). Family psychoeducation and schizophrenia: A review of the literature. *Journal of Marital and Family Therapy, 29,* 223–245.

McFarlane, W. R., Lukens, E., Link, B., Dushay, R., Deakins, S. A., Newmark, M., et al. (1995). Multiple family groups and psychoeducation in the treatment of schizophrenia. *Archives of General Psychiatry, 52*(8), 679–687.

Mueser, K. T., & Glynn, S. M. (1999). Behavioral family therapy for psychiatric disorders (2nd ed.). Oakland, CA: New Harbinger.

Pharoah, F. M., Mari, J. J., & Streiner, D. L. (1999). Family intervention for people with schizophrenia (Cochrane Review). *The Cochrane Library,* Issue 4. Oxford, UK: Update Software.

Pilling, S., Bebbington, P., Kuiipers, E., Garety, P., Geddes, J., Orbach, G., et al. (2002). Psychological treatments in schizophrenia: I. Meta-analysis of family intervention and cognitive behaviour therapy. *Psychological Medicine, 32,* 763–782.

Pitschel-Walz, G., Leucht, S., Bauml, J., Kissling, W., & Engel, R. R. (2001). The effect of family interventions on relapse and rehospitalisation in schizophrenia—a meta-analysis. *Schizophrenia Bulletin, 27,* 73–92.

Randolph, E. T., Eth, S., Glynn, S. M., Paz, G. G., Shaner, A. L., Strachan, A., et al. (1994). Behavioural family management in schizophrenia: Outcome of a clinic based intervention. *British Journal of Psychiatry, 164,* 501–506.

Schooler, N. R., Keith, S. J., Severe, J. B., Matthews, S. M., Bellack, A. S., Glick, I. D., et al. (1997).

Relapse and rehospitalization during maintenance treatment of schizophrenia: The effects of dose reduction and family treatment. *Archives of General Psychiatry, 54*(5), 453–463.

Szmukler, G., Kuipers, E., Joyce, J., Harris, T., Leese, M., Maphosa, W., et al. (2003). An exploratory randomised controlled trial of a support programme for carers of patients with a psychosis. *Social Psychiatry and Psychiatric Epidemiology, 34,* 411–418.

Tarrier, N., Barrowclough, C., Haddock, G., & McGovern, J. (1999). The dissemination of innovative cognitive-behavioural psychosocial treatments for schizophrenia. *Journal of Mental Health, 8,* 569–582

Tarrier, N., Barrowclough, C., Porceddu, K., & Fitzpatrick, E. (1994). The Salford Family Intervention Project for Schizophrenic relapse prevention: Five and eight year accumulating relapses. *British Journal of Psychiatry, 165,* 829–832.

Tarrier, N., Barrowclough, C., Vaughn, C. E., Bamrah, J. S., Proceddu, K., Watts, S., et al. (1988). Community management of schizophrenia: A controlled trial of a behavioural intervention with families to reduce relapse. *British Journal of Psychiatry, 153,* 532–542.

Tarrier, N., Barrowclough, C., Vaughn, C. E., Bamrah, J. S., Proceddu, K., Watts, S., et al. (1989). The community management of schizophrenia: A controlled trial of a behavioural intervention with families to reduce relapse: A 2 year follow-up. *British Journal of Psychiatry, 154,* 625–628.

Telles, C., Karno, M., Mintz, J., Paz, G., Arias, M., Tucker, D., et al. (1995). Immigrant families coping with schizophrenia: Behavioral family intervention v. case management with a low-income Spanish-speaking population. *British Journal of Psychiatry, 167,* 473–479.

Vaughn, K., Doyle, M., McConaghy, N., Blaszczynski, A., Fox, A., & Tarrier, N. (1992). The Sydney Intervention trial: A controlled trial of relatives' counselling to reduce schizophrenic relapse. *Social Psychiatry Psychiatric Epidemiology, 27,* 16–21.

Xiong, W., Phillips, M. R., Hu, X., Wang, R., Dai, Q., & Kleiman, A. (1994). Family based intervention for schizophrenic patients in China: A randomised controlled trial. *British Journal of Psychiatry, 165,* 239–247.

Zastowny, R. R., Lehman, A. F., Cole, R. E., & Kane, C. (1992). Family management of schizophrenia: A comparison of behavioural and supportive family treatment. *Psychiatry Quarterly, 63*(2), 159–186.

Zhang, M., Wang, M., Li, J., & Phillips, M. R. (1994). Randomised control trial family intervention for 78 first episode male schizophrenic patients: An 18 month study in Suzhou, Japan. *British Journal of Psychiatry, 65*(Suppl. 24), 96–102.

CHAPTER 23

COGNITIVE-BEHAVIORAL THERAPY

ANTHONY P. MORRISON

In recent years, the generic cognitive model (Beck, 1976) has been applied to our understanding and treatment of psychosis. This model suggests that the way we interpret events has consequences for how we feel and behave, and that such interpretations are often maintained by unhelpful thinking biases and behavioral responses. It also suggests that these interpretations are influenced by the core beliefs we form as a result of life experience. Several cognitive models of psychosis and psychotic symptoms or experiences (Chadwick & Birchwood, 1994; Garety, Kuipers, Fowler, Freeman, & Bebbington, 2001; Morrison, 2001) have suggested that the way that people interpret psychotic phenomena rather than the psychotic experiences themselves accounts for distress and disability. Several comprehensive treatment manuals describe the application of such models in greater detail (Chadwick, Birchwood, & Trower, 1996; Fowler, Garety, & Kuipers, 1995; Kingdon & Turkington, 1994; Morrison, Renton, Dunn, Williams, & Bentall, 2003).

The cognitive approach to understanding psychosis that is outlined in this chapter focuses on both the development of psychotic experiences and the maintenance of such experiences and their associated distress (Morrison, 2001). This approach suggests that it is the culturally unacceptable nature of appraisals that determines whether a person is viewed as psychotic; in relation to trauma, it may be that the transparency of the link between the traumatic event and the content and form of (subsequent difficulties or "symptoms") psychotic experiences contributes to this process. For example, someone who describes vivid perceptual experiences as being related to past physical or sexual assault is likely to be regarded as experiencing behavior consistent with a flashback experience in posttraumatic stress disorder (PTSD), whereas if he or she reports that the experiences are real, current, and unrelated to the past, then he or she is likely to be regarded as experiencing psychosis. It is also possible that the cognitive and behavioral consequences of life experiences may make people vulnerable to psychosis. Negative beliefs about the self, the world, and other people (e.g., "I am vulnerable" and "Other people are dangerous") are associated with psychosis. Positive beliefs about psychotic experiences, and procedural beliefs that encourage the adoption of paranoia as a strategy for managing interpersonal threat (e.g., "Paranoia is a helpful survival strategy"), may also be related to life experiences (including trauma), and have been shown to be associated with the development of psychosis. It is likely that psychotic experiences are essentially normal phenomena that occur on a continuum in the general population, and it appears that catastrophic or negative appraisals of such psychotic experiences result in the associated distress. It is hypothesized that psychotic experiences and distressing appraisals are maintained by cognitive and behavioral responses (e.g., selective attention, thought suppression, and safety behaviors), as well as by emotional and physiological responses and environmental factors. This model is represented graphically in Figure 23.1.

STRUCTURE, PROCESS, AND PRINCIPLES OF COGNITIVE THERAPY FOR PSYCHOSIS

Cognitive therapy for psychosis is based on the same principles that were outlined for standard cognitive therapy for emotional disorders (Beck, 1976): that cognitive therapy (CT) is collaborative, problem-oriented, and educational, involving guided discovery and the inductive method. CT is also time-limited, based on a cognitive model of the disorder in question, and on idiosyncratic case formulations derived from the model. The structure of CT for psychosis also parallels the structure of standard CT. Therefore, sessions start with a review of current mental state and feedback from the previous session, followed by the setting of an agenda, which is performed collaboratively by the patient and therapist. The agenda typically involves a review of the previous week's homework task(s), one or two discrete session targets based on the model or formulation (usually one such item is sufficient), followed by the assignment of new homework, feedback, and a summary of the current session. Time should be allocated to each agenda item and a timekeeper agreed upon by patient and therapist. It is important that the agenda is not followed unthinkingly; rather, it is intended as a guide to ensure productive use of the limited time available.

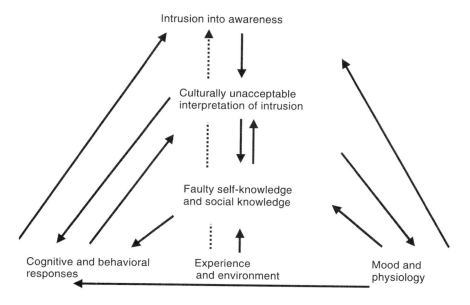

FIGURE 23.1. A cognitive model of psychosis. From Morrison (2001). Copyright 2001 by Cambridge University Press. Reprinted by permission.

The aims of CT for psychosis are worth considering. The primary aim of CT for psychosis is to reduce the distress experienced by people with psychosis and to improve their quality of life. The aim of CT is not necessarily to reduce the frequency of distressing psychotic symptoms; rather, it is to help patients to achieve the goals they have set in relation to the problems they have identified. CT for panic disorder does not aim to eliminate body sensations, and CT for obsessive–compulsive disorder does not attempt to eliminate intrusive thoughts; instead, the aim is to help people generate less upsetting appraisals of these experiences. CT for psychosis works similarly, focusing on generation of less distressing explanations for psychotic experiences rather than attempting to eliminate these experiences. Indeed, CT should recognize that psychotic experiences may well serve a function for the person. The variable targets for treatment are negotiated with the patient and often include problematic appraisals of, and responses to, psychotic experiences. It may be that this results in decreased levels of conviction, frequency, preoccupation, and distress relative to psychotic experiences; however, the main aim is to change the person's relationship to psychotic experiences, making them less troublesome. In essence, the intervention in CT focuses on whatever is put on the problem list.

The process of CT for psychosis begins with establishment of the patient's trust and a sound therapeutic relationship; without this, it is unlikely that CT will be effective. Assessment and the identification of problems and goals occur early on in the process, and these elements can facilitate the development of a good working alliance. CT then involves the development of an idiosyncratic case conceptualization, based on a cognitive model, that guides the selection of treatment strategies. These strategies are implemented and evaluated, and the outcome data of interventions are used to modify the formulation, if indicated. The process ends with relapse prevention in an attempt to consolidate and maintain treatment gains. Each of these stages is now described in detail in relation to a specific (hypothetical, for purposes of confidentiality) case based on several real cases, and illustrates many of the common issues in delivering CT for psychosis.

ASSESSMENT

Clinical assessment of a person with psychosis is very similar to a cognitive-behavioral assessment of a nonpsychotic patient. After setting the scene, and explaining confidentiality and the practicalities of therapy, it is often helpful to begin with an analysis of a recent problematic incident. The aim of this is to generate useful information in understanding the development and maintenance of problems, and in suggesting change strategies. The main purpose of an assessment is to generate information that can be used to develop a case conceptualization. The cognitive model of psychosis should, therefore, guide the process of assessment. The therapist should ask questions to identify problematic events or intrusions, and subsequently interpret these and the patient's emotional, behavioral, cognitive, and physiological responses. Specific factors to focus on include culturally unacceptable interpretations, selective attention, control strategies, positive beliefs about psychotic phenomena, imagery in relation to psychotic phenomena, and metacognitive beliefs (thoughts about thought and thought processes). It is also important to examine environmental factors that may be involved in the maintenance of the problem (e.g., the kind of neighborhood in which a person lives, housing, and financial situation).

Andrew was a 30-year-old man who had developed psychosis 5 years earlier, following a period of significant stress at work (he was a clerical assistant for the police). He currently lived at home with his mother and did very little during the day. He had received a diagnosis of paranoid schizophrenia, had been taking antipsychotic medication for the last 5 years with little benefit (and some side effects, e.g., weight gain and sexual dysfunction), and was referred for CT by his mental health care team. He heard voices of "spirits" that call him names and were abusive and often threatening toward him. He was preoccupied with tactile phenomena in which he felt that the spirits were poking, prodding, and pushing him (often to try to make him do something against his will). In addition, he believed that the spirits put sexual thoughts into his mind. The specific aspects of assessment, formulation, and treatment are illustrated with reference to Andrew in subsequent sections.

Problem Maintenance

It is common to begin with an assessment of problem maintenance by examining a recent incident in terms of events, thoughts, feelings, and behaviors, with therapist and patient collaboratively searching for meaningful links among these factors. This kind of analysis of a recent time when a patient was distressed by a psychotic experience (e.g., hearing voices) is likely to provide information about how the patient makes sense of these experiences and how this makes him or her feel.

Andrew believes that the voices he hears are spirits, who are trying to make him do bad things; this makes him feel scared and angry. This has obvious clinical implications: If he interprets the voices as a sign that he is special, or as a dead friend who is advising him, then he is likely to feel happier about the experience. The interpretation of the voices, combined with the emotional response, is likely to determine what he does in relation to the voices. This framework is also applicable to delusional beliefs, which may be unusual explanations for common phenomena such as anxiety-related sensations (e.g., Andrew misinterprets tingling and numbness as the spirits touching and poking him).

Event	Thought	Feelings	Behavior
Voices	It's the spirits.	Distress	Isolates himself
Physical sensation	The spirits are poking me.	Frustration	Throws something

It is also important to assess other aspects of problem maintenance, including the current environment. Andrew does very little during the day, is socially isolated, and has many arguments with his mother, all of which appear to contribute to his psychotic experiences and episodes of losing his temper.

Problem History and Development

It is important to assess relevant early experiences that may have contributed to the development of a patient's current difficulties. Life events in childhood contribute to the development of core beliefs and dysfunctional assumptions or rules that guide behavior and the selection of information-processing strategies. Particular events that are worth assessing include childhood sexual and physical abuse, emotional abuse and neglect, social isolation, and bullying. This is especially important in patients with psychosis given the high prevalence of such experiences in this population (Read, 1997). Similar experiences in adulthood should also be examined. A general assessment of family life, cultural and spiritual upbringing, school experiences, and friendships should also be performed, and life events and current circumstances at the onset of the problems should also be considered.

Andrew was brought up as a Catholic at home with his parents (he was an only child). His father had mental health problems, and was frequently physically and emotionally abusive to both Andrew and his mother. Andrew described his childhood as relatively happy but reported having trouble with his work at school and having no close friends. A neighbor sexually assaulted Andrew when he was 10 years old, which he reported to his parents; however, although they suggested that Andrew avoid being alone with that person in future, they did not take any further action, and Andrew was unsure whether they believed him. He left school with several qualifications and got a job as a clerical assistant for the police shortly thereafter. Andrew reported that his father died from cancer at about the same time, and that he had mixed feelings: He was upset but also relieved. He described enjoying his work for the police, which he felt was a worthwhile career, but he had quit the job due to a stressful workload and victimization by a new boss who had recently taken over the unit in which he worked.

The influence of life experiences on the development of self- and social knowledge should be considered. Assessment should include an analysis of clients' core beliefs, which are unconditional statements about themselves, the world, and other people (e.g., Andrew believed "I am vulnerable," "I am useless," "Other people cannot be trusted," and "The world is dangerous"). The conditional beliefs or rules that people adopt to compensate for these core beliefs should also be assessed. These often occur in the form of "if–then" statements; for example, Andrew believed, "If I put others' needs before my own, then I will be safe." The compensatory strategies that are the behavioral expressions of these rules should also be identified (e.g., subjugating personal needs).

Procedural beliefs, which guide the selection of information-processing strategies, should also be assessed (Wells & Matthews, 1994). Procedural beliefs that are particularly relevant to people with psychosis include beliefs about the utility of paranoia and suspiciousness (e.g., Andrew believed that "staying on your toes keeps you safe"), beliefs about unusual perceptual experiences (e.g., Andrew believed that "having odd experiences can make life more interesting"), and beliefs about unwanted thoughts (e.g., Andrew believed, "All of my thoughts must be good thoughts" and "I must try to control my thoughts at all times").

Problem and Goal List

As stated earlier, one of the aims of assessment within CT is the development of a shared list of problems and goals. Problem description at the start should be quite general, and be phrased in a more specific manner after additional information is gained. The goals that are set in relation to the problems should then be developed collaboratively.

Andrew's exhaustive problem list was as follows:

> Voices/spirits (including thought insertion and being touched)
> Weight gain
> Overmedication
> Get back to work
> Stigma of diagnosis
> Low mood and self-esteem
> Frustration

The problem list was discussed and specific, measurable, achievable, realistic, and time-limited (SMART) goals were set in relation to each problem. For example, Andrew wanted to "get rid of the spirits," referring to the voices and experiences of being touched. In relation to this aim, we operationalized the goal in terms of distress, preoccupation, or belief in the psychotic experiences, first setting an initial goal in relation to finding out more about the phenomena. In relation to his desire to go back to work, we tried to operationalize this in small steps (e.g., applications, voluntary work, part-time work or courses, etc., leading to the ultimate goal). His desire to lose weight was operationalized with a proximal goal (and linked to investigating medication reduction options).

The establishment of a shared list of problems and goals that can then be collaboratively prioritized is a central part of CT and is invaluable in engaging patients (whether they are psychotic or not).

CASE CONCEPTUALIZATION

Once assessment has been conducted, and problems and goals agreed upon, the process moves on to the development of a shared case formulation. There are several levels at which a person's difficulties can be formulated. Basic formulations can be easily constructed, summarizing recent incidents in the format of event–thought–feeling–behavior cycles, as mentioned earlier, and these miniformulations can incorporate information about triggering events, maintenance cycles, and safety behaviors.

Another level of formulation is the developmental or historical case conceptualization, which provides a more comprehensive account. This type of formulation incorporates early experiences and life events, and the impact that these have had on core beliefs, procedural beliefs, dysfunctional assumptions, and compensatory strategies, in addition to data from five systems (cognitive, behavioral, emotional, physiological, and environmental) regarding current maintaining factors. The cognitive model of psychotic symptoms suggests that the cultural acceptability of interpretations determines whether someone is viewed as psychotic, and that these interpretations are influenced by life experiences and beliefs. It also suggests that the initial interpretation of psychotic experiences, and the way people respond to such experiences, determines whether the experiences cause distress and recur. This model of psychosis is also easily translated into an idiosyncratic case conceptualization that can explain the development and maintenance of psychosis (see Figure 23.2 for Andrew's example).

INTERVENTIONS

Once the therapist and patient collaboratively develop a case formulation, strategies for change can be chosen on the basis of what is likely to achieve success quickly or to affect most significantly the person's quality of life. These options can be collaboratively discussed by the patient and therapist. Most change strategies can be described as verbal and behavioral reattribution methods, and each is considered in relation to working with Andrew.

Verbal Reattribution

Advantages and Disadvantages

It is important to consider the advantages and disadvantages of a particular belief or experience prior to attempting to change a belief, even if the belief is associated with distress. Distressing psychotic experiences that are associated with positive beliefs can be identified through a process of questioning and making inferences from the formulation,

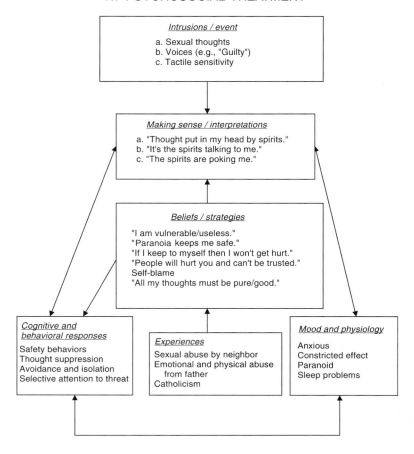

FIGURE 23.2. Andrew's case conceptualization. Tactile sensitivity

which can then be checked out with the patient. These kinds of beliefs may include the advantages of being paranoid, such as safety and excitement, or the benefits of hearing voices, such as receiving advice or having someone to keep one company. Common positive beliefs about hallucination include beliefs about the benevolence of voices and perception of the voices as providing companionship or relaxation. The origins of psychotic experiences should also be explored within this context, because psychotic experiences or unusual beliefs may have been functional at some stage as coping or survival strategies.

Paranoia was clearly helpful to Andrew given that he was brought up in an abusive environment, and it was arguably helpful more recently in relation to the bullying from his boss. Similarly, there is evidence to suggest that voices frequently evolve as a coping response to trauma (Romme & Escher, 1989), and that Andrew's voices, which were initially helpful and positive, only became distressing over time.

If significant advantages are identified, then these should be evaluated with regard to current utility, alternative sources of available benefits, and the relative weighting of advantages and disadvantages. It may be that work is required to provide an alternative way to achieve the benefits before dealing with the problematic aspects of the psychotic experience.

Andrew receives significant benefit from believing that the spirits puts his sexual thoughts into his head, since his religious beliefs suggest that it would be wrong (and possibly evil) for him to experience such thoughts. Andrew and the therapist may need to discuss this prior to any further evaluation of this experience, and it may be that education about intrusive thoughts, a survey among Andrew's peers, or a discussion with an enlightened priest may be of use.

At times, it is necessary to recognize that the benefits of a psychotic experience are outweighed by the disadvantages, and that proving the advantages may not be achievable or realistic; in such cases, patients should be enabled to make their own decision and be supported as much as possible in relation to their environment. In most cases, however, it is either possible to provide an alternative way to achieve the benefits, or the advantages are outweighed by the disadvantages. If a decision is reached to proceed, then therapist and patient can continue to evaluate, and possibly change, the belief or reduce the frequency of occurrence or distress associated with the experience.

Evidential Analysis

A standard procedure in CT is to examine the evidence for and against a particular thought or interpretation of events. This process begins with the identification of a specific thought or belief to be considered and some discussion of what can be construed as evidence (e.g., a feeling that something is true is unlikely to be viewed as evidence in a courtroom). Two columns can then be used to collate evidence for and against the particular belief.

> In relation to Andrew's beliefs that the spirits are putting sexual thoughts into his head, the therapist should elicit the evidence. Socratically, using questions such as "What makes you think that this is true?" and "Is there anything that is incompatible with your belief?" Consideration of modulating factors can also be helpful in generating evidence, as can questions related specifically to the content of the belief. This process can identify further psychotic experiences or beliefs that can also be evaluated using similar techniques (e.g., Andrew's belief regarding the voices being spirits).

Evidence **for** "Spirits are putting sexual thoughts into my head"	Evidence **against** "Spirits are putting sexual thoughts into my head"
• It feels like they are doing this. • They are not the kind of thoughts that I would have. • It happens when the spirits' voices are talking to me.	• Feelings can be misleading. • The thoughts happen when the voices are not there. • It happens more often when I am stressed. • Other people have sexual thoughts. • It does not happen when I am listening to music.

Generation of Alternative Explanations

The generation of alternative explanations is another useful strategy to help reduce the distress associated with psychotic experiences. Delusional ideas and beliefs about voices are open to examination, and it is important to help people to consider a wide variety of possible explanations for their experiences, if they are distressed by their current explanation. Brainstorming exercises and the consideration of what other people have suggested, or would suggest, can facilitate this process. The alternative explanations that are generated should be rated for degree of belief or conviction on an ongoing basis, and recent problematic situations and moderators can be evaluated in relation to consistency with each explanation. This process can be applied to general beliefs or specific incidents.

> Andrew was encouraged to consider alternative explanations for phenomena such as the voices, his sexual thoughts, and the tactile phenomena. It can be helpful to include highly unlikely alternatives in addition to more plausible explanations, because humor can help develop the therapeutic relationship and lighten the tone in therapy. This process may yield a list such as the following:
>
> *The voices that I hear are due to . . .*
> Initial belief: The spirits wanting to persecute me   80%
> A form of mental illness   25%
> A reaction to stress and trauma   50%
> An unusual thought process   20%
> I am imagining the voices   10%
> Bereavement   0%
> The voices are being beamed at me from outer space   0%

It can be very helpful to place each of these explanation into a pie chart to ensure that the total adds up to 100%; in such circumstances, it is useful to leave the most distressing explanation(s) until last.

Normalization

The use of normalizing information can help to combat the negative effects of stigma, reduce distress, and provide information to facilitate the generation of alternatives. Such information often includes facts and figures about the prevalence of psychotic experiences and beliefs in the general population; for example, 5% of the population hear voices at any given time (Tien, 1991). When providing such information, calculating the implications for the prevalence in one's own country can increase the impact that results. For example, in the United States, nearly 15 million people hear voices, many of whom will never have contact with psychiatric services. This kind of information can be extremely liberating for people who believe they are the only persons with such experiences, or that such experiences automatically mean that they are crazy.

Information about the links between life events and specific psychotic experiences can also be helpful in reducing distress and providing an alternative explanation for hallucinations and delusions.

> There is evidence to suggest that Andrew's auditory hallucinations are linked to experiences such as childhood trauma and bereavement, and that psychotic experiences are related to urban living. Andrew was asked to read as a homework assignment one week a good summary of the normalizing approach to the understanding of psychosis (Kingdon & Turkington, 1994); in the subsequent session, he asked the therapist for more information about some of these factors, and as a result his conviction that the voices were related to stress and childhood trauma increased.

Encouraging patients to gather their own normalizing information can also be a useful approach.

When asked whether he was aware that other people experienced sexual thoughts and images, and how often this might occur, Andrew said that he was sure that whereas some people did, most people could prevent this from happening, and that "good" people would not have such thoughts very often. Andrew was reluctant to conduct a survey, and his restricted social network made this difficult anyway. Thus, it was agreed that Andrew's therapist would conduct a survey (anonymously) among colleagues on his behalf (Andrew believed that most people working for the health service would be "good"). Needless to say, Andrew was surprised by the results and began to reassess his unhelpful beliefs about the meaning of having unwanted sexual thoughts.

Imagery

Recent research has demonstrated that people with psychotic experiences have recurrent images associated with them (Morrison et al., 2002).

Andrew experienced a vivid mental image of the perceived source of his voices, seeing several "spirits" of people he knew, including his dead father. Such images can be a useful way to access personal meaning and core beliefs, and can be modified to become less distressing or powerful. For example, discussing the imagery of his father made Andrew reconsider the possibility that the voices might be related to bereavement in some way, and he began to notice similarities between the content of the voices and the kind of things his father used to say to him.

Core Beliefs and Content of Voices

Core beliefs, such as "I am vulnerable" or "Other people cannot be trusted," can be evaluated and changed using the techniques just outlined. They are also amenable to other strategies, such as historical tests (searching for information from any time in the past that is inconsistent with the belief), use of criteria continua (operationalizing factors such as vulnerability and rating self or others on the resulting continua), and positive data logs (Padesky, 1994).

Andrew was encouraged to identify events in his life (considered in 3-year "chunks") in which he had successfully managed to be safe from harm and avoid danger. These examples were then considered, and factors that appeared to have helped were identified (e.g., having a person available when a small child to whom Andrew could turn for help, and having been assertive during his initial years at work). He was then encouraged to try to utilize these factors in his current situation and keep a positive data log of the results.

Beliefs about Traumatic Experiences

Given the high prevalence of trauma in patients with psychosis, it is likely that treatment strategies developed for patients with PTSD and dissociative experiences may be helpful. Such strategies include examining the idiosyncratic meaning, or the sequelae, of the trauma and developing an explanatory narrative for the trauma to aid contextualization in memory (Ehlers & Clark, 2000).

Andrew was helped to reexamine the meaning of his childhood trauma, modifying the main problematic appraisals related to the sexual assault and its consequences. The therapist encouraged Andrew to reevaluate his belief that "I'm not normal and never will be" using guided discovery and Socratic questioning, such as "I might have struggled with these experiences, but they are normal reactions to severe trauma and I am learning to cope with them." Andrew had also thought, "I should have stuck up for myself," but this was reappraised as "Nobody my age could have fought off an adult." Andrew also utilized pie charts for his feelings of guilt and self-blame, listing other factors that contributed to the assault (e.g., the neighbor's sexual attraction to young boys, the proximity of his house, being left alone at such a young age, and having been an only child). Finally, as an alternative to his initial core belief "I'm vulnerable," he generated an alternative explanation: "I'm no more vulnerable than anyone else; in fact, I'm a resilient person who has coped with a lot." Andrew's new belief was held with little conviction, but it was built up over time.

Behavioral Reattribution

The use of behavioral strategies within a cognitive framework are arguably the most effective way to achieve belief change and reduction of distress. Behavioral experiments are a vital component of CT, and safety behaviors that are used to prevent the feared outcomes associated with psychosis can be particularly important to address. Each of these aspects is considered in greater detail in relation to Andrew.

Behavioral Experiments

The use of behavioral experiments is central to effective CT for psychosis, and beliefs about voices and delusional ideas are frequently translatable into testable hypotheses that can be investigated collaboratively by patient and therapist. Behavioral experiments should be designed very carefully to ensure a no-lose outcome. Predictions should be stated in a concrete way, and the possible results should be reviewed in advance to ensure that the outcome is meaningful and will not be dismissed or accommodated within the patient's problematic belief system. Examples of behavioral experiments include the use of activity scheduling to evaluate beliefs about the consequences of activity or lack of pleasure (which can be helpful for negative symptoms), or exposure to feared situations to evaluate beliefs about voices or paranoid ideas.

Safety Behaviors

Safety behaviors, first identified in relation to anxiety disorders, are behaviors adopted to prevent a feared outcome (Salkovskis, 1991); these can be problematic for people when they prevent disconfirmation of the catastrophic beliefs about the feared outcome. Empirical studies have demonstrated the presence of such behaviors in people with psychotic experiences. Examples of such safety behaviors include avoidance of particular places, thought control strategies, hypervigilance and selective attention, and idiosyncratic strategies to prevent psychosis-related fears. Voices that produce anxiety are typically associated with safety behaviors.

Andrew sometimes believes that the voices of the spirits will make him harm someone else, such as his mother. He adopts various safety behaviors, such as trying to suppress the voices, resisting them, and trying not to be in the same room as his mother. Such safety behaviors can be manipulated to demonstrate their counterproductive effects, and are amenable to being omitted in behavioral experiments to evaluate the relevant beliefs. For example, an experiment was devised in which Andrew was asked to operationalize the timescale in which the spirits could make him attack his mother. He decided that this would occur within 10 minutes, if he did not resist the voices by these means. Considerable time was spent using verbal reattribution methods and a review of evidence regarding any actual incidents in which he had attacked her (of which there were none) to allow experimentation to feel safe (to both patient and therapist). He then decided that an appropriate test of this belief would be to try to stay in the same room as his mother when the voices were trying to make him attack her, allowing the voices to come without trying to suppress them, and simply responding by saying internally that he had no desire to hit her, and that he never had. He successfully practiced this in a role play in the session, then negotiated a therapist-assisted experiment in which he would do as planned, but with the therapist present in a family session that included his mother. Following these successes, Andrew felt sufficiently safe to do this on his own, and found that he had no trouble resisting the voices' commands. This series of experiments resulted in a sustained decrease in both conviction and distress associated with the beliefs about the spirits.

Negative Symptoms

Many negative symptoms of psychosis, including apathy, withdrawal, flat or blunted affect, anhedonia, and poverty of speech are conceptualizable as safety behaviors. Such symptoms are frequently assumed to be the result of a biological syndrome or deficit state, but many of these experiences can be understood using a cognitive case conceptualization.

> Andrew reported having developed flat affect as a deliberate survival strategy to avoid the feared outcome of physical punishment or humiliation from his father in childhood. His isolation and social withdrawal appeared to be the result of avoiding potential social contacts that he was concerned would harm or evaluate him negatively because of his mental health problems. He was also worried that he might attack other people as a result of the voices. It is also important to consider other possibilities for the causes of negative symptoms, such as overmedication, depression, anxiety, or the consequences of substance abuse.

ADJUSTMENT AND RECOVERY

Once people with psychosis have recovered from the distress associated with their psychotic experiences, many other factors should be examined and are potential targets for psychological intervention using CT. Such difficulties should also be considered at the beginning of CT, because many people prioritize problems that are traditionally viewed as "comorbid" as being more distressing than their experience of psychosis.

PTSD is a common problem for people with psychosis, which is no surprise given the prevalence of traumatic life events in people with psychosis. Depression and hopelessness are also common responses to an episode of psychosis, and such problems are clearly appropriate targets for CT. Emphasis on promoting personal recovery should also be incorporated within CT for people with psychosis, and the development of personal goals and valued social roles should be encouraged. It is also important to facilitate access to appropriate education or employment.

> Andrew was encouraged to reevaluate his concerns about the stigma of a diagnosis of schizophrenia given information regarding the common occurrence of experiences such as hallucinations, the lack of evidence supporting the violent stereotypes of people with psychosis, and the likelihood of recovery. He also addressed his weight gain

with a combination of reducing his medication, seeing a dietician, and instigating an exercise program. He addressed his desire for a more meaningful life by seeking career guidance in relation to work opportunities (both paid and voluntary), and by activity scheduling (in relation to both pleasure and achievement) to increase his opportunities for social reinforcement. Andrew was also encouraged to "reclaim" his former self by reinstating previously valued activities.

RELAPSE PREVENTION

Core beliefs and conditional assumptions, as well as positive beliefs about psychotic experiences, may be conceptualized as vulnerability factors for relapse. The therapist can address these factors at this stage of therapy, providing that the patient consents, using the strategies outlined earlier. For example, Andrew's beliefs about vulnerability and his positive beliefs about the utility of paranoia were considered in this way. In addition, a blueprint of therapy is very useful. The therapist was provided with a summary of what had occurred in therapy, and Andrew prioritized strategies that he would use should he experience difficulties in the future. Evidence also suggests that CT for people exhibiting early warning signs of relapse is feasible and can reduce relapse rates by 50% (Gumley et al., 2003). It is also important to help people distinguish between a lapse and relapse, and to ensure that they do not overcatastrophize the emergence of early signs, which could potentially fuel the development of a relapse.

EVIDENCE FOR EFFECTIVENESS OF CT

Recent studies examining CT for schizophrenia-like psychoses have shown that it is effective in reducing residual positive symptoms on an outpatient basis, and in maintaining these gains at follow-up. CT has been shown to be superior to other psychological treatments, such as supportive counseling and treatment as usual involving case management and antipsychotic medication, and routine psychiatric care. A recent meta-analysis concluded that CT is an effective treatment for persistent psychotic symptoms, that the effects of CT are robust over time, and that dropout rates are low (Zimmerman, Favrod, Trieu, & Pomini, 2005). Therefore, it appears that CT methods can be used to promote symptom reduction and reduce time spent in the hospital, and relapse prevention. In the United Kingdom, this has led to the recommendation that CT be delivered routinely as part of the treatment package offered to people with a diagnosis of schizophrenia.

KEY POINTS

- Psychosis is amenable to conceptualization as relatively normal experiences with understandable emotional and behavioral consequences due to the appraisal of and response to such experiences, rather than as an illness.
- A shared case formulation is important for engaging the patient and allowing collaborative selection of treatment strategies.
- A shared list of problems and goals aids engagement and provides a map to target such treatment strategies.
- Standard cognitive and behavioral change methods are effective in reducing the distress associated with psychotic experiences.
- All patients with psychosis should be offered access to cognitive-behavioral therapy.

REFERENCES AND RECOMMENDED READINGS

Beck, A. T. (1976). *Cognitive therapy and the emotional disorders*. New York: International Universities Press.

Chadwick, P., & Birchwood, M. (1994). The omnipotence of voices: A cognitive approach to auditory hallucinations. *British Journal of Psychiatry, 164*, 190–201.

Chadwick, P. D., Birchwood, M. J., & Trower, P. (1996). *Cognitive therapy for delusions, voices and paranoia*. Chichester, UK: Wiley.

Ehlers, A., & Clark, D. M. (2000). A cognitive model of posttraumatic stress disorder. *Behaviour Research and Therapy, 38*(4), 319–345.

Fowler, D., Garety, P., & Kuipers, E. (1995). *Cognitive-behaviour therapy for psychosis: Theory and practice*. Chichester, UK: Wiley.

Garety, P. A., Kuipers, E., Fowler, D., Freeman, D., & Bebbington, P. E. (2001). A cognitive model of the positive symptoms of psychosis. *Psychological Medicine, 31*, 189–195.

Gumley, A. I., O'Grady, M., McNay, L., Reilly, J., Power, K., & Norrie, J. (2003). Early intervention for relapse in schizophrenia: Results of a 12-month randomised controlled trial of cognitive behaviour therapy. *Psychological Medicine, 33*, 419–431.

Kingdon, D. G., & Turkington, D. (1994). *Cognitive-behavioural therapy of schizophrenia*. Hove, UK: Erlbaum.

Morrison, A. P. (2001). The interpretation of intrusions in psychosis: An integrative cognitive approach to hallucinations and delusions. *Behavioural and Cognitive Psychotherapy, 29*, 257–276.

Morrison, A. P., Beck, A. T., Glentworth, D., Dunn, H., Reid, G., Larkin, W., et al. (2002). Imagery and psychotic symptoms: A preliminary investigation. *Behaviour Research and Therapy, 40*, 1063–1072.

Morrison, A. P., Renton, J. C., Dunn, H., Williams, S., & Bentall, R. P. (2003). *Cognitive therapy for psychosis: A formulation-based approach*. London: Psychology Press.

Padesky, C. A. (1994). Schema change processes in cognitive therapy. *Clinical Psychology and Psychotherapy, 1*, 267–278.

Read, J. (1997). Child abuse and psychosis: A literature review and implications for professional practice. *Professional Psychology: Research and Practice, 28*, 448–456.

Romme, M., & Escher, A. (1989). Hearing voices. *Schizophrenia Bulletin, 15*, 209–216.

Salkovskis, P. M. (1991). The importance of behaviour in the maintenance of anxiety and panic: A cognitive account. *Behavioural Psychotherapy, 19*, 6–19.

Tien, A. Y. (1991). Distribution of hallucinations in the population. *Social Psychiatry and Psychiatric Epidemiology, 26*, 287–292.

Wells, A., & Matthews, G. (1994). *Attention and emotion*. London: Erlbaum.

Zimmermann, G., Favrod, J., Trieu, V. H., & Pomini, V. (2005). The effect of cognitive behavioral treatment on the positive symptoms of schizophrenia spectrum disorders: A meta-analysis. *Schizophrenia Research, 77*, 1–9.

CHAPTER 24

SOCIAL SKILLS TRAINING

WENDY N. TENHULA
ALAN S. BELLACK

In this chapter we describe one of the most promising and empirically supported approaches to improvement of role functioning and quality of life for people with schizophrenia: social skills training (SST). Although the phenomenology of schizophrenia is highly heterogeneous, common characteristics of the illness can generally be classified into four domains: positive symptoms, negative symptoms, cognitive impairment, and social dysfunction. Social dysfunction has been found to be very common in people with schizophrenia. The deficits are stable over time and relatively independent of other domains of the illness (e.g., social impairment persists even during periods when other symptoms have remitted). They are also resistant to treatment with antipsychotics, including new-generation medications. Social deficits in patients with schizophrenia include difficulty initiating and sustaining conversations, and inability to achieve goals or have their needs met in situations requiring social interactions. Ultimately, these impairments manifest themselves in profound difficulties in role functioning. For many patients with schizophrenia, poor social functioning, odd interpersonal behavior, and stigmatizing experiences, in combination with social anxiety, contribute to isolation, inadequate social support, and functional impairment, which in turn serve to diminish patients' opportunities to develop and improve their social skills. Skills deficits account for a significant portion of variance in ability to fulfill social roles and in quality of life.

The social skills model provides a basis for understanding social function and dysfunction in schizophrenia, and the development of SST. This model posits that social competence is based on a set of three component skills: (1) social perception, or *receiving* skills; (2) social cognition, or *processing* skills; and (3) behavioral response, or *expressive* skills. *Social perception*, the ability to read or decode social inputs accurately, includes accurate detection of both affect cues, such as facial expressions and nuances of voice, gesture, and body posture, and verbal content (what the interpersonal partner is saying) and contextual information. *Social cognition* involves effective analysis of the social stimulus, integration of current information and historical information (e.g., what the partner has done in previous interactions and one's experience in similar social situations), and planning an effective response. *Behavioral response* includes the ability to generate effective verbal content, to speak with appropriate paralinguistic characteristics, and to use suitable nonverbal behaviors, such as facial expression, gestures, and posture. Effective social behavior requires the smooth integration of these three component processes to meet the demands of specific social situations.

The use of the term *skills* in the model is intended to emphasize that social competence is based on a set of *learned* abilities rather than traits, needs, or other intrapsychic processes. Conversely, ineffective social behavior is often the result of *social skills deficits*. Research suggests that virtually all social behaviors are *learnable* (i.e., they can be modified by experience or training), and an extensive body of literature supports the social skills model, including the utility of conceptualizing social dysfunction as a function of skills deficits.

Social dysfunction is hypothesized to result from three circumstances: when the individual does not know how to respond appropriately, when an individual does not use skills in his or her repertoire when needed, or when appropriate behavior is undermined by socially inappropriate behavior. Each of these circumstances appears to be common in schizophrenia. *First,* there is good reason to believe that people with schizophrenia do not learn key social skills. Children who later develop schizophrenia in adulthood have been found to have subtle attention deficits in childhood that may interfere with the development of social relationships and the acquisition of basic social skills. Schizophrenia often strikes first in late adolescence or young adulthood, a critical period for mastery of adult social roles and skills, such as dating and sexual behaviors, work-related skills, and the ability to form and maintain adult relationships. Many individuals with schizophrenia gradually develop isolated lives, punctuated by periods in psychiatric hospitals or in community residences that remove them from their non-mentally-ill peer group, provide few opportunities to engage in age-appropriate social roles, and limit social contacts to mental health staff and other severely ill persons. *Second,* cognitive impairment, especially deficits in social cognition and executive processes, interferes with both social perception and social problem solving.

The social skills model postulates that functional outcomes can be improved by enhancing social skills and/or ameliorating skills deficits with a structured behavioral intervention: SST. As such, and given that improving social role functioning and quality of life has been a major goal of treatment and rehabilitation for schizophrenia, SST can play an important role in the treatment of persons with schizophrenia.

DESCRIPTION OF SST

SST is a treatment procedure that has been developed to address social problem-solving skills deficits directly, with the goal of enhancing social functioning. The basic technology we present for teaching social skills was developed in the 1970s and has not changed substantially in the intervening years. SST interventions are tailored to meet the real-life, current-day difficulties that affect the social experiences of each participant, but several common core elements are present regardless of the specific skills being taught. These core elements are presented and described here. In general, SST is a highly structured educational procedure that employs didactic instruction, breaking skills down into discrete steps, modeling, behavioral rehearsal (role playing), and social reinforcement.

With each new skill, the therapist provides an introduction in which he or she discusses the rationale for teaching the skill and presents the steps of the skill. The steps of each skill are presented to the patients, both in handouts and on a large display (e.g., whiteboard or easel) during each session. Complex social repertoires, such as making friends and dating, are thus broken down into discrete steps or component elements, analogous to the way a music teacher would break down a difficult piece of music into simpler segments. For example, initiating conversations requires first gaining the other person's attention via introductory remarks ("Hi, is this seat taken?"; "Excuse me, does the number 2 bus stop here?"), asking general questions (e.g., "How have you been?" "Do you come here often?"), following up with specific questions (e.g., "Did you see the game last night?"), and sharing information with *I* statements (e.g., "I think . . . ," "I feel . . . ," "I like . . . "). Nonverbal and paralinguistic behaviors are similarly segmented (e.g., making eye contact, shaking hands, nodding one's head). Participants are first taught to perform the elements of the skill, then gradually learn to combine them smoothly through repeated practice, shaping, and reinforcement of successive approximations.

The primary modality through which participants learn to combine the elements of a skill is to role-play simulated conversations. After the therapist provides instructions about the steps of the skill, then models the behavior to give the participant an opportunity to observe how it is performed, the participant engages in a role play with the therapist. Behavioral demonstration prior to having the patient role-play the skill helps make the skill concrete for the patient and often works better to convey the message than a verbal description alone. For example, in discussing the step of making eye contact, the therapist might demonstrate how it would look if he or she were trying to talk to the patient but actually looking down at the ground. Behavioral demonstration is especially helpful for lower functioning patients who show signs of cognitive impairment.

For the role play, the therapist identifies a social situation that is relevant to the patient and in which the skill might be useful. After the patient performs the role play, the therapist and other patients (if SST is being done in a group) provide feedback and positive reinforcement, followed by suggestions for how the participant's performance might be improved. Positive feedback from therapists and group members provides social reinforcement and shapes behavior in subsequent role plays. The goal is always to provide positive feedback about the role play, no matter how good or bad the person's performance. In this context, the therapist can then suggest that the participant try something different or pay special attention to a step that was missing in the previous role play. Maintaining a positive approach to feedback is essential to maximize successful learning of the skill. The following example demonstrates how important positive feedback is in a role play involving conversation skills:

What to do: Richard completes the role play, forgetting a step. The therapist says, "Richard, that was a really good role play. You did a really great job making eye contact. I could really tell that you were talking to me! I also heard you say good-bye when you were finished with the conversation. That was terrific. Let's try that same role play again. This time, after you make eye contact and say hello, I want you to pay special attention to Step 2. Do you remember what Step 2 is, Richard? That's right. It's 'Ask a general question.' Now which general question do you want to use in the role play? OK, you are going to say, 'How are you?' That's a great one to use. So let's do it again, and this time, after you make eye contact and say hello, you are going to ask, 'How are you?' and then you are going to give your reason for leaving, and say good-bye. Let's try it now."

What not to do: Richard completes the role play, forgetting a step, and the therapist says, "OK, Richard, you did the role play but you forgot Step 2. This time, remember to do Step 2."

The sequence, role play followed by feedback and reinforcement, is then repeated until the patient can perform the skill adequately. Generally, each patient should be engaged in at least three to four role plays of each behavior. There is a strong emphasis on behavioral rehearsal and overlearning of a few specific and relatively narrow skills that can then be enacted relatively effortlessly. This serves to minimize the cognitive load for decision making during stressful social interactions and increase the chances that the patient will use the skills taught outside the clinic setting. In training, typically conducted in small groups (up to eight patients), patients take turns role playing for three to four trials at a time, and providing feedback and reinforcement to one another. Role plays should be done in the most realistic manner possible. This means that facilitators should be familiar with vocabulary that is most often used in the role-play situations. Asking for specifics when developing role-play scenarios with group members is one way to gain this sort of information.

Handouts and written prompts are used to minimize demand on patients' memory and to maximize their success on the skill. The use of homework assignments is encouraged to maximize opportunities for generalization of newly acquired skills. Specific SST curricula have been developed for a variety of skills within the domains of conversation, assertiveness, conflict management, romantic relationships, medication management, HIV prevention, employment, and drug refusal skills. The general training model can be adapted and used to teach essentially any social skill.

EVIDENCE SUPPORTING SST

Several parallel versions of SST have been developed, manualized, and evaluated. The SST literature has not compared these clinical variations, but a number of common key elements employed in the majority of randomized trials yielded positive results and are therefore regarded as highly important, if not essential. As indicated earlier, training is characteristically conducted in small groups. The contents of training programs are organized into curricula, such as work-related skills, medication management (how to communicate with health care providers), dating skills, and safe-sex skills. Training duration can range from four to eight sessions for a very circumscribed skill, and up to 6 months to 2 years for a comprehensive skills training program. Regardless of duration, training sessions are typically held two to three times per week. Training is structured so as to minimize demands on neurocognitive capacity. Extensive use is made of audiovisual aids, with instructions presented in handouts and on flipcharts or whiteboards, as well as orally and on videotapes. Material is presented in brief units, with frequent repetition and review, and patients are regularly asked to verbalize instructions and plan what they will say before engaging in role play. An attempt is made to produce *overlearning*, so responses can be elicited relatively effortlessly in the environment (i.e., with minimum demand on analytical and problem-solving skills). Individuals delivering SST are generally bachelor's or master's level clinical staff, and two therapists are employed whenever possible (one to direct the session, and the other to serve as role-play partner). Skills training is generally conducted on an outpatient basis, but it can be implemented in long-term inpatient settings as well; acute admissions generally do not afford enough time for useful training. Given the challenge of generalization from training to *in vivo* application, SST should focus on skills that are *currently* relevant to the client's life rather than skills that might one day be useful.

Wide variability in methodology, outcome criteria, assessment instruments, and subject populations in different trials make the SST literature somewhat difficult to review.

The many studies that compare SST and *treatment as usual* are rarely described sufficiently to determine whether group differences reflect clinically significant effects of SST or poor results for the comparison groups. Other studies have developed new control treatments for comparison purposes, but these also make comparisons difficult. Outcome criteria have included symptoms, relapse, behavioral skill, and community functioning. Skills ratings have included diverse role-play tests, some of which closely parallel what was taught in treatment, and many of which have uncertain relationships to social role functioning in the community. Until very recently, assessment of community outcomes relied on patient self-report, with only a few studies securing reports from significant others or other informants (e.g., work supervisors). No studies that we are aware of have conducted *in vivo* observations to determine the extent of generalization, which remains the most critical question for evaluating the effectiveness of SST. Subject populations have ranged from very impaired, long-term inpatients to acute inpatients, to stabilized outpatients seen in a variety of clinical settings. Training content and duration also have varied considerably, and have occasionally combined SST with other interventions, including cognitive rehabilitation, case management, family therapy, and pharmacotherapy. Medication effects have rarely been controlled or examined in combination with SST and frequently have not even been described.

Nevertheless, several trends emerge from the three decades of SST research. SST is clearly effective at increasing the use of specific behaviors (e.g., eye contact, asking questions, voice volume) and improving function in the specific domains that are the primary focus of the treatment (e.g., conversational skill, ability to perform on a job interview). SST techniques have also become a standard component of interventions for a variety of behavioral problems in which social skill is a component, such as teaching substance abusers how to refuse drugs, and teaching people at risk for HIV how to negotiate for safe sex. The specific contribution of skills training in these approaches has generally not been experimentally teased out, but it is widely assumed to be effective when the treatment package has proven to be successful. However, the one critical question that has not been clearly answered either in specific SST programs or when SST is bundled into other treatments is the extent to which learning in the clinic translates into either specific behavioral changes or generally improved role functioning in the community.

A survey of the SST literature identified eight narrative reviews and four meta-analyses published in peer-reviewed (English language) journals since 1990, including four articles published since 2000 (Bellack, 2004). Each review employed different inclusion criteria, and covered from five to 68 articles. Only one meta-analysis (Pilling et al., 2002), which had several methodological limitations (e.g., covered a small number of studies, did not adjust for study quality or sample size), concluded that SST was not substantially effective. The other reviews led us to the following conclusions regarding the empirical support for SST interventions: First, SST is not substantially effective for reducing symptoms or preventing relapse. This finding is not surprising given that SST does not directly target either of these domains. SST would only be expected to affect symptoms or relapse rates to the extent that it teaches skills that help to reduce social failure that would otherwise cause sufficient stress to exacerbate symptoms. This diathesis–stress model depends on several mediating factors that are themselves unproven (e.g., that social failure produces sufficient stress to precipitate relapse). Second, SST has a reliable and significant effect on behavioral skills that can be maintained for up to 2 years. Third, SST has a positive impact on social role functioning, although the findings for this outcome domain are not entirely consistent. The results are better for defined skills areas (e.g., medication management, HIV prevention skills, work-related social skills) than for more general measures of social functioning. Fourth, SST appears to have a positive effect on patient satisfaction and self-efficacy: Patients feel more self-confident in (targeted) social situations after training. SST is clearly a teaching technology that is effective and well received by both patients and clinicians. These general findings are reflected in the 2003 Schizophrenia Patient Outcomes Research Team (PORT) recommendation for treatment of schizophrenia (Lehman et al., 2004): Patients with schizophrenia should be offered skills training, the key elements of which include behaviorally based instruction, modeling, corrective feedback, contingent social reinforcement, and homework assignments.

TREATMENT GUIDELINES

Tailor the Training to Your Patients

There are several considerations in how best to individualize SST for each patient. Not only is it important that the skills training content be current, relevant, and useful in the patient's life, but it is also critical to maximize learning by adapting the training to the functional and cognitive impairment levels of participants.

Which Skills to Teach

It is important to teach skills that the patients view as relevant to their lives and realistically useful to them. This makes it more likely that patients not only learn the skills during SST sessions but also use them in their daily lives. Generalization to "real life" is unlikely if the skills being taught are not directly applicable to patients' lives. For example, it does not make sense to teach dating skills to a group of long-term inpatients who have no opportunity to pursue romantic relationships. Similarly, patients who express no interest in working do not benefit from learning work-related social skills, such as job interview skills or how to ask their work supervisor for feedback about job performance.

Patient Functional Level

Patient ability to function should be assessed, and sessions can be adjusted based on the level of functioning. In this sort of assessment the therapist makes judgments—both clinical and behavioral—about the individual's abilities. The therapist looks at the following areas when making these judgments:

- How effectively does the individual perform the skill when it is first modeled?
- How quickly does the individual learn to perform a skill after it is first modeled?
- Can the individual stay focused on all of the steps of a multistep skill?

In general, therapists should gear SST toward relatively low-functioning patients. For persons who are quick to learn, who engage more easily, and who have greater ability to deal with abstractions, therapists should use clinical judgment to increase the complexity of the material (e.g., difficulty level of role-play situations). On the other hand, with individuals who are difficult to engage due to symptomatology or other factors, and/or who have difficulty attending to the material being presented, the focus should remain on learning the basics of the skill. The therapist does this by simplifying the exercises and working hard to keep the individual engaged by asking him or her to repeat session material and relating to his or her individual experiences. It is almost always better to err on the side of oversimplification than to overreach. High-functioning patients tell therapists when they have oversimplified too much. In contrast, low-functioning patients do not tell therapists when the material is over their heads.

Cognitive Impairment

The problems of seriously mentally ill patients in terms of memory, attention, and higher-level problem solving have been repeatedly demonstrated and must be taken into consideration in SST. Asymptomatic patients with schizophrenia can appear to maintain lucid conversations, seem to learn and understand well, and respond affirmatively to questions even if they do not understand. Whether they do not remember, are easily distracted, or are thinking so concretely that they cannot transpose ideas from situation A to situation B, patients often lack the capacity to learn from continuities across situations. The only effective solutions that we have found for this dilemma are (1) to impose as much structure as possible and minimize demands on abstraction (use prompts and handouts, identify simple commonalties across situations for the person to focus on, and keep instructions very simple and straightforward) and (2) to practice, practice, practice (the more automatic the response in a social situation, the less demand on working memory and analysis). Also, we do not ask participants whether they understand; rather, we ask them to demonstrate their understanding through role playing and explaining things to other patients.

Make Sessions Interactive

The emphasis in SST is on teaching and collaboration rather than lecturing. Thus, the therapist must direct the conversation back to the patient as much as possible. Therapists should stimulate participant input by asking for relevant examples and for participants' understanding of things. Note that this interactive strategy must also be tailored for each individual. Some participants, especially those who are low functioning, have a lot of difficulty with open-ended questions and high-level interactions. Thus, interactions must be tailored to meet the needs and capabilities of each individual. If unbalanced participation becomes a problem at any time during the group sessions, it is useful to establish a routine by beginning with a volunteer and soliciting a response from each member of the group in succession. It is important, however, that clients know that it is OK for them to "pass" if they do not wish to make a contribution during the group sessions.

Maintain a Positive Stance

One key to making SST work well is to be consistently positive and reinforcing. Most people with serious mental illness have long histories of failure and frustration. SST is one place that they can be assured of success, because (1) the level of demand is geared to their capacity, not to some abstract or unreachable standard; and (2) communications are always positive, emphasizing what they have done well, not what they have done poorly. SST trainers help participants set goals, explain behavioral contingencies, and reward participants' use of newly acquired skills in the real world. It is our hope that by making this reinforcement more explicit, we may also help patients to improve some of the social deficits caused by negative symptoms (e.g., avolition, social withdrawal).

Handouts

Handouts outlining the steps of each skill provide a concrete focus for patients. Therapists should refer to the handouts throughout the training and draw participants' attention to the handouts as needed. Therapists can ask the participants to read material off of the handout, if it is clear that they can read. For example: "What's the first step in asking for feedback about your job performance? Can you read it for me?" They can also take handouts home with them, which may increase the chances that they will practice the skills outside of SST sessions.

Use Examples, Illustrations, and Modeling

Therapists should make ample use of examples, metaphors, or relevant stories to illustrate particular concepts or ideas generated by participants whenever possible. For example, in designing a role play during a conversation skills session for a person who says that she does not really talk to people that live in her apartment building, but that there is a person who moved in down the hallway to whom she would like to talk, the therapist could set up the role play as an interaction between the group member and the person who moved in down the hallway. Use of examples that are concretely tied to participants' lives allows them to see the relevance of how they might use the skill. Similarly, therapist and/or group member's modeling of the skills allows participants to see how they might use the skills in their own lives.

Encourage Participants to Practice Skills between Sessions

Homework practice between sessions enhances the generalization of skills from the therapy sessions to clients' real-world experiences and gives them the opportunity to see first-hand how the new skills can improve their relations with others, social functioning, and so forth. Homework assignments developed at the end of each session can then be reviewed at the beginning of the following session. This sets up the expectation that patients use the skills taught in session outside of the clinic and gives them the opportunity to receive therapist feedback about ways they can improve application of the skills to real-life situations. It is best to develop the homework collaboratively, in such a way that the participant is able to practice the skill between sessions and has a high likelihood of successfully completing the assignment.

Do Not Work in Isolation

Participants in SST are likely to be receiving antipsychotic medications and to have a caseworker, therapist, or other clinician involved in their care. Therapists should keep in touch with their colleagues and find out when a participant has been put on a new medication or has received a major change in dosage. It is important to learn how he or she is doing in other settings (e.g., Is this a particularly bad time for a patient? Is he or she exhibiting prodromal signs of relapse?). Of special note is whether the participant is giving the therapist but not others a hard time or vice versa. Similarly, what is going on in the person's life outside of the clinical setting? Are there conflicts at home? As a general rule, generalization of the effects of training is enhanced to the extent that the skills one teaches are (1) relevant to the person's immediate environment, and (2) reinforced by the environment.

KEY POINTS

- Impairments in social skills and social competence are key features of schizophrenia that play a major role in disability.
- Social competence is based on a set of three component skills (social perception, or receiving skills; social cognition, or processing skills; and behavioral response, or expressive skills), which can be ameliorated by SST.

- SST is a highly structured educational procedure that employs didactic instruction, breaking skills down into discrete steps, modeling, behavioral rehearsal (role playing), and social reinforcement to teach social behaviors.
- SST is a structured teaching approach in which the key element is behavioral rehearsal, not conversation about social behavior and motivation.
- SST is an evidence-based practice with strong empirical support.
- SST is tailored to each individual, and fosters personal choice and growth in a manner consistent with the consumer recovery model.

REFERENCES AND RECOMMENDED READINGS

Bellack, A. S. (2004). Skills training for people with severe mental illness. *Psychiatric Rehabilitation Journal, 27*(4), 375–391.

Bellack, A. S., Mueser, K. T., Gingerich, S., & Agresta, J. (2004). *Social skills training for schizophrenia: A step-by-step guide* (2nd ed.). New York: Guilford Press.

Benton, M. K., & Schroeder, H. E. (1990). Social skills training with schizophrenics: A meta-analytic evaluation. *Journal of Consulting and Clinical Psychology, 58,* 741–747.

Dilk, M. N., & Bond, G. R. (1996). Meta-analytic evaluation of skills training research for individuals with severe mental illness. *Journal of Clinical Psychiatry, 64,* 1337–1346.

Glynn, S. M., Marder, S. R., Liberman, R. P., Blair, K., Wirshing, W. C., Wirshing, D. A., et al. (2002). Supplementing clinic-based skills training with manual-based community support sessions: Effects on social adjustment of patients with schizophrenia. *American Journal of Psychiatry, 159,* 829–837.

Hayes, R. L., Halford, W. K., & Varghese, F. T. (1995). Social skills training with chronic schizophrenic patients: Effects on negative symptoms and community functioning. *Behavior Therapy, 26,* 433–439.

Lehman, A. F., Kreyenbuhl, J., Buchanan, R. W., Dickerson, F. B., Dixon, L. B., Goldberg, R., et al. (2004). The Schizophrenia Patient Outcomes Research Team (PORT): Updated treatment recommendations 2003. *Schizophrenia Bulletin, 30*(2), 193–217.

Liberman, R. P. (1995). *Social and independent living skills: The community re-entry program.* Los Angeles: Author.

Liberman, R. P., Blair, K. E., Glynn, S. M., Marder, S. R., Wirshing, W., & Wirshing, D. A. (2001). Generalization of skills training to the natural environment. In H. D. Brenner, W. Boker, & R. Genner (Eds.), *The treatment of schizophrenia: Status and emerging trends* (pp. 104–120). Seattle, WA: Hogrefe & Huber.

Liberman, R. P., Wallace, C. J., Blackwell, G., Kopelowicz, A., & Vaccaro, J. V. (1998). Skills training versus psychosocial occupational therapy for persons with persistent schizophrenia. *American Journal of Psychiatry, 155,* 1087–1091.

Marder, S. R., Wirshing, W. C., Mintz, J., McKenzie, J., Johnston, K., Eckman, T. A., et al. (1996). Two-year outcome of social skills training and group psychotherapy for outpatients with schizophrenia. *American Journal of Psychiatry, 153,* 1585–1592.

Mueser, K. T., & Bellack, A. S. (1998). Social skills and social functioning. In K. T. Mueser & N. Tarrier (Eds.), *Handbook of social functioning in schizophrenia* (pp. 79–96). Needham Heights, MA: Allyn & Bacon.

Pilling, S., Bebbington, P., Kuipers, E., Garety, P., Geddes, J., Martindale, B., et al. (2002). Psychological treatments in schizophrenia: I. Meta-analyses of randomized controlled trials of social skills training and cognitive remediation. *Psychological Medicine, 32,* 783–791.

CHAPTER 25

COGNITIVE REHABILITATION

TIL WYKES

Unlike other therapies described in this book, cognitive rehabilitation is novel and has not yet been minutely examined. There is no consensus from its proponents on the language to describe the therapies or what their constituent parts should be. The underlying theory of how it works differs from one academic group to another, with suggestions about both compensating and repairing the cognitive system. But despite all these differences, many training packages do look similar, even if the emphasis within each package is different. The outcomes have been positive even this early in development, and high-quality randomized controlled trials have shown that the effects are not due to nonspecific therapeutic variables (Bell, Bryson, Greig, Corcoran, & Wexler, 2001; Bellack, Gold, & Buchanan, 1999; Wykes & Reeder, 2005; Wykes et al., 2003), which is why cognitive rehabilitation is included here. But to understand the place of the therapy within the field of rehabilitation, this chapter has a slightly different structure, with the background of the therapy leading to a description of the therapy as currently developed, but with the promise of an integrated approach in the future.

ARE COGNITIVE IMPAIRMENTS IMPORTANT IN SCHIZOPHRENIA?

The early descriptions of schizophrenia by Kraepelin and Bleuler emphasized the cognitive difficulties at the heart of the diagnosis of schizophrenia. Although there is still some dispute about whether these are static or deteriorating impairments, it is clear that they are also present during and, for some people, between acute episodes (e.g., McGhie & Chapman, 1961). There is also evidence from studies of children at high risk of developing schizophrenia, as well as populations of conscripted young people and birth cohorts, that people who later develop schizophrenia have lower overall premorbid cognitive capacity than those who do not develop the disorder. Although the majority of people with a diagnosis of schizophrenia show impairments, the decrements differ in magnitude across the population; some people seem little affected, and a few achieve high intellectual recognition (e.g., Dr. William Chester Minor, who in the 19th century contributed to an early version of the *Oxford English Dictionary* while a patient in an English lunatic asylum).

The detailed investigation of cognitive difficulties in the past decade has concluded that there are general deficits in multiple functions of attention, learning, and memory. In particular, executive functions, which include planning and strategy use, have been shown to be deficient. Although measuring differences between cognitive functions depends on the sensitivity of the tests, the general consensus is that memory difficulties are pervasive and specific. In other words, they are present even when there are no obvious abnormalities in overall cognitive function.

Severe cognitive impairments are not only important to service users but also have been shown to have a crucial association with functional outcomes, such as getting or keeping a job. They are also linked to the cost of mental health care. This relationship is often stronger than that with positive symptoms. But perhaps the clincher in the need to focus rehabilitation efforts on cognition is that there is now clear evidence that cognitive difficulties interfere with rehabilitation efforts in multiple domains of functioning. Cognition not only interferes with everyday life but it also limits functional outcomes over long periods of time and hinders the rehabilitation of specific functioning (Green, Kern, Braff, & Mintz, 2000; McGurk & Mueser, 2004; Wexler & Bell, 2005).

DEVELOPING THERAPIES FOR COGNITIVE DIFFICULTIES

This slowness of therapy development was due largely to the assumption that cognitive impairments were immutable, based on observations of largely unvarying cognitive difficulties over the course of the disorder. It was also proposed that these difficulties were neurological problems similar to frontal lobe lesions. Because there was little positive evidence for the effects of therapy on cognition in patients with frontal lobe lesions, this pessimism was transferred to schizophrenia and, when care moved from institutions to the community, had the effect of concentrating rehabilitation efforts on teaching specific life skills.

The initial boost to the development of therapy for cognitive problems came from an unexpected source: research on the immutability of cognitive difficulties (Goldberg, Weinberger, Berman, Pliskin, & Podd, 1987). One major U.S. study purported to show that it was impossible to teach inpatients with chronic schizophrenia how to carry out a particular neuropsychological test, the Wisconsin Card Sorting Test (WCST), which measures flexibility of thought. In the results of this study, shown in Figure 25.1, it is clear that training was not successful in improving performance until the participants were provided with specific, card-by-card instructions. However, as soon as this learning support was removed, performance returned to baseline and was no different in the group that had just repeated the test five times. This study produced a boost in research, leading to a line of inquiry that attempted to find out whether any type of instruction would have longer lasting effects; in other words, the experiments were designed to test the null hypothesis that cognition was immutable. Although many studies supported immutability, a few showed that it was possible under some conditions not only to improve performance but also to produce durable improvements. These results produced the vital bit of therapeutic optimism, and a new psychosocial rehabilitation technology was born.

WHAT SHOULD BE A TARGET FOR COGNITIVE REHABILITATION?

Cognitive difficulties cover a broad range and show interindividual variation. Clearly, an intervention designed to have the most impact on a person's life needs to be targeted, but

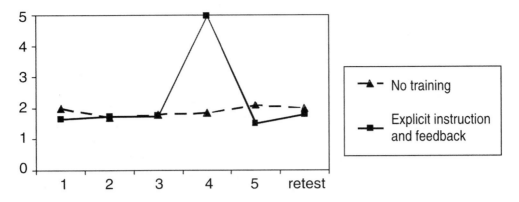

FIGURE 25.1. WCST performance with and without training. From Goldberg et al. (1987). Copyright 1987 by the American Medical Association. Adapted by permission.

these targets may differ among different real-life functions. So far the targets have been highly correlated with particular functional outcomes. Obviously this may be a gross error, because it is not clear that a change in an associated cognitive ability necessarily produces a change in function, but at least this seems to be a sensible starting point.

There are difficulties in comparing different cognitive measurements and different ways of measuring functional outcome. The most comprehensive reviews have concluded that memory and executive functions are important in predicting overall functioning, and that some basic functions, such as sustained attention, also show some relationships, although this may be a result of poor executive control. These difficulties have also been highlighted in rehabilitation programs. Supported employment programs can compensate for low-level impairments but are only partially effective at compensating for memory and executive functions (McGurk, Mueser, & Pascaris, 2005). Different cognitive problems also affect rehabilitation at different times during a program. Sustained attention, response inhibition, and idiosyncratic thinking have been found to be important in the initial stages of a work rehabilitation program, but after the engagement phase, attention, verbal memory, and psychomotor speed became better predictors of within-program performance. This does fit with what is known about the rehabilitation programs themselves. In the beginning there is a need for concentration on instructions, but later practice and speed of response are important in becoming expert in the relevant tasks.

To design the most efficacious cognitive rehabilitation program requires answers to a number of questions that can only be derived from empirical investigation:

- Can we change functioning by improving one cognitive factor, or do we need improvement across a range of cognitive abilities?
- How much improvement is enough? Improving cognition by a smidgen may have dramatic effects on functioning, but this seems unlikely. What seems more likely is that a threshold of cognitive improvement is necessary.
- Does improvement depend on the magnitude of the impairment? For instance, would it be easier to show effects with less improvement in those with the most cognitive difficulties or vice versa?
- Are there personal characteristics that make cognitive change more or less likely?
- Will the same cognitive functions that are associated with outcomes statically be associated with dynamic improvements?

None of these questions has received a conclusive answer, but that should not deter us from developing cognitive rehabilitation. Rather, the development of such a technology will provide answers to the questions and allow the advancement of both theory and practice.

EVIDENCE FOR SUCCESSFUL COGNITIVE REHABILITATION

It seems that three types of theory are cited when cognitive rehabilitation programs are described. The first is the notion of *restitution*, in which the use of a particular cognitive function is repeatedly practiced, whereas in *compensation*, patients are provided with alternative strategies to achieve goals. In the last approach, *learning theory*, behavioral procedures, such as shaping and modeling, are used to improve functioning. In fact, it is not clear that any program does anything differently based on any theory. These are all post hoc explanations for the results of clinical trials.

Single-Test Interventions

These interventions were designed to provide highly controlled comparisons of short interventions for particular tests of cognitive flexibility, memory, and attention. The results indicate that there is considerable room for optimism, and that it is possible to improve cognition. This corpus of studies also benefited the development of successful training programs in an unusual way. Published peer-reviewed data also include reports of negative effects of training paradigms. These data can be used to prevent failure in our participants. The main outcomes are that continued practice at some tasks may increase performance on that task, but there is little generalization to other, similar tasks. Too much information is detrimental to performance in some people, and training programs that focus only on increasing motivation divert attention away from the key task requirements. Some forms of training, such as errorless learning (reducing the error rate when teaching the task), scaffolding (providing tasks in which effort is required but the solution still lies within the person's range of competence), and verbal monitoring (overtly rehearsing the task rules and strategies for solution) were found to be successful. Positive and durable improvements with these techniques have been found for executive functioning, memory, and sustained attention, but the evidence for sustained attention tends to be task-specific.

Clinical Interventions

The second generation of studies progressed from attempts to influence performance on a single test to the rehabilitation of a variety of cognitive functions that might affect real-life functioning. Again, positive results have been found for the improvement of cognition, although the effect sizes are considerably reduced. Figure 25.2 shows the range of effect sizes in three meta-analyses and also distinguishes different types of training, with rehearsal-based training showing less of an effect than training strategic processing. The confidence interval for the effect of rehearsal learning crossed zero, suggesting that this is not even a robust effect.

There have now been more than 15 randomized controlled trials of cognitive training to improve cognition, and these show moderate effect sizes (0.45),[1] identical to those

---

[1] *Effect size* is here defined as the mean difference between treatment and control condition divided by the standard deviation of the measure employed.

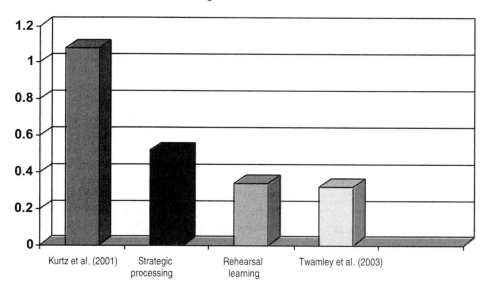

FIGURE 25.2. Average effect sizes for cognitive outcomes following CRT from meta-analyses. From Krabbendam and Aleman (2003). Copyright 2003 by Springer-Verlag. Reprinted by permission.

of cognitive-behavioral treatments. All but one meta-analysis has shown a positive effect so there does seem reason to exploit this therapy (Krabbendam & Aleman, 2003; Kurtz, Moberg, Gur, & Gur, 2004; Twamley, Jeste, & Bellack, 2003). But improving cognition is not under dispute. The real question is, do these cognitive improvements have an effect on real-life functioning? There is evidence of modest effects on positive and negative symptoms (effect size for overall symptom severity = 0.26), and more robust effects for social functioning (0.51). There are also some emerging data that cognitive remediation affects the number of hours worked. Most importantly many of these effects are durable. For instance 58% people who receive cognitive remediation and work rehabilitation were still in paid employment 12 months after the end of treatment, whereas only 21% of those who received work rehabilitation alone were still at work at this time (Wexler & Bell, 2005).

So there is evidence of positive effects on functioning outcomes. This assumes that remediation acts on cognition, and that this improvement leads to changes in real-life functioning. But the empirical data now point to a different model, one in which improvements in cognition have to be moderated by cognitive rehabilitation, because even when cognition improves in the control group, there is little evidence of improvement on functioning; in addition, nonresponders to cognitive remediation have less chance of improving their functioning. The effect on outcome seems to depend solely on the cognitive improvements produced by cognitive rehabilitation.

TYPES OF COGNITIVE REHABILITATION

What is cognitive rehabilitation? This question has come rather late, because it is the most difficult to answer. Cognitive rehabilitation has been led by pragmatic studies that attempt to demonstrate individuals' cognitive improvement. The training programs adopted have face validity, but there have been many different approaches:

- Individual or group treatment
- Computer-driven presentation or paper-and-pencil tasks
- Therapist presentation or automated presentation (or both)
- Frequency of therapy—either weekly or intensive daily sessions
- Type of training (rehearsal or strategic processing)

Every combination of factors has been used, making it almost impossible to differentiate between successful and unsuccessful characteristics. But because there are some distinct choices, some of these general models are described.

Operant Conditioning

This type of treatment is based specifically on learning theory and incorporates the differential reinforcement of successive approximations of behavior or shaping. Rather than waiting for a complete behavior to occur before offering reinforcement, reinforcement is provided for successive approximations or steps toward the final behavior. This type of training has been used with the most severely disabled patients, and there is evidence of both complex (abstract thinking) and simple (sustained attention) positive outcomes. Changing the environmental contingencies may therefore have a role to play in cognitive rehabilitation (e.g., Silverstein, Menditto, & Stuve, 2001).

Environmental manipulation has been taken even further in a program called cognitive adaptation training. Participants in this program, following a neuropsychological assessment, are provided with an environment that compensates for their specific cognitive impairments. For example, signs are placed on the bathroom wall about cleaning teeth; complete sets of clothes are provided for each day of the week; and daily rations of money are provided. In this case, there is no expectation of training particular behaviors, so that exercises may be carried out independently. The assumption is that the environmental manipulation will continue to guide behaviors and to reduce response choices that often have a detrimental effect on performance. The evidence for the efficacy of this particular therapy includes improvements in both symptoms and social functioning. Environmental control is, however, gross, and this may not be acceptable to all service users or health care professionals.

Integrated Psychological Therapy

Integrated psychological therapy (IPT) was one of the first programs to include a specific cognitive domain. There are five subprograms each of which has both social and cognitive elements in differing amounts. The subprograms are cognitive differentiation, social perception, verbal communication, social competence, and interpersonal problem solving. The explicit cognitive subprogram (cognitive differentiation) addresses a variety of cognitive abilities, such as attention and conceptualization abilities. Activities are run in a group, in which training is didactic. This method of training provides social contact that may also boost social functioning.

This therapy has been subjected to rigorous evaluation; although most patients show some improvement in cognitive ability, the specific improvements differ between studies and depend on the level of experimental control (Spaulding, Reed, Sullivan, Richardson, & Weiler, 1999).

Cognitive Enhancement Therapy

This therapy amalgamates both group and partner working. It uses task materials often from those used to treat brain injury, as well as a comprehensive approach to work therapy. Initially the therapist provides two patient partners with experience of computer presentations of tasks involving attention or memory skills. The therapist, as well as patient partners, help to guide the use of the computer, providing positive reinforcement and suggestions about ways to approach the tasks. In addition, participants also attend groups in which they present and discuss information on how they might solve individual social or work problems. After 3 months of computer training, participants also enter larger groups of six to eight people. The group program takes an additional 6 months and comprises exercises that focus on "gistful" interpretations of information, such as summing up an article in a newspaper to another person. Unlike most treatment programs for inpatients, this program is aimed at higher functioning patients (i.e., "stable outpatients").

The evaluations of cognitive enhancement and a similar program specific to supported employment both indicated positive effects for cognition and specific functioning outcomes, such as number of hours worked. What this type of training offers is an immediate transfer of training into the functioning domain, which is likely to increase the generalization of cognitive improvements from the specific cognitive rehabilitation therapy (CRT) part of the program (Hogarty et al., 2004).

Educational and Remediation Software Programs

Two types of software have been used in computer presentations: (1) that designed to treat head injury and (2) educational software that is easily available and designed to be engaging. Both sets of programs are based on models of practice, and individuals progress through the various levels of the program. Currently there is no specific theoretical guidance on the presentation or inclusion of particular tasks. Rather they are chosen for their face validity, their appeal (in the case of educational software) and their comprehensiveness, in terms of the underlying skills required. Software designed for educational use has not only been tested for its efficacy but it also provides the opportunity to control task levels and to introduce complex problem-solving and concept formation tasks. The tasks have some ecological validity, although, of course, much of the presentation can be too child oriented.

Computerized training has shown mixed effects, with some studies showing generalization and durability and others showing no between-group effects and no differential improvement compared to other types of cognitive skills therapy. The effects on functioning are also mixed. The difficulty with the use of this therapy is that it is quite possible for the therapist to be involved and have high levels of contact, or for the participant to interact only with the computer. Higher levels of initial contact with a therapist may be responsible for cognitive improvement, because the therapist can respond with sensitivity and flexibility to the strengths and difficulties of the participant. There is little current evidence on the efficacy of computer- versus therapist-driven therapy, because most programs studied have included supervision from a clinical specialist. It seems likely that such a person will be necessary, at least until a computer can suggest that a break and a cup of tea are needed.

Executive Skills Training

Several programs have been developed in this area, but the best-known one, initially designed in Australia, comprises three modules: cognitive flexibility, memory, and planning. Each of the 40 or so hour-long sessions contain different paper-and-pencil tasks, all of which had relevance to specific cognitive processing problems. The cognitive flexibility module includes a range of tasks that required engagement, disengagement, and reengagement of various cognitive information sets. Memory is targeted by a range of set maintenance, set manipulation, and delayed response tasks. Finally, planning involves tasks for set formation and manipulation, reasoning, and strategy development. The focus here is on both the development of new and efficient information-processing strategies and practice of these strategies in new contexts and with different forms of information (e.g., verbal and visual). This emphasizes the generalization from task to task within the training protocol. Tasks are easy but can be adapted to higher functioning participants, so that the tasks require some effortful processing, which is known to be helpful for cognitive training.

The randomized controlled trial data show changes with this form of therapy in both cognition and social functioning. In particular, this form of training has shown improvements in patients' memory abilities that were durable 6 months after the end of therapy.

Medication

Cognitive rehabilitation is also being approached from the viewpoint of medication to restore function. Double-blind, randomized controlled trials have shown that there are small effects of antipsychotic medication on cognition. More recently, drug therapies have been developed that specifically target the cognitive system rather than being a side effect of current medications for positive symptoms. Although these possible cognitive enhancers may offer an initial boost to the cognitive system, it seems likely that psychosocial rehabilitation will also be required. One metaphor for this is mending a broken bone. Although it is possible to set the bone in place for it to grow, it is also necessary to provide some physiotherapy to improve functioning and to develop the bone structure further. This is perhaps how cognition-enhancing drugs will be used within the comprehensive set of rehabilitation techniques that mental health services will offer. Their use with cognitive rehabilitation techniques will be synergistic rather than a replacement for psychosocial techniques.

A MODEL FOR THERAPY

What is needed is a theoretical model for therapy development, and currently few exist. As discussed earlier, most theories were provided post hoc and have not been supported by current data. They are mostly descriptive and give little guidance for the development of the most efficacious therapy. Most of the attention has been given to the types of cognition that predict poor functioning, with little consideration of what cognitive abilities would be required to carry out real-life actions. Clare Reeder and I have considered what is required for cognition to be transferred into actions. Figure 25.3 shows our model, which contains a new component, *metacognition*. We categorize actions into those that are routine (i.e., are specified by cognitive schema as soon as the goal or intention has been defined) and nonroutine (i.e., not completely specified by a cognitive schema). Most actions are not routine. For example, if I intend to make a meal, I need to decide what kind of meal I would like to make, to look in a recipe book, to consider what ingredients are available, and so on. I must reflect upon my intention, my goals, my past experience, and the way in which these interact with the current circumstances to select a certain set of appropriate actions that will allow me to achieve my goal. This ability to reflect upon and regulate one's own thinking is referred to as *metacognition*. It is the key to carrying out nonroutine actions successfully. This has profound effects on what we need to include in a cognitive rehabilitation program. Improvements in cognitive processes have a direct effect on routine actions because they improve the efficiency of cognitive schemas. But, these same improvements may not have an effect on nonroutine actions because metacognitive skills are also needed. To ensure improvement in nonroutine actions, metacognition, as well as cognition, must be a target.

To target metacognition one needs to include opportunities for the participant to reflect on current goals, strategies, and rewards. This means that one should not provide a cognitive strategy as if it were a precise number of steps. Patients need to understand the positive value of effortful processing, to be encouraged to modify and personalize a general heuristic, and to be given opportunities and incentives. General problem-solving schemas must lead to the development of broad cognitive schemas that may be used in a variety of settings. The therapist must allow reflection and teach different approaches explicitly, because they may not arise by chance and just mentioning them (as may happen in a computer program) is not always effective. It seems likely that a dependence on practice does capitalize on chance learning, and this is not the most efficient method of improving metacognition. Participants should be encouraged to articulate their cognitive and motivational processes during learning and problem solving, because this promotes metacognitive processing and knowledge.

Another added factor in the model is the notion of *transfer*, which is not a new concept, but it has been recently defined as the ability to use knowledge, experience, motivations, and skills in a new situation. The role of CRT is to train for this essential transfer, if functioning is to improve. A focus on specific task-related routines does not facilitate transfer, and a huge number of routines suited to every occasion need to be taught individually if cognitive rehabilitation is to lead to everyday behavior improvements. The development of broad, generic schemas has the most utility and may be facilitated by the use of multimedia learning environments and by helping people to connect verbal explanations to visual representations.

In summary, our model of cognitive rehabilitation should include instruction, not mentioning; the flexible use of a range of strategies, not ritualistic adherence to specific strategies in a rigid manner; and the development of broad, generic schemas, not behavioral routines that are not easily transferable between situations.

A CLINICAL MODEL OF CRT

CRT aims to provide the participant with a comprehensive cognitive structure to reduce stimulus overload and facilitate efficient cognitive processing. A detailed description of the process of therapy is given in Wykes and Reeder (2005). The current therapy involves paper-and-pencil tasks that help people to consider thinking strategically and to approach tasks in the most efficient way. The three parts of the manual stress engagement of cognitive flexibility, memory, and planning. The tasks are initially very simple and gradually increase in difficulty to ensure that information-processing strategies can be developed and then practiced. Within the therapeutic session, the responsibility for providing a cognitive structure at first lies with the therapist, but it is gradually surrendered to the participant as his or her skills improve. It is possible that this is where computerized therapy may fit, in the secondary part of therapy, when the engagement and strategic processes have been instantiated. Teaching people to adapt flexibly and efficiently to novel situations is achieved through provision of different sorts of tasks that use similar sets of strategic skills. These skills then are not context-bound but allow for the development of a new style of thinking that can be used in all aspects of the participant's life.

Finally, and most important for transfer, through therapist prompts and discussions about their use, we emphasize how the skills might be used in the real world. These trans-

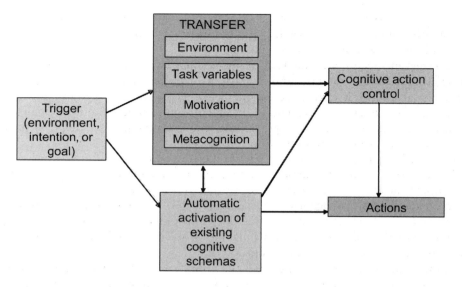

FIGURE 25.3. A model for cognitive remediation therapy.

fer skills need to be reinforced further by integrating them into different rehabilitation or life skills programs by other rehabilitation specialists. The general principles for successful generalization need to be followed in a comprehensive rehabilitation service to enable clients to achieve their full potential. We can now be much more optimistic about realizing this potential given the development of these new cognitive rehabilitation technologies. This type of therapy has been adopted in the cognitive enhancement models and seems to be of benefit.

TREATMENT GUIDELINES

1. *Initial assessment.* Investigate the range of severity of cognitive difficulties and strengths.

2. *Identify personal goals.* Cognitive rehabilitation needs to involve participants and improve motivation by the incorporation of cognitive activities that lead directly to the achievement of a personal goal.

3. *Therapeutic environment.* Provide a structured environment initially that reduces distraction.

4. *Therapeutic relationship.* The therapeutic relationship reduces social demand, instills a sense of being valued, and provides a forum to offer positive feedback about healthy cognitive behavior (thus promoting self-esteem).

5. *Individual tailoring of sessions.* Tailor sessions to an appropriate length, depending on mood, mental state, level of fatigue, and so forth, and include a variety of tasks that make varying demands in terms of the types of skills required and the level of complexity.

6. *Learning.* Learning should be constructive and reflective rather than passive, but be guided by the therapist using modeling and shaping, Socratic questioning, and multimodal practice.

7. *Use scaffolding.* "Scaffolding" is a metaphor for the way in which the educator provides the necessary supports, then takes them away over time.

8. *Errorless learning.* People with diagnoses of schizophrenia learn more quickly if they make few errors, because it is difficult to differentiate in memory between behaviors that produce a correct response and those that produced errors.

9. *Developing successful strategies.* Use verbalization, chunk material, and reduce the task to a series of subtasks.

10. *Generalize to everyday activity.* During sessions, link the cognitive strategies to real-life actions and encourage the generation of such situation descriptions by the participant. Then, use all possible supports in the person's environment to help him or her use cognitive skills in the real world.

KEY POINTS

- Cognitive difficulties are prevalent and are related to functional outcome in schizophrenia.
- Therapies have been developed to improve thinking styles and particularly CRT.
- CRT, an umbrella term, covers a number of different therapies that have varying levels of therapist input and varying levels of success.
- Cognition improved following CRT targeted therapy, has been durable, and can lead to improvements in functional outcome.
- To improve gains in functioning, therapies need to be based on theories of the relationship between cognition and action.
- The theory proposed includes a new form of cognition–metacognition that is necessary for gains in cognition that transfer into actions in the community.
- Future therapies need to concentrate on the transfer phase, in which the participant uses the skills learned in therapy in the real world.

REFERENCES AND RECOMMENDED READINGS

Bell, M., Bryson, G., Greig, T., Corcoran, C., & Wexler, B. E. (2001). Neurocognitive enhancement therapy with work therapy: Effects on neuropsychological test performance. *Archives of General Psychiatry, 58,* 763–768.

Bellack, A. S., Gold, J. M., & Buchanan, R. W. (1999). Cognitive rehabilitation for schizophrenia: Problems, prospects, and strategies. *Schizophrenia Bulletin, 25,* 257–274.

Goldberg, T. E., Weinberger, D. R., Berman, K. F., Pliskin, M. H., & Podd, M. H. (1987). Further evidence for dementia of the prefrontal type in schizophrenia—a controlled study of teaching the Wisconsin Card Sorting Test. *Archives of General Psychiatry, 44,* 1008–1014

Green, M. F., Kern, R. S., Braff, D. L., & Mintz, J. (2000). Neurocognitive deficits and functional outcome in schizophrenia: Are we measuring the "right stuff"? *Schizophrenia Bulletin, 26,* 119–136.

Hogarty, G., Flesher, S., Ulrich, R., Carter, M., Greenwald, D., Pogue-Geile, M., et al. (2004). Cognitive enhancement therapy for schizophrenia: Effects of a 2-year randomized trial on cognition and behavior. *Archives of General Psychiatry, 61,* 866–876.

Krabbendam, L., & Aleman, A. (2003). Cognitive rehabilitation in schizophrenia: A quantitative analysis of controlled studies. *Psychopharmacology, 169,* 376–382.

Kurtz, M. M., Moberg, P. J., Gur, R. C., & Gur, R. E. (2004). Approaches to cognitive remediation of neuropsychological deficits in schizophrenia: A review and meta-analysis. *Neuropsychology Review, 11,* 197–210.

McGhie, A., & Chapman, J. (1961). Disorders of attention and perception in early schizophrenia. *British Journal of Medical Psychology, 34,* 103–113.

McGurk, S., & Mueser, K. (2004). Cognitive functioning, symptoms, and work in supported employment: A review and heuristic model. *Schizophrenia Research, 70* 147–173.

McGurk, S., Mueser, K., & Pascaris, A. (2005). Cognitive training and supported employment for persons with severe mental illness: One-year results from a randomized controlled trial. *Schizophrenia Bulletin, 31,* 898– 909.

Silverstein, S. M., Menditto, A. A., & Stuve, P. (2001). Shaping attention span: An operant conditioning procedure to improve neurocognition and functioning in schizophrenia. *Schizophrenia Bulletin, 27,* 247–257.

Spaulding, W. D., Reed, D., Sullivan, M., Richardson, C., & Weiler, M. (1999). Effects of cognitive treatment in psychiatric rehabilitation. *Schizophrenia Bulletin, 25,* 657–676.

Twamley, E. W., Jeste, D. V., & Bellack, A. S. (2003). A review of cognitive training in schizophrenia. *Schizophrenia Bulletin, 29,* 359–382.

Wexler, B., & Bell, M. D. (2005). Cognitive remediation and vocational rehabilitation for schizophrenia. *Schizophrenia Bulletin, 31,* 931–941.

Wykes, T., Reeder, C., Williams, C., Corner, J., Rice, C., & Everitt, B. (2003). Are the effects of cognitive remediation therapy (CRT) durable?: Results from an exploratory trial in schizophrenia. *Schizophrenia Research, 61,* 163–174.

Wykes, T., & Reeder, C. (2005). *Cognitive remediation therapy for schizophrenia: Theory and practice.* London: Routledge.

CHAPTER 26

VOCATIONAL REHABILITATION

DEBORAH R. BECKER

The rate of unemployment for people with serious mental illness, and schizophrenia in particular, is approximately 85%. Employment provides a means for earning income, structuring daily schedules, building relationships, having opportunities to use personal talents and interests, and achieving recognition. Through employment, people increase their independence and inclusion in community life. Development and validation of supported employment have made work a realistic option for people with schizophrenia. Furthermore, in addition to increasing income, work helps to reduce disability, isolation, boredom, stigma, and discrimination.

HISTORICAL BACKGROUND

Historically, mental health practitioners have discouraged people with schizophrenia from engaging in activities that are stressful, fearing their inability to cope and the worsening of symptoms. This protective clinical approach that focuses on deficits has fostered social exclusion. In this way, people have been discouraged from assuming normal adult roles, and the expectations and stress of everyday, real-world living. Instead, clients interested in work have been directed to try intermediate steps, such as sheltered workshops, prevocational work crews, agency-run businesses, transitional jobs managed by the mental health agency, and volunteer jobs. These stepwise work experiences are characterized by low expectations, close supervision, and work readiness criteria, and rarely lead to competitive work.

In the early 1980s, Paul Wehman and colleagues at Virginia Commonwealth University described an approach that helps people with developmental disabilities find competitive jobs directly and provides the necessary training and support once the person is employed, circumventing the traditional lengthy prevocational training and assessment. This approach, called *supported employment*, is defined by competitive work that pays at least minimum wage in integrated settings with others who do not necessarily have disabilities and is consistent with the person's strengths, abilities, and interests. Supported employment is designed for people with the most significant disabilities and provides follow-along supports. Supported employment has been modified for people with psychiatric disabilities and differs from traditional vocational services in several key characteristics, as summarized in Table 26.1.

THE SUPPORTED EMPLOYMENT MODEL

Individual placement and support (IPS) is the most comprehensively described and studied approach to supported employment for people with serious mental illness. In this model, mental health practitioners encourage all people to consider competitive employment and do not screen out people based on readiness criteria, history of substance abuse, criminal activity, or symptom severity. Practitioners ask clients about their expectations about employment, which encourages clients to consider work and the role it can play in their lives. Going to work might make one client feel like an "ordinary person." For another client, work might be important because it can increase the money available to support his or her children. Not all people with schizophrenia want a competitive job, but work should be an individual choice, and people should not be excluded from access to vocational services by mental health providers. People with schizophrenia are eligible for supported employment services when they express an interest in working.

An interested client is paired with an employment specialist to seek a competitive job that is consistent with the person's experiences, skills, and interests. The employment specialist first arranges for the person to access personalized benefits counseling to learn about work incentives and how working will impact his or her benefits.

The job search occurs soon after a client expresses interest in working and at a pace that he or she determines. Some people have clear job choices and want to apply for jobs immediately. Others want to proceed less quickly and learn about work opportunities by visiting different job sites. The goal is *competitive employment*, which is defined by part-time or full-time jobs in the community that are open to anyone, including people without disabilities, and that pay at least minimum wage. The wage should be equivalent to the wage and level of benefits paid for the same work performed by other workers.

The employment specialist meets regularly with other members of the treatment team (e.g., psychiatrist, mental health worker, and therapist) to coordinate service plans. Some practitioners on the team may not be part of the mental health agency. For example, federal or state vocational rehabilitation (VR) counselors are an additional resource.

TABLE 26.1. Comparison of Vocational Services

	Evidence-based supported employment	Traditional vocational services
Eligibility	Client choice	Screened for job readiness
Vocational focus	Competitive employment	Range including sheltered work, work crews, volunteer, time-limited jobs, competitive employment
Determinants of competitive job type	Client preferences	Pool of entry-level jobs
Follow-up support	Ongoing	Time-limited
Service location	Community	Segregated settings
Staffing pattern	Integrated mental health and vocational services	Parallel mental health and vocational services

VR counselors can purchase services, work-related equipment and supplies, provide guidance and counseling, and specialized knowledge about medical problems and local employers. Practitioners from other agencies are invited to be part of the team and, together with the client, help with the planning.

The employment specialist and other members of the treatment team provide individualized support as long as the person wants and needs assistance. It is through expectations, hope, and support that people move forward in their lives.

RESEARCH EVIDENCE

Extensive research demonstrates the effectiveness of supported employment. In quasi-experimental studies, 5-day treatment programs and one sheltered workshop were converted to supported employment. Day treatment services were discontinued and the staff was reassigned to employment specialist positions. The results were similar in all sites: large increases in the employment rates at the converted sites, and virtually no change in employment rates at the control sites. There were no negative outcomes, such as increased hospitalization or program dropout. Overall, clients, families, and staff have liked the change. Some clients, however, have reported that they miss the socialization opportunities of the day treatment program. With peer support centers, started in part as a response to this concern, the results were even more dramatic when employment services of a sheltered workshop were transformed to IPS-supported employment. Competitive employment outcomes increased from a rate of 5–50%.

The strongest scientific evidence that a practice is effective is a randomized controlled trial. To date, there are 16 randomized controlled trials of supported employment (Figure 26.1) (Bond, 2007). In 15 out of 16 studies, supported employment resulted in increased employment outcomes. Supported employment was compared to sheltered work, stepwise

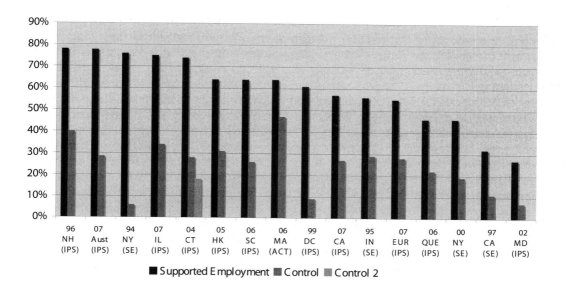

FIGURE 26.1. Employment rates in 16 randomized controlled trials of supported employment.

approaches, psychosocial rehabilitation, brokered vocational services, and skills training. Overall, there was a threefold difference in employment outcomes (60 vs. 24%, respectively).

Research has shown that competitive employment outcomes are higher in supported employment than in comparison programs, regardless of gender, age, diagnoses, minority status, work history, and urban and rural locations. A monthly employment rate of 40% for people participating in supported employment services is achievable. With increased attention on outcome results, agencywide employment data are recommended.

Most clients in supported employment programs work in part-time jobs. Starting a job at 10 hours per week and gradually increasing the number of hours is not uncommon. Jobs are typically entry-level positions and are consistent with the person's experiences. People report more job satisfaction and have longer tenure when they work in jobs that are consistent with their preferences. Ending a job by quitting, without having secured another job, or being fired, has been associated with interpersonal difficulties at work. People with schizophrenia often transition through two or three jobs before working a job long term, similar to people without disabilities.

Most studies have been short term (i.e., 18–24 months). At least three supported employment research studies with long-term follow-up (i.e., 8–12 years) have shown that people with serious mental illness are developing work careers. In two of these studies, 71% of the people had worked over half the follow-up period, and 47% were working in a competitive job at the time of the follow-up interview.

The effects of work on nonvocational outcomes are less clear. There is some evidence that people working in competitive jobs have higher ratings of self-esteem, satisfaction with finances and leisure, and better symptom control than people who work in sheltered settings, or who work minimally.

PRACTICE GUIDELINES FOR SUPPORTED EMPLOYMENT

There are seven principles of evidence-based supported employment.

1. *The client determines eligibility.* No one who wants to work is excluded. Clients often overcome barriers when they identify competitive employment as their goal. Practitioners sometimes are surprised when people for whom they had no work expectations have successful job experiences.

Setting up a simple referral system encourages all people to consider work in their lives. Client access to informational brochures in waiting areas makes work visible in the mental health agency. Working clients are invited to speak with other clients and practitioners about their experiences.

2. *Benefits counseling is part of the employment decision-making process.* Individualized benefits planning gives people the information needed to make informed decisions. In two studies (D. Bailey, personal communication, March 3, 2005; Tremblay, Xie, Smith, & Drake, 2004), people who received benefits counseling worked more and earned more money compared to people who did not receive benefits counseling. Fear of losing benefits (e.g., Social Security Income, Social Security Disability Insurance, Medicaid health insurance) is the most common reason that people with serious mental illness are reluctant to start a job. In most cases, people are better off financially if they work and take advantage of work incentives. Setting up such a system allows all clients to access benefits counseling when they consider working.

3. *Supported employment is integrated with treatment.* Rehabilitation is an integral component rather than a separate service of mental health treatment. Good communication is the key to provide seamless services. Employment specialists join treatment teams

and participate in regular treatment meetings (i.e., weekly) to coordinate services. Practitioners provide information about how clients manage their illness, which helps to determine the types of jobs and work settings that will support recovery. Employment specialists' information about how a person is functioning at work informs treatment decisions. Ways to provide integrated services include co-locating offices (i.e., employment specialists and mental health practitioners that share office space or have offices next to each other), maintaining an integrated client record, communicating frequently, and participating in treatment team meetings.

4. *Competitive employment is the goal.* Employment specialists assist people in finding competitive jobs that are integrated in regular job settings. The position is "owned" by the client and is not set aside for people with disabilities. The client receives work supervision and wage payment directly from the employer rather than from the mental health or rehabilitation agency. The mental health agency allocates sufficient funds for supported employment services and makes competitive employment a priority.

5. *The job search starts soon after a client expresses interest in working.* People are assisted in finding jobs directly, and are not asked to participate in lengthy prevocational training and assessment. Employment specialists spend several weeks meeting with clients and collecting information to develop a vocational profile to identify job types and work settings. Employment specialists initiate discussions with clients about whether to disclose to an employer information about their illness in relation to working. The client and employment specialist devise a plan to find the desired job and to determine their respective responsibilities in the job search. Some clients have difficulty making contact with employers and choose to have the employment specialist take the lead.

A central part of the employment specialist's job duties is to develop relationships with employers. Employment specialists build a network of employers to help make good job matches that meet the needs of employers and clients. Employment specialists network with everyone they know (e.g., treatment team members, board members, family members, friends, friends of friends, community members, other employers) to identify job leads that are consistent with client preferences.

6. *Follow-along supports are continuous.* Many people are able to find jobs but have difficulties maintaining them. Individualized support provided by the client's support network continues for a time period that fits individual needs. The treatment team helps to identify supports for starting a job, doing a job over time, having a problem on the job, and ending a job. Most supports are provided away from the job site.

Job accommodations may help to improve a person's job performance. For example, a person who has fearful thoughts when near a lot of people, can be helped by relocation of his or her work station. The cost of job accommodations for people with serious mental illness is usually minimal.

The employment specialist assists the client who is ending a job in planning for the next work experience by incorporating information about previous work experiences to update the employment plan and moving forward.

7. *Client preferences are important.* All aspects of supported employment are individualized. Decisions about types of work, work settings, amount of work, disclosure, job finding, and job support are made by the individual. Employment specialists help clients to identify jobs that are consistent with their skills, experiences, and interests. Therefore, jobs are varied and may be found in diverse settings.

In addition to following the evidence-based principles of supported employment, agencies develop a culture that values work, healthy risk taking, access to information, and self-help. Supported employment services are provided through a team approach in which all practitioners have a role in supporting people in their work efforts.

KEY POINTS

- Many people with schizophrenia want to work in regular community jobs with competitive wages.
- Supported employment has a strong research base.
- Individualized and comprehensive benefits planning enables people to make informed decisions about working, and leads to more people working and earning more wages.
- The goal is a competitive job that is "owned" by the person and based on his or her preferences, experiences, and skills.
- The job search begins soon after a client expresses an interest in working, and at a pace that is comfortable for that person.
- Individualized job supports are provided by the employment specialist and the mental health treatment team for as long as necessary.

REFERENCES AND RECOMMENDED READINGS

Anthony, W. A., & Blanch, A. (1987). Supported employment for persons who are psychiatrically disabled: An historical and conceptual perspective. *Psychosocial Rehabilitation Journal, 11*(2), 5–23.

Bailey, J. (1998). I'm just an ordinary person. *Psychiatric Rehabilitation Journal, 22*(1), 8–10.

Becker, D. R., & Bond, G. R. (Eds.). (2004). *Supported employment implementation resource kit.* Rockville, MD: Center for Mental Health Services, Substance Abuse and Mental Health Services Administration. Available online at *www.mentalhealth.samhsa.gov/cmhs/communitysupport/toolkits/employment/*

Becker, D. R., & Drake, R. E. (2003). *A working life for people with severe mental illness.* New York: Oxford University Press.

Becker, D. R., Drake, R. E., & Naughton, W. J. (2005). Supported employment for people with co-occurring disorders. *Psychiatric Rehabilitation Journal, 28*(4), 332–338.

Becker, D. R., Torrey, W. C., Toscano, R., Wyzik, P. F., & Fox, T. S. (1998). Building recovery-oriented services: Lessons from implementing IPS in community mental health centers. *Psychiatric Rehabilitation Journal, 22*(1), 51–54.

Bond, G. R. (2004). Supported employment: Evidence for an evidence-based practice. *Psychiatric Rehabilitation Journal, 27*(4), 345–359.

Bond, G. R. (2007). *Review of randomized controlled trials of supported employment for people with severe mental illness.* Unpublished manuscript, Indiana University–Purdue University, Indianapolis.

Bond, G. R., Becker, D. R., Drake, R. E., Rapp, C. A., Meisler, N., Lehman, A.F., et al. (2001). Implementing supported employment as an evidence-based practice. *Psychiatric Services, 52*(3), 313–322.

Bond, G. R., Drake, R. E., & Becker, D. R. (in press). An update on randomized controlled trials of evidence-based supported employment. *Psychiatric Rehabilitation Journal.*

Bond, G. R., & Jones, A. (2005). Supported employment. In R. E. Drake, M. R. Merrens, & D. W. Lynde (Eds.), *Evidence-based mental health practice: A textbook* (pp. 367–394). New York: Norton.

Bond, G. R., Resnick, S. G., Drake, R. E., Xie, H., McHugo, G. J., & Bebout, R. R. (2001). Does competitive employment improve nonvocational outcomes for people with severe mental illness? *Journal of Consulting and Clinical Psychology, 69,* 489–501.

Cook, J., & Razzano, L. (2000). Vocational rehabilitation for persons with schizophrenia: Recent research and implications for practice. *Schizophrenia Bulletin, 26,* 87–103.

Gowdy, E. A., Carlson, L. S., & Rapp, C. A. (2003). Practices differentiating high-performing from low-performing supported employment programs. *Psychiatric Rehabilitation Journal, 26,* 232–239.

MacDonald-Wilson, K., Rogers, E. S., Massaro, J., Lyass, A., & Crean, T. (2002). An investigation of reasonable workplace accommodations for people with psychiatric disabilities: Quantitative findings from a multi-site study. *Community Mental Health Journal, 38*(1), 35–50.

Torrey, W. C., Mead, S., & Ross, G. (1998). Addressing the social needs of mental health clients when day treatment programs convert to supported employment: Can consumer-run services play a role? *Psychiatric Rehabilitation Journal, 22*(1), 73–75.

Tremblay, T., Xie, H., Smith, J., & Drake, R. (2004). The impact of specialized benefits counseling services on Social Security Administration disability beneficiaries in Vermont. *Journal of Rehabilitation, 70,* 5–11.

Twamley, E. W., Jeste, D. V., & Lehman, A. F. (2003). Vocational rehabilitation in schizophrenia and other psychotic disorders: A literature review and meta-analysis of randomized controlled trials. *Journal of Nervous and Mental Disease, 191,* 515–523.

Wehman, P., & Moon, M. S. (Eds.). (1988). *Vocational rehabilitation and supported employment.* Baltimore: Brookes.

CHAPTER 27

ILLNESS SELF-MANAGEMENT TRAINING

KIM T. MUESER
SUSAN GINGERICH

Illness self-management is a broad set of strategies aimed at teaching people with schizophrenia how better to manage their illness in active collaboration with professionals, family members, and other supporters. The short-term goals of teaching illness self-management are to reduce relapses and rehospitalizations, and to improve coping with persistent symptoms to maximize functioning and subjective well-being. The long-term goals of teaching illness self-management are to promote greater independence, better role functioning (e.g., work, school, parenting), more rewarding social relationships, and a stronger sense of purpose and self-confidence. These long-term goals are often referred to as *recovery*, even when they occur in the context of persistent symptoms.

PRINCIPLES OF ILLNESS SELF-MANAGEMENT

The principles of illness self-management are derived from the *stress–vulnerability model* of schizophrenia. According to this model, the origins and course of schizophrenia are determined by the dynamic interplay among biological factors, the environment, and personal coping efforts. Specifically, the symptoms and associated impairments of schizophrenia are assumed to have a biological basis, determined by genetic and other biological factors (e.g., obstetric complications), that may interact with social–environmental stress (e.g., life events such as the death of a loved one or being the victim of a crime; living in a hostile, critical social environment). If sufficient biological vulnerability exists, schizophrenia will develop regardless of the extent of exposure to environmental stress, whereas, in other cases, stress may trigger the disorder in vulnerable individuals. Once schizophrenia has developed, symptoms, relapses, and functioning are influenced by *biological*, *environmental*, and *psychological* factors.

In terms of biological factors, *medication* can reduce the biological vulnerability that underlies the disorder. *Drugs and alcohol*, on the other hand, can increase biological vulnerability, either by affecting the brain directly, or by lessening the protective effects of medication. *Environmental stress* can trigger symptom relapses and impair functioning. On the other hand, *coping efforts* (e.g., skills for reducing anxiety, solving problems, and decreasing tension) can reduce the effects of stress, thus protecting individuals against relapses. Finally, *social support* can also reduce the effects of stress by either removing stressors or helping individuals cope with them more effectively.

Based on the stress–vulnerability model, teaching illness self-management skills to people with schizophrenia is guided by several overarching goals:

- Increase medication adherence to reduce biological vulnerability.
- Reduce substance use.
- Reduce stress through stress management and involvement in meaningful activities.
- Improve coping skills.
- Improve social support.

RESEARCH EVIDENCE FOR SPECIFIC ILLNESS SELF-MANAGEMENT PRACTICES

Reviews of research on teaching illness self-management skills have identified five specific practices that improve the course of schizophrenia: psychoeducation, behavioral tailoring, a relapse prevention plan, and coping and social skills training.

Psychoeducation involves providing factual information about the nature of schizophrenia and the principles of its treatment, using a combination of teaching strategies, such as didactic presentations and review of educational materials. Research on psychoeducation indicates that clients acquire and retain critical information about their illness and its treatment. Although such information alone tends to have a limited impact on the course of illness, it is an important ingredient for clients' informed decision making about their treatment.

Research on improving adherence to antipsychotic medication regimens has evaluated a variety of different strategies. The strongest empirical support is for *behavioral tailoring*, which has been shown to help people take their medication more regularly. This strategy involves teaching clients how to incorporate taking medications into their daily routines to minimize the common problem of forgetting to take them.

Developing a *relapse prevention plan* includes working with the client (and significant others, when available) to identify the early warning signs of relapse, and devising a plan to monitor and to respond to those signs. Implementing relapse prevention plans is effective at preventing relapses and rehospitalizations. Relapse prevention is frequently employed in individual and family interventions for schizophrenia.

Coping skills training involves teaching clients how to use coping strategies to minimize the effects of persistent symptoms. Such training uses the principles of social learning theory, including modeling, rehearsal, feedback, and home practice. For example, a clinician might model using "positive self-talk" to respond to negative voices, then ask the client to practice it. Research indicates that coping skills training reduces the severity and distress of persistent symptoms, such as auditory hallucinations, and improves people's ability to function in spite of the symptoms.

Social skills training involves teaching interpersonal skills using the same social learning principles we just described. Research indicates that skills training effectively improves the quality of social relationships, especially when there are concerted efforts to ensure that skills are generalized into the client's natural environment. Improved social relationships and support can buffer the negative effects of stress on relapse and rehospitalization.

CLINICAL GUIDELINES FOR ILLNESS SELF-MANAGEMENT

This section provides practical guidelines for teaching illness self-management skills. The following guidelines incorporate the evidence-based illness self-management strategies described earlier and also include suggestions based on clinical experience.

- Establish motivation.
- Provide psychoeducation.
- Improve medication regimen adherence.
- Reduce drug and alcohol abuse.
- Develop a relapse prevention plan.
- Teach stress reduction techniques.
- Develop coping strategies for persistent symptoms.
- Enhance social support.

Establishing Motivation for Illness Self-Management

Somewhat surprisingly, not all clients with schizophrenia are motivated to learn how to manage their illness more effectively, even those with persistent symptoms or frequent relapses. Some clients feel demoralized and helpless about their lives, and do not believe that they can recover from their illness. Others may lack insight into having schizophrenia, or any kind of mental illness, and do not view symptoms and relapses as part of a disorder. Still others feel that because they have participated in various mental health programs over the years without seeing results, they do not care to invest the effort of participating in yet another program.

The first step toward teaching self-management is to instill motivation for change. Although this may take time, it is well worth the effort, because without feeling motivated, clients are often reluctant to participate in illness self-management programs, or they drop out soon after enrolling. Motivation to improve illness self-management may be developed by first exploring what clients would like to change in their lives and discussing their personal viewpoints on *recovery*. It can be helpful to conceptualize recovery as personally meaningful changes in areas such as relationships with others, working or returning to school, independent living, control over personal finances, and participation in enjoyable leisure activities. Recognizing changes that clients would like to make in their lives naturally leads to identifying personal goals in those areas. Motivation for learning illness self-management can then be harnessed by exploring how preventing relapses, staying out of the hospital, and minimizing persistent symptoms can help clients achieve those goals.

Providing Psychoeducation

Clients benefit from learning basic information about schizophrenia, including how it is diagnosed, its symptoms, the stress–vulnerability model, the principles of treatment, and the role of medications. Clients do not have to believe they have schizophrenia to benefit from learning about the disorder, nor does the clinician have to convince clients that they have it. Many clients are relieved to learn they have a specific disorder for which effective treatments are known. For clients who are resistant to the term *schizophrenia*, it can be helpful to explain that it is simply a way of describing a group of symptoms that commonly occur together. If the client still does not accept the diagnosis, the clinician should explore other terms or phrases that may be more acceptable to the client, such as *mental illness*, *nervous condition*, *chemical imbalance*, or simply "these kinds of problems " or "the experiences you've been having."

Information about schizophrenia needs to be taught in a lively, interactive style that provides the client with frequent opportunities to relate the information to his or her own experiences. The clinician pauses frequently and asks questions to make sure the client understands the materials and to help him or her identify personal examples relevant to the information. Educational handouts about schizophrenia, its causes, and its treatment are available from a variety of sources (e.g., Gingerich & Mueser, 2002) that can facilitate teaching and be shared with significant others, such as family members.

Improving Medication Adherence

Poor adherence to antipsychotic medication is an important contributor to relapse and rehospitalization. Problems with adherence are not easy to detect, and a combination of approaches is usually most effective. Unexplained relapses and rehospitalizations, or severe symptoms in a client who has previously been successfully stabilized on medications, may be indications that he or she is not taking the medication as prescribed. Clients' self-reports of medication adherence are often inaccurate, although reports of nonadherence may be more accurate than reports of adherence. The reports of significant others or residential staff members about the client's medication adherence are sometimes more accurate, although they depend on frequent contact with the client and may be subject to the same biases as self-reports. The most accurate way of evaluating adherence is to count the client's pills to determine the percentage of missed dosages of medication, although even this can be challenging (accounting for free samples, liquid medications, etc.).

A number of strategies are useful for improving medication adherence. First, clients benefit from *basic information* about the effects of medication on reducing symptoms and preventing relapses, as well as the common side effects that may discourage adherence. Second, motivation to take medications should be developed by exploring how reducing symptoms or hospitalizations can help clients accomplish their personal goals. Some clients benefit from constructing a list of the pros and cons of taking medication.

Once clients understand the role of medications more fully and are motivated to take them, several methods may be used to improve adherence. One of the simplest strategies, *behavioral tailoring*, involves taking medication at the same time as another daily activity, such as brushing teeth or watching a favorite TV program. *Simplifying the medication regimen* by working with the prescriber to reduce the number of medications taken throughout the day can facilitate adherence. Teaching clients how to use *pill organizers* ("pill boxes") can make it easier for them to keep track of whether they have taken their medications. *Alarms*, including those available on some watches and cell phones, can be helpful to remind clients when it is time to take medication.

Finally, clients who have had consistent problems with medication adherence despite efforts to implement the strategies we have described may benefit from taking medication in an injectable depot form. Many clients see the value of taking medication but have difficulty taking oral medication regularly. Discussing the merits of taking injectable medications can make the client aware of a viable alternative to oral medication that is consistent with the goals of illness self-management.

Reducing Drug and Alcohol Use

Second to medication nonadherence, substance abuse is the most potent precipitant of relapse and rehospitalization. Alcohol and drug use problems are common in schizophrenia, with about 50% of clients having substance abuse or dependence at some point in their lives. At least part of this high susceptibility appears to be due to an increased sensitivity to the effects of alcohol and drugs. Therefore, providing information about how substances can provoke symptoms and reduce the protective effects of medication is beneficial to all clients, especially those who have recently developed the disorder and may have not yet developed problematic patterns of use.

Substance abuse treatment should be addressed in the context of the overall clinical management of schizophrenia rather than by referral to another agency or provider. By integrating treatment for substance abuse into the overall mental health care (i.e., "dual disorders" or "co-occurring disorders"), clients can be motivated to reduce or stop using substances to better manage their illness and make progress toward personal goals. However, successful substance abuse treatment must also address the various reasons people with schizophrenia use substances. For example, clients often use substances to help them cope with symptoms, to socialize, to have fun, to distract themselves from problems, and (for those with substance dependence) to provide a routine that structures their daily lives. Clients can achieve a sober lifestyle if treatment addresses these motives by helping them learn strategies for coping with persistent symptoms, develop alternative socialization outlets and new recreational pursuits, and involvement in other meaningful activities in their lives, such as work or school. More information on the treatment of substance abuse for persons with schizophrenia is provided by Kavanagh (Chapter 44, this volume).

Developing a Relapse Prevention Plan

Symptom relapses usually occur gradually over time and are preceded by the emergence of early warning signs. These signs may be subtle behavioral changes (e.g., concentration problems, social withdrawal, increased anxiety or depression) or the reemergence of symptoms previously in remission (e.g., hallucinations). Monitoring early warning signs and taking rapid action when the signs are detected (e.g., temporarily increasing the dosage of antipsychotic medication) can often avert full-blown relapses.

When developing a relapse prevention plan with the client, it is helpful to involve a significant other, such as a family member. Significant others are often aware of early warning signs that clients are not aware of. In addition, they are often in a good position to help the client take necessary action steps, such as contacting the treatment team.

The following are core components of developing a relapse prevention plan:

1. Identify triggers of previous relapses, such as specific stressful situations.
2. Identify two or three specific early warning signs of relapse based on a discussion of the past one or two relapses.
3. Develop a system for monitoring the early warning signs of relapse.
4. Determine an action plan for responding to early warning signs of relapse, including who should be contacted.
5. Write down the plan, including the specific early warning signs that are being monitored and the telephone numbers of any important contact people.
6. Rehearse the plan in a role play, post the plan in a prominent location, and give copies to anyone with an assigned role in the plan.

Questionnaires containing the early warning signs of relapse and worksheets for developing a relapse prevention plan can be found in the work of Gingerich and Mueser (2002; Mueser & Gingerich, 2006).

Teaching Stress Reduction Techniques

As noted earlier, stress can precipitate symptom relapses. However, living a full and rewarding life invariably involves some exposure to stress, so rather than telling clients to *avoid* all stress, it is important to teach them strategies to *manage* stress. Prior to teaching stress management, it is helpful to talk with the client about what situations or events he or she finds stressful, and how to recognize the signs of stress (e.g., rapid breathing, racing heart, muscular tension, confusion, anxiety). Awareness of when one is experiencing stress can serve to cue a person to use stress reduction techniques.

The same methods used to teach stress management in the general population are also effective in people with schizophrenia, including relaxed (deep) breathing, positive self-talk, progressive muscle relaxation, and imagery. The specific combination of these basic elements can be determined individually for each client. Examples of relaxation exercises may be found in popular books by Gingerich and Mueser (2002; Mueser & Gingerich, 2006).

In addition to learning relaxation exercises, it can also be helpful for clients to get involved in meaningful, but not overly demanding, structured activities. Lack of meaningful stimulation can be stressful and precipitate symptom relapses. Involvement in meaningfully structured activities, such as part-time work, school, sports, volunteer programs, or a local club, can engage clients in a positive, constructive manner that gives them a sense of meaning and purpose in their lives.

Developing Coping Strategies for Persistent Symptoms

Many clients experience persistent symptoms, such as hallucinations, anxiety, and depression, in spite of taking their antipsychotic medications regularly. These symptoms often lead to distress and interfere with functioning. Learning to use coping strategies can reduce the negative effects of persistent symptoms.

When persistent symptoms are distressful or lead to problems in functioning of which the client is aware, he or she usually feels motivated to learn more effective coping strategies. In the absence of distress or functional impairment, the clinician can explore with a client how symptoms may interfere with personal goals (e.g., hearing voices may interfere during job interviews) to motivate the client to learn coping strategies. Coping strategies may be taught by using the following steps:

1. Identify persistent symptoms. Work on one symptom at a time, and elicit from the client a detailed description of the nature of that symptom.
2. Teach the client to self-monitor the symptom on a daily basis. Keeping track of the frequency and intensity of the symptom can both increase the client's awareness of it and help him or her to identify situations in which it is more versus less problematic.
3. Identify current coping strategies used by the client and strengthen those that are helpful through additional practice in sessions and by developing plans to practice the strategies at home.
4. Select a new coping strategy collaboratively with the client, demonstrate it, en-

gage the client in practicing it in the session, and develop a plan for the client to practice it on his or her own. Examples of coping strategies for different symptoms are provided in Table 27.1. Work on one strategy at a time, and build up the client's experience by practicing it in increasingly more challenging situations.

5. Review the client's efforts to implement the new coping strategy, troubleshooting as needed. Coping strategies may need to be modified to make them more effective for an individual client.

6. Try to develop at least two coping strategies for each problematic symptom. Research shows that clients with multiple coping strategies report more success at managing their persistent symptoms.

Enhancing Social Support

Two types of strategies may be useful for increasing the social support of people with schizophrenia. First, social skills training can be used to teach critical interpersonal skills for meeting people, having conversations, getting close to people, and improving the quality of social relationships. More information about social skills training for schizophrenia is provided by Tenhula and Bellack (Chapter 24, this volume).

Second, clients can be encouraged to participate in programs at peer support agencies, where they can develop relationships with other individuals with mental illness. There are several advantages of peer support programs as a source of social support. Be-

TABLE 27.1. Examples of Coping Strategies for Common Symptoms

Symptom	Strategies
Hallucinations	• Increasing one's activity by exercising, listening to music, humming, starting a conversation with someone, or doing a task • Calmly and firmly telling the voices to stop • Using positive self-talk by telling oneself something such as "Take it easy" or "I can handle this" • Taking a break from an overstimulating situation
Anxiety	• Using relaxation techniques, such as deep breathing or progressive muscle relaxation • Talking with a supportive person about one's feelings • Identifying a specific situation that makes one feel anxious and making a plan to do something about it (e.g., if anxious about an application deadline, setting up a date and time to work on the first part of the application) • Working with a clinician to expose oneself *gradually* to situations that create anxiety
Depression	• Scheduling pleasant events on a daily basis • Increasing one's activities by starting with small attainable goals and building in rewards for following through • Correcting unhelpful thinking patterns, such as overgeneralizing, jumping to conclusions, and overpersonalizing • Dealing with sleep problems by getting up and going to bed at the same time every day, avoiding naps, limiting intake of caffeine, and reading or relaxing just prior to bedtime
Negative symptoms	• Identifying an activity that one used to enjoy (e.g., hobbies, sports, music, or artwork) and trying it again • Breaking down goals into small, manageable steps • Gradually increasing daily structure, including meaningful activities • Focusing on the present, not the past

Note. From Mueser and Gingerich (2006). Copyright 2006 by The Guilford Press. Adapted by permission.

TABLE 27.2. Examples of Illness Self-Management Programs

Program	Content	Approximate length and format	Distinguishing characteristics

Illness management and recovery (Gingerich & Mueser, 2005b); downloadable at *www.samhsa.gov*	• Defining what recovery means to the individual
	• Setting personal recovery goals
	• Ten educational modules:
	  • Recovery Strategies
	  • Practical Facts about Mental Illness
	  • Stress–Vulnerability Model
	  • Building Social Support
	  • Using Medication Effectively
	  • Drug and Alcohol Use
	  • Reducing Relapses
	  • Coping with Stress
	  • Coping with Problems and Symptoms
	  • Getting Your Needs met in the Mental Health System
		8–10 months of weekly or twice-weekly sessions; individual or group format	• Emphasis on setting and achieving personal recovery goals
			• Clinicians trained to use motivational, educational, and cognitive-behavioral strategies, and social skills training techniques
			• Clients practice skills in sessions and as part of home assignments
			• Introductory video and practice demonstration video
			• Client manual and clinician manual
			• Clients encouraged to involve family members and other supporters

Personal therapy (Hogarty, 2002)	Clinician helps client with • Developing a treatment plan • Learning about schizophrenia • Resuming tasks and responsibilities • Developing strategies for coping with stress and symptoms • Improving social skills	1 year of weekly sessions, up to 2 years of sessions every other week; individual format	• An individual psychotherapeutic approach • Clinicians use a combination of techniques, including coping skills training and social skills training • Family involvement encouraged
Social and independent living skills (Liberman, et al., 1993); modules can be purchased at *www.psychrehab.com*	Eight modules: • Medication Self-Management • Symptom Self-Management • Recreations for Leisure • Basic Conversation Skills • Community Reentry • Workplace Fundamentals • Substance Abuse Management • Friendship and Intimacy	3–4 months of weekly sessions per module (24–32 months to complete all 8 modules); group format	Trainers' manuals • Client workbooks • Videos for each module where skills are demonstrated • Clients practice the skills in session and do related home assignments • Clinicians primarily use social skills training techniques
Team Solutions (Scheifler, 2000); downloadable at *www.treatmentteam.com*	Ten modules: • Understanding Your Illness • Understanding Your Symptoms • You and Your Treatment Team • Recovering From Mental Illness • Understanding Your Treatment • Getting the Best Results from Your Medicine	4–5 months of weekly sessions; usually in group format, but can also be provided to individuals	• Introductory video • Trainer's manual • Well-developed and easy-to-read educational booklets for clients • Focuses primarily on providing education

(continued)

TABLE 27.2. (*continued*)

Program	Content	Approximate length and format	Distinguishing characteristics
	• Helping Yourself Prevent Relapse • Avoiding Crisis Situations • Coping with Symptoms and Side Effects • Managing Crisis and Emergency Situations		
Wellness Recovery Action Plan (WRAP; Copeland, 1997); materials can be purchased at *www.mentalhealth recovery.com*	Participants develop a personal WRAP plan with seven components: • Creating a Daily Maintenance Plan • Identifying Triggers, Early Warning Signs, and Signs of Potential Crisis • Developing a Crisis Plan • Establishing a Nurturing Lifestyle • Setting up a Support System and Self-Advocacy • Increasing Self-Esteem • Relieving Tension and Stress	Usually provided in 2-day workshop; follow-up is sometimes included	• Primarily taught in workshop conducted by trained peer facilitators • Written materials available • Focuses on healthy habits • Tends to avoid providing information about specific disorders • Participants receive support and inspiration from leaders and each other • Participants develop a WRAP plan that they refer to on a regular basis • Strong self-help component

cause they are mainly operated by people with mental illness, clients do not have to deal with stigma when developing relationships with others at peer support programs. Also, peer support agencies usually offer a range of social, recreational, and work activities specifically designed to foster the development of social bonds (e.g., inexpensive meals, community trips, support groups, work activities at the program). In addition, peer support agencies often offer clients opportunities to learn more about how to manage their psychiatric illness, and provide role models of people who have learned how to take charge of their lives. Finally, because participation in peer support programs involves giving support to other people, many clients find the experience of helping others to be as powerful, or even more powerful than being helped. Actively helping and supporting others provides tangible evidence that the client has something to offer others, which can boost feelings of self-esteem and worth. More information about peer support programs is provided by Frese (Chapter 30, this volume).

STANDARDIZED ILLNESS SELF-MANAGEMENT PROGRAMS

A number of illness self-management programs are available for people with schizophrenia. Although the programs overlap in content, each also has its unique features, and clients may benefit from participating in more than one program. Five standardized and widely available illness self-management programs are described in Table 27.2. These programs can be provided in a variety of settings, including inpatient and outpatient settings, peer support centers, day treatment and residential faiclities, and on assertive community treatment teams. Each person with schizophrenia should have the opportunity to learn about his or her illness and to take an active role in treatment and in recovery. Therefore, mental health facilities providing services for people with schizophrenia should offer an illness self-management program as a routine component of their basic services.

KEY POINTS

- People with schizophrenia are capable of learning how to manage their illness in collaboration with professionals and significant others.
- Motivation to learn illness self-management strategies can be harnessed by helping clients establish personal goals, then exploring with them how improved illness management can help them achieve their goals.
- The stress–vulnerability model of schizophrenia provides a general framework for improved illness self-management and includes fostering medication adherence, reducing substance abuse, reducing stress, increasing social support, and improving coping with stress and symptoms.
- Psychoeducation about the nature of schizophrenia and the principles of its management is critical to informing clients about their choices and involving them in shared decision making about their treatment.
- Insight into having schizophrenia is not a prerequisite to learning illness self-management skills, nor is acceptance of the diagnosis necessary.
- Empirical research supports several practices for improving illness self-management, including behavioral tailoring for medication adherence (fitting medication into the client's daily routine), relapse prevention training, social skills training to improve social support, and coping skills training to handle stress and persistent symptoms.
- A variety of standardized illness self-management programs have been developed, each with unique but overlapping components with other programs.
- Peer support programs provide alternatives to traditional mental health services for opportunities to learn illness self-management strategies from other individuals with mental illness.

REFERENCES AND RECOMMENDED READINGS

Bellack, A. S., Mueser, K. T., Gingerich, S., & Agresta, J. (2004). *Social skills training for schizophrenia: A step-by-step guide* (2nd ed.). New York: Guilford Press.

Copeland, M. E. (1997). *Wellness Recovery Action Plan*. Brattleboro, VT: Peach Press.

Copeland, M. E., & Mead, S. (2004). *Wellness Recovery Action Plan and peer support: Personal, group and program development*. Dummerston, VT: Peach Press.

Gingerich, S., & Mueser, K. T. (2002). *Illness management and recovery*. Concord, NH: West Institute. Also available online at *www.samhsa.gov*

Gingerich, S., & Mueser, K. T. (2005a). *Coping skills group: A session-by-session guide*. Plainview, NY: Wellness Reproductions.

Gingerich, S., & Mueser, K. T. (2005b). Illness management and recovery. In R. E. Drake, M. R. Merrens, & D. W. Lynde (Eds.), *Evidence-based mental health practice: A textbook* (pp. 395–424). New York: Norton.

Hasson-Ohayon, I., Roe, D., & Kravetz, S. (2007). A randomized controlled trial of the effectiveness of the illness management and recovery program. *Psychiatric Services, 58,* 1461–1466.

Hogarty, G. E. (2002). *Personal therapy for schizophrenia and related disorders: A guide to individualized treatment*. New York: Guilford Press.

Liberman, R. P., Wallace, C. J., Blackwell, G., Eckman, T. A., Vacccaro, J. V., & Kuehnel, T. G. (1993).

Innovations in skills training for the seriously mental ill: The UCLA Social and Independent Living Skills modules. *Innovations and Research, 2,* 43–59.

Mueser, K. T., Corrigan, P. W., Hilton, D., Tanzman, B., Schaub, A., Gingerich, S., et al. (2002). Illness management and recovery for severe mental illness: A review of the research. *Psychiatric Services, 53,* 1272–1284.

Mueser, K. T., & Gingerich, S. (2006). *The complete family guide to schizophrenia: Helping your loved one get the most out of life.* New York: Guilford Press.

Mueser, K. T., Meyer, P. S., Penn, D. L., Clancy, R., Clancy, D. M., & Salyers, M. P. (2006). The illness management and recovery program: Rationale, development, and preliminary findings. *Schizophrenia Bulletin, 32*(Suppl. 1), S32–S43.

Mueser, K. T., Noordsy, D. L., Drake, R. E., & Fox, L. (2003). *Integrated treatment for dual disorders: A guide to effective practice.* New York: Guilford Press.

Roe, D., Penn, D. L., Bortz, L., Hasson-Ohayon, I., Hartwell, K., Roe, S., et al. (2007). Illness management and recovery: Generic issues of group format implementation. *American Journal of Psychiatric Rehabilitation, 10,* 131–147.

Salyers, M. P., Godfrey, J. L., Mueser, K. T., & Labriola, S. (2007). Measuring illness management outcomes: A psychometric study of clinician and consumer rating scales for illness self management and recovery. *Community Mental Health Journal, 43,* 459–480.

Scheifler, P. L. (2000). *Team solutions: A comprehensive psychoeducational program designed to help you educate your clients with schizophrenia (instructors guide and patient workbooks).* Indianapolis, IN: Eli Lilly and Company.

Tarrier, N. (1992). Management and modification of residual positive psychotic symptoms. In M. Birchwood & N. Tarrier (Eds.), *Innovations in the psychological management of schizophrenia* (pp. 147–169). Chichester, UK: Wiley.

Zygmunt, A., Olfson, M., Boyer, C. A., & Mechanic, D. (2002). Interventions to improve medication adherence in schizophrenia. *American Journal of Psychiatry, 159,* 1653–1664.

CHAPTER 28

GROUP THERAPY

JOHN R. McQUAID

For approximately the past 50 years, effective treatment of schizophrenia has depended on pharmacotherapy. However, many clinicians and researchers have also recognized the limits of medication in facilitating functional outcomes for patients. Investigators have therefore explored the use of adjunctive treatments, including group therapy, to improve the outcomes of patients with schizophrenia. In this chapter I first discuss theoretical and pragmatic issues of using group treatments for patients with schizophrenia. I then describe interventions that inform group therapies for schizophrenia and the integration of those interventions into cognitive-behavioral social skills training (CBSST), a newly developed group intervention for schizophrenia.

CHALLENGES IN THE TREATMENT OF PSYCHOSIS WITH PSYCHOSOCIAL INTERVENTIONS

Schizophrenia, by its very nature, is difficult to treat via talk therapy. Positive psychotic symptoms (e.g., delusions and hallucinations) impair patients' accurate perception of their environment. Delusional thinking leads to the misinterpretation of stimuli (e.g., perceiving innocuous glances from others as evidence of a plot), and hallucinations provide misleading data (e.g., a voice telling the patient that there is a plot). Negative symptoms such as anergia, anhedonia, and disinterest in interpersonal relationships can interfere with the likelihood of patients with schizophrenia engaging in behaviors that can improve either their symptomatology or their level of functioning. Negative symptoms can particularly undermine psychosocial interventions that are predicated on behavioral principles. If a patient finds no activity rewarding, then it is difficult to initiate, and even more difficult to maintain, the behavior.

Beyond the symptoms of psychosis, individuals with schizophrenia often have extensive deficits in cognitive processing that reduce their ability to perceive or encode disconfirming or corrective information and to learn functional skills. Some studies indicate that cognitive impairments in areas of abstraction and cognitive flexibility are better predictors of poor functional outcomes for patients with psychosis than positive or negative symptoms.

Psychotic symptoms also generate a series of secondary difficulties. Patients with psychotic disorders, relative to the general population, have higher rates of physical health problems and disability, as well as alcohol and substance dependence. Patients with schizophrenia also tend to have very poor social networks and financial resources. This combination of symptoms, cognitive impairments, and associated health and psychosocial impairments make schizophrenia one of the most disabling disorders, physical or psychological. These patients have deficits in all the major resources needed to engage effectively in therapy.

However, within the context of a shift from hospitalization to community-based care in the 1970s, many patients with schizophrenia ended up being responsible for a much higher level of self-care than they could provide for themselves. The resulting high rates of poverty, homelessness, and physical illness among those with severe mental illness are continuing challenges today. Current clinical research has moved beyond the original models of psychotherapy for psychosis, which attempted to reduce symptoms through talk therapy informed by psychoanalytic conceptualizations of psychosis. New models, drawn from scientifically informed theories of psychopathology and human behavior, focus on a range of potential outcomes reflecting the heterogeneous nature of schizophrenia.

Is Group Therapy a Reasonable Intervention for Schizophrenia?

Because of a greater awareness of patient needs, group interventions (including classes and skills training, as well as psychotherapy) are becoming widely used for treatment of schizophrenia. Unfortunately, although there is a growing body of evidence for the efficacy of both group and individual modalities for schizophrenia, there are no direct comparisons between individual and group modalities. Nonetheless, there are several reasons to emphasize the development of group treatments.

In general, group treatment is considered a more efficient way to provide services to patients. In simple terms, group treatment allows a single therapist to serve more than one patient at the same time. The actual cost-effectiveness is unclear, because groups may be less effective than individual therapy. However, there are additional benefits inherent to group structure.

One of the most important aspects of group treatment is the ability of patients to benefit from the observation of others. Effective treatments, such as social skills training (SST), facilitate and capitalize on observational learning opportunities. Group therapy provides a chance for patients to model skills, then observe as other patients practice these skills. In addition group members can share experiences with other patients, and give and receive feedback. Perhaps as importantly, groups actually provide social contacts and social feedback to patients who otherwise may have few such opportunities. Patients who are otherwise isolated can interact with other patients who, to some extent, have similar experiences. Practically, this means patients have more opportunities to practice skills they are learning in a supportive environment.

Groups are limited, however, in several important ways. Most obviously, patients get less individualized attention. Some patients, particularly those with paranoid symptoms, may find group settings aversive. Others with grandiose symptoms or poor ability to attend to social cues may be disruptive within a group, interfering with the learning process of others. These limitations suggest several principles to consider when designing group treatments.

• *Provide targeted structure.* Most current, evidence-based group treatments for schizophrenia emphasize therapeutic structure. This includes use of manualized treatments, heavy emphasis on psychoeducation, use of clearly defined skills training exercises, and defined courses of treatment (e.g., programs with a set number of sessions with specific agendas). By increasing the structure of treatment, the clinician helps to compensate for both the cognitive deficits and the negative symptoms. In addition, skills-based interventions (e.g., cognitive-behavioral therapy) show significantly better long-term outcomes than less structured supportive therapy.

• *Incorporate individualized treatment plans.* Although structure aids learning, a competing requirement for matching treatment to the specific needs of patients is particularly clear when one considers both the wide variety of symptom manifestations, and the broad range of functional impairments in patients. Successful treatments are characterized by the application of specific exercises to help patients develop unique treatment plans. For example, cognitive-behavioral interventions for psychosis often include exercises to identify "warning signs" of symptom exacerbation that are unique to each individual, then to define treatment plans to intervene if the warning signs occur. SST incorporates role plays of specific situations that patients anticipate they will face. By its nature, group interventions limit the ability of treatment to be matched to a specific patient's needs; therefore, interventions need to be designed to account for this limitation.

• *Provide a multimodal intervention.* Research suggests that patients with psychosis tend to have multiple deficits, and that specific skills training in one area does not necessarily lead to improvements in other areas. Therefore, it is preferable for treatments to provide a broad range of effective interventions that are appropriate to patients' needs.

This need must be balanced with the concern that a skills training treatment with too many components may be either unfocused or too superficial. Therefore, an intervention must be applicable to a range of problems and incorporate a variety of techniques, but do so in a relatively concise and coherent manner.

• *Facilitate a trusting relationship.* Paranoia and ideas of reference can severely interfere with the ability of patients to benefit from group. If a patient is more concerned about the motives of the clinician than the material of the group, it is very hard for him or her to participate. Alternatively, negative symptoms may present obstacles to engagement with other group members and group leaders. Therefore, in the context of group, therapists need to incorporate common listening skills to provide a sense of safety to patients and facilitate their connection to the group.

In summary, effective interventions need to provide enough structure to keep patients with limited resources on task, focused, and involved in the intervention. Some level of individualization is needed to increase the likelihood that a patient will benefit. The intervention needs to be broad enough to address the variability among patients with schizophrenia, and the therapeutic relationship needs to be nurtured.

REVIEW OF RELEVANT INTERVENTIONS

With these considerations in mind, three interventions are particularly relevant for considering group treatment for schizophrenia: cognitive rehabilitation (CR), social skills training (SST), and cognitive-behavioral therapy (CBT). These interventions are reviewed in other chapters in this volume, so the focus here is on the application of these techniques in the context of a group format.

Cognitive Rehabilitation

Mounting evidence suggests that CR interventions can effectively benefit patients with psychosis. These interventions can be classified into three categories. *Restorative* interventions use task training to improve an area of cognitive deficit (e.g., repetitive practice of a card sorting task with corrective feedback to improve cognitive flexibility). *Compensatory* strategies adjust for the patient's cognitive limitations by teaching ways to cope with deficits (e.g., learning to use notebooks and calendars to plan and schedule, learning problem-solving skills). *Environmental* strategies involve modifying patients' environments to better match their level of cognitive functioning (e.g., having simple reminders about tasks posted in the bathroom). Whereas all three sets of interventions have some evidence of support, compensatory strategies and, to some extent, environmental strategies are most relevant to group processes.

The primary purpose for incorporating CR interventions in group therapy is to facilitate other aspects of the treatment. Particularly for education and skills-based treatments, compensatory strategies can be critical for providing patients the necessary skills to engage in the treatment.

Social Skills Training

Social skills training, as the term implies, emphasizes training patients in appropriate social cues, including nonverbal communication, assertive verbal communication, active listening, and problem solving. SST is based on social learning theory, and emphasizes both direct practice and observational learning. Treatment includes a heavy reliance on role plays and feedback on performance. The therapist videotapes role plays and reviews them with patients. Each patient receives feedback from both the therapist and other group members. By having the therapy in a group modality, patients learn by both observing and giving feedback to their groupmates, as well as practicing on their own.

Cognitive-Behavioral Therapy

Cognitive-behavioral therapy for schizophrenia was developed initially as a treatment for reducing psychotic symptoms. CBT for psychosis is based on the assumption that cognitive processes in schizophrenia share a continuum with normal cognition; that is, the delusional content is not pathological (all people can report having unusual thoughts); rather, it is limited ability to question the delusion that is problematic. The intervention was therefore designed to teach patients the skills of examining beliefs and developing alternative explanations for experiences, including psychotic symptoms. As the intervention has been applied to patients with psychosis, additional target goals have been added, including facilitation of rewarding activities, medication adherence, social interactions, and vocational goals. Most interventions have been studied in an individual format, although there are some promising studies of CBT in a group modality as well.

CBT for psychosis differs from CBT for other disorders in several ways. Treatment for psychosis tends to have a longer course (greater than a year, compared to 12–20 weeks for major depression) in part due to the greater emphasis on developing the therapeutic relationship. Therapists treating patients with schizophrenia are much less directive initially in treatment (particularly in an individual model), and more flexible in terms of treatment structure, to facilitate the development of a trusting relationship.

At its most basic level, CBT teaches patients to view their thoughts as hypotheses, to gather evidence as to whether those hypotheses are true, and to generate new, more accurate hypotheses. Techniques include learning to record thoughts, to identify the relationship of thoughts to feelings and actions, to identify alternative thoughts, and to gather evidence on the accuracy of the beliefs.

A MODEL COMBINING CR, SST, AND CBT: CBSST

Overview

As the name implies, cognitive-behavioral social skills training (CBSST) integrates CBT and SST in a group therapy intervention. The primary goal of the combined treatment is to build on the strengths of SST in achieving functional outcomes, and to enhance treatment response by using CBT and compensatory strategies to address cognitive factors that interfere with patients' effective engagement in the treatment. The manual comprises three eight-session modules: *Changing Your Thinking* (cognitive interventions), *Asking for Support* (communication), and *Solving Problems*. Patients begin the treatment at the first session of any module, then complete all three modules twice, for a total of 48 weekly treatment sessions. Each session is 2.5 hours long, including a half-hour lunch break that is an integral part of the treatment. During the break, patients and group leaders practice interpersonal skills in a more "real-world" environment.

To facilitate participation of new members, the first session of each module includes an orientation section in which patients introduce themselves to each other and learn about the treatment model of the therapy. This allows patients to join the group every 8 weeks, dramatically reducing the potential wait time compared to a traditional closed group. At the same time, patients receive a more extensive orientation to the treatment than would be available in a traditional open group, and the fact that orientation is built into the group structure minimizes disruption to the skills training.

Each session includes multiple compensatory strategies to aid learning and memory. In fact, many of the standard CBT and SST components are in part CR techniques, including the use of role plays to train cue recognition, structured problem solving, and use of forms to record data (e.g., thoughts and associated emotions). Cognitive therapy and problem-solving training interventions are designed to improve the ability of patients to observe and to examine their thinking and planning, which in turn may improve cognitive flexibility, inductive reasoning, and abstract thinking. In addition, CBSST incorporates several additional compensatory strategies. All patients receive a group manual that includes not only the materials but also the tracking forms specific to each session and spaces for notes. They also receive laminated cards that list specific skills, and remind them how and when to use the skills. In class the group leaders present information using multiple modalities, including writing on a dry-erase board, using posters, having patients read from the manual, as well as lectures and group discussion. There is an emphasis on repetition and eliciting paraphrasing comments (i.e., summaries of the therapist's statements) from patients to assess their level of understanding and to aid development of therapeutic alliance. Exercises in the manual include developing action plans to respond to anticipated needs (e.g., the name and number of the patient's doctor, along with what to do if the patient is experiencing symptoms associated with relapse). Throughout the manual, simple mnemonics are used to help patients remember tasks. For example, the thought challenging technique is called "the three C's," which stands for catch the thought, check it, and change it. Finally, during the group patients receive reinforcement (including verbal praise and tokens acknowledging success) for responses that represent an improvement over previous efforts, however small. The incorporation of these strategies is intended to facilitate engagement in treatment and to improve skills acquisition.

Goal Setting

At entry to treatment, regardless of the module, patients meet individually with a therapist to identify goals. The patient defines his or her goals (e.g., starting a relationship, getting a job), and the therapist provide guidance in terms of making the goal as specific and quantifiable as possible. The therapist then helps the patient to identify specific steps in achieving the goal. This is particularly important when goals are extremely ambitious. The therapy goals are written into the patient's manual and used in relation to all other interventions learned in each module. Throughout the course of treatment, patients are encouraged to review and update their goals based on what they have learned in treatment, and on any changes in their living environment.

Module Content

Changing Your Thinking

The focus of this module is on the development of cognitive restructuring skills. In treatments for other disorders (e.g., major depression or anxiety disorders) cognitive restructuring is used to modify cognitions that lead to the distressing target affect. The goal of learning cognitive restructuring in CBSST is somewhat broader. One of the key characteristics of psychotic thought process is that thinking is fixed, and patients have poor insight into the nature of their cognitions. Patients engage in many common cognitive distortions (overgeneralization, selective attention, emotional reasoning), then hold these beliefs with extreme confidence, regardless of external evidence. Although these patterns are most obvious in terms of psychotic beliefs or attributions about the nature of hallucinations, these same cognitive biases can have implications for more mundane aspects of functioning (e.g., beliefs about competence to take a bus or to speak to a treatment provider).

The Changing Your Thinking module provides patients with extensive practice in cognitive restructuring skills, which include recognizing cognitive processes, assessing the effect of the cognitions on emotion and behavior, and modifying thoughts that interfere with desired outcomes. Patients first learn that cognitions, emotions, and behavior all influence one another, and the rationale that modifying cognition can therefore modify emotions and behavior. Patients are then taught the three C's mnemonic to remind them of the three tasks of cognitive restructuring. Separate sessions are dedicated to practice of each of the C's. For the "check it" component, patients learn to identify common cognitive distortions, and to engage in behavioral experiments to get evidence with which to judge the accuracy of thoughts. To change thoughts, patients learn to generate alternative explanations based on the evidence from behavioral experiments.

The model is applied to nearly every experience of the patient, including beliefs about symptoms, treatment, their relevant treatment goals, and the group process itself. Patients in groups for schizophrenia, who often have had very negative learning experiences, may have unhelpful beliefs about the intervention or their ability to do the activities. Prediction of the future ("It won't be fun"), negative beliefs about competence ("I can't do anything"), and beliefs associated with psychotic symptoms ("The Devil will punish me") can reduce the likelihood of the patient successfully achieving a goal. When new materials are assigned, patients are encouraged throughout the manual to identify thought content, and if those thoughts interfere with active engagement in treatment, patients are coached in interventions to increase their likelihood of successfully completing the task. By applying cognitive techniques, patients both increase the likelihood of engaging in the task and gain additional practice with the skills.

Although cognitive therapy is often seen as educational rather than as a means to address relationship issues, therapists use cognitive techniques to help patients notice their thoughts about the group itself. The primary emphasis of the thought challenging model is to encourage patients to observe their thinking in all settings, and the group setting can be a particularly potent environment for teaching patients about both the influence of their thoughts on mood and behavior, and the consequences of changing their beliefs.

Asking for Support

This module, which draws heavily from SST, provides patients with skills in identifying warning signs of symptom exacerbation, then trains patients in communication skills. The primary emphasis is on effective communication in situations related to treatment (e.g., talking with a doctor), but patients also apply the skills as relevant to their goals and other relationships.

The primary intervention in the module is the use of role plays of specific situations, with feedback from therapists and other group members. Patients have opportunities to practice both scripted role plays and role plays based on their goals, and they are given very detailed instructions on both nonverbal (e.g., maintaining eye contact, appropriate facial expression) and verbal (e.g., use of "I" statements, expression of emotions, making a specific request) skills. This includes having a posterboard present in the room that lists the specific skills relevant to the role play. The role plays are videotaped and played back in group, so that patients can critique their own performance and receive feedback from others in the group.

In the context of the module, each patient develops a plan to respond to an exacerbation of symptoms. The plan includes identifying a support person who can help the patient recognize his or her symptoms and signing an agreement to listen to that support person's feedback, if the patient's symptoms become worse. The patient also practices discussing the symptoms with his or her case manager (if the patient has one) and physician.

Communication skills training is often the most difficult component of the treatment. For many patients, speaking in front of the group and on camera is initially quite anxiety provoking. One advantage of the modular enrollments is that more experienced group members who have previously participated in that section of the course can share their experience with new members and help to reduce their anxiety. In addition, the group leaders can use cognitive restructuring techniques to address patient concerns about participating in the exercises.

Solving Problems

The Solving Problems module draws from both SST and CBT techniques. Patients learn basic problem-solving skills using the acronym: SCALE—Specify the problem, Consider all possible solutions, Assess the best solution, Lay out a plan, and Execute and evaluate the outcome. Goals and problems are identified in session, then the patient completes a worksheet for the problem, covering each point on the form. The goals of the patient guide the problems targeted. In addition, all patients work through the SCALE model on common problems, such as recurrent symptoms. The primary goal is to train patients to be able to apply the model to any topic.

Individual differences in effective reinforcement, abilities, symptoms, and goals require that treatment be as individualized as possible in the context of a group structure. To address these points, each module is structured first around education about the theme of the module, followed by skills in assessing the topic. Participants then learn interventions for modifying the behavior, and the final session of the module provides additional practice. In each session, exercises are designed to aid group members in identifying their specific goals and relevant interventions. As participants gain more experience, they are encouraged and coached in generating modifications to the interventions in the manual to meet their own specific goals.

KEY POINTS

- Research indicates that patients with psychotic symptoms can benefit from group therapy interventions.
- Strengths of group interventions include efficiency, the opportunity for observational learning, and exposure to socialization.
- Limitations of group models include reduced individualization of treatment, the possibility of a patient's disruptive behavior interfering with the learning of others, and the aversiveness of group settings to some patients with psychosis.
- Current efficacious interventions for patients with psychosis include CR, SST, and CBT.
- CBSST is an integrative group therapy model that incorporates components from other empirically validated treatments.
- Group interventions can be designed to emphasize the strengths and to mitigate the limitations of group process by incorporating appropriate structure, providing individualized treatment plans, using a multimodal approach to treatment, and emphasizing the development of the therapeutic relationship.

REFERENCES AND RECOMMENDED READINGS

Bellack, A. S., Mueser, K. T., Gingerich, S., & Agresta, J. (2004). *Social skills training for schizophrenia: A step-by-step guide* (2nd ed.). New York: Guilford Press.

Benton, M. K., & Schroeder, H. E. (1990). Social skills training with schizophrenics. A meta-analytic evaluation. *Journal of Consulting and Clinical Psychology, 58,* 741–747.

Granholm, E., McQuaid, J. R., McClure, F. S., Auslander, L., Pervoliotis, D., Patterson, T., et al. (2005). A randomized controlled trial of cognitive behavioral social skills training for middle-aged and older outpatients with chronic schizophrenia. *American Journal of Psychiatry, 162,* 520–529.

Kingdon, D. G., & Turkington, D. (2004). *Cognitive therapy of schizophrenia.* New York: Guilford Press.

McQuaid, J. R., Granholm, E., McClure, F. S., Roepke, S., Pedrelli, P., Patterson, T. L., et al. (2000). Development of an integrated cognitive-behavioral and social skills training intervention for older patients with schizophrenia. *Journal of Psychotherapy Practice and Research, 9,* 149–156.

Pilling, S., Bebbington, P., Kuipers, E., Garety, P., Geddes, J., Martindale, B., et al. (2002a). Psychological treatments in schizophrenia: II. Meta-analysis of randomized controlled trials of social skills training and cognitive remediation. *Psychological Medicine, 32,* 783–791.

Pilling, S., Bebbington, P., Kuipers, E., Garety, P., Geddes, J., Orbach, G., et al. (2002b). Psychological treatments in schizophrenia: I. Meta-analysis of family interventions and cognitive behaviour therapy. *Psychological Medicine, 32,* 763–782.

Sensky, T., Turkington, D., Kingdon, D. G., Scott, J. L., Scott, J., Siddle, R., et al. (2000). A randomized controlled trial of cognitive-behavioral therapy for persistent symptoms in schizophrenia resistant to medication. *Archives of General Psychiatry, 57,* 165–172.

Twamley, E. W., Jeste, D. V., & Bellack, A. S. (2003). A review of cognitive training in schizophrenia. *Schizophrenia Bulletin, 29,* 359–382.

Wykes, T., Parr, A. M., & Landau, S. (1999). Group treatment of auditory hallucinations. Exploratory study of effectiveness. *British Journal of Psychiatry, 175,* 180–185.

CHAPTER 29

SUPPORTED HOUSING

PRISCILLA RIDGWAY

S*upported housing* is a general term used since the mid-1980s to describe approaches that combine housing assistance and individualized supportive services for people with serious psychiatric disabilities. Supported housing increases access to permanent, socially integrated, decent, safe, and affordable housing, and directly provides and links people to the intensive home- and community-based support services that they often need to stabilize their lives. This approach is intended to improve the social integration and quality of life of people with psychiatric disabilities, to reduce the problems they have in achieving a stable living situation, and to increase their potential for achieving successful rebound and recovery.

THE NEED FOR SUPPORTED HOUSING

Severe and prolonged psychiatric disorders affect about 1.75–2.0% of the adult population. For various reasons, attaining and maintaining a safe, decent, and affordable place to live is a serious challenge for many people with such disabilities. This section explores the basis of the need for supported housing.

Supported Housing as a Response to Unnecessary Institutionalization

Many people with prolonged psychiatric disabilities remain unnecessarily institutionalized in state hospitals, residential care facilities, custodial nursing homes, and board and care settings because of the lack of decent community-based housing and support options. Supported housing models were initially developed at a time when the general failure to focus on housing and support were acknowledged to contribute strongly to unnecessary institutional care for up to one-third of all people in psychiatric hospitals.

Now that fewer long-term psychiatric beds exist, tens of thousands of people with psychiatric disabilities are inappropriately jailed for minor offenses, in settings where they generally lack access to adequate treatment. Many thousands continue to be unnecessarily housed or "transinstitutionalized" in custodial, quasi-institutional settings, such

287

as nursing homes, board and care homes, and other residential care facilities, or are confined to skid row urban areas, a process that has been called *ghettoization*. Supported housing seeks to end the social segregation of people with psychiatric disabilities in unnecessarily restrictive settings and to improve housing options, so that people are not forced to live in substandard conditions.

Supported Housing as a Response to Epidemic Homelessness

People with prolonged psychiatric disabilities have a disproportionately high risk of homelessness according to epidemiological studies, and are greatly overrepresented among the population living in shelters and on U.S. streets. Research findings vary widely on the proportion of the homeless population that experiences serious psychiatric problems, ranging from 20 to over 90% of any given homeless study population, as assessed by clinical ratings, self-report, or other methods. Significant psychiatric history or current impairment is commonly found among 20–30% of homeless study cohorts.

People with psychiatric disabilities have at least a tenfold excess risk of homelessness above that of the general population. It is estimated that 1 in 20 adults who experience severe psychiatric disabilities is homeless in the United States. Once homeless, people with psychiatric disabilities fare very poorly, even when compared to other people who are homeless. They experience worse physical health, have fewer subsistence needs met, poorer objective and subjective quality of life, and higher rates of victimization than do others, and are more likely to live on the streets and remain homeless longer.

Why do people with severe psychiatric problems carry such a high risk for homelessness? Disproportionate homelessness has been attributed to lack of adequate social planning under the policy of deinstitutionalization, the lack of transfer of resources from state hospitals to communities, and inadequate development of community-based residential programs. Psychiatric disabilities contribute to the problem through the life-disrupting, episodic nature of many major psychiatric disorders; the lack or loss of daily living skills due to serious impairment; the high incidence of co-occurring substance abuse disorders; and the heightened vulnerability to stress and social isolation that often typify the lives of those with such disabilities. Studies have shown that multiple foster care or institutional placements during youth strongly correlate to later diagnosis of psychiatric disorder and to homelessness.

These risk factors result in the need for a range of supportive services and specialized reasonable accommodations if people are to succeed at community living. Unfortunately, housing assistance programs, mental health services, and social service programs generally remain fragmented and difficult to negotiate. Differing eligibility criteria across mental health, substance abuse, social services, and public housing programs further contribute to the problem.

Social-structural concerns are also blamed for widespread homelessness. These problems include increased competition for a declining number of affordable housing units and the general lack of affordable housing for people with low incomes. People with serious psychiatric disabilities are among the poorest of the poor. Their personal income is often limited to Supplemental Security Income (SSI)—the Federal entitlement program that provides an income to people who are assessed to be permanently disabled. This subsistence allotment generally does not exceed 25% of local median incomes. Studies of housing affordability reveal no housing market in the United States where a person on SSI can afford a modest efficiency or one-bedroom apartment, using Federal income–housing-cost standards. People who rely on SSI for their income are too poor to obtain decent housing without other forms of assistance.

Housing discrimination is another piece of the puzzle that explains the vastly disproportionate homelessness among people with psychiatric disabilities. Discrimination based on stigma remains rampant, despite nondiscrimination mandates established in law under the Americans with Disability Act. Racial disparities also exist and can compound the problem; for example, African American mental health consumers experience more days homeless, have poorer housing conditions, and find it harder to attain housing, even when they have a rental subsidy.

Supported Housing as Fulfilling a Basic and Universal Human Need

Supported housing can be seen as meeting a universal, normal, basic, human need for a decent and safe place to live; a sense of home; and a feeling of belonging within a community. A sense of home is crucial to positive mental health, in that home provides us with a basic sense of safety and security, personal privacy, and orientation within geographical space. Home serves as a container for personal belongings, acts as an extension of our identity, and is the environment where we undertake most daily self-care routines and engage in close social, familial, and intimate relationships.

Supported Housing as the Basis for Effective Treatment and Recovery

Supported housing has been found to be a critical support for effective mental health treatment. Qualitative research reveals that people with psychiatric disabilities believe housing is a basic support for mental health recovery, and that the lack of safe, decent housing strongly hinders recovery. Research shows that the acquisition of decent housing provides a turning point that allows people to begin to work on their recovery, and to set and achieve other life goals. Provision of housing support has also been shown to keep people actively engaged in treatment.

THE RESPONSE TO UNMET HOUSING NEEDS

Custodial Care or Shelter Living

Prior to the mid-1980s, the de facto response to unmet housing needs was provision of custodial settings, which were found to reduce functioning and to increase the risk of premature mortality over time. Reviews of studies of custodial residential programs do not demonstrate positive consumer outcomes.

A second de facto approach is the provision of basic shelter. This stopgap measure is unresponsive to the needs of people with psychiatric disabilities, and can actually be iatrogenic (illness-engendering) in its effect. Shelter living has been shown to cause social breakdown and to promote psychopathology. Ethnographic research indicates that people with psychiatric disabilities who are homeless are often locked into a life of chronic dislocation, and are forced to undertake unproductive rounds of full-time help-seeking efforts to meet their subsistence needs, a process that does not result in acquisition of a permanent place to live.

The Residential Continuum

Prior to the development of supported housing, the dominant model for residential services was residential treatment arrayed along a continuum of care. The design of such a continuum includes an array of specialized residential facilities, such as quarter- and half-way houses. Each option within the range of facilities along the continuum was to provide a tightly bundled set of services based on a generalized level of functioning or the needs of prototypical residents. The person with a psychiatric disability was to transition across facilities as he or she gained in functional capacity, with each setting offering reduced levels of services and structured activity, until the individual could succeed at "independent living" and had no further need for support.

The continuum model has been critiqued on several bases, including the idea that preset options and service packages are frequently at odds with housing preferences and service needs expressed by mental health consumers. Residential environments often remain socially segregated and are frequently institutional in character; they serve as formal program sites rather than as people's homes. Chronic dislocation is often promoted through transitional models that place artificial time limits on stays, resulting in chronic dislocation and disruption of social support networks. Most local mental health systems lacked a full array of programs, and the limited options within the residential continua often became bottlenecked. Most systems of care completely lacked the "last step"—permanent affordable housing. People either became stuck or recycled through programs options.

Repeated reviews of large numbers of studies of transitional and residential continuum model programs have revealed that such programs do not lead to success in stable housing, and that there is no advantage conferred by stays in residential treatment prior to a move into permanent supported housing.

Although the linear residential continuum model has largely been abandoned as a driving model in the field, a wide range of residential programs and "supportive housing" continues to exist, and such options continue to be developed in many mental health systems. Supportive housing options can be differentiated from supported housing, because they often require participation in, or force compliance with, mental health treatment; are based on professional placement rather than on consumer housing preferences; often offer varying types and intensities of bundled services tied directly to the housing rather than flexibly meeting individual needs; and frequently house only people with psychiatric disabilities at a given site, rather than promoting social integration. Often such settings have many restrictive rules, and reserve the right to select and discharge people based upon considerations other than typical tenant rights and responsibilities. Settings that are considered "supportive housing" are wide ranging, from very large congregate residential care facilities, with hundreds of beds that are institutional in character, to small- to medium-size group homes, and specialized SRO (single room occupancy hotels) with on-site staff and services. Supportive housing options also include supervised or congregate apartments that may share many of the characteristics of permanent supported housing.

THE SUPPORTED HOUSING APPROACH

A supported housing approach generally assists each person with a psychiatric disability to (1) express preferences about housing and support services; (2) select and acquire decent, safe, and affordable housing; and (3) succeed at community living with the assistance of a loosely linked, flexible, individualized set of supportive services and reasonable accommodations that are provided in natural home- and community-based settings.

The basic ideas and principles underpinning a supported housing approach include the following:

- Housing is a basic need, and having a place to live is a basic right for people with psychiatric disabilities.

- People with serious psychiatric disabilities should have choices and options. With support, they can successfully choose, acquire, and maintain a place to live.
- People should have the right to choose their housing from those options available to others in the community; housing options should be consistent with local housing styles and types, or "mainstream" housing options. People should be able to choose where and with whom they want to live.
- Even people with severe disabilities and problems in functioning, and those who are "most difficult to serve," can be successful in an intensive, flexible supported housing approach. Such an approach is not just for those who seem to have a high degree of readiness or capacity for independent living.
- People should be socially integrated into neighborhoods and communities rather than socially segregated based on their disability status.
- People should be supported in normal social roles, such as tenant and community member.
- People should have control over their activities and lifestyle.
- Housing options should be safe, of decent quality, and meet standards for affordability.
- There should be a separation between the delivery of services and housing, so that housing is the person's personal living situation or home, rather than a program environment or treatment setting.
- People should not be forced to accept a preset service package to attain or retain a place to call home; instead, support services should be individualized, voluntary, and consumer-driven. The type and intensity of services should be variable, based upon each person's changing needs and choices. People can be successfully integrated into the community if they are supported adequately, with an individualized set of highly flexible support services that change as their needs change. There should be no requirement for participation in mental health program activities linked to housing.
- Supports and services should be available as long as they are needed, with no restriction on how long people can keep their housing. Housing subsidies and support services should be ongoing rather than time-limited or transitional.

There was rapid growth in supported housing programs in 1980s. Supported housing services are provided through a variety of approaches. Studies reveal that the primary support services provided in such programs are intensive case management, supportive counseling, independent living skills training, crisis intervention and prevention, social and recreational services, client advocacy, support services to families and relatives, and assessment and diagnostic services. Some programs rely heavily upon attendant care services to provide highly intensive levels of in-home support to people with serious disabilities. Services are primarily provided in the participant's home, or other community settings, rather than in psychosocial programs, clinics, or offices. Some programs also included self-help and peer support groups to create a sense of community and to engender mutual support among people living in their own apartments.

THE GROWING EVIDENCE BASE ON SUPPORTED HOUSING FOR PEOPLE WITH PSYCHIATRIC DISABILITIES

Studies of the Impact and Efficacy of Supported Housing Programs

The research knowledge base on the effectiveness of supported housing has grown over the last two decades through successive rounds of research and demonstration programs.

The research knowledge base also includes studies of housing and psychiatric disorders, housing and supports, case management approaches linked to housing subsidies, homelessness assistance, and Housing First programs that serve people with psychiatric disabilities and active substance abuse.

Several reviews have synthesized the supported housing research evidence base. Most of the studies revealed positive outcomes associated with supported housing, better outcomes for supported housing compared to prior housing situation–homelessness–standard options, and better or equal outcomes compared to other residential program options. A few studies indicated somewhat more positive effects for comparison models, but these effects may have been related to a large differential in the resources attached to supported housing rather than an enriched comparison condition; to crossover conditions; and to specific housing market factors, such as the association between racial disparities and the time it takes to exit homelessness/acquire housing. Studies generally show that supported housing performs equally well or better than much more costly residential options.

A variety of outcome domains have been used to assess the effectiveness of supported housing programs. Outcome variables often include attainment of housing; increased community tenure; reduced homelessness; and reduction in the use of socially segregated settings, such as hospitals, shelters, and jails.

• *Reduced homelessness, housing attainment, and residential stability.* Several supported housing studies indicate great reductions in homelessness of more than 50%, and up to 80 or 90% within 1 year. Supported housing greatly increases residential stability. Studies reveal that stable housing among formerly homeless individuals ranged from about 50% in 1 year to nearly 90% over a 5-year period. These findings are generally much higher than housing stability rates for comparison conditions. Some studies have shown that residential stability for some people takes some time to achieve.

• *Reductions in recidivism to hospitalization.* Supported housing reduces recidivism to psychiatric hospitalization. Reductions in magnitude of 50% of hospital bed day use were found in several studies.

• *Reduced jail stays.* Supported housing has been found to reduce or even eliminate jail days in "difficult to serve" study populations.

• *Symptom reduction.* A few studies relate supported housing to reductions in psychiatric symptoms.

• *Increased functioning.* Some studies indicated increases in social functioning for people in supported housing over time, whereas others indicated no significant change in functioning.

• *Increased life satisfaction.* Increases in life satisfaction have been found in studies of supported housing.

• *Improved subjective and objective quality of life.* Some studies have demonstrated improved quality of life with supported housing.

• *Sense of home.* Over time, with the development of stability, privacy, sense of identity, physical comfort, domesticity, and support, people in supported housing programs have been found to develop a sense of home.

Related Research on the Importance of Consumer Choice and Preferences

Research on consumer housing and support preferences was first undertaken in the mid-1980s. Studies undertaken in many areas across the country revealed the same basic findings: People with psychiatric disabilities strongly prefer normal housing and supports rather than congregate residential services approaches. People want to live alone or with another person, or persons, of their choice, rather than in groups of people with psychiatric disabilities. They want a variety of support services to call upon, but they do not want to live in staffed settings. Consumer preferences are in marked contrast to typical clinician recommendations that emphasize placement in much more structured and restrictive settings. Some research has assessed the impact of preferences on outcomes. Residential stability and life satisfaction markedly increase when consumers perceive that they have choices, and when their housing and support preferences are honored.

THE EMERGING EVIDENCE BASE ON "BEST-PRACTICE"-SUPPORTED HOUSING SERVICES

This section reviews some of the elements of "best practice" in supported housing. These so-called "active ingredients" were identified in a meta-analysis of supported housing literature (Ridgway & Rapp, 1997). This analysis revealed that effective supported housing includes core elements associated with supportive services and housing assistance. Best-practice guidelines for supportive services often includes some form of intensive case management that involves the following:

- Workers should carry small caseloads (1:8–1:10) for consumers labeled "most difficult to serve" and up to 1:20 for others with psychiatric disabilities.
- There should be the capacity for frequent contacts (up to several times per week, especially during an initial settling in period).
- Workers should directly provide support services rather than broker services.
- Services should be provided *in vivo* (in the person's housing or other natural community setting).
- Support services delivery may use alternative models (e.g., either a team approach or individual workers who carry a small caseload).
- Workers should have explicit goals to increase residential stability, to improve quality of life, and to reduce homelessness and hospitalization.

The Importance of the Helping Relationship

Some research on supported housing reconfirms the importance of the helping relationship. A strong alliance with the worker was associated with significant reduction in the number of days people spent homeless, to moderate improvements in quality of life and satisfaction ratings, less isolation, greater housing satisfaction, and greater sense of empowerment. A few studies have found that the strength of the worker–consumer alliance is not related to outcomes.

Best-Practice Guidelines for Housing Assistance

The research shows that effective supported housing combines supportive services with housing assistance that includes the following elements:

- Rental subsidies are provided.
- Consumer housing preferences are honored.

- There is provision of direct assistance in obtaining housing and establishing a home.
- Consumers control personal space and are accorded personal privacy.
- There is an emphasis on supporting the person in achieving success at typical tenant roles and responsibilities.

Rental subsidies allow people to experience shortened hospital stays, to exit homelessness faster, to maintain involvement with mental health services, and to improve the quality of the housing that they attain. The lack of rental assistance keeps people homeless longer and extends hospital stays. Unfortunately, the low rent levels allowed under Federal rental subsidy programs often do not allow people to live in neighborhoods with high-quality housing, and people often have to contend with unsafe neighborhoods, even when their rent is subsidized. Over time people do attain a sense that their supported housing environment is their home.

Effective housing development strategies lie beyond the scope of this chapter, and information is contained in technical assistance documents rather than in formal peer review literature. Housing finance has its own language, and mental health agency staff members must master technical housing development techniques and language to participate effectively in expanding the availability of low-income housing options.

While many mental health agencies have become involved in low-income housing development or advocacy, a clear separation of housing management and service delivery is encouraged in a supported housing approach. This separation ensures that (1) housing is the person's home rather than primarily a service environment; (2) typical guidelines concerning tenant responsibilities are followed rather than being confounded with clinical issues; (3) tenant rights and evictions are handled properly; (4) stigma is avoided, and participation in community life is more fully supported, and (5) unethical dual relationships do not arise.

Who Can Be Successfully Served in Supported Housing?

Many studies to date have indicated that supported housing is effective even for people who are considered "most difficult to serve"—including people with severe disorders and multiple recent involuntary hospitalizations. Approximately half of all people with psychiatric disabilities who are homeless also have a substance use disorder. Dual diagnosis has been found to make housing stability more difficult to achieve, increases the risk of homelessness, and lengthens the time people are homeless. People with substance abuse are more likely to leave supported housing, sometimes in the early days or weeks after entry.

Housing and supports are seen as critical resources that support effective dual-diagnosis treatment. Specialized approaches that have been advocated involve active engagement, crisis intervention, persuasion, relapse prevention, and adequate housing. Some ethnographic research indicates that stable supported housing is causally associated with diminishment of problematic substance use over time. Such research indicates that access to decent housing is one quality-of-life factor that serves to reduce substance abuse in persons who were formerly homeless.

One form of supported housing has been found to be highly effective for persons with a dual diagnosis of mental disorder and substance abuse, even though the program does not demand abstinence as a precondition for tenancy. The Pathways to Housing or Housing First program model (Tsemberis & Eisenberg, 2000) does not demand that people undergo treatment or achieve abstinence from drugs or alcohol use prior to placement in mainstream housing. Instead, people are housed in their own apartments, directly off the street or out of shelters. They are served with a modified assertive community treatment (ACT) case management program. Outcomes indicate that 88% of participants remain stably housed at 5 years. This program is being replicated in hundreds of sites around the country.

One challenge in the provision of supported housing concerns the problem of loneliness and social isolation. A few researchers examining social connectedness have identified social isolation as a pitfall of scattered-site housing approaches. Others have found social isolation to be a general problem among people with psychiatric disabilities; loneliness has been found to be a common experience among those living in a variety of other housing options, including shared housing and congregate residential facilities. Nonetheless, there is clearly a need to address development of an adequate social support network and meaningful community connections as one important aspect of helping people with serious psychiatric disabilities achieve successful community integration.

SUPPORTED HOUSING AND SOCIAL POLICY

Supported housing advances several important social goals, such as the community integration mandate under *Olmstead v. L. C.* (119 S. Ct. 2176, 1999) Supreme Court decision, and goals that promote the development of consumer-directed care and meet the unmet need for housing that were identified in a variety of Federal Task Force reports and the President's New Freedom Commission. This approach also serves to fulfill the current mission statement of the Federal Center for Mental Health Services (CMHS) "to ensure a home and a life in the community for everyone" with psychiatric disabilities.

Supported housing advances the doctrines of least restrictive alternative, or most integrated setting, and nondiscrimination as exemplified in *Olmstead*. The case concerns the right of the class of mentally disabled persons to live in the most integrated and least restrictive setting that appropriately meets their needs, rather than being held unnecessarily in socially segregated environments. The Supreme Court ruled that unnecessary social segregation of people with mental disabilities constitutes discrimination under the Americans with Disabilities Act, and further, that institutional life perpetuates unwarranted assumptions about people with disabilities and curtails everyday life activities, such as family relationships, social contacts, work, educational advancement, and cultural enrichment. The argument that a state lacks sufficient resources to provide community-based alternatives was found to be an inadequate defense or justification of prolonged institutionalization. The Court found that states must have some means to demonstrate nondiscrimination to protect themselves from legal action. States must develop specific means, such as having an effective working plan, to create a range of alternatives for the care and treatment of individuals with mental disabilities, and must demonstrate through some means, such as a waiting list that moves at a reasonable pace, that people who are unnecessarily institutionalized are moving into less restrictive settings in an equitable manner.

Each state is required to involve consumers and families in developing a state *Olmstead* plan; to prevent future unwarranted institutionalization and social segregation; to ensure the availability of a range of alternative services that will end social segregation and integrate people with mental disabilities into the community; and to assist people with disabilities to make informed choices about how their needs can best be met. Although the *Olmstead* case does not speak directly to the issue of homelessness, it can reasonably be argued that supported housing sharply reduces the use of more restrictive institutional settings, hospitals, and jails, and is therefore an effective less restrictive alternative. Olmstead also demands *avoidance of future unnecessary institutionalization* among those not previously institutionalized.

The National Association of State Mental Health Program Directors (NASMHPD; 1989) has had a supported housing policy for nearly 20 years. The initial policy stated:

> All people with long-term mental illness should be given the option to live in stable, affordable, and safe housing, in settings that maximize their ability to function independently. Housing options should not require time limits for moving to another housing option. People should not be required to change living situations or lose their place of residence if they are hospitalized. People should be given the opportunity to actively participate in the selection of their housing arrangements from among those living environments available to the general public. Although public mental health systems need to exercise leadership in the housing area, addressing housing and support needs is a shared responsibility and requires coordination and negotiation of mutual roles of mental health authorities, public assistance and housing authorities, the private sector, and consumers them selves.
>
> Necessary supports, including case management, on-site crisis intervention, and rehabilitation services, should be available at appropriate levels and for as long as is needed by persons with psychiatric disabilities regardless of their choice of living arrangements. Services should be flexible, individualized, and provided with attention to personal dignity. Advocacy, community education and resource development should be continuous.

Several states have formal supported housing policies or housing assistance programs that fund bridge rental subsidies that support people with psychiatric disabilities in normalized rental housing until they are able to attain a Federal rent subsidy. Research shows that supported housing helps to balance the system of care, can be delivered at a cost less than that of formal residential programs, and actually costs less than maintaining a person with a psychiatric disability in a state of homelessness.

KEY POINTS

- A large number of people with serious psychiatric disabilities are unnecessarily institutionalized, jailed, or homeless because they lack access to decent, affordable housing and supportive services.
- There is no housing market in the United States in which a basic apartment is affordable to a person living on SSI.
- Sense of home plays several crucial roles in achievement of positive mental health.
- Supported housing is an important basis for effective treatment and turnaround to recovery.
- Even people who have severe disabilities, severe problems in functioning, dual diagnoses, and those considered "most difficult to serve," can be served successfully in supported housing.
- Residential stability and life satisfaction markedly increase when people perceive they have choices, and when their housing and support preferences are honored.
- People with serious psychiatric disabilities can successfully live in the community if they are supported adequately with a combination of housing assistance and individualized, intensive, flexible supportive services that change as their needs change.
- Supported housing increase people's community tenure and sharply reduce homelessness, use of psychiatric hospitals beds, and days in jail.
- Best practice involves small caseloads, the capacity for frequent contacts, and the direct provision of supportive services in the person's housing or other natural community setting.
- Supported housing advances the social policy of community integration.

REFERENCES AND RECOMMENDED READINGS

Allen, M. (2004). *Fact sheet: Just like where you and I live—Integrated housing options for people with mental illnesses*. Washington, DC: Bazelon Center for Mental Health Law. Available online at *bazelon.org/issues/housing/infosheets/integratedhousing/htm*

Carling, P. J. (1990). Major mental illness, housing and supports: The promise of community integration. *American Psychologist, 45*(8), 969–975.

Carling, P. J., & Ridgway, P. A. (1987). Overview of a psychiatric rehabilitation approach to housing. In W. A. Anthony & M. A. Farkas (Eds.), *Psychiatric rehabilitation: Turning theory into practice*. Baltimore: Johns Hopkins University Press.

Cooper, E., & O'Hara, A. (2002). *Priced out in 2002: Housing crisis worsens for people with psychiatric disabilities*. Boston: Technical Assistance Collaborative.

Culhane, D., Metreaux, S., & Hadley, T. (2001). *The impact of supported housing for homeless persons with severe mental illness on the utilization of the public health, corrections and public shelter systems: The New York/New York Initiative*. Philadelphia: University of Pennsylvania, Center for Mental Health Policy and Services Research.

Hogan, M. F., & Carling, P. J. (1992). Normal housing: A key element of a supported housing approach for people with psychiatric disabilities. *Community Mental Health Journal, 28*, 215–226.

Hopper, K., Jost, J., Hay, T., Welber, S., & Haugland, G. (1997). Homelessness, severe mental illness and the institutional circuit. *Psychiatric Services, 48*(5), 659–665.

Hutchings, G. P., Emery, B. D., & Aronson, L. P. (Eds.). (1996). *Housing for persons with psychiatric disabilities: Best practices for a changing environment*. Alexandria, VA: National Association of Mental Health Program Directors (NASMHPD), National Technical Assistance Center for State Mental Health Planning (NTAC).

Livingston, J. A., Gordon, L. R., King, D. A., & Srebnick, D. S. (1991). *Implementing the supported housing approach: A national evaluation of NIMH supported housing demonstration projects*. Burlington, VT: Trinity College, Center for Community Change through Housing and Support.

National Association of State Mental Health Program Directors (NASMHPD). (1989; revised, 1996). *Position statement of the National Association of State Mental Health Program Directors on housing and supports for people with psychiatric disabilities*. Alexandria, VA: Author.

Nelson, G., & Smith, F. H. (1997). Housing for the chronically mentally disabled: Part II. Process and outcome. *Canadian Journal of Mental Health, 6*(2), 79–91.

Newman, S. J. (2001). Housing attributes and serious mental illness: Implications for research and practice. *Psychiatric Services, 52*(10), 1309–1317.

Newman, S. J., Reschovsky, J. D., Kaneda, K., & Hendrick, A. M. (1994). The effects of independent living on persons with chronic mental illness: An assessment of the Section 8 Program. *Millbank Quarterly, 72*(1), 171–198.

Parkinson, S., Nelson, G., & Horgan, S. (1999). From housing to homes: A review of the literature on housing approaches for psychiatric consumer/survivors. *Canadian Journal of Community Mental Health, 18*(1), 145–164.

Ridgway, P. A., & Rapp, C. A. (1997). *The active ingredients of effective supported housing: A research synthesis*. Lawrence: University of Kansas, School of Social Welfare, Office of Mental Health Research and Training.

Ridgway, P. A., Simpson, A., Wittman, F. D., & Wheeler, G. (1994). Home-making and community-building: Notes on empowerment and place. *Journal of Mental Health Administration, 21*, 407–418.

Ridgway, P. A., & Zipple, A. M. (1990). The paradigm shift in residential services: From the linear continuum to supported housing. *Psychosocial Rehabilitation Journal, 13*(4), 11–31.

Rog, D. J. (2004). The evidence on supported housing. *Psychiatric Rehabilitation Journal, 27*(4), 334–344.

Shern, D. L., Felton, C. J., Hough, R. L., Lehman, A. F., Goldfinger, S., Valencia, E., et al. (1997). Housing outcomes for homeless adults with mental illness: Results from the Second-Round McKinney Program. *Psychiatric Services, 48*(2), 239–241.

Srebnick, D. S., Livingston, J., Gordon, L., & King, D. (1995). Housing choice and community success for individuals with serious and persistent mental Illness. *Community Mental Health Journal, 31*(2), 139–152.

Tanzman, B. (1993). An overview of surveys of mental health consumers' preferences for housing and support services. *Hospital and Community Psychiatry, 44*, 450–455.

Tsemberis, S., & Eisenberg, R. F. (2000). Pathways to housing: Supported housing for street-dwelling homeless individuals with psychiatric disabilities. *Psychiatric Services, 51*(4), 487–493.

CHAPTER 30

SELF-HELP ACTIVITIES

FREDERICK J. FRESE III

My personal experiences with schizophrenia have been published elsewhere (Frese, 1993, 2000, 2004). In brief, over 40 years ago, in early 1966, when I was first hospitalized with schizophrenia, the world for those of us with serious mental illness was very different from the way it is now. At that time psychodynamic thinking still dominated psychiatric care. Sigmund Freud's picture, as well as his books, was usually prominently on display in most psychiatrists' offices.

Antipsychotic medications, then called *major tranquilizers*, had only recently become available, and there were no medications to help ameliorate their anguishing side-effects. The heyday of lobotomies, when over 5,000 of these operations were performed annually on persons with mental illness in the United States, was beginning to pass, but these procedures were still being administered in some parts of the country (Valenstein, 1986). And electroshock treatments were regularly being administered to persons with schizophrenia. I personally observed the threat of their use employed as a patient control mechanism far too frequently.

In the decade after my initial hospitalization, I found myself at different times as an unwilling inpatient in various military, Veterans Administration, county, state, and private hospitals, in some six different states. During these various adventures, I was almost completely unaware of any activities that could be characterized as self-help for mentally ill persons. The one experience with self-help that I did experience during those difficult times occurred when I was in a private psychiatric hospital in the Cleveland area in 1974. I was asked if I would be interested in attending an Alcoholics Anonymous (AA) meeting that was being held on the hospital grounds. Although I did not consider myself to have a drinking problem, an assertion with which my therapist said he agreed, I did take the time to attend one of these AA meetings. I remember feeling that I had very little in common with the other attendees, and, as a result, I did not attend again. But I do remember wondering whether some sort of similar group might someday be available for persons with serious mental illnesses who did not have alcohol or other substance abuse problems.

Despite living with schizophrenia and being subject to periodic breakdowns during the past four decades, I have been able to carve out a career for myself as a psychologist, serving persons who, like myself, live with one or another form of serious mental illness.

In this capacity, as both a recipient and a provider of mental health services, I have had the opportunity to observe tremendous changes in the care of persons with serious mental illness. During my four-decade-long career, the primary locus of this care has shifted from the hospital to the community, medications have greatly improved, and, increasingly, a general feeling has arisen that those of us with these conditions are expected to recover. Of the many changes that have occurred, certainly one of the most consequential has been the rise of various forms of participation of mentally ill persons, and their family members, in the process of their own care. Although it is probably a broader use of the term than the manner in which it has traditionally been employed, in this chapter, I use the term *self-help* to refer to the various aspects of how mentally ill persons and their families have come to participate in the recovery process. In reviewing these efforts I focus on three ways of viewing these self-help activities.

First, I discuss the traditional, more restricted, use of the self-help concept, that is, situations in which persons with the condition take responsibility, individually or with the assistance of others, for engaging in activities that are expected to enhance their ability to cope with their conditions and, they hope, contribute to their well-being and recovery.

Second, I address activities in which such persons address individual and collective activities aimed at not only improving their abilities to cope with their conditions but also advocating for societal improvements in how mentally ill persons are perceived and treated.

Third, I address efforts whereby persons with mental illnesses organize so that they themselves increasingly take charge of treatment and recovery activities.

Finally, I make some brief comments about a recent government-sponsored effort to evaluate the effectiveness of self-help activities.

GROUPS FOCUSING ON SELF-CARE AMONG PERSONS WITH SIMILAR CONDITIONS

The term *self-help* has traditionally been employed to describe efforts by groups of recipients of health services to care for themselves, operating with varying degrees of independence from the traditional health care provider system. AA is often pointed out as an example of one such large, successful, self-help entity. This group, founded in Akron, Ohio, by a local surgeon and a New York stock broker, is probably the largest and most successful self-help group. AA has over 2 million members and over 1,000 groups in some 150 countries. AA groups usually meet once or twice a week. The primary purpose of AA is to have members stay sober and for alcoholics to achieve sobriety. Importantly, AA does not affiliate with other organizations or take stands on controversial issues. It takes no formal advocacy role.

Although AA limits its activities to persons with alcoholism, similar groups have been established for persons with mental and emotional illnesses. Perhaps the oldest of such organizations is GROW (2006), originally established in Australia in 1957, by a small group of former mental patients who had been attending an AA meeting. Its program is based on a 12-step model and, similar to AA, is anonymous in its membership. Originally known as Recovery, it changed its name in 1975. Shortly thereafter, in 1978, GROW started offering residential services. In addition to having numerous branches throughout Australia, GROW currently has over 130 branches in Ireland, as well as additional groups in New Zealand, Canada, Mauritius, and the United States. It is described on its website as a community of persons working toward mental health through mutual help, and as a 12-step program of recovery. GROW facilitates meetings of small groups (five to nine people) who have experienced depression, anxiety, or other forms of mental breakdown. GROW groups generally meet on a weekly basis.

Emotions Anonymous (EA; 2006), another organization for persons with mental health difficulties, is also patterned along the lines of AA. This "fellowship" comprises people who come together in weekly meetings for the purpose of working toward recovery from emotional difficulties. EA was founded in St. Paul, Minnesota, in 1971. As of 1996 there were over 1,200 EA chapters in 39 countries, including the United States. EA claims to be of value for persons with a diversity of emotional difficulties, but it does not mention schizophrenia or psychoses per se. Like AA, the EA program incorporates the 12 Steps, Traditions, Concepts, and Promises familiar to most AA members.

Still more recently established and also in the AA tradition, Schizophrenics Anonymous (SA; 2006) is a self-help support organization specifically tailored for people with schizophrenia. SA was started in Michigan in 1985. The SA website states that the organization has grown to over 70 groups across the United States and Canada, with groups also in Brazil and Mexico. Its website also indicates that these groups "offer fellowship, support, and information." They focus on recovery, using a six-step program, along with medication and professional help. They have weekly meetings, guest speakers, a phone network, and a newsletter.

Mental health–oriented self-help groups that do not specifically follow the AA model have also been formed. Shortly after the founding of AA, one of these entities was established in Chicago. Recovery, Inc. describes itself as a self-help mental health program, active since 1937. As opposed to the AA posture of being totally independent of professional services, Recovery, Inc. states that it designed to work in conjunction with mental health services, and that it orients its programming around the direction of the late psychiatrist Abraham Low. Recovery, Inc. is not a 12-step program, and unlike AA, does not require members to submit to the will of a higher power. As indicated on the Recovery, Inc. website, "Many patients might benefit from recovery: All types of anxiety disorders, depression, psycho-physical disorders, and stress of psychological symptoms. Those suffering from manic depression and schizophrenia can benefit after some medical treatment" (Recovery Inc., 2006). However, Recovery, Inc. does not identify persons by diagnostic categories, referring to all its members as "nervous people" or "nervous patients." Several hundred Recovery, Inc. groups are in operation throughout North America and other parts of the world. These groups meet on a weekly basis.

Whether these self-help groups work separately or in conjunction with professional providers, with a few recent exceptions, they have tended to avoid attempts to engage in political or advocacy activities.

On the other hand, one important self-help group in the mental health arena that very explicitly engages in political/advocacy activities is the Depression and Bipolar Support Alliance (DBSA; 2006). Originally named the National Depressive and Manic Depression Association, the DBSA claims to be the nation's leading patient-directed organization focusing on depression and bipolar disorder. DBSA has a grassroots network of more than 1,000 patient-run support groups across the country, with more than 55,000 people attending its peer-led support groups every year. DBSA works closely with professionals, and treatment adherence is a major goal for participants. It has an impressive 65-member Scientific Advisory Board that comprises leading researchers and clinicians in the field of mood disorders. Unlike AA and Recovery, Inc., the DBSA does engage in ongoing advocacy efforts on behalf of its membership, lobbying, and providing testimony to Congress on issues such as research funding, insurance parity, confidentiality, and integrated treatment for individuals with a dual diagnosis.

ADVOCACY-ORIENTED SELF-HELP EFFORTS

In addition to the self-help groups organized with the primary objective of helping persons with mental illnesses care for themselves, in the wake of the early civil rights movement in the United States, there emerged groups of persons who were meeting and organizing with the explicit purpose of attempting to change society, with a particular focus on changing the mental health system, as opposed to focusing on their own self-improvement and well-being (Frese, 1998).

Like African Americans, Hispanic Americans, women, and (later) other groups that had traditionally been ostracized, excluded, and/or abused by mainstream American society, in the 1960s persons diagnosed with serious mental illnesses also began to recognize the advantages of organizing with an eye toward establishing a more dignified place for themselves in society. Persons with mental health conditions began to demand an end to discrimination and that society begin to treat them as fellow human beings.

Despite the extreme stigma associated with our having been recipients of psychiatric services, some of us began to establish ongoing contact with one another, at first in local groups with names such as the Insane Liberation Front (founded in Portland, Oregon, in 1970), and the Mental Patients' Liberation Project in New York City and the Boston Mental Patients' Liberation Front (both founded in 1971). The first national meeting of these human rights groups, held in Detroit in 1973, was called the Conference on Human Rights and Psychiatric Oppression (CHRPO). At these CHRPO conferences held annually through 1985, activists began to strategize about how to achieve more dignity and freedom from a mental health system that was viewed as demeaning—a system wherein patients were given few rights and subjected to some of the most cruel and misguided "treatments" imaginable (Valenstein, 1986). One early publication that captured the sentiments of many of these advocates was the volume *On Our Own*, by Judi Chamberlin (1978), who had been involuntarily hospitalized and diagnosed with schizophrenia. In reaction to her experiences, she produced one of the earliest manifestos spelling out how things might be changed for the better. She portrayed organized psychiatry as a self-serving guild that oppressively sacrificed consumers' needs and had little basis in science. A major thrust of her thesis was to suggest the establishment of services for the mentally ill that would be run by the patients themselves. These services were to attend to people's needs as the patients defined them, not "to enforce arbitrary standards of correct behavior" (p. 199).

During this time the Community Support Program (CSP), a small division of the National Institute of Mental Health (NIMH), began to take notice of the activities of these early advocates. In 1985, CSP began funding national gatherings for recovering persons, called Alternatives. The first such conference was held in Baltimore, Maryland. Alternatives conventions began to replace the CHRPO gatherings and to include many persons in recovery who tended to be less militant than the earlier activists. Two separate national organizations rapidly formed. The more militant group initially named its organization the National Association of Mental Patients (NAMP), later changed to the National Association of Psychiatric Survivors (NAPS). They chose the term *survivor*, because they saw themselves as survivors of an overbearingly oppressive system, much the same way people had survived the Nazi Holocaust during World War II. This group put forth a call for a self-help model totally divorced from that of the traditional mental health establishment. This effort included the production of a 24-chapter manual that laid out strategies for how self-help organizations could become organized and operate (Zinman, Harp, & Budd, 1987). This volume was later expanded and updated in a book edited by Zinman and Harp (1994).

It is important to understand that those who call themselves survivors focus their activities primarily on rights as opposed to treatment per se. They see themselves as having been relegated to a position as second-class citizens living under a system of laws that allowed involuntary commitment laws to deny them their liberty. They see the psychiatric system as one that disempowers those it is claiming to help. They oppose any form of forced, coerced, or assisted treatment. They deny that there is any scientific basis for the brain disease model of mental illness. They see themselves as following in the footsteps of earlier liberation movements, particularly blacks pursuing civil rights and the women's movement for equality (Chamberlin, 1978).

Given their focus being on rights, it is not surprising that the survivors frequently work cooperatively with civil rights lawyers and legal rights groups. They tend to be very active with the National Association for Rights Protection and Advocacy (NARPA), the Bazelon Center for Mental Health Law (formerly the Mental Health Law Project), and the Protection and Advocacy entities funded by Center for Mental Health Services (CMHS), a division of the Substance Abuse and Mental Health Services Administration (SAMHSA).

Today the initiatives set in motion by these early activists are embodied by groups with names such as Mind Freedom and the Support Coalition International.

The other group of self-helpers that arose from the organizational split in 1985 generally refers to its members as "consumers." Originally the consumers established a rather large organization, the National Mental Health Consumers' Association (NMHCA), but this group has not been active since the late 1990s. Despite the recent inactivity of NMHCA, consumers, like those individuals identifying themselves as survivors, continue to fight stigma and discrimination, but they are additionally much more comfortable seeing themselves as persons in recovery and in need of treatment. The consumers tend to be perceived as less radical or "antiestablishment" than the survivors and, as a result, can frequently be seen working in partnership with organized psychiatry and other traditional mental health provider groups.

Whereas the uniting mantra of the survivor groups tends to be "No forced treatment," the shibboleths of consumer groups are more likely to include slogans such as "Nothing about us without us" and "Advocacy is the best therapy."

COMBINED FAMILY–CONSUMER EFFORTS

A self-help group that has arisen during the past three decades, which many view as being the most effective of all the mental health advocacy groups, is the NAMI organization. The acronym NAMI originally stood for the National Alliance for the Mentally Ill, but in 2005, the organization changed its official name to the National Alliance on Mental Illness.

Originally founded by a group of mental health activists who came together in Madison, Wisconsin, in 1979, NAMI was comprised primarily of family members of adults with serious mental illnesses such as schizophrenia and bipolar disorder. NAMI grew very rapidly, to the point that it recently claimed to have over 210,000 members and over 1,100 affiliates. Unlike some of the consumer- or survivor-only advocacy groups, NAMI calls for improved treatments and services, in addition to its fight against discrimination and stigma. In this effort, like DBSA, NAMI works closely with professional provider groups, particularly with research-oriented and community-based psychiatrists.

NAMI's activities in the past few years have increasingly focused on the problems of the mentally ill in the criminal justice system. NAMI has become an integral part of crisis intervention team (CIT) training for police officers, which generally comprises 40 hours of classroom and experiential training delivered by consumers, family members, mental health professionals, and experienced police personnel. Upon completion of the training, CIT graduates tend to be the officers who will respond to police calls involving persons with mental illness. These CIT programs have become very popular recently, with the states of Ohio, Illinois, and Florida now conducting several dozen such programs each year. Most other states also have established varying numbers of these CIT training programs. These police training programs almost always involve presentations by persons in recovery from serious mental illness.

Another innovation in the area of criminal justice that is strongly supported by NAMI has been the recent establishment of mental health courts. First established in Fort Lauderdale, Florida, in 1997, there are now over 100 such courts in the United States. These courts vary somewhat from jurisdiction to jurisdiction, but essentially they allow a person with mental illness to be placed in a treatment program rather than being incarcerated as a consequence of their behavior.

In addition to its advocacy work, the hundreds of NAMI affiliates across the country hold weekly or monthly self-help, care-and-share groups, in which both family members and consumers engage in the traditional group support activities.

Also during the past few years, NAMI has started working closely with the Veterans Health Administration (VHA) in advocacy and in educational and program delivery roles. NAMI members have worked closely with the VHA's legislatively established Seriously Mentally Ill (SMI) Committee. In May 2005, largely in response to the work of the SMI Committee, the VHA published the Comprehensive VHA Mental Health Strategic Plan. The document is organized along the lines of the President's New Freedom Commission (NFC) on Mental Health report (2003). Like the NFC report the Comprehensive VHA Mental Health Strategic Plan calls strongly for a transformation of the mental health delivery system, so that it becomes consumer and family driven, and focused on recovery.

One example of a self-help program established within the VHA in recent years has been the Vet-to-Vet program. In 2001, Vet-to-Vet Peer Support was established by Moe Armstrong, then a member of the National NAMI Board of Directors (BOD) and chair of the NAMI BOD's Veterans Subcommittee. With the help of Robert Rosenheck and Sandra Resnick, the Vet-to-Vet program was started as a research project funded by the VHA to evaluate satisfaction of peer support. Vet-to-Vet is a form of educational peer support program based on various materials recognized by the mental health profession. At the Vet-to-Vet sessions, those materials are read and discussed. The Vet-to-Vet model was taken from one first established in Massachusetts in 1997 by Moe and Naomi Armstrong as the Peer Educators Project, with the motto "Each One, Reach One, Teach One." This form of educational peer support, a partnership model established in the mental health system, has employment supervision from both staff and peers. Research on the effectiveness of the Vet-to-Vet program has been recently published.

NAMI has another, similar program for consumers who are not veterans. This program, called Peer-to-Peer, is run directly by the NAMI organization. The NAMI Peer-to-Peer Recovery Education Course is conducted for 2 hours per week for a 9-week period. These courses are taught by teams of three trained peers/teachers, or "mentors," who themselves are in recovery from serious mental illness. Information provided in the course focuses on relapse prevention, advanced directives, activities designed for calming, focused thinking, and enhanced awareness (National Alliance on Mental Illness, 2005).

Still another consumer-to-consumer, self-help educational program with ties to NAMI is BRIDGES, a peer education program coauthored by psychiatrist/consumers Beth Baxter and Sita Diehl, both active members of NAMI in Tennessee. BRIDGES, an acronym for Building Recovery of Individual Dreams and Goals through Education and Support, is a 10-week course, also taught by persons in recovery from serious mental illness. The focus of the BRIDGES course is on thought, mood, and anxiety disorders; dual diagnoses; various "principles" of support and tools for recovery; medications; spirituality; and advocacy techniques. The course is currently offered in several hundred locations throughout the United States.

A similar, widely known consumer-operated educational program, the Wellness Recovery Action Plan (WRAP) program (Copeland, 1999), is not affiliated with NAMI. Like the NAMI associated programs, WRAP sessions are conducted by persons in recovery from serious mental illnesses, but they are of shorter duration than the BRIDGES and Peer-to-Peer programs, generally lasting only a few hours for overview sessions or 2 days for traditional WRAP sessions. WRAP provides structured training wherein each participant develops his or her own plan to maintain wellness. In this plan, referred to as the "toolbox," one is instructed on how to use the tools to identify and deal with triggers, early warning signs, and so forth.

EVIDENCE OF EFFECTIVENESS

Regarding the effectiveness of the advocacy aspects of self-help activities, there can be little doubt that the activities of persons in recovery from mental illness and their family members have had a substantial impact on the mental health system. During the past 40 years, consumers and family members have helped bring us to the point of transforming the mental health system, so that it becomes consumer and family driven, and focused on recovery. This embodies measures to ensure that persons with mental illness are afforded humane, dignified, and increasingly effective treatment, and that consumer and/or family representatives have input into all phases of mental health research and treatment initiatives.

Another question, of course, is whether persons with mental illness are in fact benefiting from these self-help activities. Research in this area has been somewhat limited, but at least one major, recent research effort has addressed this question.

SAMHSA's CMHS supports the meaningful participation of mental health consumers/survivors in all aspects of the mental health system, including the planning, design, implementation, policy formulation, and evaluation of mental health services. Campbell (2005) reported on a SAMHSA-funded, multisite study, begun in 1998, in which the well-being of some 1,827 adult persons in recovery who participated in three types of consumer-operated services was compared to that of similar subjects who received traditional services only. The three types of consumer-operated services were four drop-in centers, two mutual support programs, and two educational/advocacy programs. Results indicated significant improvement in well-being for the participants in only two of the drop-in center programs, but no improvement for participants in the consumer-operated services programs compared to those in the traditional programs overall.

Although this recent SAMHSA-sponsored research effort has not produced the evidence many were hoping for with respect to the efficacy of self-help groups, consumer and family advocates continue to remain optimistic that self-help is of significant benefit to the persons in recovery from serious mental illness who choose to participate in these programs.

KEY POINTS

- The term *self-help* originally referred to the activities of groups of persons with similar disorders who organized to assist to one another in their recovery efforts.
- There are many different types of self-help groups for persons with behavioral health disorders.

- Some self-help groups follow a 12-step model, similar to that developed by AA. Other groups employ different models.
- Beginning in the 1960s, some mental health self-help groups began taking on roles as advocates.
- In recent years self-help/advocacy groups have increasingly been developing specialized programs aimed at assisting persons in recovery from behavioral disorders.
- Research on the effectiveness of self-help efforts so far has been limited and has produced mixed results.

REFERENCES AND RECOMMENDED READINGS

Campbell, J. (2005, December). *Effectiveness findings of the COSP multisite research initiative grading the evidence for consumer driven services.* Chicago: UIC NRTC Webcast.

Chamberlin, J. (1978). *On our own: Patient-controlled alternatives to the mental health system.* New York: Hawthorn.

Copeland, M. E. (1999). *Wellness Recovery Action Plan.* West Dummerston, VT: Peach Press.

Depression and Bipolar Support Alliance. (2006). Retrieved September 22, 2006, from *www. dbsalliance.org*

Emotions Anonymous. (2006). Retrieved September 22, 2006, from *www.emotionsanonymous.org*

Frese, F. J. (1993). Cruising the cosmos: Part 3. Psychosis and hospitalization: A consumer's recollection. In A. B. Hatfield & H. P. Lefley (Eds.), *Surviving mental illness: Stress, coping, and adaptation.* (pp. 67–76). New York: Guilford Press.

Frese, F. J. (1998). Advocacy, recovery, and the challenges of consumerism for schizophrenia. *Psychiatric Clinics of North America, 21,* 233–249.

Frese, F. J. (2000). Psychology practitioners and schizophrenia: A view from both sides. *Journal of Clinical Psychology, 56*(11), 1413–1426.

Frese, F. J. (2004). Inside "insight"—a personal perspective on insight in psychosis. In X. Amador & A. David (Eds.), *Insight and psychosis* (2nd ed., pp. 351–358). London: Oxford University Press.

GROW. (2006). Retrieved September 22, 2006, from *www.grow.ie*

National Alliance on Mental Illness. (2005, Spring). NAMI's Peer-to-Peer course set to expand. *NAMI Advocate,* pp. 4–5.

New Freedom Commission on Mental Health. (2003). *Achieving the promise: Transforming mental health care in America* (*Executive Summary,* DHHS Publication No. SMA-03-3831). Rockville, MD: Department of Health and Human Services.

Recovery, Inc. (2006). Retrieved September 22, 2006, from *www.recovery-inc.org*

Resnick, S. G., Armstrong, M., Sperrazza, M., Harkness, L., & Rosenheck, R. A. (2004). A model of consumer–provider partnership: Vet-to-Vet. *Psychiatric Rehabilitation Journal, 28*(2), 185–187.

Schizophrenics Anonymous. (2006). Retrieved September 22, 2006, from *www.sanonymous.com*

Valenstein, E. S. (1986). *Great and desperate cures: The rise and decline of psychosurgery and other radical treatments for mental illness.* New York: Basic Books.

Zinman, S., Harp, H. T., & Budd, S. (1987). *Reaching across: Mental health clients helping each other.* Riverside: California Network of Mental Health Clients.

Zinman, S., & Harp, H. T. (1994). Reaching across: II. Maintaining our roots/the challenge of growth. Available from the California Network of Mental Health Clients at *main@california clients.org*

PART V

SYSTEMS OF CARE

CHAPTER 31

CLINICAL CASE MANAGEMENT

MARGARET V. SHERRER
THOMAS O'HARE

This chapter addresses a critical component of effective treatment for schizophrenia in community settings: clinical case management. The chapter begins with a description of clinical case management, with an emphasis on the variability in how these services are delineated and implemented within a broad range of treatment settings. Next, the core functions of clinical case management services are presented, followed by a brief summary of what is known about treatment effectiveness based on outcome research to date. Finally, clinical guidelines for case management are offered, with some recommendations for future directions in training, education, and evaluation of case management services.

Often referred to as the "glue" that holds services together, clinical case management is central to effective service delivery for people with schizophrenia. In its inception, case management focused primarily on brokering and coordinating services, with little or no emphasis on the direct provision of clinical interventions. Over the past two decades, however, case management skills have been broadened considerably to include an array of strategies to enhance client functioning through the coordination of complex interventions and improvement of access to other social, material, and environmental resources. This role often requires a broad scope of knowledge concerning comprehensive assessment and treatment needs, as well as a good degree of professional initiative, leadership, and communication skills to make interdisciplinary services and bureaucratic systems work in concert for clients. Beyond mere "brokering" of services, case management has come to be seen as essential for coordinating multiple services and enhancing instrumental and social supports critical to the successful treatment of schizophrenia. Continuity of care has become a guiding principle for case management approaches, thus avoiding the fragmentation of services that can undermine even the most effective therapeutic interventions.

The case management movement began to evolve in the 1970s as a response to a National Institute of Mental Health (NIMH) mandate that each state must provide community-based services for people with severe and persistent mental illness. With the creation of the Community Support Program (CSP) in 1977, case management was identified as crucial to addressing the unmet treatment needs of community-based clients who had been discharged from long-term care in institutions and hospitals. Case management takes different forms, including assertive community treatment (ACT) teams and a range of community treatment programs with varying levels of intensity and frequency of client contact. To be most effective, case management services should be delivered within a multidisciplinary team that can provide assertive outreach, 24-hour coverage, and long-term, open-ended treatment in clients' natural environment. Client caseloads may be shared (as with ACT teams) or a case manager may be the sole point of contact for a specified number of clients (this model is sometimes referred to as "standard case management"). Caseload sizes also tend to vary with lower client-to-staff ratios (10:1 as opposed to 25:1 or higher) preferred for people with schizophrenia, who are likely to require more intensive services to achieve and maintain independent living in the community.

CORE FUNCTIONS OF CLINICAL CASE MANAGEMENT

In describing the core functions of clinical case management, this section is organized into five categories: (1) promoting client engagement and involvement in treatment; (2) acting as primary client contact within the community mental health agency; (3) brokering of services; (4) advocacy and liaison functions; and (5) psychotherapeutic work. These functions are summarized in Table 31.1 and described below.

Promoting Client Engagement and Involvement in Treatment

At the outset, case managers must initiate and create a working alliance that emphasizes trust and collaboration. In forging a strong working alliance, appropriate treatment boundaries must be established; this deserves special note, because case managers interact with clients in a wide variety of personal settings within clients' natural environment, including their homes, workplaces, and in meetings with family members and significant others, to name only a few. Because case management relationships may be viewed by clients as more intimate than those with other helping professionals, increased vigilance about therapeutic roles and boundaries may be warranted, especially with clients who are more socially isolated and might easily perceive the helping role as something akin to friendship.

As with many people with severe mental illness, clients with schizophrenia are not likely to engage in services of their own accord; therefore, assertive outreach—reaching out to clients in their natural environments—is essential for maintaining regular contact. Case managers also should assist clients in identifying personal goals, individual strengths, and perceived obstacles that should be considered in assessment and treatment planning. This is covered more fully in the section on psychotherapeutic work.

Acting as Primary Client Contact within the Community Mental Health Agency

In standard case management models in which caseloads are not shared, initiating and/or facilitating case discussions regarding client care at treatment team meetings is often the responsibility of the assigned case manager. Maintaining regular communication on individual client progress with team leaders and treating psychiatrists also is essential to continuity of care. In most systems, the case manager ensures that the client's medical record

TABLE 31.1. Clinical Case Management Activities

Promoting client engagement and involvement in treatment

- Creating a working alliance.
- Assisting in assessment and treatment planning across all client domains.
- Setting and maintaining appropriate treatment boundaries.
- Assertive outreach—reaching out to clients in their natural environments to maintain regular contact.
- Assisting client in identifying personal goals, individual strengths, and perceived obstacles that should be considered in treatment planning.

Acting as primary client contact within the community mental health agency

- Initiating and/or facilitating case discussions regarding client care at treatment team meetings.
- Maintaining regular communication on individual client progress with the team leader and treating psychiatrist.
- Ensuring that the client's medical record is kept current with all required documentation, including treatment plans, clinical updates, and progress notes.

Brokering of services

- Benefits assistance (Social Security Disability, food stamps, and other entitlements).
- Coordinating medical care (regular medical and dental care; referral for other medical specialists as needed, including encouragement to follow through on medical testing and treatment when indicated).
- Assisting clients in obtaining legal representation when needed.
- Promoting follow through with all outside referrals for benefits and services.

Advocacy and liaison functions

- Working with landlords to help clients maintain housing when problems arise.
- Supporting and assisting clients in navigating the criminal justice system.
- Helping to safeguard client rights.
- Acting as a liaison in psychiatric or medical facilities when a client is in need of hospitalization.

Psychotherapeutic work

- Comprehensive assessment and treatment planning.
- Medication and symptom monitoring.
- Crisis planning and emergency response.
- Teaching life skills to promote client independence (budgeting, money management, cooking, shopping, housekeeping, parenting, use of public transportation).
- Psychoeducation (e.g., signs and symptoms of schizophrenia, negative effects of co-occurring substance abuse, influence of stress on course and severity of mental illness).
- Coping and social skills training.
- Illness management and recovery.
- Supportive counseling.
- Family education and support.
- Coordinating and/or providing specialized services for clients with co-occurring substance use disorders.
- Social integration (helping to fortify and expand natural social supports/community involvement).
- Vocational assistance (frequently coordinated with supported employment specialist).

is kept current, including all required documentation, such as treatment plans, clinical updates, and progress notes.

Brokering of Services

The impact of social and environmental pressures (e.g., homelessness, poverty, discrimination) on the psychological well-being of individuals with schizophrenia is compelling. Beyond the provision of mental health treatment, case management involves brokering of needed services, including housing, benefits, medical care, and legal assistance. Failing to provide effective coordination of services or ignoring social and environmental needs may preclude solid, long-term outcomes with even the most skillfully delivered treatment interventions. Although many psychosocial difficulties can be effectively addressed through a supportive relationship and cognitive-behavioral coping skills, these methods often are not robust enough to overcome the environmental pressures and barriers that weigh down clients with schizophrenia.

Topping the list is assistance with securing and maintaining safe, affordable housing. Practitioners and researchers have long understood that persons with schizophrenia experience difficulties maintaining steady residences. In addition, when homelessness is associated with the loss of familial and social support, there appears to be greater risk of depression. Therefore, homelessness must be understood as a pronounced stressor associated with the loss of critical social and emotional supports.

Financial stability is likely to depend on ongoing benefits assistance such as Social Security Disability, food stamps, and other entitlements. In these instances, case managers are called upon to assist clients in navigating the bureaucratic systems and promote client follow through on application procedures. Knowledge of how entitlement programs work is essential.

Coordinating needed health care (regular medical and dental examinations, referral for other medical specialists as needed, including encouragement to follow through on medical testing and treatment when indicated) is another important case management function, one that frequently involves keeping the treating psychiatrist apprised of important medical findings through the facilitation of formal interagency correspondence documenting outside health care.

Given that clients with schizophrenia may be involved in the criminal justice system, case managers may be called upon to link a client with legal representation when needed; they may also need to work closely with parole officers or other court-appointed personnel who may be monitoring the client.

Advocacy and Liaison Functions

Case managers frequently take on the role of advocate or liaison in assisting clients to achieve independent living. For example, case managers may act as an advocate on behalf of their clients in addressing landlord concerns that, if unresolved, might result in eviction from housing. In many cases, it may be necessary to intervene with employers to help meet client vocational goals. Case managers often accompany their clients to court hearings and other legal proceedings, supporting and assisting clients in navigating the criminal justice system. In helping to safeguard client rights, case managers may work in conjunction with the state mental health advocate in cases of discrimination that violate the Americans with Disabilities Act (ADA). Last but not least, case managers may serve as liaisons in psychiatric or medical facilities when clients are in need of hospitalization or a specialized treatment program not provided by the client's mental health agency.

Psychotherapeutic Work

Ideally, case managers are well versed in the range of evidence-based practices for people with schizophrenia covered elsewhere in this book. These include collaborative psychopharmacology, ACT, family psychoeducation, social and other coping skills training, supported employment, illness management and recovery, and integrated treatment for co-occurring substance use disorders.

As a first step, case managers are expected to undertake comprehensive assessment and treatment planning across all client domains, often working in tandem with psychiatrists, nurses, clinicians, and vocational specialists.

In the assessment phase, it is important to collate data from multiple sources, including other mental health professionals, primary physicians, counselors, community members, law enforcement, and family members. Discharge summaries documenting prior episodes of care in other treatment settings should be reviewed thoroughly. Clinical case managers should be concerned with the following areas for ongoing assessment and psychosocial interventions:

- *Mental status* (e.g., psychiatric symptoms, including hallucinations, delusions, disorganized thinking, depression, anxiety, social withdrawal and motor retardation, and blunted affect, among others).
- *Highly stressful or traumatic events* (e.g., rape and other assaults, sudden losses) that may require modification in service delivery or referral for specialized posttraumatic stress disorder (PTSD) treatment.
- *Use of medications and other substances* (e.g., type and number of medications, compliance with prescribed regimen, use of medications without prescription, quantity, frequency of alcohol and other drug use, and consequences associated with their use).
- *Social functioning in interpersonal relationships* (e.g., family, friends) and extended relationships (e.g., number and types of social supports, quality of connectedness with others in the community, or signs of isolation and withdrawal).
- *Ability to negotiate daily living activities* (e.g., shopping, laundry, hygiene).
- *Access to and use of environmental resources* (e.g., housing, transportation, housing and safety concerns).
- *Money management and gainful vocational activity* (e.g., job/education).
- *Monitoring of general health status* (and facilitating primary care and dental care, including specialists for identified medical conditions).
- *Leisure activities.*
- *Spiritual and/or religious beliefs.*
- *Legal concerns* (civil and criminal).

A detailed functional analysis that includes an examination of the day-to-day experiences of the client during a "typical week" may reveal circumstances under which the client is likely to do particularly well or to experience stressors that may be associated with crises or deterioration in well-being. Potential problems may include conflict with family members, acquaintances, workmates, or others in the community; depression or anxiety associated with trauma-related symptoms (e.g., flashbacks, reexperiencing); abuse of alcohol or other drugs; or exacerbation of symptoms due to medication noncompliance. These difficulties can easily escalate into serious crises that may require emergency intervention, police involvement, or hospitalization.

Whether created by an individual case manager or as part of a treatment team, a client's treatment plan should reflect the goals of the client, not merely the treatment goals established by the team. This should be done in a collaborative fashion, ensuring that the treatment plan and clinical reviews accurately reflect the client's wishes in treatment, including a plan to be followed if he or she is in crisis.

There should be considerable flexibility and tailoring of services and intervention strategies to suit the particular client's needs and goals. Psychotherapeutic work performed by case managers typically includes *medication and symptom monitoring; crisis planning and emergency response; teaching of life skills to promote client independence* (budgeting, money management, cooking, shopping, housekeeping, parenting, use of public transportation); *psychoeducation* (e.g., signs and symptoms of schizophrenia, the negative effects of co-occurring substance abuse, influence of stress on course and severity of mental illness); *coping and social skills training; supportive counseling; family education and support; coordinating and/or providing specialized services for co-occurring substance use disorders;* and *social integration*—helping to fortify and expand clients' natural social supports and community involvement.

Given that people with schizophrenia tend to have very limited social networks, enhancing social supports is a critical function of case management. The quality of social supports is associated with a number of factors, including a sense of self-efficacy and personal empowerment. Social supports can be either naturally occurring or orchestrated as part of formal case management interventions. Enhancing social supports may take many forms, ranging from encouraging clients to try out mutual-help groups, such as Alcoholics Anonymous; facilitating the development of a consumer group for persons with mental illness; or linking clients with church and other groups of interest. Case managers may have to help clients optimize the potential benefits from social supports by helping them to improve their social skills.

Case managers are in a unique position to provide social skills training in the community, including demonstration and practice of selected skills and positive reinforcement for utilizing skills appropriately. Certainly, enhancing social skills in persons with schizophrenia is challenging, and results vary based on the client's level of social deficit, as well as the seriousness of co-occurring problems, such as substance abuse. Rather than broad-based efforts, case managers might focus on one or two specific circumstances in which the client would likely benefit most from improvement (e.g., engaging in light conversation on the job or reducing argumentative interactions with acquaintances in the client's social club environment).

Teaching self-monitoring skills to clients enables them to begin to link certain adverse circumstances or experiences with the potential for relapse, and perhaps to identify emotional upset, discouragement, suicidal thoughts, anger, conflict or other troubling experiences as a "warning signal" to seek social supports or to contact someone on their mental health team to reduce the likelihood of further problems. Case managers also can identify areas of opportunity where clients can practice their social skills and stress management skills to reduce the likelihood of crises and enhance their sense of self-efficacy, confidence, and overall well-being.

EVIDENCE SUPPORTING CLINICAL CASE MANAGEMENT

There is relatively little outcome research specific to clinical case management due in part to the ambiguity in distinguishing clinical case management from other, similar derivations of the ACT model (e.g., intensive community treatment, continuous treatment teams). In reviewing both the descriptive and the outcome literature, one encounters a variety of what can generically be referred to as "clinical skills" embedded in various case management models, with the exception of a straightforward brokering-type case management, in which various services are procured and loosely coordinated for the client. Clinical case management activities are not consistently represented in the literature, but they seem to include some or all of the following: relationship building and therapeutic engagement processes; psychosocial assessment; psychoeducation with individuals and families; skills training in the community via modeling and *in vivo* practice; substance abuse counseling; and so forth. Less is known about the level of training in clinical case management skills or the level of expertise with which these skills are applied.

Nevertheless, when case management models that include some clinical skills are compared with service brokering models, evidence suggests that they do result in modestly superior outcomes that include reduced hospitalizations and improved psychosocial functioning. To illustrate, one experimental comparison by Morse and colleagues (1997) demonstrated differential outcomes between an ACT program and broker-style case management. In the ACT program, practitioners cultivated a positive working relationship with clients, emphasized practical problem solving, enhanced community living skills, provided supportive services, assisted with money management, and facilitated transportation. By contrast, in brokering, case managers purchased services from various agencies and helped clients to develop treatment plans. ACT provided considerably more services overall (including housing, finances, health and support) and resulted in greater client satisfaction and better psychiatric ratings. However, no differences emerged with regard to substance abuse outcomes. As is typically the case in ACT programs, staff-to-client ratios were much smaller (about one-eighth) than that in the brokering case management condition. Thus, it is hard to determine in this exemplar and in similar studies whether the better outcomes for ACT were the result of more services, different services, or qualitatively better service delivery.

Considerable limitations in most of the research on case management interventions in general include the aforementioned lack of clarity in model conceptualization, along with inadequate sample size, lack of pretreatment data on clients, problems with random assignment of cases, high rates of attrition, limited use of standardized measures, violations of statistical assumptions, lack of multivariate analysis, poor distinctions among treatment conditions, and lack of attention to intervention fidelity (i.e., faithfulness to the practice model).

Notwithstanding these limitations, tentative conclusions about the effectiveness of clinical case management can be drawn. Case management shows positive outcomes in clients' lower hospital stays overall, increased social contact and social functioning, increased satisfaction with life, some reduction in symptoms (perhaps through medication compliance), increased family and patient satisfaction, improved social functioning, and better adjustment to employment and independent living. Although tying specific dimensions of clinical case management to specific outcomes is difficult, a few reports offer evidence that the therapeutic relationship between the case manager and the client may be a key factor that accounts for the modest superiority of clinical case management over broker-style approaches.

TREATMENT GUIDELINES FOR CLINICAL CASE MANAGEMENT

If one extrapolates from controlled outcome research on clinical practices with the seriously mentally ill, it is reasonable to hypothesize that much can be done to improve the effectiveness of clinical case management through the incorporation of some of the following treatment strategies:

1. Engagement and motivational enhancement skills.
2. Nurturing a sound therapeutic relationship.
3. Crisis intervention.

4. Conducting comprehensive psychosocial assessments (e.g., mental status, psychosocial, substance abuse, and material/social supports).
5. Offering psychoeducational services to individuals and families regarding mental illness, substance abuse, and the importance of medication compliance.
6. Designing and implementing monitoring and evaluation strategies.
7. Using standardized measures.
8. Employing standard problem-solving skills.
9. Using role play, rehearsal, and corrective feedback to improve specific behavioral deficits.
10. Providing skills training, graduated exposure, and practice in the community to improve overall psychosocial functioning and generalize behavioral competencies.

The challenge of clarifying and improving clinical case management must include development of a curriculum of skills that can be incorporated into the role of case manager. Feasibility depends on commitment to a number of structural service issues, including training, supervision, ongoing monitoring and evaluation, and the use of fidelity measures to maintain treatment quality. These steps also make clinical case management programs more amenable to much-needed controlled outcome research.

The scope of therapeutic services provided by clinical case managers is likely to vary considerably across treatment systems. The actual clinical functions performed by clinical case managers may be a controversial issue given that many of the psychotherapeutic interventions described in this chapter may be seen as the domain of master's- or doctoral-level clinicians. However, not all treatment teams have graduate-level trained specialists at their disposal, and the services provided by these clinicians may be limited, leaving the ongoing direct care largely to assigned case managers.

Practically speaking, it is likely that much of the therapeutic work with seriously mentally ill clients falls to the staff member who has the most frequent contact with clients, the case manager. However, there are considerable obstacles to effective incorporation of clinical skills into routine case management activities. Case management is stressful and generally low-paying work, often resulting in high staff burnout and rapid employee turnover. These problems put strain on the treatment delivery system and are detrimental to client care, which depends on stable, responsive, ongoing services provided by compassionate caregivers. Understandably, clients often become discouraged when their assigned workers repeatedly terminate employment. The client is, yet again, faced with establishing another relationship of unknown duration. This scenario tends to be less problematic on ACT teams that share caseloads, which encourages clients to interact with multiple staff members; however, less intensive case management programs may assign only one worker as the single contact point for a larger caseload of clients. These interruptions in the continuity of care are likely to increase client relapses and treatment costs.

Recruiting, training, and retaining highly skilled case managers require considerable effort from administrative and supervisory staff. Optimally, clinical case managers should be given ongoing training, support, and regular clinical supervision to foster effective therapeutic skills, to monitor client progress, to deal with challenging clients, and to guard against professional burnout. The role of clinical case manager often becomes a delicate balancing act that involves providing services for clients, meeting productivity demands, advocating for various purposes, documenting services, and conducting other administrative tasks. Therefore, teaching effective time management strategies should be considered in the training and supervision of case managers. Nevertheless, despite these recommendations, additional incentives, such as assistance with graduate education, may be required to retain skilled case managers in the mental health system. Mental health agencies and state universities might consider forming consortiums to encourage skilled case managers to advance professionally and remain in community support programs in managerial and supervisory roles, so that they may train and supervise the next generation of clinical case managers. In conclusion, despite the challenges of incorporating clinical skills into the traditional case management role and retaining experienced workers, clinical case management interventions, when used judiciously and assertively, can powerfully enhance treatment protocols for clients with schizophrenia. Clinical case management has the potential to be not only the key integrating element in a complex system of care but also the main catalyst for improving clients' psychosocial well-being and long-term recovery.

KEY POINTS

- Case managers play a vital role in coordinating multiple services and improving access to the social, material, and environmental resources deemed necessary for clients with schizophrenia to achieve independent living in the community.
- *Continuity of care* should be a guiding principle in case management approaches for treatment of schizophrenia to avoid fragmentation of services that can undermine even the most efficacious therapeutic interventions.
- Optimal case management services should be delivered by a multidisciplinary team that can provide assertive outreach, 24-hour coverage, and long-term, open-ended treatment in clients' natural environments.
- Core functions of case management include promoting client engagement and follow through in treatment; acting as the primary client contact; brokering of services; advocacy and liaison functions; and providing a wide array of psychotherapeutic interventions.
- Case managers should be well-versed in the range of evidence-based practices for people with schizophrenia; clinical interventions and services should be flexible and tailored to suit each client's particular needs and goals for recovery.
- Administrators and supervisory staff members should ensure that case managers receive ongoing training, support, and clinical supervision to foster effective therapeutic skills, to maintain professional treatment boundaries, to reduce job burnout, and to curb high staff turnover.

REFERENCES AND RECOMMENDED READINGS

Carey, K. B. (1998). Treatment boundaries in the case management relationship: A behavioral perspective. *Community Mental Health Journal, 34*(3), 313–317.

Grech, E. (2002). Case management: A critical analysis of the literature. *International Journal of Psychosocial Rehabilitation, 6,* 89–98.

Harris, M., & Bergman, H.C. (1987). Case management with the chronically mentally ill: A clinical perspective. *American Journal of Orthopsychiatry, 57,* 296–302.

Hromco, J. G., Lyons, J. S., & Nikkel, R. E. (1997). Styles of case management: The philosophy and practice of case managers. *Community Mental Health Journal, 33*(5), 415–428.

Kanter, J. (1989). Clinical case management: Definitions, principles, components. *Hospital and Community Psychiatry, 40,* 361–368.

Morse, G. A., Calsyn, R. J., Klinkenberg, W. D., Trusty, M. L., Gerber, F., Smith, R., et al. (1997). An experimental comparison of three types of case management for homeless mentally ill persons. *Psychiatric Services, 48,* 497–503.

Mueser, K. T., Bond, G. R., Drake, R. E., & Resnick, S. G. (1998). Models of community care for severe mental illness: A review of research on case management. *Schizophrenia Bulletin, 24*(1), 37–74.

Mueser, K. T., Noordsy, D. L., Drake, R. E., & Fox, L. (2003). *Integrated treatment for dual disorders: A guide to effective practice.* New York: Guilford Press.

O'Hare, T. (2005). Schizophrenia. In T. O'Hare, *Evidence-based practices for social workers: An interdisciplinary approach* (pp. 56–102). Chicago: Lyceum Books.

Scott, J. E., & Dixon, L. B. (1995). Assertive community treatment and case management for schizophrenia. *Schizophrenia Bulletin, 21*(4), 657–668.

Williams, J., & Swartz, M. (1998). Treatment boundaries in the case management relationship: A clinical case and discussion. *Community Mental Health Journal, 34*(3), 299–311.

Ziguras, S. J., & Stuart, G. W. (2000). A meta-analysis of the effectiveness of mental health case management over 20 years. *Psychiatric Services, 51*, 1410–1421.

CHAPTER 32

STRENGTHS-BASED
CASE MANAGEMENT

CHARLES A. RAPP
RICHARD J. GOSCHA

C*ase management* has traditionally been viewed as an entity (usually a person) that coordinates, integrates, and allocates care within limited resources. The primary functions have been seen as assessment, planning, referral, and monitoring. The notion is that a single point of contact is responsible for helping people with psychiatric disabilities receive the services they need from a fragmented system of care. The assumption is that people who receive these benefits and services will be able to live more independently in the community and that their quality of life will improve. The unadorned *broker* model of case management has been shown in multiple studies to be an ineffective model of practice. Enhanced case management models, such as assertive community treatment, and clinical and strengths-based models, have emerged over the last 25 years.

The strengths model of case management was developed by a team at the University of Kansas School of Social Welfare beginning in the early 1980s. It has gone through almost 25 years of development, refinement, testing, and dissemination. This chapter summarizes the research, theory, principles, and methods of the strengths model. It also provides a case example for a glimpse of the model in practice and to help distinguish the practice from more traditional problem- or pathology-based approaches.

RESEARCH ON THE STRENGTHS MODEL

Nine studies have tested the effectiveness of the strengths model in people with psychiatric disabilities. Four of the studies employed experimental or quasi-experimental designs, and five used nonexperimental methods. Positive outcomes have been reported in the areas of hospitalizations, housing, employment, reduced symptoms, leisure time, social support, and family burden.

In the four experimental studies, positive outcomes outweighed by a 13:5 ratio the outcomes in which no significant difference was reported. In none of the studies did clients receiving strengths case management do worse. The strengths model research results have also been remarkably resilient across settings. Consistency has been shown even within studies. Three of the studies had multiple sites with different case managers, supervisors, and affiliations, with a total of 15 different agencies.

The two outcomes areas in which results have been consistently positive are reduction in symptoms and enhanced quality of community life. The three studies (two experimental and one nonexperimental) using symptoms as a variable all reported positive outcomes. This included findings that people receiving strengths model case management reported fewer problems with mood and thoughts and greater stress tolerance and psychological well-being than the control groups. Although the studies used a variety of measures, which we term *enhanced quality of community life* (e.g., increased leisure time in the community, enhanced skills for successful community living, increased social supports, decreased social isolation, and increased quality of life), people receiving strengths model case management had enhanced levels of competence and involvement in terms of community living. Eight of the nine studies using these types of measures reported positive outcomes that were statistically significant.

Other outcomes that seem to be strong indicators of the effectiveness of strengths model case management include reduced hospitalization (three out of six studies showing positive outcomes), vocational (two out of two showing positive outcomes), and housing (two out two showing positive outcomes).

THE PURPOSE AND THEORY OF STRENGTHS

The purpose of case management in the strengths model is to assist people to recover, reclaim, and transform their lives by identifying, securing, and sustaining the range of resources—both environmental and personal—needed to live, play, and work in a normal interdependent way in the community. A case manager works to "identify, secure, and sustain" resources that are both external (i.e., social relations, opportunities, and resources) and internal (i.e., aspirations, competencies, and confidence) rather than to focus only on external resources (brokerage model of case management) or internal resources (psychotherapy or skills development). It is the dual focus that contributes to the creation of healthy and desirable niches that provide impetus for achievement and life satisfaction.

The strengths theory posits that a person's quality of life, achievement, life satisfaction, and recovery are attributable in large part to the type and quality of niches that he or she inhabits. These niches can be understood as paralleling a person's major life domains, such as living arrangement, work, education, recreation, social relationships, and so forth. The quality of the niches for any individual is a function of his or her aspirations, competencies, and confidence, and the environmental resources, opportunities and people available.

Recovery as an outcome is a state of being to which people aspire. It comprises two components, the first of which concerns an individual's self-perceptions and psychological states. This includes hopefulness, self-efficacy, self-esteem, feelings of loneliness, and empowerment. The second component closely resembles community integration. In short, people should have the opportunity to live in a place they can call home, to work at a job that brings satisfaction and income, to have rich social networks, and to have available means for contributing to others. It also means avoiding the often spirit-breaking experiences of forced hospitalization, homelessness, or incarceration.

Recovery as an outcome involves achieving certain psychological states and a degree of community integration. In life, the two are closely entwined. An increased sense of hope can contribute to having more friends or pursuing a job. Increased confidence may lead to enrolling in school. Similarly, obtaining a job may lead to increased feelings of self-efficacy and empowerment. Having an enjoyable date may enhance one's self-esteem.

At the core, the desired outcomes are people's achievements based on the goals they set for themselves. Although these are highly individualized goals, people do seem to group them into finding a decent place to live or attaining employment and/or an opportunity to contribute, education, friends, and recreational outlets. In other words, people with psychiatric disabilities want the same things that other people want. In addition, because they often experience psychiatric distress, people with psychiatric disabilities want to lessen this distress and avoid psychiatric hospitalization. Like other people, they want choices and the power to decide among their options. Together, these outcomes comprise the quality of one's life and are achievement or growth oriented. Clients do not speak often of adaptation, coping, or compliance as desired outcomes; rather, they speak of jobs, degrees, friends, apartments, and fun.

PRINCIPLES OF THE PRACTICE

The following six principles are derived from the theory. The principles are the transition between the theory, which seeks to explain people's success in life, and the specific methods that assist people toward that end. The principles are the governing laws or values, or tenets, upon which the methods are based.

1. *People with psychiatric disabilities can recover, reclaim, and transform their lives.* The thousands of first-person accounts of recovery and the results of longitudinal research in several countries lead one to conclude that the capacity for growth and recovery is already present within the people we serve. Our job as case managers is to create conditions in which growth and recovery are most likely to occur.

2. *The focus is on individual strengths rather than pathology.* The work is focused on what the client has achieved, what resources have been or are currently available to the client, what the client knows and talents he or she possesses, and what aspirations and dreams the client holds. The focus on strengths rather than pathology, weaknesses, and problems enhances the motivation and the individualization of the people with whom we work.

3. *The community is viewed as an oasis of resources.* Although the community may contribute to a person's distress, it may also be the source of well-being. The community provides life's opportunities, supportive social relations, and necessary resources. Our work is devoted to identifying and acquiring the community resources necessary for achievement.

4. *The client is the director of the helping process.* A cornerstone of the strengths perspective of case management is the belief that it is the person's right to determine the form, direction, and substance of the case management help he or she is to receive. People with psychiatric disabilities are capable of this determination, adherence to this principle contributes to the effectiveness of case management. Case managers should do nothing without the person's approval, involving him or her in decisions regarding every step of the process. Adherence to this principle enhances empowerment and motivation, and facilitates a strong partnership between the consumer and the case manager.

5. *The primary setting for the work is the community.* Case management occurs in apartments, restaurants, businesses, parks, and community agencies. An outreach mode of service delivery enhances the accuracy and completeness of assessments, avoids diffi-

culties in generalizing newly learned skills, increases retention of consumers in service, and provides opportunities for identifying community resources.

6. *The case manager–consumer relationship is primary and essential.* Without this relationship a person's strengths, talents, skills, desires, and aspirations often lie dormant and may not be mobilized for the person's recovery journey. It takes a strong and trusting relationship to discover the rich and detailed tapestry of someone's life and to create an environment in which a person is willing to share what is most meaningful and important—his or her passion for life.

PRACTICE GUIDELINES

Engagement

The purpose of engagement is to create a trusting reciprocal relationship between the case manager and the consumer as a basis for working together. To facilitate each consumer's recovery journey, the relationship should be a hope-inducing rather than spirit-breaking process. Examples of spirit breaking include restricting people's choices, imposing our own standard of living on people, making their decisions for them, and telling people that they are not yet ready for work, a car, or an apartment. In contrast, hope-inducing relationships are built through caring interactions, focusing on people's strengths, celebrating their accomplishments, promoting choice, helping them achieve goals that are important, and promoting a future beyond the mental health system. Engagement and the entire case management process occurs in the community, not in the mental health agency.

Strengths Assessment

The purpose of a strengths assessment is to amplify the well part of an individual by collecting information on personal and environmental strengths. The strengths assessment is organized by eight life domains: daily living situation; finances; vocation/education; social supports; health, leisure, and recreational activity; and spiritual/cultural activity. Information is organized in each life domain by the current situation, the future (desires and aspirations), and past situations. A strengths assessment, unlike many assessments, is an ongoing, continuous process. The information is gathered in a conversational manner as the case manager and consumer spend time together. It is critical that case managers collect specific information, avoiding the tendency to rely on pleasant adjectives (e.g., diligent, humorous, kind). The inquiry should focus on specific achievements, talents (playing the 12-string guitar, skill as a foreign car mechanic), and environmental resources (church choirmaster, playing gin with one's brother).

Personal Planning

The purpose of personal planning is to create a mutual work agenda between the case manager and consumer that focuses on achieving goals that the client has set. Goals are inherent to hope and indispensable precursors to achievement. The personal plan lays out the decisions that the consumer and case manager must discuss and upon which they must agree. Their decisions include the long-term goal or passion statement, specific tasks needed to pursue the goal, deciding who is responsible, and dates for task completion. The personal plan is in part a "to-do list" for both the consumer and the case manager.

Resource Acquisition

The purpose of resource acquisition is to acquire environmental resources desired by the consumer to achieve goals, to ensure his or her rights, and to increase his or her assets. Primacy is placed on normal or natural resources, not mental health services, because true community integration can only occur apart from mental health and segregated services. Therefore, work is done with employers, landlords, coaches, colleges, teachers, artists, ministers, and so forth. The identification and use of community strengths, assets, and resources are as critical as the identification and use of individual strengths.

Often, the case manager helps community resource personnel adjust to accommodate the desires or needs of a particular person. There are times, however, when adjustments are not needed in the setting or in the client, or if needed, the adjustments are very minor. This occurs when the case manager finds the "perfect niche," where the requirements and needs of the setting perfectly match the desires, talents, and at times, idiosyncrasies of the consumer.

> Harry, a 30-year old man, grew up in rural Kansas, living his whole life on a large farm. He was diagnosed with schizophrenia and entered the state psychiatric hospital. Upon discharge, Harry was placed in a group home, with services provided by the local mental health center. Although not disruptive, Harry failed to meet the group home's hygiene and cleaning requirements, did not use mental health center services, and resisted taking his medication. It was reported that Harry would pack his bags every night, stand on the porch, and announce that he was leaving, although he never left. Over the next 2 years, Harry's stay at the group home was punctuated with three readmissions to the state hospital.
>
> Although Harry was largely uncommunicative, the case manager slowly began to appreciate Harry's knowledge and skill in farming, and took seriously Harry's expression of interest in farming. The case manager and Harry began working to find a place where Harry could use his skills.
>
> They located a ranch on the edge of town, where the owner was happy to accept Harry as a volunteer. Harry and the owner became friends, and Harry soon established himself as a dependable and reliable worker. After a few months, Harry recovered his truck, which was being held by his conservator, renewed his driver's license, and began to drive to the farm daily. To the delight of the community support staff, Harry began to communicate, and there was a marked improvement in his personal hygiene. At the time of case termination, the owner of the ranch and Harry were discussing the possibility of paid employment.

CONTRASTING THE STRENGTHS ASSESSMENT AND THE PSYCHOSOCIAL ASSESSMENT

David was required to attend the day treatment program 5 days per week as a condition for residing at the program's transitional living facility. Over the past 2 weeks he had become increasingly more aggressive with staff members and other clients. He was suspended for 1 day the previous week for yelling at clerical staff members who refused to give him bus tickets. David stated that he did not want to be at day treatment, that he wanted to go to work. Staff members said that he was not "ready to go to work," but that he could demonstrate his "work readiness" by his behaviors at the day treatment program. A staff meeting was called to decide what to do with David. The prevailing thought was that he would probably need to be rehospitalized and have his medications adjusted.

In such a situation, there is a tendency to focus heavily on the "problem behavior" and to interpret particular behaviors within the framework of a person's "illness." Therefore, interventions become focused on the problem, for example, referring the person to an anger management group, adjusting medications to control behavior, hospitalizing the individual, having the person continue to show "work readiness" through prevocational classes, and so forth. The following excerpts are taken from David's actual psychosocial assessment. What is written here is one view of David, primarily from the professional's vantage point. Within the mental health system, such assessments tend to influence our perceptions of the individual and frame our interventions toward a problem or deficit reference point.

Client's name: David
Age: 42

Axis I: 295.10 Schizophrenia: Disorganized Type
Axis II: 301.7 Antisocial Personality Disorder
Axis III: High blood pressure
Axis IV: Illiteracy, unemployment
Axis V: GAF [Global Assessment of Functioning] score: 20

LIVING SITUATION

Client has been living in Wichita for 2 years. Spent first 5 months living either in either homeless shelters or on the streets. Now resides in the Sedgwick County Transitional Living Apartments with three other roommates. Does not interact much with roommates. Has been accused of taking food belonging to roommates. Becomes hostile when confronted.

Client came to Wichita via bus from Little Rock, Arkansas. Had been living in group home there for 8 years. Ran away from group home to find an uncle who, he thought, lived here in Wichita. No record of uncle living in Wichita. Transported to shelter by police after trying to spend the night at bus station.

PSYCHIATRIC HISTORY

First psychiatric hospitalization at age 17. Mother committed him after he became threatening to her. Spent 14 years in Arkansas State Hospital. Discharged in 1978 to group home. Rehospitalized 12 times between 1978 and 1986.

VOCATIONAL/EDUCATIONAL HISTORY

Cllient attended public schools until third grade. Was withdrawn by parents to be home-schooled. Client has limited reading and writing skills. Has never had paid employment. Only vocational activity has been work crew units (janitorial) at Arkansas State Hospital.

SOCIAL HISTORY

Client's father died when he was 12. Mother died when client was 33. Client has no social support network here in Kansas. Has difficulty making friends. Client has never been married.

FINANCIAL

Client receives $376 in Supplemental Security Income [SSI]. Sedgwick County Department of Mental Health is client's payee. Is not able to manage money well.

This is the situation into which a new case manager was assigned. The case manager has recently been trained in the strengths model of case management and felt conflicted relative to what he learned in training about starting where the person was at the time, allowing the person to direct the helping process, building upon a person's strengths, and the prevailing consensus of program staff that David was "decompensating" and needed an immediate involuntary intervention.

The strengths model, while not ignoring problems, shifts the focus to a more holistic view of the situation and the person. Problems are placed in a context of what might be getting in the way of individuals achieving what they want in life, or what they find particularly distressing or disabling from their experience.

The new case manager decided to begin a strengths assessment with David. He got permission from the program to take David out of day treatment for part of the day and to hang out at the mall, where they also shopped for shoes together. The strengths assessment was not conducted by sitting down in an interview, but through casual conversation as the case manager and David went about the morning activities at the mall. Figure 32.1 is the actual initial strengths assessment (later versions continued over time).

The case manager's decision was to engage David around an area that was most important and meaningful to him: his desire to go to work. "I want a job" was David's passion statement. Focusing in on David's passion for wanting a job does not mean the case manager needs to ignore any problems, difficulties, barriers or challenges. Problems, though, are put in their place within the context of something that David has motivation to pursue. What is defined as a problem is anything that is getting in the way of David being able to achieve his goal in life. David is part of defining what is problematic for him and what course he wishes to pursue. This is the essence of creating a hope-inducing environment in which David is the director of his own helping process.

Over the next few weeks, the case manager and David looked for jobs instead of going to day treatment. The strengths assessment was used to generate several employment options that might fit with David's strengths, interests, desires, and aspirations (jobs related to fishing, movies, Mexican food, etc.). David eventually got a job taking tickets at a local movie theater. What he liked most about this job was that one of the benefits was getting to go to movies free when he was not working and eating all the popcorn and soda he wanted. David found a niche in which he thrived.

As of this writing, David has now been employed continuously for 17 years, though he has had a few job changes in between (better pay, nicer theater, etc.). After spending years in the state hospital, David was only hospitalized once after getting a job, and that was for physical reasons. He did not work on improving his reading and writing skills until several years after he started working. He could read enough to recognize what movies were on people's tickets and where to send them. His motivation for eventually learning to read and write was to be able to pay his own bills. He is now his own payee. David and Tony, his roommate from the Transitional Living Apartments, eventually got their own place together. Instead of learning daily living skills from the mental health center, they learned from each other and through experience. David never attended an anger management class. His anger was never a problem outside of the day treatment program, and working and living on his own seemed to be the best medicine or therapy he could have.

Contrasting the information contained in the psychosocial assessment and the strengths assessment, one might not think it refers to the same person. What is written comes from the perceptual framework being used. In one framework, all of David's deficits and shortcomings are the focus, and interventions by staff are centered around "fixing" David. In the other, David's strengths are brought to the forefront, even in the midst

FIGURE 32.1. Strengths assessment.

Consumer's Name
David

Case Manager's Name
Rick

Currrent Status:
What's going on today?
What's available now?

Individual's Desires, Aspirations:
What do I want?

Resources, Personal Social:
What have I used in the past?

Daily Living Situation

Living in Transitional Living Apts. (I don't want to stay there, but its better than the shelter).

Likes to cook hot dogs, corn dogs, mac & cheese, burritos, etc.

Has bus card.

I want a place of my own.

I want to learn how to cook more Mexican food.

I need new shoes!

Lived in Bellview group home (hated it!—Could only watch TV until 9:00 p.m., they decided what you could watch and they told you when to go to bed).

Financial/Insurance

$376 SSI ($120 goes for rent)
$78 food stamps

Sedgwick County is my payee.

I get $50 per week for spending money.

They make me put the rest in savings (I don't need savings, I need food).

I want to be my own payee. (They are messing with my money and it's not right.)

I want to have more money to do the things I want.

Mom used to be payee until she got real sick. Transferred payeeship to Bellview. Mom used to give me extra money.

Vocational/Educational

I go to classes at day treatment: symptom management, money management, etc. (Those things don't help me at all.)

I want a job.

I want out of day program.

I used to sweep floors and clean bathrooms at ASH [Arkansas State Hospital]. I did a good job. Would sometimes wash dishes in the kitchen.

Social Supports

Tony—roommate (He pays for cable, sometimes we put our money together and rent movies).

I don't like my other roommates. They're weirdos, something's really wrong with them.

I wouldn't mind getting married. There is a girl at day program I like. She likes me too. Staff don't like it. They say you can't date in day program or TL. I'm going to ask her out when I get out of here.

Mom—she was always there for me.

Never got along with my dad.

Uncle (Bud)—we used to go fishing. He moved here to Wichita when I was a kid, but I don't know where he is now.

Cousins

Health

I'm in good health, but my teeth hurt.

Medications (primary Clozaril) make me drowsy and sometimes like I'm coming out of my head. I do better at night.

I need to get my teeth looked at. I think they might have to pull a couple.

I want to stop taking medications. I don't like the side effects.

I used to have asthma when I was a kid, but I do better now, as long as I don't try to run when it's cold outside.

(continued)

Leisure/Recreational

I like to watch TV—old westerns, Vincent Price movies. I watch any movie that is on TV.
Tony and I rent movies. He likes comedies, but I like action (It doesn't matter though).
I know a lot about movies.

I want my own TV for my room. I have enough in savings to get one, but they say I can't use it for that.
I want a VCR.

Used to go fishing a lot.
Used to have my own pole and tackle box.
Used to go to the movie house when I was a kid, sometimes with Mom, sometimes with friends.

Spirituality/Culture

My family attended First Baptist when I was young. I didn't like going to church, but I liked Sunday school.

What are my priorities?
1. *I want a job.*
2. *I want to be my own payee.*
3. *I want out of day program.*
4. *I want my own place.*

Consumer's Comments:

Case Manager's Comments:
David is a very funny guy. He tells great stories. I have also never met a person who knew so much about movies (knows who starred in just about every movie).

_____   _____   _____   _____
Consumer's Signature   Date   Case Manager's Signature   Date

of a challenging situation. What David wants in life is what drives the helping process and draws upon his natural energy and intrinsic motivation.

KEY POINTS

- The purpose of strengths model case management is to assist people to recover by identifying, securing, and sustaining the range of environmental and personal resources needed to live, play, and work in a normal, interdependent way in the community.
- The six principles of the model need to work in concert, mutually reinforcing each other.
- The consumer–case manager relationship should be a hope-inducing, not a spirit-breaking process.
- The strengths assessment amplifies the well part of an individual by collecting information on personal and environmental strengths in eight life domains.
- The strengths assessment is ongoing, conversational, and captures *specific* talents and achievements of the person.
- The personal plan acts as the mutual agenda for work between the case manager and consumer, focusing on achievement of the goals the person has set.
- Natural community resources and people have primacy over formal mental health services when acquiring opportunities, social supports, and tangible resources.
- The strengths model does not ignore problems, but rather than placing them as the center of attention, they are considered obstacles to goal attainment.

REFERENCES AND RECOMMENDED READINGS

Kisthardt, W. (1993). An empowerment agenda for case management research: Evaluating the strengths model from the consumer perspective. In M. Harris & H. Bergman (Eds.), *Case management for mentally ill patients: Theory and practice* (pp. 165–182). Longhorn, PA: Harwood Academic.

Rapp, C. A., & Goscha, R. (2004). The principles of effective case management of mental health services. *Psychiatric Rehabilitation Journal, 27*(4), 319–333.

Rapp, C. A., & Goscha, R. (2006). *The strengths model: Case management with people with psychiatric disabilities.* New York: Oxford University Press.

Taylor, J. (1997). Niches and practice: Extending the ecological perspective. In D. Saleebey (Ed.), *The strengths perspective in social work practice* (2nd ed., pp. 217–228). Boston: Allyn & Bacon.

Weick, A., & Chamberlain, R. (2002). Putting problems in their place: Further exploration in the strengths perspective. In D. Saleebey (Ed.), *The strengths perspective in social work practice* (3rd ed., pp. 95–105). Boston: Allyn & Bacon.

CHAPTER 33

ASSERTIVE COMMUNITY TREATMENT

NATALIE L. DeLUCA
LORNA L. MOSER
GARY R. BOND

Assertive community treatment (ACT) is an approach to integrated, community-based care for people with severe mental illness (SMI) who, for a variety of reasons, may not engage in traditional mental health services. ACT was developed in the 1970s by Leonard Stein and Mary Ann Test and their colleagues in Madison, Wisconsin. The original program, Training in Community Living, was later named Program of Assertive Community Treatment (PACT). For nearly three decades, PACT has been regarded as a model of exemplary mental health practice. Over that time, service models adopting some PACT principles have proliferated worldwide, with a variety of different names, such as *the full service model, assertive outreach, mobile treatment teams,* and *continuous treatment teams.* ACT is the most widely used label for programs that share core ingredients with PACT.

ACT is not a clinical intervention itself; rather, it is a way of organizing services to provide concrete help essential for the community integration of clients with SMI. This distinction is important, because it suggests that implementing the structural elements of the model alone does not ensure that high-quality clinical interventions will occur; rather, ACT programs must attend to both clinical skills development and the more familiar model specifications.

Over time, a consensus view of ACT's critical elements has been established, the majority of which distinguish ACT from traditional services. ACT relies on a multidisciplinary group of mental health professionals who employ a team approach in providing a full range of clinical and rehabilitation services to individuals with SMI living within the community. Furthermore, ACT is designed to treat individuals with SMI who have not benefited from office-based outpatient treatment. On admission to ACT programs, ACT clients typically have experienced recurring difficulties in successful community living, indicated by any combination of frequent hospitalizations, incarceration, homelessness, substance abuse, and treatment nonadherence.

DESCRIPTION OF ACT

From the beginning, Stein and Test (1980) very clearly specified the critical elements of ACT. Although ACT has been modified and extended over the past several decades, the original formulation has endured remarkably well. According to both expert consensus and observations of mature ACT teams, the following are key features of the ACT model:

• *Multidisiciplinary staffing.* ACT teams include professionals from different disciplines whose expertise is necessary to provide comprehensive services. Because of the essential role of psychotropic medications for the treatment of SMI, the psychiatrist and nurse roles are essential. All ACT teams also have a group of generalist case managers who primarily attend to activities of daily living. The ACT model has evolved over time to include specialists from different disciplines, thus helping the team to expand the range of services it can provide. Practitioners who specialize in providing housing assistance, employment services, and treatment of substance use disorders should be included on a fully staffed ACT team. Psychotherapists, psychologists, social workers, and occupational therapists may also be included. Many teams have found that employing clients in recovery as peer support specialists has provided a valuable addition to their service.

• *Team approach.* ACT teams have shared caseloads in which several team members work collaboratively with each client. The ACT team meets daily to share client updates, to coordinate services, to identify crises needing immediate attention, and to help plan ongoing treatment and rehabilitation efforts. The entire team is responsible to each client, with different team members contributing their expertise as appropriate. One advantage to the team approach is increased continuity of care over time. The team approach also appears to reduce staff burnout: Although the mechanisms are not precisely known, this benefit is thought to be due to the shared responsibility and mutual support that helps reduce strain in difficult treatment situations, and the opportunity to access team resources and its problem-solving capacity as needed.

• *Integration of services.* In most communities, the social service system is fragmented, with different agencies and programs responsible for different aspects of the client's care. Through a multidisciplinary team approach, the ACT team provides integrated services that address treatment issues (e.g., medications, physical health care, symptom control), rehabilitation issues (e.g., employment, activities of living, interpersonal relationships, housing), substance abuse treatment, practical assistance, social services, family services, and other services according to the needs and goals of each client. The advantages of integrated approaches over *brokered* approaches (i.e., referring clients to other programs for services) are well documented.

• *Low client–staff ratios.* Client–staff ratios are small enough to ensure adequate individualization of services; most guidelines suggest no more than a 10:1 ratio. In recent years it has been increasingly recognized that the client–staff ratio needs to take into account caseload characteristics. For clients with the most debilitating conditions, an even smaller ratio may be optimal, whereas for clients who are more stable, a ratio of up to 20:1 may be appropriate. When caseloads are too large, case management services are clearly ineffective.

• *Locus of contact in the community.* All members of the ACT team make home visits. Most contacts with clients and others involved in their treatment (e.g., family members) occur in clients' homes or in community settings, not in mental health offices. In the ACT model, at least 80% of contacts occur out of the office, although some types of office contact are appropriate. *In vivo* contacts—that is, interventions in the natural settings in which clients live, work, and interact with others—are more useful than interventions in hospital or office settings, as they reduce the challenges that arise when transferring skills taught in the hospital or clinic to real-world settings. In addition, assessment in real-world settings is more valid than office-based assessment, because practitioners can observe behavior directly rather than depend on client self-report. Home visits also facilitate medication delivery, problem solving, crisis intervention, and networking.

- *Medication management.* Effective use of medications is a top priority for ACT, necessitating careful diagnosis and assessment of target symptoms, well-reasoned choices of medications, appropriate dosing and duration of therapy, and management of side effects, in accordance with evidence-based practice (EBP) guidelines. ACT teams often deliver medications to clients, tailoring this assistance to the unique needs (and, to the greatest extent possible, the preferences) of the client, thus increasing appropriate use of medications.

- *Focus on everyday problems in living.* ACT teams focus on assisting clients in a wide range of ordinary daily activities and chores, depending on a client's most pressing needs (e.g., securing housing, keeping appointments, cashing checks, and shopping). Because ACT teams facilitate increased independence among clients, they also help clients learn to develop skills and supports in natural settings.

- *Rapid access.* ACT teams differ sharply from most social services in that they respond quickly to client emergencies, even when they occur after regular business hours. From the first conceptualization of this model, the goal for this program element has been 24-hour coverage. In a proactive ACT team that communicates well, staff members often find ways to anticipate and respond to potential problem situations, which helps to prevent crises from erupting. ACT teams involved in client admissions to and discharges from hospitals facilitate continuity of care.

- *Assertive outreach.* In targeting a more challenging clinical population, including clients who are unlikely to seek out help on their own and may be resistant to help when it is offered, ACT teams must develop strategies to engage reluctant clients, both in the initial stages of assessment and after enrollment. ACT teams are persistent in their offer of help; for example, they do not disenroll clients who miss appointments. Outreach efforts should focus on relationship building by establishing rapport in a manner that enhances client motivation to engage with the team, even if mental health issues are not immediately addressed. Initial outreach should include offers of tangible assistance, especially with regard to finances and housing. Some ACT teams have a client assistance fund to pay for emergency expenses, a helpful engagement tool that allows teams to be flexible and responsive to client needs.

- *Individualized services.* Treatments and supports are individualized to accommodate the needs and preferences of each client. Truly individualized services foster a personally meaningful recovery process that may be neglected in other treatment settings. Because of their broad knowledge of community resources and the wherewithal to access them, ACT teams often increase available options beyond what clients would otherwise have (e.g., increased access to housing).

- *Time-unlimited services.* In most ACT programs, rather than "graduating" from the program when their situation stabilizes, clients continue to receive ACT assistance on a long-term basis. This allows for the development of stable, trusting therapeutic relationships. This principle follows from studies suggesting that clients regress when terminated from intensive, short-term programs. As discussed below, there is growing evidence that this principle should be modified for clients who show substantial improvement.

As noted earlier, ACT is regarded to be an organizational framework for delivering services rather than a specific clinical intervention itself. Increasingly, practice guidelines for ACT have incorporated major EBPs, such as illness self-management, medication guidelines, supported employment, integrated treatment for dual disorders, and family psychoeducation. One great advantage is that ACT is completely compatible with these EBPs; in fact, preliminary work in conceptualizing and developing several of these practices first occurred within the context of ACT teams.

Implementing ACT Services

Clear program guidelines, as established by practice manuals, state standards, or other formalized means, help to define the structural foundation of an ACT team. Published standards prescribe the qualifications of practitioners who should be hired, how many clients the team should take on, and how often to provide services. Studies of ACT implementation efforts have shown that these types of structural program elements are more readily put into place than are process-oriented program elements, such as individualization of services. It is critical to include the key *structural* elements that define ACT services, but to serve clients best (particularly to facilitate recovery rather than maintenance), key *clinical* elements must be included in the process of delivering ACT. Crucial clinical practices include assessment, treatment planning, and clinical supervision. These clinical elements are discussed in more detail in the final section of the chapter.

Target Population

There is now broad consensus that it is neither practical nor necessary to provide ACT programs universally to all clients with SMI. Instead, ACT is typically reserved for a relatively small minority of clients who have not benefited from usual outpatient services. Most ACT programs target individuals with SMI who do not respond well to less intensive care modalities (e.g., who fail to keep office appointments) and are frequent users of emergency psychiatric services, especially inpatient care. ACT teams have been conceptualized in several ways with respect to admission criteria. The first is to facilitate the discharge of long-term inpatients, a strategy that has gained renewed currency with the closing and downsizing of state and provincial hospitals. A second conceptualization is to employ ACT as an alternative to admission for acutely ill patients—so-called "deflection" programs. Similarly, ACT teams have also been used as an alternative to arrest and incarceration for persons with SMI and a long history of criminal justice system involvement. The third and most common use is to maintain unstable, long-term clients (sometimes referred to as "revolving-door" clients) in the community. Some programs specialize further in outreach to clients with a dual diagnosis of mental illness and substance use disorders who are homeless, or to those entangled with the criminal justice system. It is estimated that in a well-functioning mental health system, approximately 15–20% of clients with SMI would benefit from ACT services. If the service system is deficient, more ACT teams may be required to fill service gaps. In less populated areas, the percentage of SMI clients who fit ACT admission criteria may be even lower.

Contraindications for Use

Evidence from both research and clinical practice suggests that ACT is very flexible across a wide range of clients. Its effectiveness has been reported for clients from many different cultural backgrounds. Experience suggests that ACT teams are well suited for both young adults and older adults. Differences in gender, education, and other background characteristics have not been reported as factors limiting the effectiveness of ACT.

Moreover, client background characteristics do not predict satisfaction with ACT services.

One of the appealing features of ACT is adaptability for many different types of clients who do *not* benefit from conventional services, as discussed earlier. Based on cost considerations, ACT teams are not recommended for clients who have already attained high levels of self-management of their illness. Based purely on clinical considerations, however, ACT services have been found to be beneficial to clients spanning a wide spectrum of symptom severity and disability.

Step-Down ACT Programs

As previously discussed, the ACT model was originally conceived of as a time-unlimited service. There is now greater recognition that some clients will likely graduate once they attain their recovery goals. Increasingly, program planners have adopted "tiered" case management systems in which different levels of case management intensity are aimed at different levels of client need. Transferring ACT clients to less intensive case management services appears to be more successful if the transfers are gradual and individualized. Furthermore, the "step-down" programs to which clients are transferred should follow ACT principles but provide service at a lesser intensity. There also should be flexibility in movement back and forth between different tiers for such an approach to be maximally effective.

EVIDENCE IN SUPPORT OF ACT

ACT is one of the six practices identified as evidence-based by the National Implementing Evidence-Based Practices Project. It is one of the most extensively researched models of community care for people with SMI. The evidence for the effectiveness of ACT is quite consistent across numerous reviews that have appeared in the literature. Compared to usual community care, ACT has been found to be more successful in engaging clients in treatment. Additionally, ACT substantially reduces psychiatric hospital use and increases housing stability, and moderately improves symptoms and subjective quality of life.

Mental health service planners are increasingly attentive to the need to establish program standards and monitor implementation. Based on the premise that better implemented ACT programs have better client outcomes, it becomes critical to develop methods for assessing the degree to which programs follow the ACT model. *Fidelity* is the term used to denote adherence to the standards of a program model, and a measure used to assess the degree to which a specific program meets the standards for a program model is known as a *fidelity scale*. The best known and most widely used of these fidelity scales is the Dartmouth ACT Fidelity Scale (DACTS). Several studies have suggested that more carefully implemented ACT programs have better outcomes, such as reduced number of hospitalization days, greater retention in service, and higher client satisfaction. These fidelity studies have further bolstered the argument that ACT is indeed an EBP. Notably, fidelity, as measured by the DACTS, captures mainly the structural components of the model; current plans to expand and revise this scale to include key clinical processes will allow for fuller assessment of the model.

Negative Outcomes from ACT

The ACT literature has been very consistent in suggesting an *absence* of negative outcomes. Significantly, surveys suggest that a greater number of clients receiving ACT services compared to usual services are mostly satisfied, and satisfaction with ACT services is similar for individuals of different backgrounds.

Nevertheless, it is worth noting that some critics of the ACT model argue that ACT programs are coercive or paternalistic, and that they are not based on client choice. The basis of this criticism derives mostly from anecdotes and theoretical arguments rather than empirical studies. Recent studies have attempted to examine systematically the use of coercion by outpatient teams (including ACT), both from practitioner and client perspectives. From the few existing studies examining this issue, it appears that at least a small percentage of clients served by an ACT team are formally coerced (e.g., legally committed to receive treatment) by the team at some time. However, these studies noted that clients more frequently encountered informal coercion throughout treatment, such as threats of commitment and making services or resources (e.g., money, housing) contingent on treatment compliance or abstinence from drugs or alcohol. A recent study of clients' perceptions of ACT indicated that whereas clients were positive about their ACT experience overall, some negative experiences included conflicts with staff about medications and money management, and promotion of authoritative rather than collaborative practices.

One large-scale survey that examined interventions used by ACT teams to influence client behavior found that case managers reported using techniques spanning a range of tactics from low levels of coercion (e.g., merely ignoring a behavior) to high levels of coercion (e.g., committing a client to the hospital against their will). Verbal persuasion was widely reported, whereas the more coercive interventions were reported for less than 10% of clients. Case managers used more influencing tactics with clients who had more extensive hospitalization histories, more symptoms, more arrests, more recent substance use, and who reported a weaker sense of alliance with staff. The results of an ACT client satisfaction survey suggested that clients were least satisfied on dimensions related to client choice. Moreover, complaints about ACT services are more frequent in ACT programs with low model fidelity.

Characteristics of both the ACT model (e.g., use of assertive engagement and high frequency of community-based contacts) and clients targeted for ACT services (e.g., difficult to engage in less intensive services) may heighten the potential for more coercion and less collaboration in the treatment process. Each day, ACT teams confront many thorny conflicts between clients' expressed preferences and what team members feel are the best interests of clients. Ideally, client choice is promoted, and coercion is used minimally and with discretion. By helping clients avoid hospitalization (including involuntary commitments), ACT enables them to live more normal lives and in this respect increases client choice. Moreover, ACT teams often expand the range of opportunities for clients with respect to where they can live, whether or not they can find work, and whether they have an income. Again, the extent to which ACT teams truly promote client choice may be related to their degree of fidelity to the model, as well as practitioner training and skillfulness, and agency-level culture and processes. Research in the use of coercive tactics of ACT teams and other mental health services continues to develop.

RECOMMENDATIONS FOR ACT PRACTICE

Providing ACT services first requires a strong structural framework to support the specific requirements of the model. Several basic steps to follow when implementing ACT or any EBP have been published. The steps include making systematic efforts to identify and to build consensus among key stakeholders in a community, locating appropriate funding mechanisms, identifying leadership within an organization, and developing a plan for implementation that includes training, supervision, and program monitoring. Numerous resources are emerging to help in the implementation of ACT. In recent years, detailed practice manuals have become available. In addition, the National Implementing EBP Project developed materials that aid implementation, including materials translated into Spanish. The National Alliance on Mental Illness (NAMI) has a technical assistance center to promote ACT dissemination and has given special attention to the methods for building consensus in a community among family members and clients. In the remainder of this section we present brief recommendations for the roles of different stakeholders in ACT implementation.

State mental health authorities have an important role in the success of ACT program implementation. States that have established standards to define requirements for accrediting ACT programs have done so with the intent of increasing program fidelity. Another role for state mental health authorities is to ensure stable and adequate funding. In some states this has necessitated the arduous process of revising the state Medicaid plan. A state-level technical assistance center can provide new teams with support in resource acquisition, along with ongoing consultation and training. In some cases, technical assistance centers may also help to monitor implementation progress and work with teams to develop performance improvement plans.

At the agency administrator level, careful decisions about staff hiring, especially for supervisory positions, are an important element in the success of an ACT team. ACT services are aimed at clients with high service needs and an array of complicating life circumstances. The level of clinical skill among team members should be sufficiently high to meet the challenge of providing intensive, recovery-oriented ACT services. Ongoing training specifically geared toward clinical skills development among practitioners should be a priority at all levels of any organization that offers ACT services. ACT teams work best when they admit clients at a controlled rate. Commitment from all levels of the organization, including the patience to endure the inevitable challenges and ambiguities of the start-up phase, is also necessary. Ongoing monitoring of program implementation is another critical step in successful implementation.

Support from mental health authorities at the state and local levels, along with commitment and support from agency administration, is necessary to provide a foundation for sustaining ACT services; however, equally important efforts must be made at the practitioner and team levels to ensure that high-quality ACT is implemented. A knowledgeable, empowered team leader is the linchpin of successful ACT.

A team leader should manage both clinical and administrative aspects of the team's functioning. On the administrative side, team leaders should have considerable authority with respect to both hiring decisions and taking disciplinary action when appropriate. Team leaders should be informed of relevant program model expectations and maintain service data records that document compliance with these expectations. It is helpful to work in tandem with agency billing and/or information management departments to provide regular reports of frequency and intensity of services, location of service, and other data deemed relevant to managing ACT team practice. These data are also useful in monitoring program implementation over time.

Team leaders should ensure their team's participation in monitoring efforts; external review is an excellent way to gauge program fidelity, the team's development over time, and to help establish team plans and goals for strategic improvements in service. If external review is not available, team leaders can use published resources to monitor the team's progress. Team leaders should also ensure that client outcome data are tracked and used to guide team goal setting.

A team leader is a liaison between higher administration and the frontline staff. One key responsibility is to ensure support for adequate clinical training and supervision opportunities specific to the needs of ACT team members. Identifying team needs and ensuring access to practical supports for the team, such as individual cell phones, moderated billing requirements, and personal computers, are also important duties of team leaders.

In the ACT model, a team leader must strike a balance between the considerable administrative responsibilities and his or her role as a lead clinician. It is important that the team leader model good clinical practice and remain connected to clients through some provision of direct clinical services. Additionally, the team leader should take responsibility for ensuring that all team members receive regular *client-centered supervision* (i.e., specifically focusing on clients' needs, and barriers encountered and strategies used to meet these needs). In some cases, other senior team members, such as the psychiatrist, can help share the duties of clinical supervision.

Elements of High-Quality Clinical Practice in ACT

Once the supportive structure is in place, ACT team members must work together clinically in a way that supports recovery for all clients. Regular, frequent clinical supervision provides a necessary forum for addressing persistent concerns creatively and enhancing the skills of all team members. Another strategy for enhancement of services is to promote cross-training between members of different disciplines within the team. Structured cross-training allows all team members to share their expertise, while building capacity for truly integrated service from the team as a whole. A well-established, meaningful assessment and treatment planning process can help to tie all these elements together.

When a client is referred to the ACT team, an initial 30-day assessment period is recommended. During this time, the team members work together to engage the client, while collecting relevant pieces of a comprehensive biopsychosocial assessment. This provides the starting point for ACT services, while enabling a thoughtful determination of whether ACT services are suitable for the client. It should be noted, however, that assessment within ACT is fluid and ongoing; once the initial assessment is made, additional information is always incorporated as it is learned. The comprehensive assessment should help to identify areas in which the client may benefit from ACT services. The next step is to create an individualized treatment plan.

Treatment planning should be a collaborative process between the client and the ACT team (or a subset of the team, depending on team size and areas of expertise). Ongoing engagement with each client is vital to building a meaningful working relationship. Particularly in a team-based approach to care, a treatment plan helps to ensure understanding and investment of all key players in the client's recovery journey. Thus, rather than being regarded as a paperwork burden, treatment plans are tools to be used by the team and the client to guide interventions, delineate responsibilities, and to measure progress toward goals. Working from client-centered, meaningful treatment plans helps the team to remain accountable for providing individualized services, a hallmark of the ACT model. Treatment plans should be created with the client's input, written in language and from a perspective that is meaningful to the client, and referenced and updated routinely to assess how well the team is supporting the plan for recovery. In ACT programs, whereas the clinical practices related to assessment and treatment planning have been observed to be among the most important aspects of fully realized ACT service, they simultaneously have been the most resistant aspects to change and improvement.

In summary, the ACT model is an enduring, effective method for organizing services to help clients who experience an extraordinary level of disability. To provide effective

ACT services, practitioners must not only adhere to the structural features of the model but also develop the necessary skills to deliver integrated, comprehensive treatment that promotes recovery for the clients they serve.

KEY POINTS

- ACT is a clearly defined model that, when carefully implemented, has been shown to reduce psychiatric hospitalizations greatly and increase housing stability, while moderately impacting psychiatric symptoms and quality of life.
- ACT is appropriate for individuals with schizophrenia spectrum disorders, with the most persistent and devastating levels of impairment, who have not successfully engaged with less intensive, office-based mental health services.
- Well-run ACT programs must attend to both clinical skills development and model specifications.
- The ACT organizational framework is well suited to implementation of evidence-based clinical interventions, such as illness self-management, medication guidelines, supported employment, integrated dual-disorder treatment, and family psychoeducation.
- Ongoing quality improvement efforts based on monitoring fidelity to the ACT model and valued client outcomes should be a part of any ACT team's practice.
- In providing ACT services, it is important to promote client choice, recovery, and meaningful community integration, and to be particularly sensitive to the promotion of these values when considering the intensive, assertive nature of ACT services.
- A good ACT team requires an empowered team leader, and sufficient organizational support to implement the model fully.

REFERENCES AND RECOMMENDED READINGS

Adams, N., & Grieder, D. (2005). *Treatment planning for person-centered care: The road to mental health and addiction recovery.* Burlington, MA: Elsevier Academic Press.

Allness, D. J., & Knoedler, W. H. (2003). *The PACT model of community-based treatment for persons with severe and persistent mental illness: A manual for PACT start-up* (2nd ed.). Arlington, VA: National Alliance on Mental Illness.

Assertive Community Treatment Implementation Resource Kit. (2003). SAMHSA Center for Mental Health Services. Available online at *www.mentalhealth.samhsa.gov/cmhs/communitysupport/toolkits/community/*

Backlar, P., & Cutler, D. L. (Eds.). (2002). *Ethics in community mental health care: Commonplace concerns.* New York: Kluwer Academic/Plenum Press.

Bond, G. R., Drake, R. E., Mueser, K. T., & Latimer, E. (2001). Assertive community treatment for people with severe mental illness: Critical ingredients and impact on patients. *Disease Management and Health Outcomes, 9,* 141–159.

Coldwell, C. M., & Bender, W. S. (2007). The effectiveness of assertive community treatment for homeless populations with severe mental illness: A meta-analysis. *American Journal of Psychiatry, 164,* 393–399.

Corrigan, P. W. (2002). Empowerment and serious mental illness: Treatment partnerships and community opportunities. *Psychiatric Quarterly, 73*(3), 217–228.

Coursey, R. D., Curtis, L., Marsh, D. T., Campbell, J., Harding, C., Spaniol, L., et al. (2000). Competencies for direct service staff members who work with adults with severe mental illnesses: Specific knowledge, attitudes, skills, and bibliography. *Psychiatric Rehabilitation Journal, 23*(4), 378–392.

Krupa, T., Eastabrook, S., Hern, L., Lee, D., North, R., Percy, K., et al. (2005). How do people who receive assertive community treatment experience this service? *Psychiatric Rehabilitation Journal, 29,* 18–24.

Monahan, J., Redlich, A. D., Swanson, J., Robbins, P. C., Appelbaum, P., Petrila, J., et al. (2005). Use of leverage to improve adherence to psychiatric treatment in the community. *Psychiatric Services, 56,* 37–44.

Phillips, S. D., Burns, B. J., Edgar, E. R., Mueser, K. T., Linkins, K. W., Rosenheck, R. A., et al. (2001). Moving assertive community treatment into standard practice. *Psychiatric Services, 52,* 771–779.

Rapp, C. A. (1998). The active ingredients of effective case management: A research synthesis. *Community Mental Health Journal, 34,* 363–380.

Stein, L. I., & Santos, A. B. (1998). *Assertive community treatment of persons with severe mental illness.* New York: Norton.

Stein, L. I., & Test, M. A. (1980). An alternative to mental health treatment: I. Conceptual model, treatment program, and clinical evaluation. *Archives of General Psychiatry, 37,* 392–397.

Teague, G. B., Bond, G. R., & Drake, R. E. (1998). Program fidelity in assertive community treatment: Development and use of a measure. *American Journal of Orthopsychiatry, 68,* 216–232.

van Veldhuizen, J. R. (in press). A Dutch version of ACT. *Community Mental Health Journal.*

CHAPTER 34

EMERGENCY, INPATIENT, AND RESIDENTIAL TREATMENT

MOUNIR SOLIMAN
ANTONIO M. SANTOS
JAMES B. LOHR

Although the current goal of treatment for patients with schizophrenia is to maintain clinical stability in an outpatient setting, patients often require treatment in more secure environments. These treatment venues usually take the form of emergency rooms, inpatient services, or residential programs. In this chapter we outline the primary characteristics and approaches to each of these secured-environment treatments.

EMERGENCY ROOM ISSUES IN THE TREATMENT OF SCHIZOPHRENIA

Reasons for Emergency Room Visits

There are several common reasons for patients with schizophrenia to be seen in emergency rooms. In many cases, relatively minor clinical reasons, such as running out of medication or having a recent outpatient visit canceled, are the cause of the visit; such visits may not actually be associated with a worsening of psychopathology or a change in environment, but may instead be more reflective of judgment problems or chronic, underlying paranoid ideation. It is important to keep in mind that if such visits for minor reasons are frequent for a given patient, the clinician must address these with, for example, more refills for prescriptions or connection to a system in which the patient may call in with problems. If many patients at a facility are seeking emergency visits for such issues, then the institution should consider setting up alternatives, such as a walk-in medication refill clinic, or a 24-hour hotline or "warmline" (for less critical problems).

Oftentimes, emergency room visits are for more severe problems, such as thoughts of harm or increasing paranoia and confusion. Patients in an acute crisis may become a problem for their families, friends, or even the police. They may be either unable to take care of themselves or a threat to self or others. Because of their condition, they may require monitoring on a 24-hour basis inside an inpatient unit.

In more severe cases, patients may present themselves to the emergency room with issues such as suicidal or homicidal thoughts; if this occurs, it is important to recognize and subsequently relay to the patients that their presentation to the emergency room for help actually reflects good judgment on their part. Focusing on the positive aspects of the situation is crucial, because patients are often aware that they are having a setback or exacerbation, which may be upsetting to them, and this upset alone can contribute to the overall worsening of their condition. By reframing a patient's visit to the emergency room as a reflection of his or her good judgment, the physician can be very helpful in contributing to the patient's recovery from a crisis.

However, many patients do not come to emergency settings on their own, but are instead brought by family members, board and care operators, conservators, or police. Such patients may be reluctant, confused, lacking in insight, and occasionally combative, and often are likely to require inpatient stabilization. In these challenging situations, the experience of the physician is critical to minimize the crisis effectively rather than worsen it.

Basic Approaches to Assessment and Treatment in the Emergency Room

The most important guiding principle in treatment is *safety*—for the patient and the staff. Safety begins with the physical structure and layout of the emergency room. To have a single clinician interview an acutely psychotic patient in a small room that contains sharp objects, in which the door opens inwardly (and can be shut by the patient and not easily opened from the outside), invites problems and should be avoided. There should instead be easy access for multiple staff to enter and exit, while maintaining the patient's privacy. Additionally, a system for panic alert, consisting of either buttons or switches physically placed in discreet locations, or as a part of a pager system, is critical. An appropriate code system for assaultive behavior is also essential, with a clearly identified team of individuals who have received appropriate training in the management of assaultive behavior. Although individual sites vary in the ways they deal with the possibility that a patient is carrying a weapon, a security system does need to be in place; sometimes this involves the use of metal detectors or gowning patients upon entry.

Another important goal is *stabilization* of the situation. Again, the structure of the emergency setting can play a role, because it is more difficult to stabilize patients if they are being evaluated in an area where trauma victims or other extremely intense medical issues are also being addressed. After the safety of the situation has been optimized, stabilization generally involves addressing whatever led to the exacerbation of illness or the reasons for the emergency room visit. For example, if there has been an acute change in the patient's environment or the development of a family crisis, psychosocial or family interventions alone may allow for stabilization of the situation, without a change in medication management or a need for admission to a more restrictive environment. In cases in which an exacerbation was caused by environmental issues, the structured setting of an emergency room, or simply the change from the previous environment, can sometimes dramatically contribute to the stabilization of the patient.

When dealing with patients in acute psychotic states, it is important to be aware of and take into consideration *medical causes*. There may be a tendency for clinicians to assume that an increase in psychosis simply represents a worsening in the underlying schizophrenic illness. Many patients have an exacerbation related to medical causes however (infections, thyroid problems, etc.). Therefore, a full physical examination should be performed on patients who have acute exacerbations of illness; this also includes an investigation of drug or alcohol intake, which frequently contributes to psychotic worsening. It is important to be aware that exacerbations of symptoms caused by drug and alcohol abuse, which lead to psychiatric destabilization, can sometimes be managed by simply waiting for the drug effects to dissipate.

Many patients can be rapidly stabilized in the emergency room setting, then discharged to their original environment. In some cases, stabilization can be accomplished in a few hours. However, many emergency facilities have special policies and procedures that allow for longer stays, frequently up to 24 hours, after which the patient may have to be admitted or considered for admission. Some facilities have designated areas for the purpose of longer stays that are often quieter and geographically distant from the more central medical- and trauma-oriented areas.

Psychopharmacological Management in Emergency Rooms

Patients frequently require psychopharmacological intervention, which can promote more rapid stabilization given the use of appropriate agents. In many cases, the cause for exacerbation of schizophrenic illness is related to reduced medication intake, which perhaps may be due to adherence problems, stolen medications, or the patient's inability to receive or obtain medications. Sometimes, when it is difficult to ascertain whether the patient has been adherent to a medication regimen, obtaining blood levels of medications can be useful. If a patient is on a medication that requires periodic monitoring of serum level, such as lithium or valproate, checking the level can then serve two purposes—as an indicator of both therapeutic level and adherence.

Even when the cause of symptom exacerbation is medical or psychosocial in nature, psychopharmacological intervention may be helpful in reducing symptoms and agitation. In general, antipsychotic medications are most commonly used to reduce symptoms acutely and stabilize the patient. The choice of medication is dependent on the specific issues of the patient. Often, patients who have had adherence problems may be placed once again on their initial treatment regimen, although an attempt should be made to address the cause of the nonadherence. Otherwise, high-potency antipsychotics are often used (either first- or second-generation drugs), according to either the clinical needs of the patient or any formulary restrictions of the facility.

Confidentiality and Release of Information

Patient confidentiality is an extremely important issue that should always be maintained, particularly in an emergency room environment, which can become pressured and chaotic. The American Medical Association, the American Psychiatric Association, and the American Association of Psychiatry and the Law all have ethical guidelines. As a general rule, information exchanged between the patient and the clinician is confidential. However, exceptions include situations in which the patient is a danger to self or others, expresses the intent to commit a crime, is a suspected victim of child abuse, is involved in civil commitment proceedings or court-ordered examination, or has certain medical emergencies. Facility rules and regulations may not exist for every possible situation, in which case, clinicians must use their best judgment. However, clinical decisions should be based *not* on concern for avoiding litigation, but on what is best at the time for the safety of the patient and of others, and treatment of the patient.

Although complex, the *Tarasoff* principle (*Tarasoff v. Regents of the University of California*, 1976), which is not standard for all states, provides a commonly used legal framework for decision making when third parties are being threatened (Felthous, 1999). According to the California Supreme Court decision, the principle, known as *Tarasoff* II (1976) reads:

> When a psychotherapist determines, or pursuant to the standards of his profession should determine, that his patient presents a serious danger of violence to another, he incurs an obligation to use reasonable care to protect the intended victim against such danger. The discharge of this duty may require the therapist to take one or more of various steps, depending upon the nature of the case. Thus it may call for him to warn the intended victim or others likely to apprise the victim of the danger, to notify the police, or to take whatever steps are reasonably necessary under the circumstances. (p. 2)

It is best to do as much as possible, which includes warning the intended victim *and* notifying the police. Felthous (1999, pp. 51–57) has delineated four key questions to ask in the process of evaluation for disclosures of information:

1. Is the patient dangerous to others?
2. Is the danger due to serious mental illness?
3. Is the danger imminent?
4. Is the danger targeted at identifiable victims?

Release of information is largely guided by the Health Insurance Portability and Accountability Act (HIPAA) of 1996. Information covered by the confidentiality standards comprises all clinical and all financial information related to that patient's care, including the patient's financial status. All information must be kept in a secure environment and not be taken off site except in keeping with regulations, such as a response to a subpoena or a direct transfer of patient care. Exceptions to the disclosure of information include having patient consent for release of information or certain emergency situations (in which case an attempt should be made to obtain consent as soon as possible).

Disposition

Although many patients can be discharged back to their original environment, this is frequently not feasible, and a more restrictive level of care is often necessary. The detailed individual disposition is often highly dependent on the array and availability of local services. Moreover, it is generally critical to have Department of Social Services involvement in this process. The disposition of patients with schizophrenia is a complex issue that requires health care staff to be knowledgeable about available services, about the resources that may be most relevant and beneficial to the needs of the current patient, and about how to access these programs. This frequently time-consuming process is very worthwhile in terms of reducing recidivism and maintaining stability.

INPATIENT TREATMENT OF SCHIZOPHRENIA

Voluntary and Involuntary Treatment

There are basically two types of admission to an inpatient facility—voluntary and involuntary. Some inpatient units allow voluntary admissions to the facility, in which case informed consent is required; these patients may then sign out of the hospital at any time. Following the principle of least restrictive treatment, it is often recommended that patients be offered the option of voluntary admission even when there are grounds for involuntary admission. Clinical judgment and experience is required here, and there may be differences in local rules and regulations governing these decisions. For patients with state-appointed conservators of person, the conservator can authorize admission to the hospital.

The rules for involuntary commitment, as well as for the different types of commitment and lengths of time, are set by the states, and vary from state to state. Generally, there are three reasons for commitment—danger to self, danger to others, or inability to care for oneself (grave disability). Usually several different specific time lengths for the involuntary commitment period are available. There is often one type of short-term commitment for further medical evaluation and treatment, and rapid stabilization (usually for a period of days, often 3 days), and another type that may often follow the shorter one, involving a longer period (in terms of weeks) for more comprehensive evaluation and further treatment stabilization. Of course, involuntarily committed patients still have rights, which in some cases may include the right to refuse medication. In California, for example, a special hearing is required to medicate patients who refuse treatment, even if they are involuntarily committed.

The Goals of Treatment and the Interdisciplinary Treatment Plan

The primary goals of treatment in an inpatient setting are stabilization and discharge. Discharge planning begins with the very first encounter with the patient; primary problems with clearly identifiable goals should be ascertained. At the interdisciplinary treatment planning meeting, which takes place as early as possible in the admission process, these goals should be formalized and the approaches to treatment documented. A discharge date set at this time can always be modified later, depending on clinical improvement.

The Physical Structure of an Inpatient Psychiatric Facility

Once again, an inpatient unit should be designed with safety in mind. Critical issues include visibility, access, and a generally safe environment with breakaway fixtures and other safety features. Visibility can be optimized by having a centrally located nursing station with large windows. Group rooms should be comfortable, quiet, and designed with minimal likelihood for distraction. In areas in which there are culs-de-sac or other places with poor visibility (e.g., seclusion rooms), mirrors or closed-circuit cameras can be used. Facilities that accept involuntary admissions generally have available seclusion rooms that are designed to provide minimal environmental stimulation, thus allowing for environmental stabilization of patients in acute psychiatric states. Special guidelines, regulations, and accountability practices required for seclusion vary from facility to facility but generally adhere to Joint Commission on Accreditation of Healthcare Organizations (JCAHO) standards.

Length-of-Stay Issues

One of the biggest challenges in the development of inpatient treatment programs is the need to provide a therapeutic experience despite patients' length of hospital stay, which has shortened over the years. Many facilities are still utilizing treatment models (e.g., certain forms of group treatment) designed to be administered over weeks, even though the length of stay may only be on the order of 7–10 days. The program design must take into account the various conditons of patients in a setting with fairly rapid patient turnover. Thus, group strategies oriented toward understanding medication and adherence, activities of daily living, and other relevant "here-and-now" issues are more important than in-depth dynamically based approaches that dwell on past problems. The length of stay is generally brief, so the therapies need to be brief as well. Behaviorally based approaches should be short-term in nature and focus on critical current problems.

Medical and Psychopharmacological Management

All patients admitted to an inpatient unit should have a thorough medical examination. It is not unusual to see medical conditions mask or create psychiatric symptoms, and mimic idiopathic psychiatric disorders. For example, abuse of drugs such as cocaine, methamphetamine, and phencyclidine (PCP) can result in schizophrenia-like conditions. Also, patients who receive treatment for chronic obstructive pulmonary disease (COPD) or medications such as prednisone for asthma may develop psychoses as well.

Some psychotropic medications are considered unsafe in the presence of certain medical conditions. For example, a patient with an immune disorder should not be treated with clozapine, which can cause agranulocytosis. Some antipsychotic medications affect cardiac conductivity; for this reason, an electrocardiogram (ECG) is required before initiation of such medications. After the assessment of vital signs, it is important to obtain basic lab work, urine drug screens, ECGs, and other specific tests to screen for medical disorders at the time of a psychiatric admission. Only when medical conditions have been ruled out as a direct or indirect cause of the psychiatric symptoms can the patient be diagnosed with a psychiatric disorder.

Because stabilization of patients more often than not requires polypharmacy, special attention should be given to side effect profiles and drug–drug interactions. However, it is also important to remember that many patients are admitted because they are overmedicated, often with several medications, so it is critical to evaluate completely the drug regimen and obtain appropriate blood levels of any patient admitted, and discontinue medications that may be unnecessary or detrimental to the patient.

Patients who have persistently aggressive behavior in the emergency room and in the inpatient unit often present a special challenge to treatment, and rapid stabilization is essential; this can usually be achieved with antipsychotic medications. Benzodiazepines, beta-blockers, or mood-stabilizing drugs may also be helpful and are often used in combination with antipsychotic drugs.

An important yet often neglected concept in psychopharmacological inpatient treatment is the continuing availability of drugs used during the inpatient service, after the patient has been discharged. Significant care problems can result when medications that patients begin taking on an inpatient unit are unavailable to them (because of cost or outpatient formulary restrictions) after discharge. The high cost of medication affects the accessibility of many drugs, particularly for unfunded patients. Sample medications and patient assistant programs sponsored by pharmaceutical companies are often used by community clinics to offset the high cost of psychotropic medications. Many community clinics use a drug formulary to manage pharmacy costs. Despite efforts on multiple levels, the cost of medication still has a crippling impact on providing continuing care for patients with schizophrenia. It is crucial for unfunded mentally ill patients to obtain publicly funded insurance to cover medications costs as quickly as possible, and this process should be started on the inpatient unit, if possible. Providing patients with financial assistance, such as Social Security Disability, helps them to maintain a stable living situation, which subsequently might decrease the chance of relapse and rehospitalization.

Physical Restraint and Seclusion Policies

Restraint refers to physically restraining individuals—and not chemical restraint, which is generally considered an invalid or poorly defined concept. The use of physical restraint is an acceptable treatment modality, but it should be used after all less restrictive modalities have been carefully considered. Restraints should be individualized, and the least restrictive type of restraint should be used for the shortest possible period of time, with frequent reassessment of the ongoing need for it. Acceptable uses for restraints include prevention of imminent harm to the patient or others when alternative means are ineffective or inappropriate; prevention of disruption of the treatment program, or of violence or damage to the environment; decreasing stimulation of the patient as a part of the treatment plan, or at the request of the patient, if the clinical treatment team is in agreement.

Care must be taken to ensure that the rights and dignity of the patient are upheld, and that the patient is a part of the decision-making process to the greatest extent possible. Seclusion rooms can be used for multiple purposes, including isolation and reduction of sensory stimulation of the patient for short, temporary periods (time-outs), as well as settings for the use of physical restraints. Although restraints may be administered in a seclusion room, they can also be used in other settings, as is often the case for patients with schizophrenia who are in general medical or intensive care unit settings.

Once the decision is made to utilize restraints, the process should be carried out quickly and effectively, with adequate staff present to ensure safety. The team of individuals involved should have experience and training in the relevant processes. Orders should be time-limited, and should never be administered on an as-needed basis. Observation should be frequent (or constant, in some cases), and documentation should be regular and thorough. Furthermore, documentation should provide justification for the continuing need for restraint.

RESIDENTIAL TREATMENT OF SCHIZOPHRENIA

Residential Treatment Programs

Residential programs offer a form of care that is intermediate between intense stabilization-oriented inpatient treatment and the more maintenance-oriented approaches of outpatient treatment. Thus, although the primary focus of inpatient programs is on stabilization and discharge, the focus of most residential programs is on improvement—to the point that the patient can be maintained in an outpatient setting. Therefore, a residential program offers settings with lesser levels of restriction and longer stays than an inpatient program. In fact, the increasing availability of residential programs may have been an important factor in acute psychiatric hospitalization stays being much shorter than in the past, but with equivalent or even better overall outcomes (American Psychiatric Association, 2004; Johnstone & Zolese, 1999).

Treatment of chronic mental illness in residential treatment facilities is perhaps one response to the worldwide attempt to deinstitutionalize patients with these illnesses. Institutionalization failed to give patients a proper chance in life to become productive in the community. Today, institutionalization is generally considered only a temporary solution, whereas integration into society and the community has become the crucial goal of treatment. Nevertheless, the naive idea that deinstitutionalization itself is the golden solution has failed, because it simply places a group of marginalized people back into society without preparing them. "The classical paradigm of social psychiatry postulating that dehospitalization automatically generates social integration has proven to be wrong, and that deinstitutionalization of the chronically ill and living in the community "supported by different services aiming at integration has also failed to be successful" (Eikelmann, Reker, & Richter, 2005, p. 664).

Our understanding of residential treatment is in relative infancy in comparison with that of inpatient treatment and requires considerably more research comparing different treatment approaches, as well as outcome analyses. Researchers in the Netherlands (Depla, de Graaf, van Busschbach, & Heeren, 2003) compared two models of residential living for their effectiveness. These models were placed within the residential homes for older adults. Depla and colleagues (2003) found that "dispersed housing" (patients' apartments dispersed throughout the facility) was more effective than "concentrated housing" (patients concentrated on one unit in the facility). Improvement in outcome of the dispersed housing model may have related to patients having more control over their own lives, in contrast to the concentrated housing model, which resembled more of a hospital-like setting. Depla and colleagues found that residential treatments have an advantage over psychiatric hospitals, because they "afforded more privacy, were closer to public services, and had a more diversified population" (p. 730).

Other investigators have shown that when chronically ill patients were returned to their community and were "supported by a mental health system with adequate community resources and continuity of care," they could "achieve improved life satisfaction, remain clinically stable with less medication and maintain community tenure" (Hobbs, Newton, Tennant, Rosen, & Tribe, 2002, p. 65).

General Issues Regarding Residential Treatment Facilities

Physical Structure

Most residential treatment facilities attempt to provide a comfortable, casual, more home-like environment, especially when compared to inpatient treatment facilities. In some cases, residential programs are actually located in large homes. Nevertheless, it is important to remember that these are treatment facilities, and general rules of safety and confidentiality should apply. For example, doors to patients' rooms should open outward, to prevent patients' barricading themselves inside. Additionally, an attempt should be made to control and monitor dangerous objects, such as razor blades. Also, areas with private patient information and medications need to be locked. (These considerations do not apply as much to the housing and supervised living programs described below.)

Goals of Treatment and the Interdisciplinary Treatment Plan

Although most residential programs have longer lengths of stay than inpatient programs, the need to set up specific goals of treatment and an interdisciplinary treatment plan is just as important. Without specific goals and approaches, and routine review of progress, it can become all too easy for patients simply to settle into the more home-like environments and exhibit no change, with staff members focusing more on stabilization than on improvement and eventual discharge. One of the problems to guard against is that treatment-oriented residential programs can be vulnerable to misuse, in that these programs can become just a way to house patients. Thus, specific criteria for admission and discharge need to be set up, and care must be taken to ensure that unsuitable patients are discharged from these facilities.

The Milieu

Although some residential programs are specifically designed for patients with schizophrenia, such patients frequently represent only a fraction of the population of a residential treatment facility. This can provide challenges in terms of the milieu, because patients with schizophrenia do better in environments with less expressed emotion, which is often difficult to achieve in a facility with a mixed clientele. Additionally, some patients with other diagnoses may be disturbed or frightened by patients with schizophrenia who are overtly paranoid or disorganized. Some facilities deal with this issue geographically, by placing more agitated patients in different areas of the facility, or through staffing, by having more, or more experienced, staff members take greater responsibility for the more agitated or seriously ill individuals.

Length-of-Stay Issues

Just as it is important to design inpatient programs with the length of stay in mind, so it is with residential programs. The greater lengths of stay in residential programs allow the implementation of more involved and lengthier programs in comparison with those found in an inpatient unit. Another important difference between inpatient and residential programs is that the residential program structures can make use of the more home-like environment to address daily living issues directly. Many programs have patients involved in cooking, cleaning, shopping, and other activities, and some programs have field trips, on which patients learn to make better use of available transportation modalities. Even so, specific goals should be tracked, and discharges carefully planned.

Choosing a Treatment Program

Choosing an appropriate residential treatment program can be critical in preventing deterioration of the patient's condition, avoiding hospitalization, and providing stability for the patient. Many factors affect the choice of residential treatment, such as safety, severity of symptoms, overall patient functioning, medical problems, and the ability of the patient to cooperate with treatment. Psychiatric and medical services provided by different programs vary from one setting to another. Some patients need structured and more supervised services, whereas others require limited or no supervision. Finally, to increase the chances of success, family and patient preferences should be accommodated whenever possible.

When deciding among programs, one should keep in mind that the final goal of any residential program is to enable patients to have a life in the community, even if they need considerable support for that lifestyle. Patients should be able to take responsibility for their lives, look after their food and housing needs, and manage their medications, and be given every opportunity to be creative, productive human beings. Many residential programs whose objective is to lead patients to greater independence should be person-centered. In a person-centered approach (Rogers, 1983), the individual is deemed trustworthy and is considered to know best the directions of his or her life and to be capable of making decisions that lead to a better way of living. The power of the treatment team is transferred to the patients as he or she articulates and pursues the direction his or her own life is to take. Team members effectively become sensitive consultants that through empathy and careful listening facilitate the patient's way toward independence.

Types of Residential Programs

Although there are many modalities of community residential treatment facilities, we present some of the more commonly available types of programs.

Crisis Residential Treatment Services

Crisis residential models of acute care offer examples of community mental health practices that place emphasize patient integration into the community, with the least restrictive environment possible and at low cost. With rising costs of psychiatric hospitalization, crisis residential treatment program models have become popular in some areas as an alternative to inpatient admission for certain patients. Without compromising outcome (in fact, there may be better outcome for patient satisfaction), the cost for having a patient in a crisis residential program can be as little as one-third the cost of a comparable inpatient hospitalization (Hawthorne et al., 2005).

These programs focus on psychosocial rehabilitation of patients who need crisis intervention for situations such as deterioration of psychiatric symptoms, which is often due to adherence problems or recent changes in medication regimens. Patients may also need intervention because of safety issues, such as passive suicidal and homicidal ideation in the absence of any plan of harm, and with the ability to "contract for safety" (an agreement between the patient and staff that the patient will contact staff before engaging in any behaviors harmful to themselves or others). A crisis might also be related to a relationship problem, homelessness, substance abuse, or medical problems that contribute to worsening of the psychiatric condition but are not significant enough to require hospitalization or skilled nursing care.

Admission to these programs is voluntary, and the patient should be able to participate fully in the program to receive maximum benefit. Program size ranges from a few beds to over 10 beds, and each program is generally located in a house within a neighborhood. Programs are fully staffed, 24 hours a day, 7 days a week, by mental health professionals and provide extensive services based on the biopsychosocial model, with an interdisciplinary team approach that addresses every patient's unique situation. Patients receive rehabilitation and therapeutic services such as psychotherapy, medication management, and education by therapists, psychiatrists, and nursing staff members in a structured environment. The services support individuals in their efforts to restore, maintain, and apply interpersonal and independent living skills, and to access community support systems.

Crisis residential programs provide patients with opportunities to reintegrate into the community, and they also facilitate continuation of outpatient management for both psychiatric treatment and substance rehabilitation programs. Also, these programs help patients find stable housing and financial resources, such as state and Social Security Disability. Patients are usually admitted to these programs for a period that ranges from a few days to 30 days, with length of stay determined by degree of improvement.

Adult Residential Treatment Services

Adult residential treatment programs are generally oriented toward rehabilitation and provide services in a noninstitutional, residential setting. Adult residential treatment programs offer a range of activities and services for individuals who would otherwise be at risk of hospitalization or other institutional placement. These services are available and staffed 24 hours a day, 7 days a week. They are recommended for individuals who are expected to move toward more independent living situations, or a higher level of functioning, within 3–12 months—sometimes even longer.

Adult residential treatment services are for patients who require an excellent alternative to long-term psychiatric inpatient hospitalization or more intensive services that cannot be provided on an outpatient basis. They are usually based on a biopsychosocial model, with an interdisciplinary team to address the complexity of patients' needs, including mental health, skills building, housing, psychoeducation, co-occurring substance abuse, and medication needs. They offer patients an opportunity to stabilize by introducing better routines into their lives; to learn about and increase their awareness of their illness, so that they can participate more actively in their treatment plan; to take advantage of vocational and educational opportunities; and to prepare to live independently and reintegrate into the community.

Residential treatment programs offer other levels of service besides the 24-hour staffing model. A second level of service is a less structured environment that still focuses on treatment and learning to live in a community, but with greater emphasis on acquiring skills for independent living. Skills acquisition is monitored by a treatment team that helps patients with their individualized treatment plans. Patients might participate in group activities and work together on basic tasks, such as planning meals and cooking, housekeeping chores, shopping, doing laundry, and other activities that lead to greater independence. Often there is also a greater focus on the educational or vocational needs of patients compared to that in the first level of care.

The third level is even less formally structured, with the minimal number of staff required for skills development, independent living, and self-monitoring. However, the focus on treatment continues. Patients are encouraged and supported to apply the skills they learned earlier (e.g., during the first and second levels). Additionally, staff makes sure that patients' needs are met, and that they are supported in improving their ability to become independent. At this level, attending to vocational desires and aspirations and providing education and hands-on training are primary goals.

Transitional Housing

Another type of community residential program provides nonacute short-term transitional housing, where patients with chronic mental illness can reside independently in supervised and supported houses with a direct connection to psychiatric outpatient treatment programs. Patients with psychiatric illnesses, whose lives are unstable secondary to homelessness or lack of resources, and who require frequent and comprehensive psychiatric services, are often considered good candidates for such programs. Patients who are admitted to these programs frequently also have problems with medication adherence, and may decompensate quickly without regular support and supervision. For this reason, such programs benefit from their connection to an outpatient psychiatric treatment program, where individual and group therapy are offered in addition psychopharmacology evaluation and treatment, and may be continued after patients leave the program. A case coordinator works closely with patients to utilize available community resources and build a network of support to achieve individual rehabilitation goals. These services are very helpful in providing patients with long-term support, creating a sense of connection to a community of peers, eliminating gaps in treatment, and reducing the possibility of relapse. Typically, an average stay at a transitional house is between 6 and 8 months.

Supportive Housing

The focus of supportive housing is first to find the house for the patient in need, then to provide psychiatric services (Tsemberis & Eisenberg, 2000). In an attempt to ensure stability and to prevent decompensation, supportive housing became available as a long-term, nonacute residential treatment modality that is not directly connected to psychiatric services. In comparison to patients in transitional housing, chronically mentally ill patients admitted to supportive housing programs are usually more stable, and require less structured environments and less availability of psychiatric services. However, psychiatric supportive services are easily accessible whenever there is a need to improve a patient's overall condition or to prevent deterioration. Although patients enjoy considerable autonomy and independence, they may need some supportive services. In comparison to patients in transitional housing, patients usually can stay indefinitely in supportive housing.

Board and Care Homes

Board and care homes offer affordable, supportive, long-term care services in a variety of settings, ranging from small, adult foster care homes to larger, quasi-institutional, hotel-like facilities. These facilities can be operated either privately or by charitable nonprofit organizations (Kalymun & Seip, 1990). These homes offer the widest range, in terms of numbers of patients, of all residential approaches: Some accommodate only a few patients, whereas others have more than 100 patients.

These facilities provide supervised living environments, arrangements for medical appointments, transportation, laundry and cleaning service, three meals a day, and personal assistance. Many of these homes offer care to former long-stay patients in mental hospitals and other chronically mentally ill individuals. In the absence of family support, board and care homes are a valuable alternative to homelessness and to nursing home placement among older adults with mental illness.

Care must be exercised in choosing board and care facilities. Many are excellent, but some operators, faced with financial pressures (Blaustein & Viek, 1987), reduce operating expenses to the extent that some patients may be disadvantaged. For example, less skilled (and less expensive) caregiving staff may provide inadequate levels of support. Residents often lack the power to demand adequate support, especially given the lack of alternative, affordable long-term care living environments. As a result, advocates for the mentally ill and for older adult populations have sought increased regulation and monitoring of board and care homes to ensure the safety and well-being of residents. However, little progress has been made in either passing new legislation or increasing the monitoring and enforcement of current regulations, sometimes because of the unwillingness of Federal and state government decision makers to allocate additional resources for board and care facilities.

Intermediate-Care Facilities

Intermediate-care facilities provide service for patients with chronic mental illness who have mild medical conditions that require limited nursing care (e.g., diabetes and hypertension). Thus, patients are admitted to these facilities for monitoring and nursing supervision of medical problems. At the same time, they receive psychosocial services, such as socialization activities and supportive services, as well as psychiatric medication management, to maintain stabilization and to prevent symptom relapse.

Patents can stay at the facility as long they need the provided service. However, they may be transferred to a regular nursing facility if there is a need for skilled nursing care due to worsening medical conditions. Patients may also be discharged to board and care homes when they achieve a greater degree of medical and psychiatric stability.

Nursing Homes/Skilled Nursing Facilities

Nursing homes, or skilled nursing facilities (SNFs), were designed for geriatric or chronically medically disabled patients; however, recently they have frequently been used for patients with mental illness particularly as a way to facilitate discharges from state hospitals. Because these facilities were not developed for patients with psychiatric illnesses, these patients may face many problems when they go to a nursing home, because the staff is usually not prepared to cope with and to serve them appropriately. These nursing homes may offer inadequate evaluations or limited psychiatric and psychological services (Sherrell, Anderson, & Buckwalter, 1998). Unfortunately, there appears to be little in the way of a plan to address these issues in the future.

These services are normally provided by contractors, and currently there is little systematic planning to provide services to the mentally ill. Often, there is no consistent evaluation and treatment plan, unless a family member or a staff member of the nursing home requests that service of the facility (a task that generally falls on the social director). Although some SNFs have attempted to address these issues, if these facilities are to be used for the mentally ill, they will require better developed activity programs, greater psychiatric supervision, and more consistent and thoughtful psychologically based care. Otherwise, patients may undergo psychiatric deterioration and worsening in social functioning and self-care.

Therefore, SNFs are not appropriate facilities for the psychiatric patient, because they cannot provide the services needed for adequate treatment. Most SNFs will have to undergo a thorough restructuring to provide adequate services in terms of not only treatment but also rehabilitation and reintegration to society; this does not seem likely in the near future.

CONCLUDING THOUGHTS

Our intention in this chapter has been to shed light on various ways clinicians can help psychiatric patients who require assistance in critical moments of their lives to maintain clinical stability, or who need long-term inpatient or residential treatment to become fully functioning human beings. In the past, clinical stability was often addressed by institutionalizing patients and providing them with inpatient treatment. The facilities that provided these treatments sometimes functioned more like prisons than hospitals, although they were labeled as hospitals and had some hospital-like characteristics. Having an individual with schizophrenia function and be productive in society was unimaginable, and the word *rehabilitation* was not even in the psychiatric parlance. The advent of deinstitutionalization brought new dimensions to ways that we can help patients with schizophrenia not only attain greater stability and symptom improvement but also reclaim their position in society as people with significant contributions to make to society as a whole.

All the services discussed—inpatient, outpatient, and residential—are valuable in their own ways if they are operated thoughtfully, without abuse, and with well-devised plans. On the other hand, all services have their limitations; psychiatric patients who, in years past, would have been routinely admitted to an inpatient unit are today often considered for residential facilities or even individual housing in communities with appropriate assistance. We also know that many psychiatric patients are placed in facilities that are not appropriate for them, and that have no plan or personnel prepared to cope with the complexity of services needed to care for psychiatric patients.

As we have seen, our services to psychiatric patients are still far from optimal. However, the winds of change have touched this exciting field, and the momentum seems to be growing. Improving the quality of services has created new opportunities. More research should be done to enhance psychiatric treatment and rehabilitation, and to help these patients receive the care they deserve. We anticipate that in the future the quality and effectiveness of inpatient and outpatient facilities will continue to improve. We also anticipate more fluid boundaries between inpatient and outpatient facilities, so that patients can move more efficiently from one facility to another depending on their needs and complexity of their cases. But we need more information to be able to advise families and patients regarding the suitability of a facility based on the patients' conditions.

We trust that further research and efforts will result in a deeper understanding of treatment options for schizophrenia and perhaps help to reduce the societal stigma associated with the condition. With this, we hope that people with serious psychiatric difficulties will become less isolated in a society that is better able to integrate them as contributing members of the community at large.

KEY POINTS

General

- Remember that people requiring assistance in critical moments of their lives, such as during a period of schizophrenia illness exacerbation, are very vulnerable and require a considerable focus on sensitivity and confidentiality.
- A strong and well-developed plan to face the complexities and difficulties of emergency rooms, inpatient services, and residential programs will pave the way for excellence.
- It is critical that the medical, psychopharmacological, and psychological aspects of these different kinds of intervention be addressed as soon possible by an interdisciplinary team and be updated frequently as needed.
- Many different types of programs provide an intermediate focus between emergency room and outpatient care. It is important to choose the program most appropriate to the needs of the patient and to consider changes in disposition as the patient's status changes.

Specifics

- In the emergency room, it is important to focus on safety and on the stabilization of the situation.
- Clinical decisions should *not* be made simply out of concern for avoiding litigation; rather, they should be based on what is best in terms of safety and treatment of the patient.
- Remember that discharge planning should begin with the very first encounter with the patient.
- Be mindful of the challenge of having to provide a full therapeutic experience, even during a short stay.

REFERENCES AND RECOMMENDED READINGS

American Psychiatric Association. (2004). *Practice guidelines for the treatment of psychiatric disorders. Compendium 2004.* Arlington, VA: Author.

Blaustein, M., & Viek, C. (1987). Problems and needs of operators of board-and-care homes: A survey. *Hospital and Community Psychiatry, 38*(7), 750–754.

Depla, M. F., de Graaf, R., van Busschbach, J. T., & Heeren, T. J. (2003). Community integration of elderly mentally ill persons in psychiatric hospitals and two types of residences. *Psychiatric Services, 54*(5), 730–735.

Eikelmann, B., Reker, T., & Richter, D. (2005). [Social exclusion of the mentally ill—a critical review and outlook of community psychiatry at the beginning of the 21st century]. *Fortschritte der Neurologie Psychiatrie, 73*(11), 664–673.

Felthous, A. R. (1999). The clinician's duty to protect third parties. *Psychiatric Clinics of North America, 22*(1), 49–60.

Hawthorne, W. B., Green, E. E., Gilmer, T., Garcia, P., Hough, R. L., Lee, M., et al. (2005). A randomized trial of short-term acute residential treatment for veterans. *Psychiatric Services, 56*(11), 1379–1386.

Hobbs, C., Newton, L., Tennant, C., Rosen, A., & Tribe, K. (2002). Deinstitutionalization for long-term mental illness: A 6-year evaluation. *Australian and New Zealand Journal of Psychiatry, 36*(1), 60–66.

Johnstone, P., & Zolese, G. (1999). Systematic review of the effectiveness of planned short hospital stays for mental health care. *British Medical Journal, 318,* 1387–1390.

Kalymun, M., & Seip, D.E. (1990). Assisted living with residents in mind: Conclusion of the national survey analysis. *Contemporary Long Term Care, 13*(1), 25, 28–29.

Rogers, C. R. (1983). *Freedom to learn for the 80s.* Columbus, OH: Merrill.

Sherrell, K., Anderson, R., & Buckwalter, K. (1998). Invisible residents: The chronically mentally ill elderly in nursing homes. *Archives of Psychiatric Nursing, 12*(3), 131–139.

Tarasoff v. Regents of the University of California. (17 Cal. 3d 425, 1976, 1–20).

Tsemberis, S., & Eisenberg, R. F. (2000). Pathways to housing: Supported housing for street-dwelling homeless individuals with psychiatric disabilities. *Psychiatric Services, 51*(4), 487–493.

CHAPTER 35

TREATMENT IN
JAILS AND PRISONS

ROGER H. PETERS
PATTIE B. SHERMAN
FRED C. OSHER

In 2004, over 2 million prisoners were held in Federal or state prisons and local jails, and over 3% of the U.S. adult population was under some form of correctional supervision. Jails and prisons have grown dramatically in the past 15 years as a result of a significant increase in arrests and incarceration for drug offenses, mandatory sentencing guidelines, and the erosion of public services for homeless persons, persons with mental illnesses, and the indigent. For example, the number of inmates in U.S. jails increased from 405,000 in 1990 to 691,000 in 2003, and the prison population increased from 793,000 to 1,394,000 during this period. Jails are typically operated by county sheriffs and are locally operated correctional facilities that confine persons on either a pretrial or short-term postsentence basis. Jails are usually for inmates confined for sentences of 1 year or less, whereas prisons are designed for offenders with sentences of more than 1 year, and are operated under the authority of state and Federal governments.

The increasing number of offenders with mental illness confined in jails and prisons has been of significant concern to correctional and health care administrators. Approximately 16% of inmates report major mental health problems or an overnight stay in a mental hospital, and more precise diagnostic estimates of persons with mental illnesses in jails and prisons range from 10 to 15% of the correctional populations. Rates of mental illness among offenders are significantly higher than rates among the general population. For example, 6.7% of prisoners reported a history of schizophrenia, compared to 1.4% of the general population. Over 70% of inmates with severe mental disorders have co-occurring substance use disorders. Persons with mental illnesses in jails and prisons are more likely than other inmates to have a history of physical and sexual abuse, to be unemployed prior to their arrest, to have a family history of incarceration and substance abuse, and to have a history of incarceration for violent offenses.

Factors cited most frequently as contributing to the criminalization of persons with mental illnesses include high rates of co-occurring substance use disorders; reduced access to long-term care in state mental hospitals, with the adoption of restrictive civil commitment criteria; and inadequate access to effective community support services. Research suggests that conduct disorder and antisocial personality disorder predispose individuals to both schizophrenia and substance use disorders, thus providing a link between these disorders and likely contributing to increased rates of co-occurring disorders among offenders. The tremendous increase of individuals with schizophrenia and other mental disorders in correctional settings during the past two decades has outstripped the capacity of correctional mental health services, which have experienced only nominal growth during this same period. Although only a small proportion of correctional facilities now provide a range of specialized mental health services, a larger proportion of correctional populations use these services, and inmates with mental disorders are more concentrated in facilities that offer these services.

One of the greatest challenges in working with offenders with mental health disorders involves their rapid cycling within the criminal justice system and other social service systems. In addition to their frequent contact with law enforcement, courts, and corrections systems, offenders with serious mental illness have recurrent contact with crisis mental health services and other emergency health care services in the community. These individuals are frequently homeless, have few financial or social supports, and lack vocational skills. These sites of contact afford opportunities for diversion from jail. When released from jail or prison, individuals with serious mental illnesses often have difficulty engaging in community mental health services, and are frequently released with little or no access to medications. Other barriers to community integration include lack of affordable housing, transportation, and the termination of income supports and entitlements. There is a tremendous need to provide reentry planning and linkage with community service providers for offenders with mental illness, prior to their release from custody. In many jurisdictions, pre- or postbooking diversion programs have been developed to identify persons with mental illness prior to arrest and placement in jail, and to route these individuals to appropriate services in settings outside the criminal justice system.

SPECIAL ISSUES IN PROVIDING CORRECTIONAL TREATMENT

The experience of incarceration is quite stressful and can exacerbate symptoms of psychotic disorders and other major mental illnesses, particularly among inmates with schizophrenia. For example, changes in correctional housing assignments and daily routines, noise, lack of privacy, sleep deprivation, and verbal and physical abuse may lead to worsening of symptoms and self-injurious behavior. In addition, inmates with mental illness are frequently ostracized and stigmatized by other inmates, and are often the victims of criminal behavior within the correctional setting. Jail suicide rates are approximately 50 per 100,000 inmates, which is five times higher than rates in the general population. Persons with schizophrenia have particularly high rates of suicide, making their periods of incarceration high-risk events. For these reasons, inmates with mental disorders are sometimes placed in specialized housing/treatment units.

In comparison to other inmates, individuals with schizophrenia generally experience greater difficulty in adapting to jails and prison, as indicated by more frequent infractions and confinement in disciplinary "lockup" units. Inmates who receive psychotropic medication are sometimes prevented from employment opportunities in correctional settings and from participation in work release programs. Persons with schizophrenia are also likely to remain in jail and prison longer than other inmates, and are less frequently paroled or placed on probation. They are more likely than other inmates to serve their entire sentence, and are often released from custody without adequate preparation.

Agitation; isolation from others; difficulties with eating, sleeping, and self-care; hallucinations and delusions; and difficulties in comprehending or following staff directives are frequently observed among inmates with schizophrenia. These signs and symptoms of the illness are often misinterpreted as evidence of hostility and dangerousness, disinterest, lack of motivation, or resistance to treatment. Failure to identify accurately and to understand the behavioral effects of schizophrenia often leads to inmates being cited for infractions and the use of sanctions, such as lockup in isolated confinement areas.

Inmates with schizophrenia differ widely in the type, scope, and severity of their symptoms, and the complications related to their co-occurring disorders. Many mental health disorders (e.g., trauma related to physical and sexual abuse, organic syndromes, developmental disabilities, sexual disorders, personality disorders) require specialized and intensive resources, and correctional priorities must be weighed in determining to what extent special programs are developed for these groups. Generally, the highest priority for correctional mental health services is assigned to inmates who have severe mental disorders, including schizophrenia and other major Axis I mental disorders with related impairment in psychosocial functioning. Given the wide differences in inmates' mental health and psychosocial functioning, a major challenge is to develop sufficiently comprehensive screening and assessment approaches to identify the breadth and intensity of mental health treatment services that are needed.

Differing goals and orientations among corrections and treatment staff may lead to obstacles in implementing jail and prison treatment services for inmates with schizophrenia. The most salient goals for correctional staff are to protect public safety, to allow inmates to complete legal processing (in jails), and punishment. Training correctional staff to identify signs and symptoms of schizophrenia, and to react effectively to erratic and unusual behaviors (i.e., deescalation techniques and referral to mental health services) has been found to reduce adverse incidents and sanctions in jails and prisons. Correctional staff members are not always aware of the research indicating that treatment helps to reduce recidivism, decrease in-house injuries, and protect public safety, or they may not be convinced of these findings. Joint training events and planning meetings between corrections and treatment staff are often useful in reconciling differing goals and approaches.

PROFESSIONAL STANDARDS AND TREATMENT GUIDELINES

Several sets of professional standards and guidelines for delivering mental health and substance abuse services in correctional facilities have emerged over the past three decades. These were largely influenced by the courts, beginning with the landmark case *Estelle v. Gamble* (429 U.S. 97 [1976]), in which the U.S. Supreme Court determined that inmates have a legal right to receive adequate care in correctional facilities to meet their "serious medical needs," because they are unable to obtain treatment on their own. Later Federal cases, including *Bowring v. Godwin* (551 F.2d 44, 47 [4th Cir., 1997]), ruled that inmates who have "serious medical needs" have a right to mental health treatment. The American Public Health Association (APHA), the American Medical Association (AMA), and the American Correctional Association (ACA) have all developed mental health standards and guidelines for correctional facilities. In the early 1980s, the National Commission on Correctional Health Care (NCCHC) developed another set of guidelines that are still widely used, and the American Psychiatric Association (APA) compiled a more detailed set of guidelines related to mental health services in corrections in 1989, and updated these in 2000.

The ACA, the Joint Commission on Accreditation of Healthcare Organizations (JCAHO), and the NCCHC currently provide correctional health services accreditation programs. In 2003, the ACA and the Commission on Accreditation for Corrections published the fourth edition of *Standards for Adult Correctional Institutions,* which describes minimal thresholds for mental health services in correctional settings. Recommendations include the following:

- *Mental health screening* provided within 14 days of admission to correctional facilities.
- *Mental health examination* that includes assessment of suicidal risk, violence, history of mental health and substance abuse treatment, use of psychotropic medication, and sexual abuse.
- *Outpatient services* for detection, diagnosis, and treatment of mental illness.
- *Crisis intervention* and management of acute psychiatric episodes.
- *Stabilization of mental health symptoms* and prevention of psychiatric deterioration.
- *Referral and admission to licensed mental health facilities* for offenders whose psychiatric needs exceed the treatment capability of the correctional facility.
- Development of procedures for obtaining and documenting *informed consent.*

The most recent version of the NCCHC standards (2003) addresses a broad range of mental health and substance abuse services, and provides more detailed recommendations for clinical procedures and approaches. In 2004, the NCCHC developed professional guidelines in *Treatment of Schizophrenia in Correctional Institutions,* based in part on the APA's *Practice Guideline for the Treatment of Patients with Schizophrenia* (2004), but focusing on correctional treatment issues. Recommendations to guide clinical services include the following:

- *Assessment* conducted at entry/admission to the correctional system.
- *Diagnosis* completed by a credentialed clinician that addresses subtypes of schizophrenia and considers cultural issues, and the influence of co-occurring substance use disorders.
- *Management overview* examines the severity of the disorder, as determined by current symptoms, functional impairment, mental health history, and co-occurring conditions.
- *Treatment goals and a treatment plan* that are developed to address biological, interpersonal, social, and cultural factors affecting adjustment, and reflect the phase of the disorder (i.e., acute, stabilization, and stable phase).
- *Routine services* include a mental status examination and review of side effects of psychotropic medication and level of functioning.
- *Treatment strategies* include psychopharmacological services and psychosocial services provided in group settings.
- *Continuity of care* includes discharge planning and active involvement of mental health and case management staff in planning and linkage with community service providers.
- *Environmental controls* to minimize stressors and to encourage use of behavioral principles (e.g., positive reinforcement, token economies).
- *Quality improvement* to assist in identification of inmates with schizophrenia and to measure noncompliance and other key treatment outcomes.

Additional, more comprehensive guidelines were developed (Hills, Sigfried, & Ickowitz, 2004) by the U.S. Department of Justice, National Institute of Corrections, entitled *Effective Prison Mental Health Services.* These address a broad range of clinical, management, and administrative issues, and include sections on screening and assessment, and mental health treatment; use of seclusion, segregation, and restraints; suicide prevention; treatment of female inmates; psychopharmacological interventions, transition/reentry services; and treatment of special populations such as violent offenders, sex offenders, persons with mental retardation or developmental disabilities, and older adults.

IDENTIFICATION AND TREATMENT OF SCHIZOPHRENIA IN JAILS AND PRISONS

Screening, Assessment, and Treatment Planning

As previously noted, jail and prison inmates are four times more likely than nonincarcerated individuals to have schizophrenia. Most inmates also have concurrent substance use disorders that significantly affect their treatment needs. Therefore, identification of both sets of disorders in jails and prisons is of paramount importance. Inmate mental health information is sometimes available through law enforcement reports, arrest records, or previous prison records, but in most cases, little or no archival mental health information accompanies the inmate at the point of initial incarceration. As a result, a standardized, universal, and comprehensive screening for mental health, substance abuse, and other health-related disorders should be provided by all jails and prisons.

Screening for mental health and co-occurring substance use disorders should be provided at the earliest possible point during incarceration, such as at time of jail booking or at admission/reception to the prison system. Early screening and identification facilitates the rapid stabilization of acute mental health symptoms; initiation of enhanced observation and related management procedures to prevent suicide or other self-injurious behavior, and supervised detoxification from drugs or alcohol, if needed; and engagement in intensive treatment services. Moreover, results from early identification and screening can be used to place ("classify") inmates in housing units or in particular institutions (e.g., within prison systems that include multiple institutions) to expedite involvement in specialized treatment services, and to provide close monitoring and management of behavioral problems. Classification to "special needs" units within jails and prisons also assists in preventing predatory inmates' victimization of persons with schizophrenia or other major mental disorders. Early identification of mental health disorders is of critical importance to prosecutors and the courts in evaluating public safety risk, release decisions, legal issues related to "competency to stand trial" and "sanity" at the time of the offense, and the need for treatment and community supervision. A more comprehensive psychosocial assessment typically is provided following the inmate's placement in a mental health or other specialized treatment program.

Correctional screening for mental illnesses is not an event, but a process that starts at booking and continues throughout confinement. Initial screening for mental health and co-occurring substance use disorders in jails and prisons includes observation of hallucinations, delusions, and other unusual behaviors; and review of self-reported symptoms, current and past use of medications, and history of treatment. Brief self-report screening instruments are often used in correctional settings to detect mental health disorders and substance use disorders. Evidence-based mental health screens for inmates include the Brief Symptom Inventory (BSI; Derogatis & Melisarotos, 1983), the Symptom Checklist–90 (SCL-90; Derogatis, Lipman, & Rickels, 1974), the Brief Jail Mental Health Screen (Steadman, Scott, Osher, Agnese, & Robbins, 2005), the Global Appraisal of Individual Needs (GAIN; Dennis, Titus, White, Unsicker, & Hodgkins, 2002), and the Mental

Health Screening Form–III (Carroll & McGinley, 2000). Evidence-based substance abuse screens for inmates include the Simple Screening Instrument (SSI; Center for Substance Abuse Treatment, 1994), the Texas Christian University Drug Screen (TCUDS; Knight, Simpson, & Hiller, 2002), the Alcohol Dependence Scale (ADS; Skinner, 1982), and the Alcohol and Drug Use sections from the Addiction Severity Index (ASI; McLellan et al., 1992).

The majority of female inmates and a large proportion of male inmates have a history of physical, sexual, or emotional abuse. As a result, all inmates should receive screening and assessment in this area, and the staff should be trained to provide referral to institutional and community services to address related treatment needs. An undiagnosed history of trauma often leads to misattribution of behavior (e.g., defensiveness, resistance to treatment) and may undermine inmates' engagement in traditional treatment services. A variety of brief standardized screening instruments are available to identify symptoms of trauma.

Because of the high risk of suicide by persons with schizophrenia while in custody, effective suicide prevention programs within jails and prisons are imperative. Suicide screening instruments are essential components of these programs. New York's Suicide Prevention Screening Form is one example of such a standardized screening measure. Other components of effective suicide prevention programs include the following:

- Suicide prevention training for correctional, medical, and mental health staff.
- Effective and ongoing communication with outside agencies, facility staff, and the suicidal inmate.
- Suicide resistant, protrusion-free housing for suicidal inmates.
- Structured levels of supervision for suicidal inmates.
- Timely emergency interventions following suicide attempts.
- Critical incident stress debriefing to affected staff members and inmates, as well as a multidisciplinary mortality review of suicides and serious attempts.

There are several significant challenges in conducting effective screening and assessment for schizophrenia and other, related disorders in jails and prisons. As mentioned previously, most inmates entering correctional facilities do not have much accompanying information regarding their treatment needs and treatment history (e.g., current medication use). Several communities have recently established data links between public mental health providers and law enforcement authorities to identify new arrestees in jails who have serious mental illness. Due to the disorienting effects of mental health disorders, substance abuse, or stress related to incarceration, arrestees are sometimes unreliable informants in these areas, and available correctional records describing diagnoses may be dated and inaccurate. Additionally, the majority of recently arrested inmates have used drugs or alcohol in the 48 hours prior to incarceration, creating difficulties in differentiating between the toxic effects of substances and symptoms of major mental health disorders.

Inmates are often wary of disclosing mental health or other disorders, due to the risk of being placed under close monitoring (e.g., suicide watch), in more restrictive housing units, and in intensive treatment programs. Self-disclosure of mental health or co-occurring disorders may also reduce opportunities for bail or other types of pretrial release and parole, or may create more restrictive conditions of pretrial or postsentence release. Inmates may malinger or exaggerate symptoms in correctional settings to obtain more favorable housing, to postpone or to facilitate transfer to another housing unit or facility, or to obtain medication. Yet persons with schizophrenia are unlikely to exaggerate their condition. The staff should exercise caution in attributing mental health symptoms to malingering, because misdiagnosis may lead to suicide or exacerbation of mental health disorders. Stress related to incarceration may precipitate recurrence of mental health disorders, and ongoing screening for mental health disorders should be provided by the treatment staff and correctional officers.

Because schizophrenia is a heterogeneous disorder, individualized treatment planning should be provided for all jail and prison inmates. Inmates with schizophrenia typically have a wide range of psychosocial needs that should be addressed in the treatment plan, including psychiatric stabilization and medication monitoring, chronic substance abuse, homelessness or lack of stable housing and transportation, lack of social/peer supports, and other health disorders.

Treatment Modalities

Staff members in most prisons and larger jails use formal criteria to determine whether individuals with mental disorders are placed in special housing units apart from the general inmate population. Inmates with acute symptoms of schizophrenia are often housed in special medical units that provide close supervision and monitoring. These units are frequently used for inmates whose mental disorder impairs their judgment or behavior, and creates management problems within the institution. Research indicates that specialized correctional mental health units are effective in reducing disciplinary infractions, suicide attempts, and use of crisis services, hospitalization, and seclusion.

Jails and prisons provide up to four levels of care for inmates with schizophrenia: (1) short-term acute care to stabilize symptoms and to manage crises, usually provided in single-cell special housing units; (2) long-term residential care in special housing units for inmates who have severe mental disorders and cannot tolerate traditional dormitory housing; (3) transitional or intermediate care in either short-term residential or day treatment settings to assist inmates in developing psychosocial skills prior to returning to the general institutional population; and (4) outpatient treatment and case management services dispersed throughout the jail or prison system to provide medication monitoring, and individual and group counseling, with the goal of maintaining stable mental health functioning. In addition to these graded levels of care, crisis intervention services are provided in many of the larger correctional facilities for inmates with schizophrenia who, because of acute symptoms, create a danger to themselves or others or are unable to care for themselves.

Psychosocial Treatment

Group psychosocial treatment in correctional settings provides a useful vehicle for skills training of inmates with schizophrenia and other severe mental disorders. These groups focus on problem-solving skills, adherence to medication and other illness-management skills, impairment related to interpersonal communication, cognitive deficits related to memory and attention, and motivation for treatment. Group interventions for inmates with co-occurring disorders also focus on relapse prevention and strategies to cope with the interactive effects of these disorders. Psychosocial skills training programs are quite consistent with correctional goals to facilitate integration of individuals with schizophrenia within the general inmate population. Several available evidence-based and relatively inexpensive treatment manuals provide psychosocial skills training for inmates with schizophrenia. The logistics of holding treatment groups in maximum security settings can be daunting, yet is plausible with the use of specialized containment units.

Pharmacological Treatment

The use of medication to ameliorate an inmate's symptoms of schizophrenia is an essential component of correctional mental health treatment. Medication management of schizophrenia is perhaps the most widely researched among the evidence-based practices for schizophrenia, and the range of effective medication options grows each year. The principal class of medications used in treating schizophrenia is the "antipsychotics," which can be subdivided further into typical antipsychotics (older, with common side effects including sedation and movement disorders) and atypical antipsychotics (newer, sometimes better tolerated). Older medications used to treat schizophrenia can cost $150–250 a year, whereas newer agents cost $2,000–6,000 a year. There is continued controversy over both the benefits and risks of various antipsychotics in correctional settings.

Proponents of atypical medication cite the fact that the medications are well tolerated, with relatively few unpleasant side effects. In addition, several studies in correctional settings have indicated an association between atypical medication use and decreased hostility and aggression, which in turn decreases the need for seclusion and restraint and may reduce officer and inmate injury. Clozapine has been shown to reduce rates of suicide in prison, and studies indicate that use of atypicals is associated with increased compliance rates. Opponents of atypical medications cite the increased risk of weight gain, glucose intolerance, and the enormous costs associated with these newer agents as reasons for not using them as first-line agents.

The fact that inmates present with varied treatment histories, symptom profiles, and co-occurring conditions is the basis for the APA's recommendation that psychiatrists have the ability to prescribe *any* psychotropic medication in correctional settings. Medication algorithms for schizophrenia have allowed care providers to establish multiple treatment options supported by empirical data related to effectiveness and side effects. Several correctional facilities have developed their own algorithms for the treatment of schizophrenia. The New York Forensic Algorithm Project (FAP) started with the identification of four subgroups of inmates with schizophrenia and developed four parallel intervention plans. With regard to medications, the FAP begins with the use of *any* antipsychotic medication, suggests the use of atypicals, then augmentation with other psychotropic agents, and finally recommends clozapine for inmates with refractory schizophrenia. Importantly, the FAP also recommends specific programming in certain prison environments as an adjunct to medication management.

Whatever the protocol, the correctional medication management program must be consistent with community standards that include the following:

- Prescription use should only occur in the context of an adequate psychiatric evaluation.
- Medications should only be dispensed by licensed health care professionals.
- The goal of treatment must be determined individually rather than being designed to serve institutional goals of behavior control or population management.
- Continuity in medication management between community providers and correctional providers should be maintained.

Treatment of Co-Occurring Disorders

An estimated 5–13% of jail and prison inmates have co-occurring mental health and substance use disorders. This population has pronounced biopsychosocial problems (e.g., homelessness, unemployment, HIV/AIDS) and is at elevated risk for violence and behavior problems. Inmates with significant co-occurring disorders generally do not adjust well to traditional mental health or substance abuse programs and require specialized services. A small but growing number of specialized treatment programs for co-occurring disorders are available in jails and prisons. These programs typically are located in units isolated from general population inmates, are highly intensive and structured, are longer in duration than traditional treatment programs, and feature programming that includes a dual focus on mental health and substance abuse issues. These programs are often embedded within larger substance abuse or mental health treatment units, or within "treatment prisons" that address a wide range of inmate needs. Assessment and treatment services are individualized in these programs according to the level of engagement and motivation, and psychosocial functioning of each inmate.

Therapeutic communities (TCs) have recently been adapted for inmates with co-occurring disorders and include modifications to reduce levels of confrontation; shorten group treatment sessions; provide more staff coordination and involvement in activities, and specialized groups that address medication issues, managing emotions, and criminal thinking. Research indicates that these modified TCs can significantly reduce criminal recidivism for inmates with co-occurring disorders. Specialized jail treatment and diversion programs have also been developed for inmates with co-occurring disorders. Jail diversion programs are designed to identify new arrestees with mental health disorders, and provide intensive case management and assertive community treatment to monitor their involvement in treatment.

TRANSITION PLANNING AND REENTRY INTO THE COMMUNITY

Although discharge or transition planning is a key element of professional standards for correctional mental health care, it is one of the least frequently provided services. For inmates with schizophrenia, community reintegration is fraught with complications. Access to ongoing psychiatric care may be compromised by inadequate insurance, transportation and housing, or profound cognitive impairment associated with their illness. Many inmates with schizophrenia were receiving Medicaid and other forms of public assistance at the time of their arrest. Too frequently these benefits are terminated rather than suspended and are not immediately available upon the inmate's release from correctional settings. It typically takes at least 45 days to reactivate benefits upon release. A consequence of not having benefits is that the released inmate does not have any way to pay for medication and treatment. As a result of abrupt discontinuation of treatment, many inmates experience recurrence of acute and harsh psychiatric symptoms, thereby increasing the risk for suicide, and for arrest and incarceration. Without adequate transition planning and support, successful community reintegration for inmates with schizophrenia is unlikely.

The APA lists the following "essential services" for adequate inmate transition planning:

1. Appointments should be arranged with mental health agencies for all inmates with serious mental illnesses, especially those receiving psychotropic medication.
2. Arrangements should be made with local mental health agencies to have prescriptions renewed or evaluated for renewal.
3. Mental health treatment staff should ensure that discharge and referral responsibilities are carried out by designated staff.
4. Each inmate who receives mental health treatment should be assessed to determine the appropriateness of community referral.
5. Mental health staff should participate in developing service contracts to ensure access to community-based case managers to provide continuity of service.

In addition, adequate transition planning identifies necessary housing placements and appropriate linkages to treatment services.

Although little research is available to guide transition planning for inmates with schizophrenia, the recently developed APIC model (assess, plan, identify, coordinate) identifies several important elements that are likely to improve outcomes for this group upon release from custody. These elements include correctional assessment, planning, identification, and coordination of community components required to support integration of the released inmate. The APIC model provides a reentry checklist for use in recording transition needs while an inmate is in custody.

Transition planning is of critical importance in supporting the recovery of inmates with schizophrenia, and implies a partnership between correctional and community providers. Several communities have implemented forensic assertive community treatment (FACT) models, in which evidence-based features of assertive community treatment are blended with approaches to enhance public safety. Early findings suggest that this approach may reduce hospital admissions and reincarceration.

KEY POINTS

- Inmates in jails and prisons have rates of schizophrenia that are approximately four times higher than in the general population.
- Mental health services in correctional facilities have not expanded sufficiently to meet the growing needs for these services.
- Treatment of schizophrenia in correctional settings is affected by symptom exacerbation related to the stress of incarceration, discontinuity in the prescription and administration of medications, frequent confinement in disciplinary units, and the presence of co-occurring substance abuse and other health disorders.
- Professional standards and guidelines are available to assist mental health professionals and correctional administrators in assessment, treatment, and management of inmates with schizophrenia and other mental illnesses.
- Early screening and identification of schizophrenia, other mental health disorders, co-occurring substance use disorders, and suicide risk are of critical importance in providing stabilization and engagement to treatment in jails and prisons.
- Several different modalities of treatment in jails and prison are commonly provided for inmates with schizophrenia, including short-term acute care, long-term residential services, transition or intermediate care services, and outpatient treatment and case management services.
- Medication algorithms and other specialized guidelines have been developed to assist mental health professionals in treating inmates with schizophrenia.
- Specialized treatment approaches have been developed in jails and prisons to address co-occurring mental health and substance use disorders, and these have been found to reduce criminal recidivism upon release.
- Transition and reentry services are important in providing continuity of psychotropic medications and other treatment services, stable housing, and financial entitlements, and can help prevent rapid cycling back to the criminal justice system.

REFERENCES AND RECOMMENDED READINGS

Abram, K. M., & Teplin, L. A. (1991). Co-occurring disorders among mentally ill jail detainees: Implications for public policy. *American Psychologist, 46*(10), 1036–1045.

American Correctional Association. (2003). *Standards for adult correctional institutions: Fourth edition.* Laurel, MD: Author.

American Psychiatric Association. (2000). *Psychiatric services in jails and prisons: A task force report of the American Psychiatric Association* (2nd ed.). Washington, DC: Author.

American Psychiatric Association. (2004). *Practice guideline for the treatment of patients with schizophrenia* (2nd ed.). Arlington, VA: Author.

Buscema, C. A., Abbasi, Q. A., Barry, D. J., & Lauve, T. H. (2000). An algorithm for the treatment of schizophrenia in the correctional setting: The Forensic Algorithm Project. *Journal of Clinical Psychiatry, 61*(10), 767–783.

Carroll, J. F., & McGinley, J. J. (2000). *Guidelines for using the Mental Health Screening Form III.* New York: Project Return Foundation.

Center for Substance Abuse Treatment. (1994). *Simple screening instruments for outreach for alcohol and other drug abuse and infectious diseases* (Treatment Improvement Protocol (TIP) Series, No. 11). Rockville, MD: U.S. Department of Health and Human Services.

Chandler, R. K., Peters, R. H., Field, G., & Juliano-Bult, D. (2004). Challenges in implementing evidence-based treatment practices for co-occurring disorders in the criminal justice system. *Behavioral Sciences and the Law, 22*(4), 431–448.

Dennis, M. L., Titus, J. C., White, M. K., Unsicker, J. I., & Hodgkins, D. (2002). *Global Appraisal of Individual Needs (GAIN): Administration guide for the GAIN and related measures.* Bloomington, IL: Chestnut Health Systems. Available online at *www.chestnut.org/li/gain*

Derogatis, L., Lipman, R., & Rickels, K. (1974). The Hopkins Symptom Checklist (HSCL)—a self-report symptom inventory. *Behavioral Science, 19,* 1–16.

Derogatis, L. R., & Melisaratos, N. (1983). The Brief Symptom Inventory: An introductory report. *Psychological Medicine, 13,* 595–605.

Hills, H., Siegfried, C., & Ickowitz, A. (2004). *Effective prison mental health services: Guidelines to expand and improve treatment.* Washington, DC: U.S. Department of Justice, National Institute of Corrections.

Knight, K., Simpson, D. D., & Hiller, M. L. (2002). Screening and referral for substance-abuse treatment in the criminal justice system. In C. G. Leukefeld, F. Tims, & D. Farabee (Eds.), *Treatment of drug offenders: Policies and issues* (pp. 259–272). New York: Springer. Instrument available online at *www.ibr.tcu.edu/pubs/datacoll/top10.html*

Lamb, H. R., Weinberger, L. E., & Gross, B. H. (2004). Mentally ill persons in the criminal justice system: Some perspectives. *Psychiatric Quarterly, 75*(2), 107–126.

Manderscheid, R. W., Gravesande, A., & Goldstrom, I. D. (2004). Growth of mental health services in state adult correctional facilities, 1988 to 2000. *Psychiatric Services, 55*(8), 869–872.

McLellan, A. T., Kushner, H., Metzger, D., Peters, R. H., Smith, I., Grissom, G., et al. (1992). The fifth edition of the Addiction Severity Index. *Journal of Substance Abuse Treatment, 9,* 199–213.

Metzner, J. L., Cohen, F., Grossman, L. S., & Wettstein, R. M. (1998). Treatment in jails and prisons. In R. M. Wettstein (Ed.), *Treatment of offenders with mental disorders* (pp. 211–264). New York: Guilford Press.

Morash, M., & Bynum, T. (1995). *Findings from the national study of innovative and promising programs for women offenders.* Washington, DC: U.S. Department of Justice, National Institute of Justice.

Mueser, K. T., Drake, R. E., & Wallach, M. A. (1998). Dual diagnosis: A review of etiological theories. *Addictive Behaviors, 23*(6), 717–734.

National Commission on Correctional Health Care. (2003). *Correctional mental health care: Standards and guidelines for delivering services.* Chicago: Author.

National Commission on Correctional Health Care. (2004). *Treatment of schizophrenia in correctional institutions.* Chicago: Author.

Osher, F., Steadman. H. J., & Barr, H. (2003). A best practice approach to community reentry from jails for inmates with co-occurring disorders: The APIC model. *Crime and Delinquency, 49*(1), 79–96.

Peters, R. H., & Bartoi, M. G. (1997). *Screening and assessment of co-occurring disorders in the justice system.* Delmar, NY: National GAINS Center.

Peters, R. H., & Hills, H. A. (1997). *Intervention strategies for offenders with co-occurring disorders: What works?* Delmar, NY: National GAINS Center.

Skinner, H. A. (1982). *Alcohol Dependence Scale: User's guide.* Toronto: Addiction Research Foundation.

Steadman, H. J., Scott, J. E., Osher, F., Agnese, T. K., & Robbins, P. C. (2005). Validation of the Brief Jail Mental Health Screen. *Psychiatric Services, 56*(7), 816–822.

PART VI

SPECIAL POPULATIONS AND PROBLEMS

CHAPTER 36

FIRST-EPISODE PSYCHOSIS

DONALD ADDINGTON
JEAN ADDINGTON

NATURE OF THE SPECIAL POPULATION

The focus of this chapter is on treatment for individuals experiencing a first episode of one of the disorders described in DSM-IV as schizophrenia and other psychotic disorders. These include schizophrenia, schizophreniform disorder, schizoaffective disorder, delusional disorder, brief psychotic disorder, shared psychotic disorder, substance-induced psychotic disorder, and psychotic disorder not otherwise specified.

Why Focus on the First Episode?

The first episode of psychosis has been singled out for both clinical and research reasons. Clinical reasons for giving specific attention to the first episode include diagnostic uncertainty, the negative impact of treatment delay, the increased responsiveness to treatment of positive symptoms, the potential for assisting the patient and family through education, and support and for integrating psychosocial treatments. Diagnostic issues can cause confusion for clinicians, patients, and families, because the realm of psychotic disorders includes several related disorders, not just schizophrenia. Although some of these disorders may lead to schizophrenia, others do not. From a treatment perspective, there are few evidence-based guidelines for these other disorders, such as brief psychotic disorder or substance-induced psychosis. Thus, the uncertainty generated by diagnostic systems can lead clinicians to provide or recommend inconsistent and poorly coordinated care.

Treatment delay has received much attention in the literature. All too often development of prodromal symptoms is slow prior to the first episode. During this time there are often disruptions to the normal development of interpersonal relationships and instrumental functioning. Furthermore, these young people are at risk of harm from suicide, attempted suicide, or aggression during this period. Unfortunately, clinicians often use a number of unsuccessful strategies to respond to these nonspecific symptoms and deteriorating course. The problem may be ignored or attributed to normal adolescent adjustment, or to other causes, such as mood disorders or addictions. The poor outcome from these strategies can lead frustration on the part of families and patients, and result in a lack of confidence in clinicians and treatment services. Furthermore, it has been well established in the literature that young people often have a psychosis for many months or even years before they receive adequate treatment. This delay in treatment is known as the duration of untreated psychosis (DUP). A long DUP clearly can have terrible impact on the young person and his or her family in terms of distress and coping difficulties, and an obvious negative impact on psychological and social well-being. Although not proven, a biological impact has been suggested as well. A final reason for giving the first episode specific attention is that positive psychotic symptoms in a first episode of psychosis, compared to repeated episodes, are more likely to respond to antipsychotic pharmacotherapy. Paradoxically, observations of the natural history of treated psychosis suggest that the chances of relapse are greater in the early years of the disorder.

The first episode of psychosis also has important research implications. These include studying treatment-naive patients; studying more representative populations of patients, not just those with a more severe course; understanding the natural history of the disorder; and finally, separating the effects of chronic illness from the underlying disorder.

Special Treatment Teams

Providing treatment for people experiencing a first episode of psychosis involves developing both an overall system of care and individualized treatment plans for patients and their families. The goals of the care system should be to promote early intervention and to support optimal individualized treatment for patients and families.

Interestingly, there has been much discussion about the relative benefits of establishing specialized teams to deal with the first-episode population. Organizational benefits include enhancing the knowledge and skills of the team members, as well as systematically providing professional and public education. Offering a specific program can facilitate bringing together groups of patients and their families while having the means to move patients through well-established and effective care pathways.

There may be drawbacks to special teams. There is still a limited evidence base for the advantage of specialized treatment teams versus treatment as usual. Concerns that resources are allocated to a small group of patients at the expense of services for other groups are often voiced. Of course, at the level of the individual, effective treatments for a first episode of psychosis are similar to those for persons with a more chronic course of illness. However, these specialized services can actually improve early access to services, and really make them more user-friendly for both patients and families. For these specialized first-episode services, funding often emerges as a political issue. It can be easier to argue for funds for new and innovative service delivery models in an environment in which mental health services often are not funded at levels equivalent to those for other health services. However, the absence of information based upon the evaluation of real services in the real world limits this discussion to opinion and experience.

DESCRIPTION OF TREATMENT APPROACHES

Early-psychosis treatment can be divided into services that promote early intervention and those that promote optimal care once contact has been established with the treat-

TABLE 36.1. Components of Early-Psychosis Treatment Services

Early intervention	Optimal care
Public education	3-year focus and continuous care
Gatekeeper education	Pharmacotherapy
Easy access	Case management
	Family therapy
	Integrated addictions
	Patient education

ment services (see Table 36.1). The strategies that promote early intervention and reduce the DUP require skills and knowledge that go beyond those traditionally taught to clinicians. They can, however, be learned by clinicians who are interested in broadening their skills and their outlook on the health system.

Early Intervention

There are two clinical justifications for early intervention in a first episode of psychosis. First it has been demonstrated that early treatment can reduce harm caused by social disruption and critical incidents, such as suicide attempts, that can occur during an episode of untreated psychosis. Second, there is evidence that earlier intervention can improve outcome over the first few years of the disorder. This evidence is based on a number of studies and some recent reviews. Numerous strategies aimed at reducing the duration of untreated psychosis have been reported. These strategies have been assessed, but usually in combination, which makes it difficult to know which strategies are critical.

Gatekeeper education involves the education of those professionals who have first contact with individuals who are developing a first episode psychosis. These groups most often include family physicians, as well as school and college counselors. Education usually includes making these clinicians aware of the frequency of the disorders and their clinical manifestations, and suggested methods for accessing care. This education can easily be provided by the first-episode treatment teams.

Public education, although not studied to date as a stand-alone strategy, has been offered in a number of ways. It has been part of high school education about mental health. Education about early intervention has played a major role in campaigns with a primary focus on reducing stigma or DUP. Public education programs may include television, radio, and/or cinema advertisements, and print campaigns and websites either as a first-line information sources or as a backup to other forms of public education.

Ensuring easy access to services is a third strategy for reducing the DUP. Specific strategies include central access services with a single point of access for all mental health services, including psychosis treatment services. Improving access requires removing certain barriers to care. For example, referrals do not have to come through a family physician. There is no need to exclude patients with comorbid substance abuse or mild developmental delay, or even those with past criminal convictions. In addition, providing services and information in a variety of languages further serve to improve access. Outreach teams that conduct an initial assessment of patients in their own homes have also been used, sometimes as part of crisis services, other times as a preferred service delivery model, and still other times only for those patients who are hard to reach.

Optimal Care

The optimal care for a first episode of psychosis, of course, varies considerably according to the needs of the patient. We know that a proportion of patients will achieve a full recovery, but many will continue to experience a range of difficulties, sometimes with symptom control or substance abuse, and more often than not with social and occupational functioning. These are similar to problems of patients experiencing a more chronic course of schizophrenia, but families and the patients themselves at the first episode are naive to the nature of the disorder and how to begin to negotiate available mental health services. This further underscores the need for early-psychosis treatment services to be accessible, to provide education readily to the patient and family, and to integrate the components of a comprehensive treatment plan.

Assessment

Assessing a first episode of psychosis requires a comprehensive approach to obtaining information from all possible sources. Relevant physical examinations and biological investigations are presented in Table 36.2. At this early stage, engagement of the both the patient and family is paramount. The assessment should take a developmental perspective, including an evaluation of the individual's ability to relate to others and to function in work or school throughout the different stages of development. A number of symptom and functioning domains need to be addressed. The course and relationship of the development of positive and negative symptoms of psychosis, depression, and substance abuse

TABLE 36.2. Baseline Biological Investigations

Area of investigation	Test
Substance use or abuse	• Inquiry • Toxicology screen
Cognitive function	• Neuropsychological testing
Genetic	• Family history of psychosis • Clinical screening for chromosome 22q11 deletion syndrome (with testing as indicated clinically)
Structural brain abnormalities	• Computed tomography scan or magnetic resonance imaging
Hematology	• Complete blood count
Blood chemistries	• Electrolytes • Renal function tests • Liver function tests • Thyroid function tests
Infectious diseases	• Syphilis test, hepatitis or HIV tests, if indicated
Cardiovascular	• Vital signs • Electrocardiogram
Extrapyramidal symptoms and signs	• Parkinsonism (bradykinesia, rigidity, tremor) • Dystonia • Dyskinesia • Akathisia
Body mass	• Body mass index
Blood sugar	• Fasting plasma glucose
Hyperlipidemia	• Lipid panel (total cholesterol, low- and high-density lipoprotein, cholesterol, triglycerides)

have to be assessed. The wide range of available structured and semistructured measures is an excellent way to ensure that all the domains are not only assessed initially but also monitored over time for change.

It is well known that people with schizophrenia have a reduced lifespan, and more recently, there is great concern about the metabolic side effects of pharmacotherapy. Attending to the physical needs of individuals with a first episode of schizophrenia by early assessment and ongoing monitoring during treatment should be routine. This allows for adjustment of the treatment in response to emerging problems.

Pharmacotherapy

Pharmacotherapy with antipsychotic medications continues to be central to the treatment of first-episode psychosis. The goals of pharmacotherapy have expanded and are synergistic with the goals of psychosocial treatments (to be discussed later). The main goals of pharmacotherapy include remission of positive symptoms and relapse prevention. Secondary goals include the reduction of negative and depressive symptoms, and improvements in neurocognition and quality of life.

Antipsychotics are most effective in the reduction of the positive symptoms of psychosis, and are more effective in first-episode than in multiepisode cases, with response rates in the range of 50–90% of patients achieving a positive symptom remission, depending upon the criteria used. Maintenance studies designed to establish the benefit of antipsychotics in relapse prevention show consistent and strong differences between medication treatment and placebo over 2 years, which is the longest outcome published. Naturalistic studies show relapse rates from 50 to 80% over 5 years and a five times higher rate of relapse in those who stop pharmacotherapy.

Adherence to pharmacotherapy is generally less than 50% over 1 year. This adherence is not simply due to lack of insight, although insight is a factor. Recent clinical trials in which time to medication discontinuation has been the primary outcome indicate that medications are discontinued by both clinicians and patients. Reasons include lack of efficacy and side effects. It is helpful to encourage openness about the issue and provide education about specific risks and signs of pending relapse when there is nonadherence. The goal is to maintain a good therapeutic relationship and to resume pharmacotherapy as soon as possible when the patient's psychotic symptoms return.

The issue of advising patients and families on the optimal duration of maintenance pharmacotherapy following the first psychotic episode is addressed in a number of clinical practice guidelines for the treatment of schizophrenia. Recommendations are for 1 or 2 years of pharmacotherapy after a remission of positive symptoms following a first episode of psychosis. Risk of relapse is increased by earlier onset and comorbid substance abuse.

Depression in the first episode tends to improve, along with a reduction in positive symptoms, but at a slower rate than in multiepisode patients or those with a more chronic course of illness. Insight also increases with time, which is important, because increased insight is related to adherence. As with multiepisode patients, those with negative symptoms respond poorly to pharmacotherapy. The neurocognitive deficits of schizophrenia tend to be present from the first episode. Although patients experience useful improvements in neurocognition with pharmacotherapy over the first year, they are still significantly impaired in comparison to normal control groups.

Initiating antipsychotic pharmacotherapy should begin as soon as possible and does not need to be initiated in a hospital unless safety issues require inpatient care. Provided that a medical history has been taken and there are no concerns about an organic cause of the psychosis, medications can be started before the physical examination and symptom investigations have been undertaken. The potential risks and benefits of the proposed medications should be discussed with the young person and his or her family. Initiating a medication regimen needs to be integrated into the process of engaging the patient and family into treatment. This involves developing meaningful and realistic pharmacological treatment goals for the patient. For one patient, eliminating distressing hallucinations might be the primary target. For another, improved sleep and reduced anxiety may be most salient. Negative early experiences with pharmacotherapy can have a long-term impact on adherence. Adherence is more likely when families have been involved in education and support.

First-episode patients are more sensitive than multiepisode patients to extrapyramidal side effects and are more likely to respond to lower doses. As a result, starting doses may be lower than those recommended for the general treatment of schizophrenia, and the dose may be titrated upward at weekly intervals, depending on the positive symptom response and the side effects experienced. It is important to explain such a "start low, go slow" strategy to patients and families and to ensure that safety is appropriately addressed. For the 20% of patients who cannot achieve a remission of positive symptoms with an adequate dose of antipsychotic for an adequate duration of time, clozapine should be offered as a second-line treatment.

Most clinical practice guidelines have recommended second-generation antipsychotic medications as the first-choice treatment of first-episode schizophrenia. The main benefit appears to be the lack of extrapyramidal side effects. The main drawbacks have been the increased costs compared with first-generation antipsychotics and the potential for metabolic side effects, especially weight gain. The results of recent large-scale "realistic" or pragmatic clinical trials in the United States and Europe have generally demonstrated a lack of meaningful differences in major clinical outcomes, such as time to treatment discontinuation, symptoms, and quality of life. None of these studies was conducted in first-episode patients, but randomized controlled studies in first-episode patients have not demonstrated consistent and significant differences in efficacy and safety with second-generation antipsychotics.

Psychosocial Interventions

Psychosocial interventions in schizophrenia are supported by a growing body of evidence, as summarized in recent clinical practice guidelines, and some useful general guidelines have been articulated. Such interventions should be seen as necessary, complementary treatments to improve clinical symptoms, functional outcome, and quality of life, and to provide support for patients, their families, and caregivers. Common comorbid conditions, such as substance abuse, anxiety disorders, and depression, are also appropriate targets for psychosocial interventions. Psychosocial interventions are best implemented when acute symptomatology has been reduced to the extent that the patient can successfully engage in treatment. They should be adjusted to the stage of the illness and the needs of patients and their families. Listening and attending to the patient's concerns not only develops empathy, rapport, and a good therapeutic relationship but it can also improve engagement and adherence to treatment. Several studies support the effectiveness of psychosocial treatments for psychotic illnesses; however, not all of these studies have been replicated in patients with first-episode psychosis, indicating a clear need for increased studies. Psychosocial interventions for schizophrenia can target broad or narrow outcomes. They can provide emotional support, enhance skills for functional recovery, or alter illness processes such as symptoms, addictions, or relapse.

The evidence base for psychosocial interventions in early psychosis comes from three sources: clinical practice guidelines and evidence-based reviews of treatments for multi-episode schizophrenia, specific studies of interventions in the first episode of schizophrenia, or from programs that provide comprehensive treatment. The first source is most relevant for the patient with early psychosis who presents with clearly established schizophrenia. The second source can provide guidance on interventions for which a specific evidence base exists for this population. The third source can provide evidence of the acceptability and feasibility of delivering such programs in the real world. These sources can also develop standards and benchmarks for delivering services to individuals with first-episode psychosis and their families.

Case Management

Case management was designed to ensure that patients' individualized treatment programs meet their needs, and developed to address difficulties in negotiating the treatment system and to compensate for patient deficits. Although many models of case management have been described, the type of case management in everyday practice is not clear-cut, because most case managers use a blend of brokerage and clinical case management. Case management is generally provided for individuals with severe and persistent mental disorders. In a population with first-episode psychosis, a number of individuals do not meet such criteria. Nonetheless, the cognitive impairments in the first-episode population are comparable to those of individuals with multiepisode schizophrenia, and overall these patients' levels of functioning do not return to levels comparable to those of the general population. These two factors make case management a justifiable resource for this population. In addition, many patients may not attend clinics due to illness-related factors such as paranoia, social and language differences in immigrant populations, or lack of social supports due to poverty or substance abuse. These factors may all require a more active outreach approach to case management in the form of assertive community treatment (ACT) at the extreme end of a service continuum. ACT combines team-based and outreach approaches to case management. ACT teams have a high staff-to-patient ratio (i.e., 1:10). They have been investigated for treatment of more difficult to engage patients with psychotic disorders, with problems such as substance abuse and social breakdown leading to homelessness. ACT programs have been found to be effective in reducing hospital readmission rates and improving housing and occupational functioning, as well as service satisfaction and quality of life. These programs neither lead to any differential improvement in clinical state nor change the overall costs of care.

Family Intervention

Family interventions in schizophrenia are the most consistently effective psychosocial interventions in schizophrenia research. However, one of two studies of families of individuals with first-episode psychosis did not confirm the benefits found in the majority of studies. The main result of a meta-analysis of 25 intervention studies was that the relapse rate can be reduced by 20% if relatives are included in the treatment of patients with schizophrenia. If family interventions continued for longer than 3 months, the effect was particularly marked. Furthermore, different types of comprehensive family interventions had similar results.

The goals of working with families during patients' first-episode psychosis are generally broader than those in relapse prevention, and include maximizing the adaptive functioning of the family, and minimizing disruption to family life and the risk of long-term grief, stress, and burden. Family members must be collaborators in this process. The issues for families of patients with a first episode of psychosis differ from those in families of patients with multiepisode psychosis (see Table 36.3). Diagnostic ambiguity and uncertainty are major issues, which means that education must be less specific than that for individuals with a more clearly established course. Furthermore, families that may have no prior experience in dealing with someone with a psychosis may be less willing to seek outside support.

One model for working with families, called the recovery stage model, is based on the course of recovery for a person experiencing their first psychotic episode. The model has four stages: (1) managing the crisis, (2) initial stabilization and facilitating recovery, (3) consolidating the gains, and (4) prolonged recovery. Each stage has specific interventions and clearly defined goals. Briefly, the primary goal in the first stage of treatment is crisis management, which involves engaging the family and developing a good working relationship. Individual families are provided support and education about psychosis. The second stage focuses on stabilizing the patient and family, and facilitating recovery. Families are offered both individual and group treatment at this stage. In the third stage, the family worker helps family members integrate the information and skills they learned in the previous stages into their daily lives. In the final stage of treatment, families are prepared to transition into appropriate, long-term treatment programs. Note that in each phase of treatment, families identified as high-risk for difficulties are offered additional interventions and support. Lengths of the stages vary depending on the needs of the family and the patient's rate of recovery. Typically, the crisis stage may last a few months, followed by a 3- to 12-month recovery stage and a 12-month consolidation stage.

A 3-year follow-up of a large Canadian sample of families of individuals with first-episode psychosis describes several clinically relevant issues, including the undoubtedly high levels of family distress. This distress has been demonstrated to improve significantly for many families after 1 year. However, families with more severe distress often took 2 years to recover. In considering the psychological well-being of the families, it was actually family members' appraisals of the impact and consequences of the illness that were most associated with their psychological well-being, not the severity of the illness. Furthermore, in this study, more than 80% of available families participated. These results indicate that family interventions are beneficial and can be effective in real clinical situations, and that engaging the family during the patient's first psychotic episode is advantageous.

Family interventions can be provided in two ways: to individual families or to groups. The interventions can be provided by either a special family worker or by case managers as part of a range of services for the individual patient. There is little research evidence to guide the choice of interventions. There is some evidence that family groups can become long-term self-supporting organizations, but it is not clear what proportion of the population of families can be engaged in groups. Providing each family with a specific family worker who makes outreach visits to family homes has been shown to engage the families of 70–80% of patients. Both family education and support provided by an in-

TABLE 36.3. Issues for Families of Early-Psychosis Patients

Issues for families	Treatment implication
Diagnostic ambiguity	Focus on individual family unit
Inexperience	Focus on issues
Lack of external support	Education accepts ambiguity

dividual family worker, or by one trained to run family groups, have been shown to be effective in research studies; it is not known how effective family interventions are when provided by a case manager.

Cognitive-Behavioral Therapy

Cognitive-behavioral therapy (CBT) is gaining recognition as a potentially effective treatment for improving outcome among patients with schizophrenia, with several randomized controlled trials (RCTs) demonstrating the effectiveness of CBT for individuals with established illness. These data have led to its being recommended for the treatment of patients with persistent symptoms at evidence level B in the Canadian Clinical Practice Guidelines for Schizophrenia and at level A in the Schizophrenia Clinical Guideline on Core Interventions in Primary and Secondary Care. The U.K. guidelines also recommend CBT to improve insight (evidence level B) and in the management of poor adherence (evidence level C). The U.K. guidelines define *CBT for schizophrenia* as a discrete psychological intervention that encourages recipients to establish links among their thoughts, feelings, and actions with respect to the current or past symptoms, and allows recipients to reevaluate their perceptions, beliefs, and reasoning related to the target symptoms. CBT for schizophrenia involves at least one of the following: (1) recipients' monitoring of their own thoughts, feelings, and behavior with respect to the symptoms; (2) promotion of alternative ways of coping with the target symptoms; and (3) reduction of stress. There are few studies of CBT in early psychosis, but there is no reason to suppose that the most robust finding of an impact of CBT on symptoms refractory to pharmacotherapy would not apply to the 20% of patients who do not achieve a remission of their first episode of psychosis.

A detailed review of specific studies of CBT in first-episode psychosis suggests that cognitive therapies are acceptable in early psychosis. Although some studies have examined treatments during the acute phase of the psychotic illness, advantages over routine care have been small and time-limited. Furthermore, routine care is generally effective in the acute first episode, leaving less room for added improvements. In contrast to the use of cognitive therapy as a general treatment for a first episode of psychosis, a more targeted approach has been taken in a number of studies that have examined the impact on relapse prevention, adherence, and the treatment of comorbid problems, such as substance use, anxiety, and depression.

The results from clinical trials of CBT for psychosis and the need to develop psychosocial interventions for patients with first-episode psychosis make CBT a compelling treatment to consider as an integral part of early-psychosis services. However, more research into its effectiveness is clearly warranted. In addition, research needs to consider the skills required for therapists, and the integration of cognitive therapies with other treatment modalities. Few mental health therapists will have received any training in cognitive therapy for psychosis. For therapists trained in cognitive therapy for depression or anxiety, differences in techniques allow for the cognitive impairments of schizophrenia, stigma, or loss. The key techniques include (1) developing a therapeutic alliance based upon the patient's perspective, (2) developing alternative explanations of schizophrenia symptoms, (3) reducing the impact of positive and negative symptoms, and (4) offering personally relevant models to address medication adherence.

Group Therapy

There have been no randomized controlled studies of group therapy in first-episode schizophrenia, and research in the schizophrenia field in general is limited. Group therapy is a therapeutic intervention that can complement other interventions, such as individual and family work. Because a group leader may choose from a range of theoretical models that might best meet the identified needs and goals of clients, he or she needs to know and understand the practical application of the range of theories underlying group programs. *Group process* describes the "life" of the group—that is, what is happening in the group and how this changes over time. Group processes include aspects such as phases of group development, communication patterns, group composition, energy level, group roles, themes, and leadership style. Group processes are a function of group dynamics (the behavior of people within a group context). Group process can be considered from both an individual and a group perspective—that is, seeing the group "as a whole" and considering it an entity in and of itself. Skills and knowledge are needed to manage any group. Groups can provide targeted interventions that increase adherence or reduce substance abuse. Additionally the therapist should consider key, implicit factors of any group work, such as universality, instillation of hope, cohesion, altruism, interpersonal learning, imitative behavior, socialization, catharsis, and corrective recapitulation of the primary family group.

Group therapy for multiepisode schizophrenia has been demonstrated to be effective for increasing medication adherence, although replication studies have not necessarily confirmed these results. In addition, group therapy has been shown to be effective for comorbid addictions and for social skills training, both of which are indicated for individuals with specific problems, namely, addictions and social deficits.

Integrated Addictions Treatment

Several reports from first-episode programs have reported high levels of comorbid substance use. Integrated treatment of addictions and psychosis, recommended as the optimal approach for dealing with comorbid schizophrenia and addictions, is supported by the majority of clinical practice guidelines. Although, there is little specific research on this issue, there is no reason to think that this should not apply to the early-psychosis population. There is evidence from comprehensive treatment programs that comorbid addictions can improve with time. The issue of treating comorbid addictions is particularly important for the first-episode population, because it is easy to dismiss a first presentation of psychosis as a drug-induced psychosis, which often leads to a recommendation for addictions treatment only. Because the majority of individuals with addictions never develop a psychosis, it seems appropriate to refer routinely those who do to an early-psychosis treatment service.

The critical components of integrated programs for psychosis and addictions include screening; motivational interventions; a comprehensive, long-term, staged approach; provision of help to clients in acquiring skills and supports to manage both illnesses and to pursue functional goals, and assertive outreach, when required.

Work and Education Rehabilitation

Studies of vocational programs in schizophrenia have demonstrated the efficacy of supported employment programs. There have been limited studies in early psychosis. For many of these individuals, education is a more appropriate goal than employment. Some patients who seek employment may qualify for disability benefits, which may include access to formal organizational processes for graduated return to work or limited work. Others may more appropriately be referred to supportive employment programs if they are unable to find and retain employment without assistance.

Supported employment facilitates competitive work in integrated work settings for individuals with the most severe disabilities, for whom competitive employment has not traditionally occurred, and for those who, because of the nature and severity of their disability, need ongoing support services to perform their job. Supported employment provides assistance such as job coaches, transportation, specialized job training, and individually tailored supervision. Recent studies indicate that the provision of ongoing support services for people with severe disabilities significantly increases their rates of employment retention.

Return to education is best achieved through a graduated process at an initially less intense level than that prior to the psychosis. Different jurisdictions provide varying degrees of support or accommodation for persons with disabilities, including disabilities that result from mental disorders. It is important for case managers to be familiar with the resources available within the local educational institutions and to work collaboratively with them.

Suicide Prevention

Studies of pathways to care indicate that many patients attempt suicide in the early stages of psychosis, prior to diagnosis and treatment. Indeed for a proportion of patients the suicide attempt is the presenting problem that identifies the underlying disorder. An inconsistent finding in studies is that patients in the early years of the illness have an increased risk of suicide and attempted suicide. However, both prior depression and suicide attempts are robust predictors of suicide and attempted suicide. Furthermore, depression, a common early sign of psychosis, is a greater problem during recovery from first-episode than from multiepisode psychosis. Results from an RCT and real-world services support the contention that early-psychosis programs reduce the rate of attempted suicide.

Recovery from psychosis has received more attention recently, because it is apparent that remission of positive symptoms often is not accompanied by a full functional recovery. It is appropriate that this should be considered an important issue for the treatment of early psychosis. There are two approaches in thinking about the term *recovery*: The first is a pragmatic, research-based approach that seeks to establish criteria for level of functioning and absence of symptoms. The second use of the term does not include symptomatic and functional recovery, but it does include concepts such as awareness of the toll the illness takes, recognition of the need to change, insight as to how this change can begin, and the determination it takes to recover. Both are valid uses of the term, and a few studies have demonstrated that these concepts appear to be mutually reinforcing. Attention to both the biomedical and the psychosocial aspects of treatment are required for both approaches.

DELIVERING SERVICES TO PATIENTS WITH EARLY PSYCHOSIS

Early-psychosis treatment services are provided wherever patients present with first-episode psychosis. Such services may be easy or difficult to access, coordinated or fragmented, and sensitive or insensitive to the specific needs of these patients and the families who support them. There is a debate as to whether such services should be provided by specialized teams or as part of routine mental health services. Specialized programs exist around the world and have been mandated in the United Kingdom and in Ontario, Canada's largest province. Most of these services deliver some or all of the evidence-base services described earlier. Specialized programs are a way for health providers to organize and deliver services to a group of patients; they are not discrete treatment packages that are separate from other mental health services. Mental health services for individuals with an early psychosis should be organized to provide timely, necessary, and appropriate services for the defined population, whether within a specialized program or as part of general services. The debate over specialized programs is in part about competition for resources for patients, and in part a scientific debate about the necessary and sufficient evidence-based services a provider needs to deliver. Absent from this debate has been a set of broadly accepted performance measures by which early-psychosis services can be evaluated. Establishing standards and norms for performance measures for such services, however they are delivered, would put the focus on outcomes rather than on the organization of services.

KEY POINTS

- Improved services for first-episode psychosis require strategies to promote early intervention and optimal care.
- Much of the evidence base for components of early-psychosis treatment services comes from research on schizophrenia services; some of it from specific trials in early psychosis, and some from early intervention programs.
- Services derived from the treatment of patients with multiepisode psychosis need to be adapted to this population.

REFERENCES AND RECOMMENDED READINGS

Addington, D., Mckenzie, E., Addington, J., Patten, S., Smith, H,, & Adair, C. (2005). Performance measures for early psychosis treatment services. *Psychiatric Services, 56*(12), 1570–1582.

Addington, J., & Addington, D. (2006). Phase-specific group treatment for recovery in an early psychosis programme. In J. O. Johannessen, B. V. Martindale, & J. Cullberg (Eds.), *Evolving psychosis: Different stages, different treatments.* Hove, UK: Routledge.

Addington, J., McCleery, A., & Addington, D. (2005).Three-year outcome of family work in an early psychosis program. *Schizophrenia Research, 79*(1), 77–83.

American Psychiatric Association. (2004). *Practice guideline for the treatment of patients with schizophrenia* (2nd ed.). Arlington, VA: Author.

Canadian Psychiatric Association Working Group. (2005). *Clinical practice guidelines: Treatment of schizophrenia. Canadian Journal of Psychiatry, 50*(13, Suppl. 1), 1S–56S.

Dickerson, F. B., & Lehman, A. F. (2006). Evidence-based psychotherapy for schizophrenia. *Journal of Nervous and Mental Disease, 194*(1), 3–9.

Drake, R. E., Essock, S. M., Shaner, A., Carey, K. B., Minkoff, K., Kola, L., et al. (2001). Implementing dual diagnosis services for clients with severe mental illness. *Psychiatric Services, 52*(4), 469–476.

Drake, R. E., Mueser, K. T., Brunette, M. F., & McHugo, G. J. (2004). A review of treatments for people with severe mental illnesses and co-occurring substance use disorders. *Psychiatric Rehabilitation Journal, 27*(4), 360–374.

Haddock, G., & Lewis, S. (2005). Psychological interventions in early psychosis. *Schizophrenia Bulletin, 31*(3), 697–704.

Jones, P. B., Barnes, T. R., Davies, L., Dunn, G., Lloyd, H., Hayhurst, K. P., et al. (2006). Randomized controlled trial of the effect on quality of life of second- vs first-generation antipsychotic drugs in schizophrenia: Cost Utility of the Latest Antipsychotic Drugs in Schizophrenia Study (CUtLASS 1). *Archives of General Psychiatry, 63*(10), 1079–1087.

Lieberman, J. A., Stroup, T. S., McEvoy, J. P., Swartz, M. S., Rosenheck, R. A., Perkins, D. O., et al.

(2005). Effectiveness of antipsychotic drugs in patients with chronic schizophrenia. *New England Journal of Medicine, 353*(12), 1209–1223.

Marshall, M., Lewis, S., Lockwood, A., Drake, R., Jones, P., & Croudace, T. (2005). Association between duration of untreated psychosis and outcome in cohorts of first-episode patients: A systematic review. *Archives of General Psychiatry, 62*(9), 975–983.

McGorry, P. D., Edwards, J., Mihalopoulos, C., Harrigan, S. M., & Jackson, H. J. (1996). EPPIC: An evolving system of early detection and optimal management. *Schizophrenia Bulletin, 22*(2), 305–325.

Melle, I., Johannesen, J. O., Friis, S., Haahr, U., Joa, I., Larsen, T. K., et al. (2006). Early detection of the first episode of schizophrenia and suicidal behavior. *American Journal of Psychiatry, 163*(5), 800–804.

Melle, I., Larsen, T. K., Haahr, U., Friis, S., Johannessen, J. O., Opjordsmoen, S., et al. (2004). Reducing the duration of untreated first-episode psychosis: Effects on clinical presentation. *Archives of General Psychiatry, 61*(2), 143–150.

Mueser, K.T., Bond, G. R., Drake, R. E., & Resnick, S. G. (1998). Models of community care for severe mental illness: A review of research on case management. *Schizophrenia Bulletin, 24*(1), 37–74.

National Collaborating Centre for Mental Health. (2003). *Schizophrenia full national guideline on core interventions in primary and secondary care* (Report No. 1). London: Gaskell.

Penn, D. L., Waldheter, E. J., Perkins, D. O., Mueser K. T., & Lieberman, J. A. (2005) Psychosocial treatment for first-episode psychosis: A research update. *American Journal of Psychiatry, 162*(12), 2220–2232.

Resnick, S. G., Rosenheck, R. A., & Lehman, A. F. (2004). An exploratory analysis of correlates of recovery. *Psychiatric Services, 55*(5), 540–547.

Robinson, D. G., Woerner, M. G., Delman, H. M., & Kane, J. M. Pharmacological treatments for first-episode schizophrenia. *Schizophrenia Bulletin, 31*(3), 705–722.

Royal Australian and New Zealand College of Psychiatrists. (2005). Royal Australian and New Zealand College of Psychiatrists clinical practice guidelines for the treatment of schizophrenia and related disorders. *Australian and New Zealand Journal of Psychiatry, 39*(1–2, 1–30.

Scott, J. E., & Dixon, L. B. (1995). Assertive community treatment and case management for schizophrenia. *Schizophrenia Bulletin, 21*(4), 657–668.

Twamley, E. W., Jeste, D. V., & Lehman, A. F. (2003). Vocational rehabilitation in schizophrenia and other psychotic disorders: A literature review and meta-analysis of randomized controlled trials. *Journal of Nervous and Mental Disease, 191*(8), 515–523.

CHAPTER 37

TREATMENT OF THE SCHIZOPHRENIA PRODROME

BARNABY NELSON
ALISON YUNG

THE PRODROME, PREPSYCHOTIC INTERVENTION, AND THE PERSONAL ASSESSMENT AND CRISIS EVALUATION (PACE) CLINIC

This chapter outlines a treatment approach specifically designed for young people identified as being at imminent or "ultra high risk" (UHR) of developing a psychotic disorder—that is, as possibly being in the prodromal phase of a psychotic disorder. This approach has been developed at the Personal Assessment and Crisis Evaluation (PACE) Clinic in Melbourne, Australia, the first clinic to provide a clinical research service for this group.

From the outset, it is important to note that although the title of this chapter refers to the "schizophrenia prodrome," the focus of discussion is on the prevention of frank or full-blown psychotic disorder rather than on schizophrenia as a discrete illness. The first psychotic episode is the target, which is regarded as a more proximal and therapeutically salient target than schizophrenia. Schizophrenia is a subtype of psychotic disorder to which some individuals progress after a first psychotic episode, but it is not an inevitable result of this first episode.

The possibility of treating psychotic disorders during the prodromal phase is an alluring prospect for a number of reasons. The prodromal phase is characterized by a considerable array of psychiatric symptoms and disability, including self-harming and other health-damaging behaviors. A substantial amount of the disability that develops in psychotic disorders accumulates prior to the appearance of the full positive psychotic syndrome and may even create a ceiling for eventual recovery. In addition, recent studies have indicated that at some point in the transition from prodromal phase to full-blown psychotic disorder, alterations in brain structure (and presumably function) occur. If the prodrome is recognized prospectively and treatment is provided at this stage, then existing disability may be minimized, recovery may be possible before symptoms and poor functioning become entrenched, and the possibility of preventing, delaying, or ameliorating the onset of diagnosable psychotic disorder arises. Neurobiological changes that occur around the time of onset of full-blown psychotic disorder might also be prevented, minimized, or reversed. Thus, the prodromal phase presents two possible targets for intervention: (1) current symptoms, behavior, or disability, and (2) prevention of further decline into frank psychotic disorder.

Aside from these two treatment aims, there are a number of other benefits of treatment of people during the prodrome. Individuals experiencing this early phase of the disorder may engage more quickly with treatment than those who present late, when psychotic symptoms are entrenched, social networks are more disrupted, and functioning has further deteriorated. Additionally, the individual may be more likely to accept treatment if full-blown psychosis does emerge compared to the individual who has been unwell for a longer time before seeking assistance. This may be especially so given that the person is likely already to have developed a therapeutic relationship with a treating team. Effective treatment can be provided rapidly if the person does develop psychosis, possibly avoiding the need for hospitalization and minimizing the deleterious effect of extended untreated psychosis. Finally, prepsychotic intervention offers the chance to research the onset phase of psychotic illness, which may provide insight into the core features of the psychopathology and psychobiology of psychosis.

However, intervention during the prodromal phase is an approach that carries risks as well as benefits. The most salient of these is the issue of *false positives*, which are individuals who are identified as being at risk of developing a psychotic disorder, but who in fact are not destined to develop a psychotic disorder. These individuals may be harmed by being labeled as being at high risk of psychosis and may receive treatment unnecessarily. Clearly, it is difficult to distinguish these patients from those identified as being at risk of developing a psychotic disorder and who would indeed have developed a psychotic disorder if some alteration in their circumstances (e.g., a treatment intervention, stress reduction, cessation of illicit drug use) had not prevented this from occurring. This latter group has been termed the *false false-positive* group. These issues highlight the retrospective nature of the concept of the psychotic prodrome: Onset of frank psychosis cannot be predicted with certainty from any particular symptom or combination of symptoms; the fact that an individual was "prodromal" can only be asserted once frank psychosis has emerged. Thus, the PACE Clinic introduced the term *at-risk mental state* (ARMS) to refer to the phase prospectively identified as the possible precursor to full-blown psychosis.

Given the lack of specificity of many prodromal symptoms of schizophrenia and other psychotic disorders, strategies are needed to increase the accuracy of prediction of psychosis from the presence of an ARMS. The PACE Clinic adopted a "close-in" strategy to identify this population, using a combination of established trait and state risk factors for psychosis with common phenomenology from the prodromal phase of psychotic disorders, as well as narrowing identification to the age range of highest risk (late adolescence and early adulthood). According to PACE inclusions rules, UHR individuals must meet criteria for at least one of the following groups: (1) *attenuated psychotic symptoms group*, individuals who have experienced subthreshold, attenuated forms of positive psychotic symptoms during the past year; (2) *brief limited intermittent psychotic symptoms group*, individuals who have experienced episodes of frank psychotic symptoms that have lasted no longer than a week and have spontaneously abated; or (3) *trait and state risk factor group*, individuals who have a first-degree relative with a psychotic disorder, or who have a schizotypal personality disorder in addition to a significant decrease in functioning during the previous year. The person must be between ages 14 and 30 years, and cannot have experienced a psychotic episode for longer than 1 week or received neuroleptic medication prior to referral to the PACE Clinic.

Early work at PACE indicated that young people meeting these intake criteria had a 40% chance of developing a psychotic episode in the 12 months after recruitment, despite the provision of supportive counseling, case management, and antidepressant medication, if required. This substantial "transition to psychosis" statistic provided good support for the validity of the PACE criteria in identifying the UHR population. Since the mid-1990s, multiple centers internationally have adopted these criteria.

Subsequent studies at PACE have included intervention trials that comprised both psychological and pharmacological treatments. These are reviewed briefly, along with the general treatment approach adopted by the PACE Clinic.

GENERAL TREATMENT MEASURES

Information Giving

The rationale for use of the clinical service needs to be explained to the patient at initial assessment. This explanation should cover the dual focus of the clinical service—treatment of current symptoms and disability, and prevention of full-blown psychotic disorder. It is possible that being labeled as high risk for psychotic disorder may lead to stigmatization of the individual, both by others and by the person him- or herself. The PACE Clinic has addressed this issue in a number of ways: The choice of name avoids any direct reference to mental health; the location of the clinic is in a suburban shopping center, a nonstigmatizing and acceptable environment for young people; information is provided sensitively, emphasizing that psychosis is not the inevitable result of UHR status, that monitoring of mental state is available, and that timely intervention is provided if symptoms worsen, and that the individual's UHR status will remain confidential; ongoing opportunities for discussion of risk and normal developmental challenges are provided; and referral to other mental health services that also emphasize early intervention and focus on recovery.

Case Management

Case management refers to helping the patient deal with practical issues, such as arranging accommodation, arranging social security payments, enrolling in education, applying for employment, and liaising with other services. Case management is provided in addition to specific psychological and pharmacological interventions. This is important, because neglecting difficulties in more fundamental aspects of daily living may have an impact on the efficacy of the therapy and increase the patient's level of stress.

Crisis Management

Although the UHR population does not meet full DSM criteria for a psychotic disorder, it is not uncommon for these patients to experience crises. Therefore, risk issues need to be taken into account. It is necessary to have emergency and after-hours services available or to be able to tell young people how to access after-hours support should they need it.

Family Interventions

Family members are often distressed and anxious about the changes they have noticed in their UHR relative. Support for these family members is helpful. Psychoeducation about being at high risk for psychosis should be provided to family members to deal with their distress and to minimize the possible negative outcome of UHR status on family functioning (e.g., pathologizing and stigmatizing the UHR individual). Parents should be provided information regarding their child's progress and treatment, as appropriate. This process needs to be sensitive to the young person's confidentiality and privacy. Additionally, it may become apparent that systemic family issues are a factor in the young person's distress and symptoms. These issues may be addressed in the clinic, or they may require referral to a more specialized family service.

PSYCHOLOGICAL TREATMENTS

Psychological treatment has been a cornerstone of the treatment provided at PACE since its inception. Both supportive psychotherapy and cognitively oriented psychotherapy have received trials at PACE. These approaches share several characteristics: Both focus on engagement and the formation of a strong, collaborative, respectful relationship between the therapist and the patient, and both aim toward the development of effective coping skills.

Supportive Psychotherapy

Although it does not specifically target psychotic symptoms, supportive therapy endeavors to provide the patient with emotional and social support, and it incorporates many of the constituents of Rogerian person-centered therapy, including empathy, unconditional positive regard, and patient-initiated process. The aim is to facilitate an environment in which the young person is accepted and cared for, and in which he or she can discuss concerns and share experiences with the therapist.

Key strategies for promoting engagement beyond basic counseling skills include offering practical help, working initially with the client's primary concerns and sources of distress, flexibility with time and location of therapy, provision of information and education about symptoms, working with family members, and collaborative goal setting. In addition to promoting change through nondirective strategies, basic problem-solving approaches are also offered. This may include helping the patient to develop skills such as brainstorming responses to situations, role play of possible solutions, goal setting, time management, and so forth. The patient is encouraged to be proactive and to monitor his or her own progress. Some degree of role playing may occur within sessions as a springboard to changes in behavior outside the sessions.

Cognitively Oriented Psychotherapy

A substantial body of evidence has indicated the benefits of psychological intervention, particularly cognitive-behavioral therapy (CBT), in the treatment of established psychotic disorders. It is also a highly acceptable, relatively safe form of treatment for patients. Given the reported benefits and acceptability of psychological treatment for people with established psychosis, a good case may be made for this intervention's value in treating individuals in the prepsychotic or prodromal phase of illness.

The assessment/engagement phase of this therapy is crucial. Patients may be confused or distressed by their symptoms, and early sessions provide an opportunity for the therapist to develop a formulation that can provide patients with some understanding of their symptoms, as well as guide the course of therapy. This early phase of therapy also provides an opportunity for the therapist to emphasize the collaborative nature of the therapy and to select appropriate interventions for the therapeutic relationship based on the client's developmental level and symptomatic presentation. The strategies for engagement are similar to those mentioned earlier for supportive therapy.

The cognitively oriented therapy developed at PACE for the high-risk group uses strategies developed for acutely unwell and recovering populations. Cognitive models approach the core symptoms of psychosis as deriving from basic disturbances in information processing that result in perceptual abnormalities and disturbed experience of the self. Cognitive biases, inaccurate appraisals, and core self-schemas further contribute to maladaptive beliefs. Cognitive therapy aims to help people to develop an understanding of the cognitive processes (including biases and maladaptive appraisals) that influence their thoughts and emotions, and to develop more realistic and positive views of themselves and events around them.

The stress–vulnerability model of psychosis informs the treatment approach. A central assumption of this model is that environmental stressors (e.g., relationship issues, substance use, lifestyle factors) are key factors in precipitating illness onset in vulnerable individuals. This implies that the implementation of appropriate coping strategies may ameliorate the influence of vulnerability. Therefore, strengthening the individual's coping resources forms a core component of the cognitive therapy offered at PACE.

Although stress management forms the backbone of this therapy, it is important to address the wide array of presenting symptoms in this population. To this end, a range of treatment modules have been developed within the cognitive therapy: *Stress Management, Depression/Negative Symptoms, Positive Symptoms,* and *Other Comorbidity.* The assessment of the presenting problem(s), and the client's own perception of his or her functioning, informs the selection of modules to be implemented during the course of therapy. Although the therapy comprises individual modules targeting specific symptom groups, it may not be appropriate to target one group of symptoms in isolation (i.e., any course of therapy, indeed, any individual therapy session may incorporate aspects of more than one module). The therapy was designed to be provided on an individual basis, but it could potentially be adapted to suit a group treatment situation. Young people can currently attend PACE for a maximum of 12 months, with session frequency varying from weekly to every 2 weeks, and even monthly in the final stages, depending on client need.

The treatment modules are described below.

Stress Management

In keeping with the stress–vulnerability model of psychosis, elements of the Stress Management module are provided to all patients. This module has the added advantage of providing an easily understood introduction to cognitive–behavioral principles, which sets the direction of future sessions. Strategies include the following:

- Psychoeducation about the nature of the stress and anxiety.
- Stress monitoring that encourages patients to record varying stress levels over specific time periods and to identify triggers and consequences of anxiety or stress.
- Stress management techniques, such as relaxation, meditation, exercise, and distraction.
- Identification of maladaptive coping techniques (e.g., excessive substance use, social withdrawal).

• Identification of cognitions associated with subjective feelings of stress or heightened anxiety, which may include the completion of relevant inventories.
• Cognitive restructuring of dysfunctional thoughts that may be maintaining anxiety/stress are countered with a more functional cognitive style (e.g., more positive coping statements, positive reframing, and challenging).

Other strategies include goal-setting and time management, assertiveness training, and problem solving.

Positive Symptoms

The strategies incorporated within this module are primarily drawn from cognitive approaches to managing full-blown positive symptoms. The goal of this module is to enhance strategies for coping with positive symptoms when they occur, to recognize early warning signs of these symptoms, and to prevent their exacerbation through the implementation of preventive strategies. The fact that the experience of positive symptoms by UHR individuals is less intense and/or less frequent than that of individuals with frank psychosis can assist in guiding UHR individuals to recognize and manage these symptoms. For example, unusual perceptual experiences may be more easily recognized as anomalous, and attenuated delusional thoughts may be more easily dismissed or challenged than more entrenched delusional thoughts. Strategies include the following:

• Psychoeducation about symptoms, including a biopsychosocial account of the origins of unusual experiences tailored to the individual patient. This can serve both to "normalize" these experiences and enhance motivation for treatment. It is important that the therapist's language be modified appropriately for this population. For instance, because these individuals have not been diagnosed with a psychotic disorder, it may not be helpful to use the term *psychosis*. Use of this term may depend on the individual's level of anxiety about the possibility of developing a psychotic disorder and his or her general cognitive level. Generally, it is most useful to adopt the language that patients use to refer to their unusual experiences. Focusing discussion on dealing with current symptoms is often more productive than concentrating on the potential negative outcomes.
• Verbal challenge and reality testing of delusional thoughts and hallucinations. An individualized, multidimensional model of beliefs relating to delusional thinking or perceptual abnormalities is developed. This model is based on issues such as the meaning that the individual attributes to the experiences, the conclusions that he or she draws from the experiences and how he or she explains them. This model is then challenged by examining its supporting evidence and generating and empirically testing alternative interpretations of experiences.
• Coping enhancement techniques, such as distraction, withdrawal, elimination of maladaptive coping strategies, and stress reduction techniques.
• Normalizing psychotic experiences. Suggesting to patients that their attenuated psychotic symptoms are not discontinuous from normality or unique to them can serve to decrease some of the associated anxiety and self-stigma.
• Self-monitoring of symptoms to enhance the client's understanding of the relationship of his or her symptoms to other factors, such as environmental events and emotional states. An important component of self-monitoring is for the patient to be alert to any worsening of symptoms, which might indicate the onset of acute psychosis.

Depression/Negative Symptoms

Negative symptoms include low motivation, emotional apathy, cognitive and motoric slowness, underactivity, lack of drive, poverty of speech, and social withdrawal. These symptoms may often be difficult to distinguish from depressive symptoms, although emotional flatness as opposed to depressed mood is often used as a key distinguishing feature. Treatment of these symptoms is incorporated into the therapy, because evidence suggests that they have a significant impact on the future course of the disorder. Additionally, negative symptoms may be easier to treat in the UHR population than in individuals with established psychosis, because the symptoms are less firmly entrenched.

Cognitive-behavioral strategies used to target negative symptoms closely resemble those developed for treatment of depression. Strategies include goal setting, activity management (both mastery and pleasure activities), problem solving, social skills training, and cognitive restructuring of self-defeating cognitions. Negative symptoms can serve a protective function in the sense of ensuring that the individual avoids potentially stressful situations that may precipitate or exacerbate positive symptoms. If there are indications that negative symptoms may be serving this protective function, then the patient is encouraged to take a slow, graded approach to increasing activity levels and challenging tasks.

Other Comorbidity

This module includes cognitive-behavioral strategies for more severe anxiety and substance use symptoms experienced by UHR patients. The most frequent comorbid problems experienced by UHR patients are social anxiety, generalized anxiety, panic disorder, obsessive–compulsive symptoms, posttraumatic symptoms, and substance use. Components of this module include psychoeducation about the comorbid symptoms and, in line with the stress–vulnerability model, the possibility of comorbid symptoms exacerbating attenuated psychotic symptoms; development of an appropriate model to explain the patient's symptoms, including consideration of his or her life experiences, coping strategies, developmental level, ongoing stressors, and available supports; and presentation of a cognitive-behavioral model of anxiety, including discussion of the relationship between cognitions, affect, and behavior. More specific strategies that may be employed, depending on the presenting problems, include management of physiological symptoms of anxiety; exposure techniques; behavioral strategies, such as thought stopping, distraction, and activity scheduling; motivational interviewing in relation to substance use; and cognitive strategies.

The first PACE intervention study demonstrated a reduction in transition rate to psychosis in the treatment group, which received a combination of low-dose antipsychotic medication and cognitively oriented psychotherapy over a 6-month treatment period, compared to the control group, which received supportive psychotherapy alone. At the end of the 6-month treatment period, nearly 36% of the control group had developed psychosis compared to 9.7% of the treatment group ($p = .026$). However, the difference between the groups was no longer significant 6 months after the cessation of treatment. Both groups demonstrated improvement on a range of measures of psychopathology and functioning after the initial 6 months. Because the treatment group received a combination of antipsychotic medication and cognitive therapy, it was not possible to determine which intervention was the most helpful. A second trial, currently underway, aims to compare low-dose antipsychotic, cognitive therapy, and a combination of the two in a placebo-controlled design. Support for the efficacy of CBT in the UHR group comes from a recent British trial, which found that cognitive therapy significantly reduced the risk of transition to psychosis in a UHR group.

PHARMACOLOGICAL TREATMENT

Antipsychotic Medication

The use of antipsychotic medication is based on its demonstrated efficacy with psychotic populations. It is thought that this might translate to the prepsychotic phase—that is, that antipsychotic medication may be useful in treatment of existing attenuated psychotic symptoms and in prevention of the emergence of frank psychosis.

The first PACE intervention trial (described previously) used low-dose risperidone (1–2 mg per day) in combination with CBT. There were few side effects reported. However, many patients were nonadherent (42%) or only partially adherent (13%) with medication. The conclusion from this trial was that it may be possible to delay the onset of psychosis, although the "active ingredient" in the treatment provided (antipsychotic medication or cognitively oriented therapy) still needs to be distilled. However, the fact that the rate of transition to psychosis remained significantly lower in the risperidone-adherent subgroup at the end of the posttreatment 6-month follow-up period compared to the control group provides some evidence for the potential efficacy of antipsychotic medication in this population. The Prevention through Risk Identification, Management, and Education (PRIME) team have recently reported a similar pattern of results with olanzapine. This study also had problems with adherence, with 32% of patients dropping out of treatment.

Opponents of this treatment approach have argued that psychosis is not necessarily harmful, and that side effects of pharmacological treatment may in fact increase an individual's morbidity without providing benefit, particularly in the false-positive subset of patients.

In recognition of the need for further evaluation of the appropriateness and efficacy of antipsychotics in the UHR population, these medications should not be considered a first treatment option for this group at present. Exceptions may include situations in which there is a rapid deterioration of mental state, in which severe suicidal risk is present and treatment of depression has proved ineffective, or when the individual is judged to be a threat to others. If antipsychotic medication is considered, then low-dose atypicals should be used. However, firm recommendations for pharmacological treatment, including optimal dose and duration of treatment, will be only be forthcoming after more research.

Other Pharmacological Agents

Although the reported studies indicate the possible benefit of antipsychotic medication in the high-risk population, it is possible that other interventions may be more appropriate for the early stages of illness. Indeed, frank psychotic symptoms may just be "noise" around an underlying disease process that might respond to something quite different from antipsychotic medication. If this is the case, then targeting attenuated psychotic symptoms in this population may result in symptomatic improvement, while the underlying disease process remains untreated and may continue to progress. Therefore, other pharmacological treatments, such as neuroprotective agents and antidepressants, have been suggested as being of potentially greater benefit in the UHR population.

The rationale for neuroprotective agents is that dysfunctional regulation of generation and degeneration in some brain areas might explain neurodevelopmental abnormalities seen in early psychosis. Neuroprotective strategies counteracting the loss or supporting the generation of progenitor cells may therefore be a therapeutic avenue to explore. Candidate therapies include lithium, eicosapentanoic acid (EPA), and glycine. Studies using lithium, glycine, and EPA are currently underway at the PACE and PRIME Clinics.

Other pharmacological interventions may also be indicated in the UHR group, depending on the young person's presentation and current problems. For instance, specific treatment for syndromes such as depression and anxiety may include medication.

RECOMMENDATIONS AND FUTURE DIRECTIONS

This chapter has provided a brief overview of the identification of the high-risk population and the current approach to its psychological and pharmacological treatment, with an emphasis on the approach used at the PACE Clinic. This area, still in its infancy, therefore requires constant evaluation. Although there is some evidence for the efficacy of the treatments we have reviewed, ongoing research will provide a clearer indication of the most effective types of psychological and pharmacological interventions, and suggest avenues for refining these interventions. Intervention research with this population should continue in the context of methodologically sound and ethical clinical trials. Larger sample sizes, with a higher proportion of "true positive"cases are required to increase validity of the findings.

Due to the early stage of research in this field, researchers need to keep an open mind about possible treatments and to be responsive to developments in related areas of research, including the treatment of established psychosis. In addition to intervention research, it is also necessary to continue attempts to determine the most potent psychopathological, neurocognitive, neurological, and biological vulnerability markers, and combinations thereof, for transition from an at-risk mental state to full psychosis. This will not only assist in increasing the accurate identification of truly prodromal individuals (i.e., minimize "false positives") but also guide the refinement of treatment interventions.

KEY POINTS

- The prodromal phase of psychotic disorder presents two possible targets for intervention: (1) current symptoms, behavior, or disability, and (2) prevention of further decline into frank psychotic disorder.
- The *prodrome* is a retrospective concept; the term *at-risk mental state* (ARMS) has been introduced to refer to the phase prospectively identified as the possible precursor to full-blown psychosis.
- The PACE Clinic introduced a "close-in" strategy to identifying the ARMS population, using a combination of trait and state risk factors.
- The treatment approach adopted by the PACE Clinic has comprised general treatment measures and both psychological (supportive psychotherapy and cognitively oriented psychotherapy) and pharmacological treatments.
- General treatment measures include information giving, case management, crisis management, and family interventions.
- Cognitively oriented psychotherapy is informed by the stress–vulnerability model of psychosis and comprises four treatment modules: Stress Management, Depression/Negative Symptoms, Positive Symptoms, and Other Comorbidity.
- Intervention trials with antipsychotic medication indicate that rate of transition to psychosis may be reduced in medication-adherent individuals.

- Although there is evidence for the effectiveness of a combination of low-dose antipsychotic medication and cognitively oriented psychotherapy in delaying rate of transition to psychosis compared to supportive psychotherapy alone, the active component in therapy still needs to be distilled.
- In recognition of the need for further evaluation of the appropriateness and efficacy of antipsychotics in the UHR population, these medications should not be considered as a first treatment option for this group at present.
- It is important to continue research into the most potent vulnerability markers for transition from ARMS to full psychosis, because this will assist in the accurate identification of truly prodromal individuals and guide the refinement of treatment interventions.

REFERENCES AND RECOMMENDED READINGS

Addington, J., Francey, S. M., & Morrison, A. P. (Eds.). (2006). *Working with people at high risk of developing psychosis.* Chichester, UK: Wiley.

Corcoran, C., Walker, E., Huot, R., Mittal, V., Tessner, K., Kestler, L., et al. (2003). The stress cascade and schizophrenia: Etiology and onset. *Schizophrenia Bulletin, 29*(4), 671–692.

McGorry, P. D., Yung, A. R., & Phillips, L. J. (2003). The "close-in" or ultra high-risk model: A safe and effective strategy for research and clinical intervention in prepsychotic mental disorder. *Schizophrenia Bulletin, 29*(4), 771–790.

McGorry, P. D., Yung, A. R., Phillips, L. J., Yuen, H. P., Francey, S., Cosgrave, E. M., et al. (2002). A randomized controlled trial of interventions designed to reduce the risk of progression to first episode psychosis in a clinical sample with subthreshold symptoms. *Archives of General Psychiatry, 59,* 921–928.

Morrison, A. P., Bentall, R. P., French, P., Walford, L., Kilcommons, A., Knight, A., et al. (2002). Randomized controlled trial of early detection and cognitive therapy for preventing transition to psychosis in high-risk individuals: Study design and interim analysis of transition rate and psychological risk factors. *British Journal of Psychiatry Supplement, 43,* s78–s84.

Morrison, A. P., French, P., Walford, L., Lewis, S. W., Kilcommons, A., Green, J., et al. (2004). Cognitive therapy for the prevention of psychosis in people at ultra-high risk: Randomized controlled trial. *British Journal of Psychiatry, 185*(4), 291–297.

Parnas, J. (2003). Self and schizophrenia: A phenomenological perspective. In T. K. A. David (Ed.), *The self in neuroscience and psychiatry* (pp. 127–141). Cambridge, UK: Cambridge University Press.

Phillips, L. J., & Francey, S. M. (2004). Changing PACE: Psychological interventions in the prepsychotic phase. In J. F. M. Gleeson & P. D. McGorry (Eds.), *Psychological interventions in early psychosis: A treatment handbook* (pp. 23–39). Chichester, UK: Wiley.

Yung, A. R., Phillips, L. J., & McGorry, P. D. (2004a). *Treating schizophrenia in the prodromal phase.* London: Taylor & Francis.

Yung, A. R., Phillips, L. J., Yuen, H. P., & McGorry, P. D. (2004b). Risk factors for psychosis in an ultra high-risk group: Psychopathology and clinical features. *Schizophrenia Research, 67,* 131–142.

CHAPTER 38

OLDER INDIVIDUALS

THOMAS W. MEEKS
DILIP V. JESTE

OVERVIEW OF LATE-LIFE SCHIZOPHRENIA

Popular images, as well as scientific discourses, regarding schizophrenia often focus on how the illness impacts young adults, but schizophrenia also affects a substantial portion of older adults. Among people over age 65, between 0.1 and 0.5% have schizophrenia compared to prevalence estimates near 1% in the general population. Despite the lower prevalence of schizophrenia compared to some other, late-life mental disorders such as dementia and depression, the health care costs for older adults with schizophrenia are quite significant, with one reported estimate of $40,000 per person per year. As the population structure of industrialized nations continues to shift toward ever-increasing numbers of older adults, and as improved health care has extended life expectancy in schizophrenia, the importance of late-life schizophrenia can be expected to grow substantially in the upcoming decades.

Before discussing the unique aspects of schizophrenia in older adults, it is helpful to consider the heterogeneity in this population. One characteristic of schizophrenia that creates important distinctions for illness course and treatment is the age of illness onset. Most older adults with schizophrenia (about 75–80%) developed the illness many years earlier, at a "typical" (i.e., early) age of onset—before age 40. This is notable, because although life expectancy is still somewhat abbreviated for persons with schizophrenia due to factors such as elevated smoking and suicide rates, many people are living with this illness well into their later years. Most of the remaining 20–25% of older adults with schizophrenia have had what is considered a "middle-age onset" (between ages 40 and 65). Only about 3% of schizophrenia cases occur after age 65, which is often termed a *very late schizophrenia-like psychosis*. This terminology reflects that schizophrenia symptoms beginning in late life may represent a distinct illness, often associated with medical or neurological abnormalities. Several distinguishing features of schizophrenia according to age of onset are outlined in Table 38.1. For instance, middle-age onset schizophrenia (compared to early, or typical, onset) generally demonstrates a higher preponderance of

TABLE 38.1. Clinical Comparisons of Schizophrenia According to Age of Illness Onset

	Early (typical) onset	Middle-age onset	Very-late onset (schizophrenia-like psychosis)
Age of onset (years)	< 40	40–65	> 65
Family history of schizophrenia	+	+	–
Frequent prodromal childhood difficulties	+	+	–
Female preponderance	–	+	++
Negative symptoms	++	+	–
Cognitive impairments	++	+	++
Abnormal brain magnetic resonance imaging	–/+	–/+	++
Require lower than usual dose of antipsychotics	–	+	++

Note. ++, usually true; +, often true; –/+, possibly observed; –, usually not true. From Palmer, McClure, and Jeste (2001). Copyright 2001 by InformaWorld. Adapted by permission.

females, more paranoid and less disorganized subtypes, better premorbid functioning, and fewer negative and cognitive symptoms.

Émil Kraepelin was amazingly ahead of his time in characterizing many aspects of the illness we now call schizophrenia; however, some important discoveries about older adults with schizophrenia over the last few decades stand in contrast to presumptions about the illness that Kraepelin termed *dementia praecox.* For many years, in accordance with this terminology of *dementia,* ideas about aging with schizophrenia were largely negative in connotation, including expectations of a progressive, downhill course in symptoms and functioning, as well as notably shorter lifespans for persons with schizophrenia compared to the general population. However, schizophrenia is not typically a "neurodegenerative" disease in the same sense as Alzheimer's or Parkinson's diseases. Certainly older adults with schizophrenia face considerable and unique challenges, but the overall message from recent years of research in this population has been one of hope for meaningful quality of life among aging persons with this disorder. The increased study of persons with schizophrenia outside of institutional settings may partially explain the more optimistic outcomes.

There is notable heterogeneity in the clinical course that schizophrenia takes over several decades, with a minority of persons experiencing the extremes of sustained remission or progressive deterioration. Psychosocial supports and early treatment are two important factors that may contribute to the relatively uncommon state of sustained remission. Nonetheless, the majority of persons with schizophrenia appear to have relatively stable to slightly improved symptom severity after the first few years of the illness. In particular, older adults with schizophrenia may experience less severe positive symptoms (i.e., delusions and hallucinations), although negative symptoms (e.g., apathy) may commonly persist. Cognitive impairment (e.g., impaired attention and working memory) is a core feature of schizophrenia and a frequent problem associated with aging in general. Thus, one might expect cognitive decline to be accentuated in aging persons with schizophrenia. Although older adults with schizophrenia generally experience more problems with cognition than do normal older adults, the *rates* of age-associated cognitive decline are similar between the two groups. Thus, on the whole, the prognosis for older adults with schizophrenia is not as bleak as previously thought. Nonetheless, it should be noted that even older adults whose symptoms improve with aging often do not achieve the same level of daily functioning or quality of life as never-affected older persons, and that treating late-life schizophrenia still requires considerable diligence and skill.

TREATMENT OPTIONS

Since the inception of chlorpromazine in the 1950s, antipsychotic medications have been a central component of schizophrenia treatment. The last several decades have witnessed a broadening array of antipsychotic medications, including the development of second-generation (atypical) antipsychotics. Atypical antipsychotics (clozapine, risperidone, olanzapine, quetiapine, ziprasidone, and aripiprazole) are classified as such primarily because they have a lower propensity than first-generation (typical) medications to cause movement disorders, such as parkinsonism (tremor, rigidity, and/or slowed movements) and tardive dyskinesia (TD). This is particularly relevant in older populations because increased age is a cardinal risk factor for developing both antipsychotic-induced parkinsonism and TD. Older adults taking antipsychotics are up to five times more likely than similar younger patients to experience these movement-related side effects. However, with the possible exception of clozapine, none of these new medications has proved to be as significant a milestone in treatment efficacy as the original discovery of antipsychotics in general. Despite its consistently demonstrated superior efficacy compared to other antipsychotics, clozapine is particularly difficult to use in older adults because of its side effect profile (e.g., agranulocytosis, anticholinergic effects, sedation, seizures, and orthostasis).

Although it is generally accepted that antipsychotic medication is indicated for older adults with schizophrenia, debate remains as to how best to choose a specific antipsychotic medication. Over the last several years, atypical antipsychotics (other than clozapine) have generally been considered first-line therapy for schizophrenia in all age groups (including older adults), with no distinction as to any single, preferred atypical agent. This status as first-line therapy has been due to well-established lower risks of movement disorders with atypical drugs, as described earlier, as well as less proven but sometimes touted better overall tolerability and efficacy for negative symptoms compared to typical agents. Regrettably, most pharmacotherapy trials for schizophrenia include a paucity of older adults. The largest randomized controlled trial specifically for older adults with schizophrenia, conducted with olanzapine and risperidone, demonstrated comparable efficacy between the two medications.

Yet recent comparisons of typical and atypical agents in general adult populations have called into question appreciable differences between these medication classes in overall treatment effectiveness. Additionally, serious risks of atypical antipsychotics in older adults treated for dementia-related psychosis and agitation have emerged, namely, a 1.6–1.7 times increased risk of death in patients with dementia taking these drugs compared to those receiving a placebo, as well as increased rates of cerebrovascular adverse events (e.g., stroke or transient ischemic attack). Whether these risks are specific to older adults with dementia, and whether they also apply to first-generation antipsychotics, remains to be determined. Certainly these risks should be thoroughly explored in future studies of older adults with schizophrenia. Although the lower risk of potentially irreversible movement disorders with atypical versus typical agents makes atypical medications an appealing choice for older adults (who are at elevated risk for such movement disorders), several atypical agents may be more problematic than older medications in causing metabolic disturbances, such as weight gain, diabetes mellitus, and hyperlipidemia. Such metabolic disorders are already common problems in older adults and are important risk factors for some of the top causes of morbidity and mortality among older adults (e.g., heart disease and stroke).

Considering all these various factors, there is not one clear and convincing first-line antipsychotic medication for older adults with schizophrenia. So how, then, does one decide on antipsychotic therapy for the older adult with schizophrenia? There is no simple answer, and all of these previously mentioned factors must be weighed in light of each individual patient's unique history. One notable difference among various antipsychotic agents that may have both clinical and systemwide relevance is cost (e.g., from the perspective of older adults on fixed incomes, or from the perspective of administrators regarding the impending difficulty in financing health care for the growing number of older adults). Aside from cost issues, the various available antipsychotic medications differ primarily in side effect profiles, though individual patients may preferentially respond to one medication or another for unclear reasons. Some of these side effect differences, as previously described, may be generalized by antipsychotic "class" (i.e., typical vs. atypical). Other differences in side effect profiles vary from one agent to another, both within and between classes, and these differences may also be important to consider when treating special subpopulations, such as older adults. For example, medications that strongly block acetylcholine receptors are generally poorly tolerated in older adults, who are especially prone to develop anticholinergic side effects such as cognitive impairment, constipation, and urinary retention. Likewise, many antipsychotic medications antagonize alpha-adrenergic receptors, sometimes resulting in postural hypotension. This side effect may be especially problematic in older adults, who often are taking antihypertensive medications that may add to this effect, and who may be prone to hypotension-related falls (with falls being a major cause of morbidity and mortality in older adults). Excess sedation and parkinsonism may also be antipsychotic side effects that contribute to falls in older adults. Antipsychotic medications also differ in their effects on cardiac conduction (e.g., QT interval prolongation). Whereas the increased rates of cardiac disease in older adults may heighten the relevance of cardiac conduction effects, the clinical significance of these different effects among antipsychotics is unknown.

Once a specific antipsychotic agent has been chosen, it is important to adjust medication dosage based on the person's age. Older adults generally respond to lower doses of antipsychotic medication and are more sensitive to the side effects. Aging brings about changes in both pharmacokinetics (e.g., reduced renal and hepatic clearance of drugs) and pharmacodynamics (e.g., dopaminergic neuronal cell loss or altered receptor density) related to antipsychotic medications. As a general rule, older adults with schizophrenia often require only 50–75% of the usual antipsychotic dose given to younger adults with the same disorder. It may be helpful in less urgent situations to begin therapy with 25% or less of the usual adult dosage, then titrate up as necessary. Certain subgroups, including the "old-old" (those over age 75) and persons with middle-age or very-late-onset schizophrenia, may respond to even lower doses (e.g., 25–33% of the usual adult dosage). The most evidence regarding effective daily doses from controlled trials exists for risperidone (ca.2 mg/day) and olanzapine (ca.10 mg/day) among relatively "young-old" adults (average age 65–70).

Although antipsychotic medications are pivotal in the treatment of late-life schizophrenia, clinicians, patients, and families often recognize their limitations. Even when they are well-tolerated and effective, antipsychotic medications may not be sufficiently effective to return older adults with schizophrenia to "normal" functioning. Also, medications have little effect on certain aspects of schizophrenia (e.g., social skills deficits, cognitive impairment). Many psychosocial interventions investigated as treatment augmentation to pharmacotherapy in general schizophrenia populations have had varying degrees of success. Examples include cognitive-behavioral therapy (CBT), psychoeducation, family therapies, vocational rehabilitation, cognitive training, social skills training, and assertive community treatment (ACT). As with medication trials, these psychosocial trials frequently include relatively few older adults. Often there is an unspoken (or even spoken) assumption about the inappropriateness of psychosocial interventions for older adults in general. Popular "wisdom," reflected in idiomatic expressions such as "You can't teach an old dog new tricks," has at times pervaded even well-intentioned clinical settings. This ageist attitude may be amplified even further when the public and clinicians consider older adults with schizophrenia.

Fortunately, in the last several years, controlled trials of psychosocial interventions specifically for middle-aged or older adults with schizophrenia have yielded promising results for improving certain functional disabilities that persist after adequate antipsychotic medication treatment. These include three manualized and empirically tested psychosocial interventions that use various forms of skills training. For example, CBSST (cognitive-behavioral social skills training), a 24-week, group-based intervention combining cognitive-behavioral techniques (e.g., examining/challenging distorted beliefs) and social skills training (e.g., practicing conversational skills) successfully improved social functioning and cognitive insight among middle-aged and older adults with schizophrenia. This treatment was adapted for cognitive difficulties associated with both schizophrenia and normal aging, and it also included instructional material that was specific to troublesome situations or beliefs commonly encountered in aging populations (e.g., challenging the belief "I am too old to learn," or problem solving around sensory impairments).

Another 24-week, modular intervention termed FAST (functional adaptation skills training) also successfully improved community functioning in middle-aged and older adults with schizophrenia. Skills addressed by this treatment include organization/planning; social skills/communication; and management of medications, transportation, and finances. A noteworthy similarity between CBSST and FAST is their emphasis on homework assignment and review, a key component originally emphasized in CBT, as developed by Beck, which has been tied to successful psychotherapy outcomes for a variety of disorders. Behavioral principles, including behavior remodeling, role playing, and reinforcement, also inform various aspects of the FAST intervention.

A third empirically tested psychosocial intervention (skills training and health management) for older adults with severe mental illnesses (including schizophrenia) likewise focuses on skills training but also includes helping patients to access preventive medical care and medical care for chronic conditions. This intervention improved social functioning and the appropriateness of medical care received. This highlights an issue that becomes increasingly prominent as persons with schizophrenia age—medical comorbidity. Because medical care for physical health in persons with schizophrenia has been notoriously inadequate for a variety of reasons (patient-, clinician-, and system-related), clinicians treating schizophrenia should be especially alert to the multitude of age-associated health problems that may accrue with time. Lifestyle habits that often accompany schizophrenia (e.g., smoking, lack of exercise, poor diet) and metabolic side effects of antipsychotic medications combine to necessitate proactive attention to physical health screening and treatment in the aging person with schizophrenia. Unfortunately, fragmentation of physical and mental health care systems may at times make psychiatrists de facto primary care physicians for persons with schizophrenia.

Another psychosocial approach successfully used in younger patients with schizophrenia is vocational rehabilitation, often through individual placement and support (IPS), a form of supported employment. Key components of supported employment are quick job placement, obtaining competitive (i.e., not specially set aside) positions, earning minimum wage or higher, unlimited time frames for vocational support efforts, and collaboration between the employer and the mental health team. Although one might assume that older adults do not need or want to have occupations, employment can have a significant positive impact on older adults' quality of life in many situations, building a sense of purpose and self-esteem. Recently an IPS intervention that resulted in significant rates (69%) of competitive, paid work among middle-aged and older adults with schizophrenia was found to be substantially better than two other forms of vocational rehabilitation. Overall, the ability of these various nonpharmacological treatments to improve the functioning of older adults, who often have been affected by schizophrenia for decades, is impressive, but there is much room to build upon these results and expand the armamentarium of psychosocial treatments for this population.

SUMMARY OF TREATMENT GUIDELINES

1. Antipsychotic medication is the mainstay of pharmacological treatment for older adults with schizophrenia. There is no consensus on which specific antipsychotic should be used as first-line therapy.

2. Patients who have been treated successfully with a particular medication that was begun at a younger age may remain on that medication (with an explanation of the relative differences in side effect profiles associated with other available medications), although the dose may need to be reduced in later life.

3. Important side effect differences to highlight (whether continuing with an existing medication or starting a new one) include (a) higher risk of movement disorders (including possibly persistent TD) with typical than with atypical antipsychotics, in an age-dependent manner; (b) possible elevated risk of metabolic disorders, such as diabetes mellitus and obesity, with certain atypical antipsychotics (e.g., clozapine, olanzapine); and (c) risk of death and cerebrovascular events when using atypical antipsychotics, if the patient has comorbid dementia (and that current relevant data about these risks in older adults with schizophrenia are scarce).

4. Medications with the most data from controlled trials specifically for older adults with schizophrenia include risperidone, olanzapine, and haloperidol.

5. Initial antipsychotic doses for older adults with schizophrenia should be 25–50% of those used in younger adults. Whereas effective doses for older adults with early-onset schizophrenia are usually 50–75% of those used in younger adults, doses may need to be only 25–33% of younger adult doses for patients with late-onset schizophrenia or with "old-old" (over age 75) patients.

6. Monitoring for medication-related side effects (irrespective of the specific medication used) should include regular evaluation for extrapyramidal symptoms and TD (e.g., using the Abnormal Involuntary Movement Scale), as well as routine monitoring of weight, blood pressure, blood glucose or hemoglobin A1C, and lipids.

7. Patients should be offered psychosocial interventions as adjunctive therapy to antipsychotic medications. The most empirically validated psychosocial treatments for middle-aged and older adults with schizophrenia include CBSST, FAST, and IPS vocational rehabilitation.

8. Other psychosocial interventions shown to help younger persons with schizophrenia might also be helpful for older adults. Examples include supportive psychotherapy, family therapy, psychoeducation, and case management/ACT.

9. Due to increasing medical comorbidity associated with aging and traditionally inadequate health care for persons with schizophrenia, clinicians should remain vigilant to ensure that older persons with schizophrenia receive appropriate treatment for active medical problems, as well as standard preventive/screening procedures (including counseling for applicable lifestyle modifications).

10. Despite the relative stability of intrinsic cognitive deficits associated with schizophrenia over time, dementia may still co-occur with schizophrenia in aging individuals;

clinicians should be cognizant of cognitive changes in patients that may signify normal aging or co-occurring disorders that cause dementia.

KEY POINTS

- A majority of older adults with schizophrenia have had the illness since they were young adults.
- New onset of schizophrenia after age 40 can occur, but it is less common and has important clinical differences than early-onset illness.
- Antipsychotic medications are useful for late-life schizophrenia, but may have more side effects in older than in younger adults, often requiring reduced doses.
- Choice of antipsychotic medication should be guided in part by an individual patient's preferences, as well as risks for different side effects.
- Psychosocial treatments, such as skills training, cognitive-behavioral techniques, and supported employment, are effective adjuncts to pharmacotherapy in late-life schizophrenia.
- Psychosocial treatments may improve residual impairments in role functioning even among persons who are responsive to medications.
- Medical comorbidity is common in older persons with schizophrenia, and mental health clinicians should facilitate proper medical care for these patients.
- The prognosis for aging individuals with schizophrenia is not as bleak as once thought, because positive symptoms often improve with age.
- Sustained remission occurs in a minority of aging persons with schizophrenia, and its likelihood may be increased by improved social support.

REFERENCES AND RECOMMENDED READINGS

Bartels, S. J., Forester, B., Mueser, K. T., Miles, K. M., Dums, A. R., Pratt, S. I., et al. (2004). Enhanced skills training and health care management for older persons with severe mental illness. *Community Mental Health Journal, 40,* 75–90.

Folsom, D. P., Lebowitz, B. D., Lindamer, L. A., Palmer, B. W., Patterson, T. L., & Jeste, D. V. (2006). Schizophrenia in late life: Emerging issues. *Dialogues in Clinical Neuroscience, 8,* 45–52.

Goff, D. C., Cather, C., Evins, A. E., Henderson, D. C., Freudenreich, O., Copeland, P. M., et al. (2005). Medical morbidity and mortality in schizophrenia: Guidelines for psychiatrists. *Journal of Clinical Psychiatry, 66,* 183–194.

Granholm, E., McQuaid, J. R., McClure, F. S., Auslander, L. A., Perivoliotis, D., Pedrelli, P., et al. (2005). A randomized, controlled trial of cognitive behavioral social skills training for middle-aged and older outpatients with chronic schizophrenia. *American Journal of Psychiatry, 162,* 520–529.

Harris, M. J., & Jeste, D. V. (1988). Late-onset schizophrenia: An overview. *Schizophrenia Bulletin, 14,* 39–55.

Jeste, D. V., Barak, Y., Madhusoodanan, S., Grossman, F., & Gharabawi, G. (2003). An international multisite double-blind trial of the atypical antipsychotic risperidone and olanzapine in 175 elderly patients with chronic schizophrenia. *American Journal of Geriatric Psychiatry, 11,* 638–647.

Jeste, D. V., Dolder, C. R., Nayak, G. V., & Salzman, C. (2005). Atypical antipsychotics in elderly patients with dementia or schizophrenia: Review of recent literature. *Harvard Review of Psychiatry, 13,* 340–351.

Jeste, D. V., Rockwell, E., Harris, M. J., Lohr, J. B., & Lacro, J. (1999). Conventional vs. newer antipsychotics in elderly patients. *American Journal of Geriatric Psychiatry, 7,* 70–76.

Marriott, R. G., Neil, W., & Waddingham, S. (2006). Antipsychotic medication for elderly people with schizophrenia. *Cochrane Database of Systematic Reviews, 25,* CD005580.

Palmer, B. W., McClure, F., & Jeste, D. V. (2001). Schizophrenia in late-life: Findings challenge traditional concepts. *Harvard Review of Psychiatry, 9,* 51–58.

Patterson, T. L., McKibbin, C., Mausbach, B. T., Goldman, S., Bucardo, J., & Jeste, D. V. (2006). Functional Adaptation Skills Training (FAST): A randomized trial of a psychosocial intervention for middle-aged and older patients with chronic psychotic disorders. *Journal of Clinical Psychiatry, 86,* 291–299.

Schimming, C., & Harvey, P. D. (2004). Disability reduction in elderly patients with schizophrenia. *Journal of Psychiatric Practice, 10,* 283–295.

Schneider, L. S., Dagerman, K. S., & Insel, P. (2005). Risk of death with atypical antipsychotic drug treatment for dementia: Meta-analysis of randomized placebo-controlled trials. *Journal of the American Medical Association, 294,* 1934–1943.

Twamley, E. W., Padin, D. S., Bayne, K. S., Narvaez, J. M., Williams, R. E., & Jeste, D. V. (2005). Work rehabilitation for middle-aged and older people with schizophrenia: A comparison of three approaches. *Journal of Nervous and Mental Disease, 193,* 596–601.

Van Critters, A. D., Pratt, S. I., Bartels, S. J., & Jeste, D. V. (2005). Evidence-based review of pharmacologic and nonpharmacologic treatments for older adults with schizophrenia. *Psychiatric Clincs of North Amercia, 28,* 913–939.

CHAPTER 39

UNDERSTANDING AND WORKING WITH AGGRESSION, VIOLENCE, AND PSYCHOSIS

GILLIAN HADDOCK
JENNIFER J. SHAW

A significant number of people who have a diagnosis of schizophrenia are difficult to engage in standard treatments for psychosis due to persistent problems of aggression and violence. Some of them reside in locked and secure environments, where opportunities to engage in "normal" activities and routines are restricted. In addition, a large proportion of people with problems of aggression and violence have treatment-resistant psychotic symptoms and problems with substance use that lead to significant challenges for service providers in determining what sort of treatment works best.

There has been much discussion as to whether people with a diagnosis of schizophrenia have a higher propensity than others to be violent or aggressive. However, research results are mixed, with some studies finding links with the diagnosis and others not. This confusion has led researchers to explore what factors might contribute to the occurrence of aggression and violence in people with severe mental illness. One consistent finding is the link between substance abuse, schizophrenia, and violence. People with schizophrenia who misuse substances show consistently higher rates of violence than non-substance-using clients. There may be a number of reasons for this higher rate. For example, it has been shown that the presence of comorbid personality disorders such as conduct disorder and antisocial personality disorder, together with substance use in this population, can contribute to higher rates of violence (see References and Recommended Readings). However, an additional reason for the higher rates of violence in people with severe mental illnesses who misuse substances might be that substance use interferes with clients' ability to engage in treatment, resulting in more persistent psychotic symptoms. This is consistent with findings that higher rates of violence have been associated with the presence of particular delusional symptoms. Particular psychotic symptoms that have been highlighted include feeling threatened or controlled by external forces or people, such as paranoid beliefs in voices, which imply control over the individual (sometimes referred to as *threat control override symptoms*). In addition to substance use, research has pointed to the importance of anger that, when coupled with psychotic symptoms, is associated with higher rates of violence and aggression. However, the link between anger and violence is not a simple one: Whereas anger can be an activator of aggression, it is neither necessary nor sufficient to induce violence, and an understanding of a violent event has to be contextualized within the environment in which the incident occurred. This is very relevant for people with psychosis, whose experience and response to anger-provoking events may be partly influenced by not only their delusional thinking but also their day-to-day life within adverse, controlling, disrespectful, and unempathic environments.

This evidence suggests that clinicians must account for the following key factors when working with people who have a psychosis and problems with aggression and violence: (1) illness factors, such as particular psychotic symptoms; (2) substance use; (3) anger; and (4) environmental factors. Any intervention is likely to require the clinician to understand the problems of aggression and violence across all of those areas, while taking into account the complex environmental, personality, and historical factors that contribute to the problem. It is helpful not to view the aggression or violence as something that is wholly located within the individual, but as the product of a complex system of constantly changing variables.

People who are aggressive and violent often reside on inpatient or possibly secure units and present with a range of complex needs compared to people living within the community. For example, although there is some variation, this group of people is likely to have had prior challenges to services in terms of anger and violence within the context of a history of chronic substance use. Because they are more likely to be "resistant" to traditional treatment approaches, these individuals' persistent psychotic symptoms or beliefs may have interfered with traditional assessments and treatments. Typical symptoms may include the presence of specific types of command hallucinations and/or delusional beliefs that interfere with engagement in services (e.g., delusionally driven catastrophic implications of discussing psychotic experiences with the staff). Additionally, it is not uncommon for clients within such secure units to be socially unsupported outside of their residential unit due to a history of gradual deterioration in interpersonal relationships and, in the case of people residing in some secure units, to be geographically displaced from their home location.

These difficulties pose challenges in maintaining a cohesive multidisciplinary approach, and present problems in the process of diagnosis and identification of the most appropriate treatment approaches. Furthermore, all therapeutic work has to occur within the context of a need to balance custodial and therapeutic agendas.

PSYCHOTHERAPEUTIC INTERVENTIONS FOR THIS POPULATION

Psychotherapeutic treatments for this group of people have not been widely described in the literature. However, recent work has suggested a number of approaches that may be helpful. For example, psychological interventions, such as cognitive-behavioral treatments in conjunction with antipsychotic medication, have been shown to reduce effectively the severity and frequency of psychotic symptoms in people with treatment-resistant psychosis. Cognitive-behavioral methods have also been successful in treating anger- and substance use–related problems in clients with severe mental health problems. It is possible to integrate these treatments to provide a comprehensive intervention that attempts to meet the complex needs of people with psychosis and violence problems.

Figure 39.1 illustrates a clinical formulation that assists in understanding, assessing, and treating people with these complex problems. As can be seen, the occurrence of violence is seen as a product of a dynamic interaction between psychosis, anger, environment, and substance use. These key factors contribute to the likelihood of violence, which occurs once a person reaches a threshold and is unable/or does not wish to restrain from violence. A good balance between providing optimum medical and psychological interventions aimed at the key factors in the model and delivering these interventions within an optimum environment is key to providing a comprehensive, multidisciplinary approach for working with people with psychosis and problems with violence and aggression.

COMMON MULTIDISCIPLINARY ASSESSMENT PROCESSES

Because inpatient environments comprise a multidisciplinary mix of mental health professionals, it is important that all members of the team work together in meeting clients' needs. It is helpful for one or two individuals to take a lead in coordinating and managing the care that clients receive.

Engagement

Often this group of people has traditionally been difficult to engage in treatment, so much attention needs to center on this difficulty before staff proceeds with complex psychological

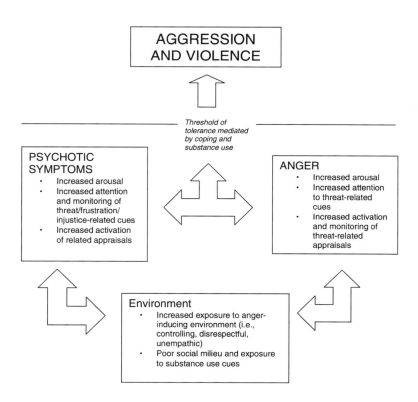

FIGURE 39.1. Clinical formulation to assist in understanding, assessing, and treating people with psychosis and problems with aggression and violence. From Haddock, Lowens, Brosnan, Barrowclough, and Novaco (2004). Copyright 2004 by Cambridge University Press. Reprinted by permission.

interventions. The individual may not wish to engage in treatment for a range of reasons: Commonly, the individual does not agree that he or she needs to be treated for mental health issues or that his or her diagnosis is correct, so the treatment he or she is being offered is incorrect. In addition, medical treatment or restraint used to manage aggressive incidents in the past may interfere with a client's willingness to engage in a dialogue about treatment with mental health staff that he or she perceives as uncaring and hostile. Psychotic beliefs may make a client suspicious of the intentions of clinicians, leading to his or her unwillingness to discuss symptoms or problems. In addition, when staff members are subjected to abuse or violence from a client, their motivation to engage that individual may be reduced due to fear of future violence or of exacerbating the client's symptoms and/or anger.

It is essential to work collaboratively with the client to overcome these issues. Motivational interviewing approaches can be extremely helpful in engaging people in treatment when they are resistant. This approach was, originally developed to help people with substance use problems engage in treatment; however, it has been shown to work very well in helping people with psychosis engage in various treatments (see References and Recommended Readings).

Comprehensive Assessment

The following assessment package may be helpful as a first step in determining the unique needs of each individual.

Assessing Psychosis

The impact and severity of psychotic and nonpsychotic symptoms can be assessed using structured interviews that allow detailed exploration of the individual's experiences. The Positive and Negative Syndrome Scale (PANSS; Kay, Opler, & Lindenmayer, 1989) can be a useful interview for exploring both psychotic and nonpsychotic experiences. It is helpful if it is conducted collaboratively as a means to help the individual describe his or her experiences, with a view toward receiving help from the clinician if necessary. The Psychotic Symptom Rating Scales (PSYRATS; Haddock, McCarron, Tarrier, & Faragher, 1999) are more in-depth interviews that help the individual to explore his or her hallucinations and delusional beliefs in detail. Questions are about the content of the experiences, and the individual's beliefs and distress in response to the experiences. These symptom-based assessments can be extremely useful in gaining a comprehensive picture of the individual's psychotic and nonpsychotic experiences, which can be used to guide treatment and to monitor progress.

Assessing Anger

1. An individual's experience of anger can be very comprehensively assessed with self-report scales. The Novaco Anger Scale and Provocation Inventory (NAS-PI; Novaco, 2003) is particularly relevant and has been used widely in forensic and nonforensic populations with psychosis. The NAS-PI is a self-report scale that asks the individual to describe him- or herself when angry, in terms of the way anger affects his or her thinking, level of arousal, and behavior (Does he or she shout, hit, keep it to him- or herself, etc.?).

2. It can also be helpful to have an external account of an individual's anger and aggression. A good assessment scale rated by ward staff is the Ward Anger Rating Scale (WARS; Novaco, 1994), designed to record staff observations of the individual's angry, threatening, or violent behavior.

Assessing Substance Use Issues

Substance use has been linked consistently with the occurrence of violence within the schizophrenia population, so it should be assessed thoroughly. Even if the individual lives in a facility with little or no access to drugs, illicit substances may still play a part in the likelihood of future violence. Many people who may have become violent only when under the influence of substances may believe that simply avoiding substances is the key to not being violent in the future. Although this may be true, not assessing problems related to violence may discount such problems until there is a greater likelihood that the person will use substances. However, if the individual is motivated, he or she may engage in a great deal of useful relapse prevention work in relation to substances. As previously discussed, the type of intervention that might be necessary depends on the individual's attitude toward substance use and his or her motivation to change, as indicated in the engagement process described earlier.

Assessing Medical and Biochemical Needs

In treating people with complex presentations, it is important to review physical health needs and to ensure that there are no medical causes for any changes in presentation or increased aggression or violence. This review includes the following:

1. A full physical examination and follow-up on any abnormalities detected.
2. A review of routine blood tests to establish whether any further tests are indicated (e.g., thyroid function tests, HIV status).
3. A review of previous electroencephalography, computed tomography, and magnetic resonance imaging scans to consider whether there are clinical indications to repeat them.

People presenting with such complex needs have often been subjected previously to various types of intervention. Medication may have been altered frequently, at times as a knee-jerk response to violence, and many clients may have been subjected to injections of antipsychotic medication against their will. It is important to perform a full assessment of previous and current pharmacological interventions. This entails a detailed analysis of the case notes and drug sheets that document the effect of changes in medication on symptoms and presentation. It is only by conducting this somewhat laborious exercise that clear patterns of improvement or deterioration emerge and inform future directions for pharmacological treatments.

Similarly, medication side effects and clients' attitudes toward medication should be assessed using standardized instruments such as the Liverpool University Side Effect Rating Scale and the Drug Attitude Inventory (Day, Wood, Dewey, & Bentall, 1995). Clients who have experienced significant side effects may be reluctant to engage in further pharmacological treatment. Education about medication and motivational approaches that may increase willingness to consider medication help clients to make informed choices about medication and encourage adherence.

Assessing the Role of Environmental Factors in the Occurrence of Violence

The context in which an act of aggression or violence takes place is extremely important and should form a major part of the assessment process. The clinician gains a good understanding of the client by examining the circumstances under which previous aggressive or violent acts took place (e.g., did they tend to occur in certain places, around certain people, or at certain times of the day?). Circumstances that are not immediately obvious may be informed by other assessments and discussions with the individual and caregivers. For example, an individual's delusional beliefs can be important in determining the situations in which he or she may feel uncomfortable or start to become aroused. People with paranoid beliefs about others may become more distressed in situations involving other people (e.g., around mealtimes, during the administration of medication). In addition, NAS and WARS items can provide clues as to the most likely situations in which an individual might become aggressive. Information may also be gathered from case notes and by questioning key staff members who witnessed or were involved in the aggression or violence. If no particular pattern appears to contribute to the occurrence of violence, then some detailed, prospective observational assessment may be helpful.

Formulating the Issues in Preparation for Intervention

The strategies we have described can be used with other appropriate assessments to gain a thorough and comprehensive view of the individual's experiences in terms of the maintenance of key problems (including psychotic symptoms) and how they relate to expression of anger, aggression, and violence. This assessment process should be an "individually tailored" evaluation of the specific difficulties the person is experiencing. The aim is to gain a history of the client and his or her illness, and an understanding of the range of current problems. Personal history taking is important and likely includes early experiences, significant experiences throughout life to date, the client's present situation, a history of the client's use of coping strategies, and how any aggression or violence fits into this. An individual's cultural beliefs in relation to the function of anger and aggression may be extremely important. For example, cultural stereotypes in relation to assertiveness and machoism may be important motivators in some people who act aggressively and may be linked closely to self-esteem. Staff members or therapists can use the assessment data to stimulate discussion about anger, aggression, or other issues to elicit these types of beliefs. This can be useful when clients are ambivalent or are in denial about issues relating to these areas.

It is not uncommon to identify problems relative to a whole range of areas, including psychosis, negative symptoms, depression, anxiety, financial problems, social and familial problems, anger, disagreements with treatment, and diagnosis. The therapist and client should negotiate priorities for formulation and assessment in one or two key areas. However, whatever the agreed priorities, the therapist should ensure that issues about aggression and psychosis are in some way incorporated into the assessment and formulation. Even when anger or aggression is not acknowledged to be problematic, it can still be discussed in the context of "normal" responses to difficult situations. The clinical formulation of psychosis and aggression described in Figure 39.1 can be used as a focus for assessment and intervention, and to devise a collaborative plan for intervention.

INTERVENTION STRATEGIES

Ensuring Optimum Medical Treatment

A review of the case notes and drug sheets, together with information gathered from the client and caregivers on "what works" best, is an essential first step. The clinician needs to consider particular treatments that may have been effective previously and/or treatments that have not been tried. Some clinicians, when treating clients with complex needs, particularly those with a history of violence and nonadherence, "play safe" and use depot injectable antipsychotic medication to ensure that the clients are definitely receiving the required dose. Unfortunately, these older types of antipsychotic drugs are more prone to produce side effects, particularly those of a neurological type. These side effects are unpleasant and, because they may be clearly visible to others, can exacerbate clients' low self-esteem and lack of confidence. The so-called "atypical" antipsychotics are pharmacologically "cleaner" drugs, with fewer distressing side effects and, with respect to the atypical clozapine, are efficacious in treatment-resistant psychosis. Moreover, in those who have been violent in the context of psychosis, olanzapine, risperidone, and clozapine have been shown to be particularly effective.

These drugs are usually administered by mouth, so they require some level of motivation and agreement from the client. It has been shown, however, that with sufficient educational and motivational work clients can make the transition to the atypicals and reliably take their medication because they notice more improvement in their symptoms and have fewer side effects.

In maximizing the impact of pharmacological treatment it is important to consider the appropriate dose of antipsychotic; indications for the use of augmentation with a second antipsychotic drug; and the pharmacological indications for the treatment of any other psychiatric condition, for example, depression. Most importantly there should be a sufficient trial of a particular treatment regimen before alternatives are considered, together with regular monitoring of changes in symptom intensity, side effects, adherence, and behavior over time.

There is no evidence for the efficacy of long-term pharmacological treatment for aggression itself, independent of the treatment of the underlying psychosis. In particular, there is no evidence that anticonvulsants, such as sodium valproate and carbamazepine, have any place in the long-term treatment of aggression. In the short-term management of violence and aggression, there is a place for the use of rapid tranquilization, but only under strict protocol arrangements and with due consideration of all other techniques for the management of aggression, including verbal deescalation, and so forth. Such rapid tranquilization protocols should be in accordance with legal requirements (especially with respect to detained clients), the consent to treatment, and emergency treatment powers and duties under the relevant mental health legislation. When the behavioral disturbance occurs in a nonpsychotic context, it is preferable initially to use only lorazepam orally, or intramuscularly, if necessary. When the behavioral disturbance occurs in the context of psychosis, an oral antipsychotic in combination with oral lorazepam should be considered to achieve early onset of calming/sedation.

Psychological Interventions

The psychological intervention should be guided by the individual formulation of difficulties/needs that the clinician and client have generated collaboratively. Areas with potential for change should be considered together and action plans devised. These are likely to be extremely idiosyncratic and to vary widely. The plans may require action by the individual client, a responsible medical officer, a social worker, or other involved caregiver or relative. When psychosis, substance use, and anger problems are identified as priorities, individual cognitive-behavioral interventions for psychotic symptoms, anger, and substance use may be helpful.

Cognitive-Behavioral Therapy for Psychosis

There is a growing acceptance of a role for cognitive-behavioral therapy (CBT) for psychosis in mental health treatment. Government guidelines in the United Kingdom recommend this as a treatment strategy for all people with schizophrenia whose symptoms do not respond to antipsychotic medication. The approach is collaborative and is aimed at improving control over symptoms and reducing the distress and disruption caused by them. CBT is usually delivered by one therapist meeting weekly with the client for about 1 hour. This can be flexible depending on the individual client. Problems with concentration sometimes mean that shorter, more frequent sessions are more acceptable.

Identifying the Focus for Therapy

The assessments described earlier should provide a really good overview of the individual's areas of concern. Where there are multiple problems, it is helpful to focus on a small number of problem areas. Using the formulation to assimilate information and provide feedback to the client may help the clinician identify where best to focus the intervention. The case description below illustrates this.

> John was 29 years old and had a 10-year history of schizophrenia. He had 10 inpatient admissions over this time period, until eventually he was admitted to a medium-secure facility following a number of violent and aggressive attacks on staff members. John readily admitted to being extremely angry about his situation. He believed that staff members (and particularly his doctor) were incompetent, and that they were not treating him for the right problem. Whereas they believed he had schizophrenia because of his strange and magical experiences, John believed that the problem was his intense anxiety, caused by his "real" strange and magical experiences. He wished to have more anxiolytic medication and to stop taking anti-psychotic medication, which, he believed, was causing multiple side effects, such as dribbling, drowsiness, and inability to gain an erection. Staff members would not listen to him, and they continued to provide treatment he did not need, so John felt that the only way to gain any control over the situation was to hit out at the staff.
>
> Because John was extremely angry with all the staff members on his unit, a slightly more "neutral" therapist, who was not part of the core ward team, was brought in to attempt to engage him. This was presented to John as an attempt at mediation between John and the staff to identify a way forward. The therapist spent several sessions just listening to John's side of the story and trying to identify the real problems that prevented John from achieving his goal to get out of the hospital and live a more normal life. After a number of sessions, the following key areas were identified:
>
> 1. John's disagreement with staff about his diagnosis and treatment.
> 2. His difficulty in controlling his anxiety.
> 3. His difficulty in controlling his anger.
> 4 His desire to use substances as soon as he was discharged. This was significant, in that ward staff members had told John that he would never be discharged unless he promised not to take drugs. John felt that cannabis helped him manage his anxiety, so he would not agree to this (and did not see why he should!).

Establishment of these key problem areas then led to an intervention package that involved a review of John's diagnosis and medication with the staff, CBT for anger and anxiety, and some work around John's beliefs and his desire to use substances. John was happy with this agreement, particularly because he was hopeful that he and the therapist could prove to the staff that he did not have schizophrenia. The intervention was carried out over 30 weekly sessions, with some additional sessions carried out jointly with the staff to ensure that the approach addressed the environmental issues. The outcome was positive, in that John felt that his feelings about his medication were being taken into account, and that people were listening to his perspective. With his anxiety and anger reduced, John was able to admit that some of his experiences were related to having schizophrenia. This allowed the therapist and staff to utilize some CBT techniques to assist with managing these experiences.

John illustrates a key issue in working with people with schizophrenia and highlights why motivation must be considered an important part of the engagement process. Individuals often need to believe that there is something in it for them to make changing their behavior worth the effort. It is common for clients' anger and aggression to play an important role for them, and giving this up may involve considerable effort. Without an important goal to motivate them, change efforts are unlikely to be successful.

Further description of CBT approaches for working with psychotic symptoms are not discussed further here. The reader is directed to more comprehensive texts (References and Recommended Readings) listed at the end of this chapter.

Strategies for Working with Anger

Comprehensive interventions for working with anger have been described fully by Ray Novaco and adapted to apply in a number of settings. The approach has been modified for working with people with active psychotic symptoms and substance use problems (see References and Recommended Readings). The approach has a number of key elements.

PSYCHOEDUCATION

Providing people with a good understanding of anger, its components, and functions is an extremely useful starting point, once they realize that their anger may be an important issue. It is important that people understand that anger is a state and is not directly linked to aggression and violence, and that anger itself may be a positive and welcome emotion. Anger can become problematic if it leads to negative consequences, such as unwanted aggression or violence, but it can also be a useful emotion to stimulate positive and useful action when necessary (e.g., running away from danger, being assertive). Helping people to become sensitive to their anger and to use it positively can be especially important, given that mental health services have previously given the message that anger is a bad thing. Information about the components of anger in terms of a CBT model may also be extremely useful in helping people to recognize their own anger and to see that there may be strategies to overcome its negative aspects.

SELF-MONITORING AND USE OF ANGER HIERARCHIES

Helping people to monitor the way their anger influences their cognitive, emotional, or physiological state and their behavior can then be an important step in devising the best interventions. People may want to keep diaries or to make a mental note of their day-to-day activities between therapy sessions, then discuss and examine these data with the therapist to investigate when their anger was not helpful and what factors fed into it (psychotic beliefs, substance use, etc.). This may make the type of solutions obvious to the individual. For example, individuals who notice that they become upset and angry whenever they have particular interactions with staff members become aware that something about the way staff members interact with them is upsetting. Staff members who are unaware of an individual's particular delusional beliefs may inadvertently behave in a way that angers the individual. This may then set the scene for work in a caregiver session that may allow the staff to handle the situation differently. At the same time, the individual can examine the cognitions that may exacerbate the anger and do some CBT work with the therapist to help to modify and reduce their impact. He or she may also become aware of how physiological arousal is adding to the distressful situation and use some strategies to reduce this arousal.

The use of a hierarchical system that pinpoints specific situations/states in which anger is problematic helps to identify salient situations in a graded fashion—ranging from situations of low anger to those in which anger is extreme. This anger hierarchy can be used to identify problematic situations and appropriate coping strategies. Individuals may also expose themselves to increasingly severe anger-provoking situations to test out new coping strategies and practice "imaginal inoculation training" to deal with difficult situations.

COGNITIVE RESTRUCTURING

Treatment usually includes some cognitive strategies for dealing with anger-related cognitions and beliefs. The anger hierarchy may help to identify thoughts and appraisals in angry situations and facilitate the search for alternative appraisals and coping strategies. Traditional cognitive strategies may be used to elicit alternative thoughts and to question conclusions in relation to inaccurate or distorted thoughts. Behavioral experiments can be used to test alternatives and to practice coping.

In addition, discussion of key beliefs in relation to the function and meaning of anger for the individual is important. This helps to identify key beliefs that may exacerbate anger in certain situations. Giving people the means to explore their ideas and attitudes toward anger and its expression highlights areas that reduce the potential for violence. Issues related to the necessity to behave violently to maintain self-worth may need to be explored, along with alternative ways to build self-worth. This might involve training individuals to be assertive without becoming violent, or building their self-esteem strategies.

INTEGRATING CHANGES INTO KEY GOALS

It is important to integrate the anger intervention into the overall formulation and to link it to key goals for the individual. Successful anger control may involve key lifestyle changes, so it may be necessary to incorporate some short- and long-term goal planning into the overall plan.

ENVIRONMENTAL ISSUES

Ensuring that the intervention takes into account the role of the environment and other people is essential; the intervention is likely to be doomed if this is not done. For some individuals, engaging in one-to-one therapy is extremely difficult, and the environment rather than individual CBT work, as described earlier, may be the main focus for therapeutic work. However, the principles of the therapeutic CBT model apply, regardless of the main focus of the intervention and assessment and formulation of the difficulties described earlier, are appropriate even if detailed assessment of the individual is not possible. Usually a particular staff member or caregiver who has most contact with the individual is identified as the coworker or facilitator of the CBT therapy. At a minimum, even people who are engaged in individual work should be involved in joint meetings with the named caregiver and the CBT therapist early in therapy, in midtherapy, and toward the end of therapy to consolidate generalization and to conform with the *Staying Well Manual* (see below). The purpose of the meetings is to ensure that the approaches used in therapy are generalized to other team members, to assess how staff attitudes and behavior interact with the individual's concerns and problems, to provide strategies that facilitate attitude and behavior change in staff members if necessary, and to ensure that changes implemented by both client and staff are agreed upon collaboratively. We find this to be a key therapeutic strategy, because many aggressive individuals are living within inpatient and secure environments feel that they have little influence and control over their treatment and the future likelihood of discharge. This is the key goal for many people during therapy, and joint meetings can be extremely helpful in promoting shared understanding between the mental health care teams and individuals.

In addition, staff members on inpatient and secure units work in an extremely challenging environment, in which they are expected to take on a dual role of "caregiver" and "restrainer" that may hinder the development of a therapeutic role with clients and lead to problems in the relationship. Opportunities to explore incorrect attitudes, beliefs, and knowledge in caregivers should be sought in a manner that is nonjudgmental and encouraging. This may be empowering for staff members who *inadvertently* behave in ways that exacerbate clients' aggressive behavior with treatment regimens that are inappropriate or unhelpful. Individual sessions can help staff members to develop alternative ways of responding to clients' aggression and violence, by becoming aware of a cognitive-behavioral formulation of clients' difficulties.

THE *STAYING WELL MANUAL* AND CONSOLIDATION OF PROGRESS

"Staying well" strategies and methods to ensure that treatment gains are consolidated and generalized should be incorporated into each client's treatment package at some point, usually toward the end of therapy. It is extremely important to consolidate these strategies into the individual's overall future care and to ensure that the approaches generalize across situations and time. The complexity of this is dependent on client progress and degree of engagement in treatment.

A typical staying well/consolidation plan includes the following:

1. A description of the key needs/problems identified during treatment.
2. A summary of individuals' understanding and formulation of their problems incorporating, where appropriate, the key areas of anger, substance use, environment, and aggression/violence.
3. A summary of approaches that have been used to address these problems, who has carried them out, and how these can be continued and developed in future
4. A description of what strategies are in place to help the individual continue to work on areas of difficulty. These may often involve identifying key personnel, who may be assigned certain tasks that extend beyond the initial, intensive treatment period. This may be a key worker or other ward staff member who agrees to take responsibility for meeting with the client regularly to monitor hot issues (distress over psychotic symptoms, anger hierarchies, etc.).
5. Plans for monitoring lapse/relapse and danger times. The individual might be encouraged to use a "traffic light" system to help him or her (and others, if appropriate) to monitor thoughts, feelings, and behaviors, and to identify when these might become

problematic. This system divides the individual's experiences into traffic light phases. A pictorial expression of the following phases can be useful to the individual to monitor how he or she is feeling.

- *Green.* The individual feels relatively OK in this state, in control of the main problem areas, and feels able to cope with everyday stresses. Strategies that help the individual to remain in the green phase are described.
- *Amber.* In this state, the individual has started to experience some exacerbation of aggressive thoughts and feelings, which may be expressed as unusual experiences or behavior. This is considered to be warning phase that stimulates some action by, or on behalf of, the individual and/or others to prevent further symptom exacerbation and to facilitate a return to the green phase.
- *Red.* This is considered the "danger" state. Identifying these signs can help to ensure that appropriate, collaboratively agreed-upon actions take place. These signs vary enormously but may necessitate a change in treatment regimen, living accommodations, staff and family actions, and so forth. Having plans for this stage firmly in place and agreed upon by the individual and the caregiving staff reduces the potential for conflict and identifies clear roles with which the individual is happy.

The complexity of this system can vary from simple descriptions to very detailed accounts. It is helpful to describe each stage in terms of the way individuals experience their feelings, cognitions, and behaviors, in line with a CBT model with accompanying strategies. These extremely idiosyncratic descriptions are based on the strategies identified during the intensive intervention period.

6. Helpful information that has been acquired during therapy. It is usual for the therapist to bring handouts/information sheets to therapy sessions. It is helpful to have these collated into the "staying well" pack, even if the individual has already received them during therapy. In addition, useful telephone numbers and contacts may be included to ensure the individual has all the resources he or she might require.

Whatever the client's stage of progress during therapy, a staying well manual can be useful. Ideally, this is compiled collaboratively and shared with key personnel. Even when a client is unwilling to work individually on a staying well plan, a manual for the staff to refer to can be helpful. Finally, it is essential that the manual be agreed upon and shared with other people, when appropriate. The client's collaboration and permission in this are important.

KEY POINTS

- Violence in severe mental illness is determined by a number of encompassing historical and predispositional factors, and environmental and clinical factors.
- The presence of personality disorders may a feature.
- Cognitive-behavioral therapy is an effective and acceptable treatment for people with severe mental illness and violence.
- Key themes to address when working with this group are engagement and motivational issues, substance use, psychotic beliefs, and anger.
- Ensuring that the intervention is formulation-driven is essential for choosing the right intervention.
- Motivational interviewing can aid engagement and help to identify whether the individual is ready and willing to change.

REFERENCES AND RECOMMENDED READINGS

Day, J., Wood, G., Dewey, M., & Bentall, R. P. (1995). A self-rating scale for measuring neuroleptic side effects: Validation in a group of schizophrenic patients. *British Journal of Psychiatry, 167*(1), 113–114.

Haddock, G., Lowens, I., Barrowclough, C., Brosnan, N., Lowens, I., & Novaco, R. (2004). Cognitive-behaviour therapy for inpatients with psychosis and anger problems within a low secure environment. *Behavioural and Cognitive Psychotherapy, 32,* 77–98.

Haddock, G., McCarron, J., Tarrier, N., & Faragher, E. B. (1999). Scales to measure dimensions of hallucinations and delusions: The Psychotic Symptom Rating Scales (PSYRATS). *Psychological Medicine, 29,* 879–889.

Hogan, T. P., Awad, A. G., & Eastwood, R. (1983). A self-report scale of drug compliance in schizophrenia: Reliability and discriminative validity. *Psychological Medicine, 13*(1), 177–183.

Kay, S. R., Opler, L. A., & Lindenmayer, J. P. (1989). The Positive and Negative Syndrome Scale (PANSS): Rationale and standardization. *British Journal of Psychiatry, 155,* 59–65.

Leucht, S., Barnes, T. R. E., Kissling, W., Engel, R. R., Correll, C., & Kane, J. M. (2003). Relapse prevention in schizophrenia with new-Generation antipsychotics: A systematic review and exploratory meta-analysis of randomized, controlled trials. *American Journal of Psychiatry, 160*(7), 1209–1222.

Miller, W. R., & Rollnick, S. (2002). *Motivational interviewing: Preparing people for change* (2nd ed.). New York: Guilford Press.

Mueser, K. T., Crocker, A. G., Frisman, L. B., Drake, R. E., Covell, N. H., & Essock, S. M. (2006). Conduct disorder and antisocial personality disorder in persons with severe psychiatric and substance use disorders. *Schizophrenia Bulletin, 32*(4), 626–636.

National Institute for Clinical Excellence. (2002). *Schizophrenia core interventions in the treatment and management of schizophrenia in primary and secondary care.* London: Author.

Novaco, R. W. (2003). *Novaco Anger Scale and Provocation Inventory.* Los Angeles: Western Psychological Association.

Novaco, R. W. (1994). Anger as a risk factor for violence among the mentally disordered. In J. Monahan & H. Steadman (Eds.), *Violence and mental disorder: Developments in risk assessment.* Chicago: University of Chicago Press.

Swanson, J. W. (2004). Effectiveness of atypical antipsychotic medications in reducing violent behaviour among persons with schizophrenia in community-based treatment. *Schizophrenia Bulletin, 30,* 3–20.

Tarrier, N., Wells, A., & Haddock, G. (1998). *Treating complex cases: A cognitive behavioral approach.* Chichester, UK: Wiley.

CHAPTER 40

HOUSING INSTABILITY AND HOMELESSNESS

ALAN FELIX
DAN HERMAN
EZRA SUSSER

As deistitutionalization proceeded in the 1960s and 1970s, the typical length of stay in psychiatric hospitals shortened dramatically, whereas the number of admissions to these institutions increased. This so-called "revolving door" reflected the inadequacy of community-based services to keep those with severe and persistent mental illness from the recurring cycle of relapse and rehospitalization. During this period, however, most localities had sufficient supplies of affordable, if not desirable, housing, such that homelessness among mentally ill people was relatively rare. Beginning in the early 1980s, economic factors, combined with a rapidly shrinking pool of inexpensive housing throughout much of the country, contributed to a dramatic rise in the number of homeless people with schizophrenia and other severe and persistent mental illnesses. Ever since, the problem of "the homeless mentally ill" has become a widespread and vexing phenomenon, capturing broad concern and ongoing attention from citizens, advocates, mental health professionals, and public officials.

In addition to its dramatic impact on morbidity and mortality, homelessness and residential instability impede the ability of mentally ill people to access and benefit from needed treatment. Furthermore, it contributes to deterioration in social functioning and attenuation of social bonds and family support. To minimize homelessness and its associated adverse outcomes, it behooves clinicians in a variety of treatment settings to develop an understanding of the relationship between severe mental illness (SMI) and homelessness, and its implications for the delivery of psychiatric and allied services.

Over the past 20 years, experience gleaned from innovative clinical programs, combined with a growing body of descriptive and intervention research, has provided a clearer yet still evolving picture of the complex needs of this population and an initial understanding of the kinds of service approaches that may be most effective. In this chapter, we first summarize findings on the prevalence of homelessness among people with SMI and the key factors associated with risk of homelessness in this population. We then discuss what is known about the effectiveness of various interventions and service approaches. Finally, we propose broad treatment guidelines based on the available data, in combination with our clinical experience.

HOW COMMON IS HOMELESSNESS AMONG PEOPLE WITH SEVERE MENTAL ILLNESS AND SCHIZOPHRENIA?

Methodological difficulties, chiefly varying definitions of homelessness and the frequent reliance on small, unrepresentative samples of mentally ill persons, have limited the reliability of many estimates of the occurrence of homelessness in the mentally ill population. However, several methodologically rigorous studies confirm that the prevalence of homelessness in persons with SMI, including schizophrenia, is distressingly high. For instance, in a study of patients admitted to a state hospital in New York, 28% of those diagnosed with schizophrenia spectrum disorders reported that they had experienced homelessness during the 3 years preceding the current hospitalization (Susser, Lin, & Conover, 1991a). In a study of persons with schizophrenia spectrum disorders who were discharged from inpatient psychiatric treatment in New York City, roughly 8% of subjects reported at least one episode of homelessness during the 3 months following discharge, a proportion that is likely an underestimate because of significant loss to follow-up (Olfson, Mechanic, Hansell, Boyer, & Walkup, 1999).

One of the most recent major studies used administrative data to estimate the period prevalence of homelessness among all service users of the public mental health system in San Diego. This study found that roughly 15% of patients with schizophrenia experienced homelessness over the course of 1 year (Folsom et al., 2005). This estimate is not inconsistent with the results from an earlier study of persons treated in the public mental health system in Philadelphia, in which 10% of persons with SMI had used the public shelter system during a 3-year period (Culhane, Averyt, & Hadley, 1997).

The elevated risk of homelessness in persons with schizophrenia and other severe mental disorders is not limited to those who have long histories of involvement in the mental health services system. For instance, in a suburban county, a study of a representative sample of persons hospitalized for the first time with psychotic disorders (including but not limited to schizophrenia spectrum disorders), found that 15% had experienced at least one lifetime episode of homelessness before or within 2 years of their initial hospitalization, and that a majority of these episodes occurred before the initial hospital stay (Herman, Susser, Jandorf, Lavelle, & Bromet, 1998).

HOW COMMON IS SCHIZOPHRENIA AMONG PERSONS WHO ARE HOMELESS?

This is perhaps the most commonly asked and frequently studied question pertaining to the nexus of homelessness and mental disorder. Nevertheless, the usefulness of many studies of this issue has been limited by both nonrepresentative sampling schemes and nonstandard diagnostic ascertainment. In addition, because it has been shown that SMI is rare among homeless persons who are housed as families (one of the fastest growing homeless subgroups), prevalence studies that include homeless families necessarily generate systematically lower estimates of SMI.

A comprehensive review of this question summarized the results of 10 studies that employed rigorous diagnostic and sampling methods to estimate the prevalence of schizophrenia in homeless persons, including research carried out in the United States and elsewhere (Folsom & Jeste, 2002). The overall prevalence of schizophrenia among the stringently designed studies ranged between 4 and 16%, with a weighted average prevalence of 11%. This, the authors note, is roughly 7–10 times higher than the prevalence of schizophrenia in the U.S. housed population. Schizophrenia tended to be more common in younger persons; in the chronically homeless; and single homeless women, who were about twice as likely as men to be diagnosed with schizophrenia.

WHAT INDIVIDUAL-LEVEL FACTORS ARE ASSOCIATED WITH HOMELESSNESS AMONG PEOPLE WITH SEVERE MENTAL ILLNESS?

What do we know amount about particular demographic, clinical, and life-history factors associated with homelessness in people with schizophrenia? Do those who become homeless have more severe disorders than their domiciled counterparts? Do they have more comorbid disorders, such as substance misuse, antisocial personality, and serious medical conditions? Are they less "adherent" to treatment? Do they have less family support? Have they had adverse childhood experiences that predispose them to adult homelessness? A number of studies have shed light on these questions.

Comorbid substance abuse appears to be an important factor associated with homelessness among persons with schizophrenia and other severe mental disorders. A case–control study of homeless versus never-homeless men with schizophrenia found that a concurrent diagnosis of drug abuse (but not alcohol abuse) was significantly associated with homelessness, whereas a companion study of women with schizophrenia found that both drug and alcohol abuse were risk factors for homelessness. The association between homelessness and substance abuse in severely mentally ill persons has also been found in a number of other methodologically rigorous studies, with drug abuse tending to be more strongly associated with homelessness than alcohol abuse (Caton et al., 1994, 1995).

Adverse childhood experiences such as family separations, abuse, and neglect have been shown to be potent risk factors for homelessness in the general population and have also been found to be associated with homelessness in persons with SMI. Perhaps the largest study of this question to date compared the prevalence of childhood adversities in severely mentally ill homeless persons and a comparison group of never-homeless psychiatric patients, and found that histories of out-of-home care and running away from home were significantly more common in the homeless group (Susser, Lin, Conover, & Struening, 1991b). Consistent with this finding, the previously mentioned Caton and colleagues (1994) study of men with schizophrenia found that the level of family disorganization during childhood (as measured by a composite scale) was significantly higher in the homeless group compared with the never-homeless comparison group. There is some evidence that, particularly among women with SMI, lack of current family support is associated with homelessness.

As in studies of the general population, race appears to be associated with the risk of homelessness among persons with severe mental disorders. The recent San Diego study we noted earlier found that African American with SMI were somewhat more likely to experience homelessness than their European American, Latino, and Asian American counterparts.

Homeless mentally ill persons are likely to suffer from serious, and often neglected, medical conditions. Homeless people are especially at risk for tuberculosis, HIV, asthma, pneumonia, bronchitis, hypertension, diabetes, and circulatory and vascular disorders.

These disorders may exacerbate an existing psychiatric disorder and complicate its treatment. Furthermore, particularly due to the side effects of antipsychotic medications, including the metabolic effects of the now widely used second-generation, or "atypical," antipsychotic medications, overall medical treatment of homeless people with schizophrenia can be quite challenging.

Many observers have documented the degree to which jails and prisons have absorbed much of the custodial function previously provided to mentally ill persons by the state hospital system. Put another way, the revolving door has shifted from the state hospital to the state prison. Homelessness among mentally ill persons is strongly associated with incarceration and other contact with the criminal justice system. This relationship is a two-way street; homelessness places mentally ill people at higher risk of arrest and incarceration, whereas arrest and incarceration place mentally ill people at higher risk of homelessness. The latter process reflects the lack of continuity of care between jails and prisons, and the outside community, and the lack of housing options for persons with SMI and criminal histories.

Interestingly, when individuals with and without mental illness have been asked for their own perceived reasons for becoming homeless, both groups point to insufficient income, unemployment, and lack of suitable housing. The presence of psychiatric or substance abuse disorders, or the lack of treatment adherence, were not recognized as risk factors for homelessness. In other words, there may be a discrepancy between a mentally ill person's perception of why he or she became homeless and other contributing factors that providers might recognize, presenting a challenge to the treatment situation.

TREATMENT APPROACHES

The Community Mental Health Act of 1963 was meant to address the outpatient needs of the thousands of chronically mentally ill individuals in the United States who otherwise might have spent years, or even lifetimes, on the wards of state psychiatric facilities. Books such as E. Fuller Torrey's *Nowhere to Go* document the failed implementation of this plan, setting the stage for the explosion in the population of people who were homeless and mentally ill, as affordable housing declined at a rate comparable to the downsizing of the state hospitals. New York City, for example, lost approximately 90% of its single-room-occupancy hotel units, and the number of hospital beds declined by roughly the same 90% from its peak in the mid-1950s through the 1980s. Lack of adequate funding and lack of appropriate services contributed to the failure of the community mental health system to provide necessary care for individuals in the more severely mentally ill population.

In discussing treatment approaches for mentally ill homeless persons, one must broaden one's view of "treatment" to include outreach, housing, and other service approaches. This section summarizes several innovative models developed to help individuals with schizophrenia who have fallen into the unfortunate grip of homelessness.

MODEL PROGRAMS AND BEST PRACTICES

We chose the model programs and best practices described below and listed in Table 40.1 because they have empirical support and have become, or are becoming, widely utilized. In describing them, we emphasize some common guiding principles of treatment along with some differences in approach that remain controversial. These program models have evolved from earlier work carried out on assertive community treatment (ACT) and a number of specialized demonstration projects for homeless persons funded via the Federal McKinney Homeless Assistance Act during the late 1980s and early 1990s.

OUTREACH AND DROP-INS

Outreach programs that attempt to engage and bring services to homeless SMI individuals on the street and in shelters are now in wide use. Research has shown that mentally ill people living on the street and in other public places tend to be more severely impaired, to have more unmet needs and less motivation to seek treatment, and to take longer to seek services than their sheltered counterparts. Street outreach techniques have been refined to emphasize a nonintrusive, client-centered approach that is an effective way to engage the most disadvantaged people.

Regardless of the setting, outreach often involves bringing services to an unwilling recipient. Effective outreach personnel must proceed cautiously and offer to meet recipients' basic needs (food, a shower, a place to sleep, help with obtaining benefits) before recommending more formal treatment. Evaluations and treatment services should be offered only when the client has indicated that he or she is ready and willing. A new approach to outreach incorporates Housing First (described in detail later in this chapter), in which rapid housing placement is offered, often prior to the client's acceptance of psychiatric and substance abuse treatment.

All outreach teams should have access to a drop-in center where individuals can come in off the street to shower, eat, get some clean clothes, and rest. The drop-in center must be a safe place where individuals are treated with respect. Once someone begins to feel safe in a drop-in center, he or she often becomes receptive to treatment and other services. However, taking medication is often the last thing on the agenda of persons living on the street. It takes a sensitive attunement to the client to know when to offer medication and at what later point to push for it. Unfortunately, some outreach teams do not work together with drop-in centers, and many drop-in centers lack the professional staff to treat people with schizophrenia. Once it becomes necessary to refer individuals from one agency to another, the potential for losing that individual back to the streets increases. Despite the existence of a developed knowledge of effective outreach techniques, providing treatment and case management services to someone on the street remains extremely difficult.

Shelter-based interventions also have been shown to be effective, bringing psychiatric and medical treatment to the shelter rather than relying on shelter residents to seek out care in the community. Because many shelter residents are reluctant to seek psychiatric treatment, "outreach" within the shelter becomes necessary.

CASE MANAGEMENT

Prior to the advent of the assertive case management approach described below, case management tended to focus on linking patients via referral to available services in the community. This approach, so-called "broker" case management, was largely ineffective for very ill patients, especially those who were homeless. A solo case manager, whose job was limited to acting as a broker between the patient and providers, was an insufficient safety net. If, for any number of practical or psychiatric reasons, a patient could not avail him- or herself of existing services, he or she would often "fall through the cracks" of the system. This became particularly evident during transitions, such as between institutional settings (shelters, hospitals, jails, and prisons) and the community, leading researchers to identify lack of continuity of care as a key weakness in the service delivery system for persons with SMI. Furthermore, many case managers were not, and still are not, trained in the therapeutic techniques of engagement, motivational interviewing, management of transference and countertransference, and termination. Without such training, therapeutic alliances are often never made, or once made, they break down irreparably. In 1980, Richard Lamb was an early advocate for this expanded role of case managers (see References and Recommended Readings).

In a head-to-head comparison of broker case management and assertive case management, the latter has been shown to be superior for homeless mentally ill persons recruited from emergency rooms and inpatient units. Other studies have looked specifically at the role of the therapeutic alliance between patient and case manager. Although the data are inconsistent, the strength of that alliance has in some cases been found to be associated with positive clinical outcomes, better life satisfaction, and reduced homelessness. Yet another study has demonstrated that for domiciled patients with schizophrenia and schizoaffective disorder, greater intensity of psychosocial rehabilitative services and greater continuity of care were associated with greater improvement in social, work, and independent living domains, and with fewer days of hospitalization. Thus, there is some hard evidence that intensive, continuous case management and rehabilitative services can prevent homelessness in patients with schizophrenia.

The two evidence-based case management models we describe below, ACT and the critical time intervention (CTI), both utilize intensive community-based case management with a team approach. The ACT team typically includes a psychiatric practitioner (psychiatrist, nurse practitioner, or physician's assistant), nurse, and social work supervisor, but may also include substance abuse counselors, rehabilitative specialists, or peer counselors. Although there are common elements to the two approaches, we describe their differences.

ASSERTIVE COMMUNITY TREATMENT

Over the past 15 years, ACT has been adapted for use with homeless individuals with SMI, often with coexisting substance abuse disorders. Key ingredients of ACT include the multidisciplinary team, along with a low number of shared caseloads; a targeted population (SMI, with or without homelessness); 24-hour services; assertive engagement while maintaining client choice and privacy; provision of services in the community, and inclusion of family, recipient, and cultural perspectives. The team should comprise individuals trained in social work, psychiatry, nursing, psychosocial rehabilitation, and rehabilitation of persons with substance abuse or mentally ill chemically addicted (MICA) persons. When working with street or sheltered populations, ACT teams must do outreach where the homeless gather, including parks, subways, bus stations, bread lines, churches, drop-in centers, and shelters. A randomized clinical trial of ACT for homeless mentally ill individuals has shown its effectiveness in improving housing, clinical, and life satisfaction outcomes.

As a long-term intervention with ongoing intensive services and broad treatment goals, ACT is an expensive yet, it has been argued, cost-effective and labor-intensive service that is suitable for some, but not all, people with persistent SMI. With a greater recognition of the role of psychiatric rehabilitation and recovery, a reduction in services over time is not only appropriate but also often desirable to the client who feels increasingly independent and empowered to meet his or her own needs. One criticism of ACT has been that some of its strong points, such as its assertive and long-term approach, may foster client dependency. An important challenge to psychiatric providers on clinical and administrative levels is to identify which consumers need longer term intensive services, and which may benefit from a time-limited intervention during a critical time, or times, in the consumer's life. Furthermore, resource limitations in some localities have caused a number of ACT teams to shift to time-limited interventions, allowing clients to "graduate" from the program, similar to CTI, described below.

CRITICAL TIME INTERVENTION

As one of the McKinney demonstration projects developed in the late 1980s, CTI adopted some of the ACT principles, yet introduced novel approaches to preventing recurrent homelessness in a time-limited (9-month) intervention. CTI assumed that there would be a "critical period" of transition from shelter life to community-based housing for a population of homeless men with SMI leaving a large New York City shelter. Like ACT, CTI utilized an assertive team case management approach that included a nurse and psychiatrist working with a primary case manager. However, CTI aimed specifically to reduce homelessness by focusing on several risk areas: medication adherence, substance abuse treatment, family psychoeducation, prevention of housing-related crises, and money management. Yet for a given client, only one or two of the most significant risk areas would become the focus of the intervention. In addition, informal, community-based skills training was ongoing throughout the phased 9-month intervention. The time-limited nature of the intervention, another departure from the prevailing philosophy of ACT at that time, necessitated a reduction in the intensity of direct services by the team over the three phases of CTI. The first phase, "Transition to the Community" is most like ACT, involving at least weekly visits and very active direct care by a CTI worker, typically an experienced but not professionally trained individual working under professional supervision. The second phase, "Try-Out," involves a stepping back by the CTI worker, a growing reliance on linkages to community supports and on the client's own skills, and active intervention by the worker only as needed. In this phase CTI is probably best described as a hybrid of assertive and linkage approaches. In the final phase, "Transfer of Care," the CTI worker mostly observes and troubleshoots to fine-tune the community linkages. In this phase, a formal termination process is crucial, perhaps marked by a shared meal and review of the client's progress.

The effectiveness of CTI has now been studied in a number of randomized clinical trials. Findings from the initial CTI study (see References and Recommended Readings) include a significant reduction in homelessness that lasted at least 9 months *beyond the intervention itself,* a reduction in negative and autistic symptoms, and evidence of cost-effectiveness. Current CTI adaptations include a variety of populations and settings, such as men and women with SMI discharged from inpatient psychiatric treatment, mentally ill persons discharged from prisons, homeless mothers with mental illness transferred from shelters into transitional housing, and homeless mentally ill veterans treated by dedicated homeless outreach teams. CTI has recently been recognized as a model program by the President's New Freedom Commission on Mental Health and by the Substance Abuse and Mental Health Services Administration.

HOUSING APPROACHES

Much debate exists as to what types of housing approaches are most effective for homeless persons with SMI and at what point in the treatment process housing should be introduced. On one side of the debate are advocates for the "continuum" approach, which includes a slow, planned progression from street to shelter to transitional residence to supportive housing and, finally, to permanent independent housing. This philosophy assumes that "housing readiness" skills are required before housing is offered. This supports an approach in which clinicians aim first to stabilize the patient through psychiatric and substance abuse treatment, build skills and obtain supports necessary for housing stability, then seek permanent housing as the final step in the process.

On the other side of the debate, an innovative approach called "Housing First" moves homeless people with SMI and sometimes those with coexisting addictions, from the street directly into housing, typically independent or shared apartments located in a normal residential (i.e., nontreatment) setting. It assumes that with adequate supports, such as a payee to see that the rent is paid and an ACT team providing home visits, practically anyone living on the street can function in permanent housing. The assumption underlying this approach is that by obtaining housing before other services, people improve significantly simply by virtue of being off the street, and they are then more amenable to other interventions, including psychiatric and substance abuse treatment.

Pathways to Housing, a New York–based organization, pioneered this approach and has reported surprisingly high housing retention rates. Others too have shown that providing access to affordable independent housing (e.g., via Federal Section 8 vouchers) is a way to honor the housing preferences of people with schizophrenia. Unfortunately, governmental support of this housing subsidy program has been inconsistent in recent years, leading, at times, to long waiting lists for these vouchers.

The Housing First approach certainly warrants strong consideration as a model for housing homeless people with SMI. Of course, for a Housing First program to succeed, a community must have available, affordable housing stock. A key element to Housing First, therefore, is actively seeking out low-income housing and maintaining good alliances with landlords in the community.

In June 2001, the New York State Office of Mental Health (NYS OMH) hosted a Best Practices Conference that included a workshop on best practices in the field of supported housing. The workshop identified several emerging best practices (see NYS OMH website at *www.omh.state.ny.us/omhweb/omhq/q0901/SuppHouse.html*) in supported housing. The NYS OMH views supported housing as an approach whose intent is to

> ensure that individuals who are seriously and persistently mentally ill may exercise their right to choose where they are going to live, taking into consideration the recipient's functional skills, the range of affordable housing options available in the area under consideration, and the type and extent of services and resources that recipients require to maintain their residence within the community. (NYS OMH website: *Supported Housing Program Implementation Guidelines,* Sec. IIA, "The Supported Housing Approach")

The recommendations for best practices in supported housing from the Best Practices Conference are summarized in Table 40.1.

INTEGRATED DUAL-DISORDERS TREATMENT

The recent development of approaches that combine services for substance abuse and severe mental disorder is one reflection of better systems integration as agencies on all governmental levels recognize the ineffectiveness of maintaining totally separate agencies that treat either mental illness or substance abuse, but not both, in an integrated way. At the

TABLE 40.1. Best Practices in Supported Housing

- Rental subsidies are provided.
- Housing is protected while the person is in crisis.
- Consumer choices and preferences are honored.
- Assistance is available in obtaining and establishing a home.
- The consumer controls his or her personal space and privacy.
- The consumer has typical tenant roles and responsibilities.
- Individual or team support services have low caseloads.
- Support is available 24/7, with frequent contact.
- Direct support and assistance are flexibly tailored and provided *in vivo*.

clinical level, recent evidence suggests that approaches in which the same clinicians treat both disorders at the same time, so-called "integrated" treatment programs, are effective in reducing substance abuse in this population.

Controversy exists regarding the effectiveness of residential programs that permit substance use (e.g., the so-called "wet house," where alcohol is permitted) for people with coexisting substance abuse and mental illness. Supporters of a harm reduction ideology argue that it is better for people with dual disorders to have a home and access to help, especially while actively using substances, than to be on the street getting high and going untreated; others believe that a so-called "zero-tolerance" to substance use is the preferred treatment approach for persons with SMI. No current, definitive empirical evidence clearly demonstrates the superiority of either approach.

TREATMENT GUIDELINES

Most of what we have discussed so far relates to the program or systems level. Yet there are important guidelines for the individual clinician working with people with schizophrenia who are homeless or vulnerable to becoming homeless. These guidelines are general and should apply to all phases of a patient's recovery, but clinicians obviously must adjust their approach to where the patients are in the course of their illness and homelessness.

1. *Meet the patients "where they're at."* We mean this both literally and figuratively. Clinicians who treat homeless people should be prepared to work outside on the street, in parks, and perhaps in subway tunnels and other public spaces. Shelters, soup kitchens, and drop-in centers are other settings to meet homeless people. When doing so, clinicians

TABLE 40.2. Treatment Models and Best Practices

- Outreach and drop-in centers
- Intensive therapeutic case management
- ACT
- CTI
- Supportive housing and Housing First
- Integrated dual-disorder (mentally ill and chemically abusing [MICA]) services

should put aside the diagnostic manual and medication arsenal, at least initially, and replace them with friendly conversation. A clinician might serve a meal, give someone a warm blanket, or try a game of ping-pong or chess to engage a person initially, before he or she becomes a "patient." The best approach is to find out what that person wants or needs and to try to offer some help in that area first. He or she might want housing, a job, someone to check a leg wound, or a chance to call a relative; meeting these needs, or at least taking initial steps to do so, likely opens the door to additional treatment. When doing a history, the clinician should first take a life history—where the person was raised, where his or her family resides now, and how he or she became homeless—before asking about symptoms and psychiatric history. The clinician tries to be warm, funny, sympathetic, and natural. Remaining professional does not require being stiff, authoritative, and distant.

2. *Street outreach providers should be flexible, aiming for gradual, nonthreatening engagement for some clients and rapid housing for others, while also being prepared to handle crises.* In addition to the slow process of engaging people who may not want help, or worse yet, who might feel threatened by it, outreach teams must be prepared to handle medical and psychiatric emergencies. Besides making an assessment of danger to self or others, a psychiatrist doing outreach must be expert in diffusing aggression, maximizing safety of all involved (patient, clinical team, passersby), and should understand how to communicate clearly and persuasively with police and paramedics. To ensure that emergency room personnel provide adequate care, a note, and ideally a staff person, should accompany the patient to the emergency room.

The Housing First approach may run counter to the gradual, cautious engagement process most outreach teams have learned to employ, but for some clients, the offer of housing may be the most powerful engagement tool. There are always some individuals with SMI for whom the street is familiar and, paradoxically, less threatening than the indoors. Therefore, outreach providers should remain flexible in their approaches, heeding our first guideline, meeting clients where "they are at" both physically and psychologically.

3. *Be a team player.* Whether part of an ACT, CTI, or outreach team, or a housing or shelter program, one cannot treat this population without the services of others. The work requires putting aside the diplomas and the ego, and embracing the satisfaction of working alongside other spirited, dedicated, and experienced staff members. Fortunately, the nature of the work often "selects" people with these qualities. One should listen to what outreach workers, peer counselors, nurses, and social workers have to say. They often have unique perspectives and experiences that psychiatric providers lack. One gives back to the team by not only providing expertise in diagnosis and treatment, but also sharing one's understanding of the psychodynamic aspects of the treatment situation. Psychiatric providers can supervise case managers, making use of their understanding of engagement, resistance, transference, countertransference, and termination. They can help manage difficult clinical situations that arise, for example, with the paranoid or borderline patient. In other words, they see themselves as more than professionals sitting in their offices, writing prescriptions, and calling 911 when necessary. If their agency expects only this, they offer to do more.

4. *Be part of the community.* Beyond a relationship with the clinical team, a psychiatric provider treating homeless people is more effective if he or she is familiar with the resources in the community, such as knowing which houses of worship serve meals or distribute clothing or getting to know the religious leaders in the community. They will appreciate having the clinician's phone number when someone comes into their house of worship and is clearly in need of psychiatric help. The psychiatric provider meets with the police and offers to help train officers. Local shop owners and residents may even become

helpful "eyes and ears" in the community. Having a good relationship with the local hospitals and pharmacies does not hurt either, nor does forming a relationship with housing providers, including independent landlords. Showing up during a crisis where a patient is housed goes a long way toward maintaining good relations with landlords and other tenants.

5. *Take a biopsychosocial approach.* The homeless population is at risk for multiple medical disorders. This, combined with poor access to care, means that many patients have untreated, sometimes advanced medical problems by the time they are discovered. Therefore, the biological aspect of care should involve referral for a comprehensive medical assessment, ideally at the same site of outreach (e.g., mobile medical van, drop-in center, shelter). However, a psychiatric provider can certainly do a preliminary assessment and laboratory screening if medical care is not readily accessible. Of course, recognizing and treating the full array of psychiatric symptoms (e.g., positive, negative, cognitive, affective, anxiety-related, and trauma-related), diagnosing substance use disorders, and prescribing appropriate medications are key aspects of the biological approach to mental illness. The psychosocial approach should involve taking a detailed psychosocial history; making a psychodynamic formulation; assessing family and other relationships; evaluating educational and work history; and understanding the role of religion, spirituality, and culture in the person's life. In addition, it involves recognizing the role of homelessness and poverty in people's lives, in the manifestations of their illness, and in their experience of treatment and rehabilitation.

6. *Consider reality.* For years, homeless individuals have been sent out of emergency rooms and inpatient units with prescriptions they cannot afford to fill and instructions that they either do not understand or that are impossible for them to follow due to their illness, poverty, or homelessness. There is no excuse for this. Treatment in any setting must take into account the patient's social circumstances. If a clinician believes a medication is the best one for a patient who lacks insurance and cannot afford it, he or she can give the patient a suitable alternative, providing samples, vouchers, or contact with a company that has an indigent patient plan. The clinician knows about public hospitals or clinics where free or very inexpensive medications can be obtained, or makes sure that a patient who needs bed rest or must elevate his or her feet has access to a bed! This might mean keeping the patient in the hospital a bit longer, or making extra calls to find a shelter, drop-in center, or emergency housing.

Many homeless people are afraid of being sedated by medication. For good reasons, they fear this will make vulnerable to street crime. Patients should be asked about this, and their concerns should be respected. As with any patient population, the clinician's aim should be to work collaboratively with the patient, using coercive means, such as involuntary hospitalization, only when safety is a real concern.

7. *Employ a harm reduction approach.* Harm reduction is an approach to patient care that stems from the substance abuse field but has broader applications. The prototype for harm reduction is needle exchange for intravenous drug users to prevent HIV and hepatitis. Harm reduction is compatible with the previous guideline emphasizing the need to consider reality and aim for a realistic level of improvement, even if it means tolerating some level of self-destructive behavior. For example, a patient who is actively using drugs might be able to avoid becoming psychotic by taking medication. Treating someone who is actively using substances involves some risk unto itself, but if, in one's judgment, the greater harm would come from not treating that person, then one should treat him or her. Too many programs exclude patients for behaviors such as active substance use or past violence. A harm reduction approach can be applied to psychopharmacology, substance abuse treatment, and even housing. The Housing First approach is one such way to apply a harm reduction approach to housing.

8. *Be a "doctor without borders."* When at all possible, the clinician should follow up with patients beyond his or her own niche. Ideally, an outreach team and drop-in center use the same psychiatric providers. It is even better if the same providers extend their services to those who are later housed. Agencies should employ programs, such as CTI and ACT, that promote enhanced continuity of care. Even when there are practical impediments to providing this level of continuity, phone calls to follow up referrals, outreach to make sure patients are receiving care, and being available to help when gaps in care become evident are all ways to help patients negotiate a complex and all-too-often fragmented system of care. Outpatient providers should routinely visit patients in the hospital and plan care jointly with the inpatient staff. Likewise, it is tremendously helpful for inpatient staff to follow up with outpatient staff after discharge to make sure all is going as planned.

9. *Be an advocate.* Implicit in some of the previous recommendations is the notion of changing the system when it does not meet the needs of individual patients. This can be done by helping patients to obtain benefits and to access appropriate medical, mental health, and legal services. And, of course, this can be done by helping patients access housing. It can also be done on the agency level by changing the type of services delivered and the manner in which they are delivered. And it can be done on the service systems level by providing expertise in court cases by testifying or offering *amicus* briefs. Other ways to influence the system of care for homeless people with schizophrenia include working alongside consumers and other advocates to fight for improved housing, treatment, and benefits. This can be done by joining committees and workgroups of professional organizations, governmental agencies, and advocacy groups, or through other means of political action.

KEY POINTS

- Homelessness and housing instability are common in people with schizophrenia.
- People with schizophrenia who become homeless tend to have one or more comorbid conditions, such as substance abuse or undiagnosed medical disorders, as well as histories of trauma, separation from family, and contact with the criminal justice system.
- The previous two points provide the rationale for a comprehensive team approach to treatment and rehabilitation of people with schizophrenia who are either homeless or at particular risk for homelessness.
- People with schizophrenia who are residentially unstable often move between the street and shelters, and various institutional settings. This recurrent cycle necessitates models that enhance continuity of care regardless of residential status.
- Psychiatrists treating this population must think and act outside the box. Effective engagement methods, use of harm reduction, and doing outreach often require psychiatrists to act in ways contrary to traditional training.
- Evidence-based practices for this population do exist and can be utilized for both primary and secondary prevention of homelessness.

REFERENCES AND RECOMMENDED READINGS

Breakey, W. R., & Thompson, J. W. (1997). *Mentally ill and homeless: Special programs for special needs.* Amsterdam: Harwood Academic.

Caton, C., Shrout, P., Dominguez, B., Eagle, P., Opler, L., & Cournos, F. (1995). Risk factors for homelessness among women with schizophrenia. *American Journal of Public Health, 85*(8), 1153–1156.

Caton, C., Shrout, P., Eagle, P., Opler, L., Felix, A., & Dominguez, B. (1994). Risk factors for homelessness among schizophrenic men: A case–control study. *American Journal of Public Health, 84*(2), 265–270.

Culhane, D. P., Averyt, J. M., & Hadley, T. R. (1997). The rate of public shelter admission among Medicaid-reimbursed users of behavioral health services. *Psychiatric Services, 48*(3), 390–392.

Falk, K., & Albert, G. (1995). *Treating mentally ill homeless persons: A handbook for psychiatrists.* New York: Project for Psychiatric Outreach to the Homeless, Inc.

Folsom, D., & Jeste, D. V. (2002). Schizophrenia in homeless persons: A systematic review of the literature. *Acta Psychiatrica Scandinavica, 105*(6), 404–413.

Folsom, D. P., Hawthorne, W., Lindamer, L., Gilmer, T., Bailey, A., Golshan, S., et al. (2005). Prevalence and risk factors for homelessness and utilization of mental health services among 10,340 patients with serious mental illness in a large public mental health system. *American Journal of Psychiatry, 162*(2), 370–376.

Herman, D. B., Susser, E. S., Jandorf, L., Lavelle, J., & Bromet, E. J. (1998). Homelessness among individuals with psychotic disorders hospitalized for the first time: Findings from the Suffolk County Mental Health Project. *American Journal of Psychiatry, 155*(1), 109–113.

Katz, S. T., Nardacci, D., & Sabatini, A. (1993). *Intensive treatment of the homeless mentally Ill.* Washington, DC: American Psychiatric Press.

Lamb, H. R., Bachrach, L. L., & Kass, F. I. (1992). *Treating the homeless mentally ill: A report on the Task Force on the Homeless Mentally Ill.* Washington, DC: American Psychiatric Association.

McQuistion, H. L., Felix, A., & Susser, E. S. (2003). Serving homeless people with mental illness. In A. Tasman, J. Kay, & J. A. Lieberman (Eds.), *Psychiatry* (2nd ed.). West Sussex, UK: Wiley.

Olfson, M., Mechanic, D., Hansell, S., Boyer, C., & Walkup, J. (1999). Prediction of homelessness within three months of discharge among inpatients with schizophrenia. *Psychiatric Services, 50*(5), 667–673.

The President's New Freedom Commission on Mental Health. (2003). *Achieving the promise: Transforming mental health care in America* (DHHS Publication No. SMA-03-3832). Rockville, MD: Author.

Rosenheck, R. A., Resnick, S. G., & Morrissey, J. P. (2003). Closing service system gaps for homeless clients with a dual diagnosis: Integrated teams and interagency cooperation. *Journal of Mental Health Policy and Economics, 6*(2), 77–87.

Susser, E., Lin, S. P., & Conover, S. A. (1991a). Risk factors for homelessness among patients admitted to a state mental hospital. *American Journal of Psychiatry, 148*(12), 1659–1664.

Susser, E., Lin, S., Conover, S., & Struening, E. (1991b). Childhood antecedents of homelessness in psychiatric patients. *American Journal of Psychiatry, 148*(8), 1026–1030.

Susser, E., Valencia, E., Conover, S., Felix, A., Tsai, W. Y., & Wyatt, R. J. (1997). Preventing recurrent homelessness among mentally ill men: A "critical time" intervention after discharge from a shelter. *American Journal of Public Health, 87*(2), 256–262.

Torrey, E. F. (1988). *Nowhere to go: The tragic odyssey of the homeless mentally ill.* New York: Harper & Row.

Tsemberis, S., Gulcur, L., & Nakae, M. (2004). Housing first, consumer choice, and harm reduction for homeless individuals with a dual diagnosis. *American Journal of Public Health, 94*(4), 651–656.

U.S. Department of Human Services, Substance Abuse and Mental Health Services Administration, Center for Mental Health Services, and Policy Research Associates. (2003). *Blueprint for change: Ending chronic homelessness for persons with serious mental illness and/or co-occurring substance use disorders* (DHHS Publication No. SMA-04-3870). Rockville, MD: Author.

CHAPTER 41

MEDICAL COMORBIDITY

INGRID B. RYSTEDT
STEPHEN J. BARTELS

Serious medical disorders are more common in persons with schizophrenia and are associated with increased disability, diminished quality of life, and early mortality. This chapter offers an overview of common medical conditions in schizophrenia, along with important considerations for effective management.

The chapter consists of two parts. The first section describes the problem (prevalence and impact of medical conditions in schizophrenia and quality of medical care), as well as potential barriers to effective medical care and health promotion. Drawing on this background, the second section of the chapter reviews in lay language four groups of medical conditions from the perspective of persons with schizophrenia (diabetes, hypertension/ heart disease, chronic obstructive pulmonary disease [COPD], and HIV/hepatitis B and C). Important self-management strategies are highlighted. Health monitoring related to antipsychotic medications is briefly reviewed.

DESCRIPTION OF THE PROBLEM

Prevalence

A variety of medical conditions are more common among persons with schizophrenia than in the general population, including diabetes, COPD, HIV/AIDS, and hepatitis B and C. Up to three-fourths of persons with schizophrenia have a co-occurring medical condition, and many of these individuals have more than one medical disorder. It is estimated that one in six persons with schizophrenia has diabetes, one in four has hypertension, and one in eight has other cardiovascular disease. Furthermore, almost one-fourth of persons with serious mental illness have COPD. Finally, infections with the hepatitis B virus (HBV), hepatitis C virus (HCV), and HIV are more common in persons with schizophrenia than in the general population. Approximately one in four persons with serious mental illness has been infected with HBV, and one in five persons with HCV. Rates of infection with HIV vary, with higher estimates approaching one-fourth of persons with schizophrenia.

Medical disorders among persons with schizophrenia frequently are related to preventable lifestyle factors, such as smoking, alcohol and drug abuse, unsafe sexual practices, obesity, poor diet, and lack of exercise. In addition, antipsychotic medications generally increase the risk for weight gain or medical illness, including diabetes. Consequently, obesity, smoking, and diabetes are important topics in primary care visits for persons with serious mental illness. When addressing lifestyle and the management of medical conditions, it is important to be aware that certain clinical features of schizophrenia (e.g., cognitive deficits and negative symptoms associated with lack of motivation and difficulty in planning and initiating behaviors) may pose additional challenges in terms of adherence. The housing, residential, and financial situation can similarly present difficulties (e.g., reduced ability to select healthy diet choices).

Impact

On average, persons with serious mental illness die approximately 10 years earlier than persons in the general population, frequently due to medical causes. In addition to premature mortality, medical conditions also have a negative impact on physical functioning and quality of life. Poor physical health and functioning are associated with reduced capacity to participate in critical life activities, including work, social relationships, leisure activities, and activities of daily living. Acquired physical disabilities, frailty, and the burden of multiple medical problems, commonly associated with old age, can in persons with schizophrenia have their onset in middle age. Sometimes the physical functioning of persons with schizophrenia resembles that of significantly older individuals in the general population.

Chronic medical conditions in the general population are frequently associated with greater use of medical services. However, persons with schizophrenia may actually have lower hospitalizations rates for procedural interventions compared to persons in the general population (e.g., related to heart disease; Lawrence, Holman, & Jablensky, 2001). There is no clear consensus in the research literature on whether persons with schizophrenia use fewer medical services (perhaps indicating inadequate health care) or greater amounts of acute medical services (possibly reflecting a more severe course of illness and poor ongoing management). Some studies identify higher rates of outpatient visits, whereas others identify lower rates. The relationship between comorbid medical illness and cost of overall care for persons with schizophrenia remains largely unexplored. However, Dixon and colleagues (2000) observed that persons with schizophrenia and diabetes have higher health care service utilization and expenditures compared to persons with schizophrenia and no diabetes.

Quality of Services

One factor that contributes to increased mortality for persons with schizophrenia is lower quality of medical services. For example, Druss and colleagues (2001) reported that persons with schizophrenia were more likely than persons without a mental illness to die after a heart attack. Their study also found that these greater rates of mortality were in part explained by lower quality care and a failure to provide the same level of guideline-based care following a heart attack for persons with schizophrenia as that provided for the general population.

Other studies indicate that persons with schizophrenia spectrum disorders receive similar or lower rates of general preventive follow-up care compared to the general population. Furthermore, it appears that persons with schizophrenia and diabetes receive fewer services related to diabetes management, even when they have more medical visits. Schizophrenia may be more strongly associated with underutilization of preventive services compared to other psychiatric diagnoses. Substance use increases the risk of underutilization of services, despite the fact that substance abuse is itself a risk factor for medical illness.

Potential Barriers

In the same manner that schizophrenia requires lifelong management, most medical conditions demand a long-term focus on lifestyle changes and medical management. However, certain features of schizophrenia make it difficult for patients to engage in healthy behaviors. For example, negative symptoms may contribute to low energy and low motivation to perform physical exercise regularly or to maintain a healthy diet. Similarly, social withdrawal may prevent persons with schizophrenia from leaving the home to engage in physical exercise or to shop for healthy foods.

A range of factors potentially prevents persons with schizophrenia from seeking necessary medical services. Cognitive and motivational difficulties associated with schizophrenia contribute to a decreased capacity to identify significant medical symptoms or to recognize that a medical condition warrants attention. Motivational difficulties and/or thought disorder associated with schizophrenia can also affect desire to engage in self-care or to follow through with recommended preventive health recommendations. In this context, medical follow-up and self-management may be especially challenging. Other potential barriers to adequate and appropriate care include problems with medication adherence and inadequate knowledge about chronic medical conditions. See Table 41.1 for a summary of potential barriers to effective medical care.

Difficulty with transportation, lack of health insurance, or other financial limitations can make follow through on medical appointments difficult. Interacting with the medical health care system can also be challenging and even overwhelming. For example, impaired social and communication skills associated with schizophrenia can directly affect the ability to call for a medical appointment and or to communicate with physicians during a medical visit. Social withdrawal, verbal or cognitive difficulties, perceived stigma, or fear may contribute to a reluctance to communicate medical symptoms clearly during an office visit. At the same time, medical providers frequently are inexperienced in dealing with schizophrenia. For example, increased preoccupation with an important physical symptom may be dismissed as a psychiatric symptom or as a part of the mental illness. Unfortunately, this failure to address medical problems appropriately is mirrored by the mental health system when mental health providers lack experience in detecting and caring for physical illnesses.

At the systems level of care, the lack of integration between mental health and medical services constitutes a major barrier. A variety of models are being evaluated in re-

TABLE 41.1. Potential Patient Barriers to Effective Medical Management

• Inadequate knowledge about the chronic disease	• Cognitive or verbal difficulties
• Negative symptoms	• Fear
• Low motivation	• Financial constraints
• Low energy	• Inadequate health insurance coverage
• Denial	• Lack of transportation
• Social withdrawal	

search studies to help address this fragmentation of services by bridging the gap between mental health and medical services. For example, a designated health care advocate who facilitates personal empowerment and access to services may be helpful for persons with schizophrenia. Other possible approaches include adapting medical disease management services specifically for persons with serious mental illness or redesigning services to provide integrated models of mental health care and medical care.

Important factors in effective management of persons with schizophrenia and medical conditions include mitigating barriers to optimal care, and increasing communication and coordination between medical providers and mental health providers. Basic knowledge about the most common medical conditions better equips mental health providers in assisting persons with schizophrenia in optimal self-management and health promotion strategies.

COMMON MEDICAL CONDITIONS IN PERSONS WITH SCHIZOPHRENIA

The following sections describe several common medical conditions in persons with schizophrenia, including diabetes, hypertension, heart disease, COPD, hepatitis B and C, and HIV, along with areas of special consideration in the self-care of these specific conditions when supporting persons with schizophrenia. The section concludes with a discussion of the significance of smoking, as well as health monitoring in connection with antipsychotic use.

Caring for Diabetes in Persons with Schizophrenia

There are two types of diabetes: type 1 diabetes and type 2 diabetes. Type 1 diabetes (previously called juvenile diabetes), which generally begins in childhood or early adulthood, is caused by an early failure by the body to produce enough insulin. Insulin is a hormone that converts sugar (glucose), starches, and other important foods into energy necessary for daily life. Type 1 diabetes is not caused by obesity or inactivity. In contrast, type 2 diabetes more frequently begins later in life and commonly occurs in overweight individuals. Persons with schizophrenia may have either type 1 or type 2 diabetes, although type 2 diabetes is much more common.

The hormone insulin helps the body metabolize sugar. With diabetes, the body frequently does not have enough insulin and is therefore unable to reduce the blood sugar level adequately after a meal. Persons with type 2 diabetes may also develop a resistance to insulin. As a result, their blood sugar (glucose) is consistently elevated and builds up in the blood rather than going into cells. Over the long run, consistently elevated blood glucose can seriously damage the eyes, kidneys, heart, and nerves of persons with diabetes. To maintain a normal blood sugar level, all persons with type 1 diabetes must take insulin. Persons with type 2 diabetes may be able to control their blood sugar with rigorous dietary changes and regular exercise. When diet and exercise do not adequately lower blood sugar, persons with type 2 diabetes must take oral medications or insulin.

Regardless of the type of diabetes, a person with diabetes has an increased risk for heart disease and stroke, as well as longer-term diabetic complications in other organ systems, including damage to the nerves that results in loss of sensation in the feet or hands, damage to the eyes that causes a progressive loss of vision, and damage to the kidney that can result in kidney failure. The risk for complications is reduced if normal or safe blood sugar levels are continuously maintained and monitored.

Diabetes requires a range of self-management activities that may be especially challenging for persons with a serious mental illness. For example, a person with diabetes needs to have good knowledge of dietary and exercise requirements, and the relationship between exercise, diet, medication, and blood sugar level. Diabetes educators can help persons with diabetes manage their illness. Individuals with schizophrenia often require more prompting, assistance in monitoring and self-administering their medications, and more self-management support compared to persons without mental illness. Consequently, establishing collaboration between the mental health case manager and medical provider or diabetes educator is important. Staff at group homes or family and friends can also be a valuable resource.

All persons with type 1 diabetes (and many persons with type 2 diabetes) monitor their blood sugar levels with a glucometer (pricking a finger to measure the current blood glucose level). The blood sugar level provides important guidance for how to adjust and fine-tune the dosage of the diabetic medication. In addition, medical providers check a specific type of blood hemoglobin called hemoglobin A1c (HbA1c) every 3–6 months to get a picture of "average" level of blood sugar over the past months. To minimize the risk of diabetic complications, it is important to keep the HbA1c measure low. When the HbA1c is above target range, medications may need to be adjusted. In addition, self-management skills should be revisited when the diabetic control is not optimal. It is important to identify approaches that enable individuals to take diabetic medications regularly, eat appropriately, and exercise more frequently. Examples of helpful enablers include written or phone-call reminders; prompting by family members or by care providers; and ongoing education, support, and reinforcement of positive health behaviors.

Some persons with schizophrenia may not have the skills or financial resources to shop for healthy foods or to prepare healthy meals. Case managers, rehabilitation counselors, nurses, and others can provide information, education, and even direct assistance in helping patients learn how to locate healthy (and low-price) foods in the grocery store and to prepare simple, nutritious meals. Those who live in group homes generally do not have the ability to choose their daily diet. In some cases, it may be necessary to engage dieticians and diabetes educators to help staff ensure that meals meet specific dietary requirements. A person with schizophrenia may also benefit from assistance in designing a personalized exercise routine that includes a schedule and instructions on where and for how long a walk should occur, or, the location of the local Young Men's Christian Association (YMCA), and how to obtain and use a membership. Exercising with a friend may be a useful and important strategy to maintain motivation.

In addition to regular visits with the medical provider, a person with diabetes should receive regular screening for potential complications of diabetes. These screening tests are designed to detect potential complications early and to allow for prompt treatment. Table 41.2 provides examples of important follow-up. Over time, diabetes can damage the blood supply to the retina (the back of the eye and the location of visual receptor cells), which can result in a condition called retinopathy. If not promptly treated, this condition can result in diminished vision and blindness. Regular dilated eye exams help detect retinal changes early. Diabetes can also damage the kidneys. Urine and blood tests are used to monitor and detect early changes in kidney function. In addition, persons with diabetes should have regular checkups to evaluate cardiovascular health, due to their increased risk of heart disease, stroke, and blood vessel disease. Finally, diabetes can cause damage to the nerves responsible for sensation or the perception of heat, cold, and pain in the feet and hands. For example, this nerve damage (called diabetic neuropathy) can make persons with diabetes unaware of injuries or minor infections of their feet, which, if undetected, can progress to life-threatening infections that result in amputations, permanent

TABLE 41.2. Diabetes Follow-Up

• Glycated hemoglobin (HbA1c)	• Lipid panel
• Blood pressure	• Foot exam
• Dilated ophthalmic exam	• Self-management education (diabetes educator)
• Urine screen	• Smoking cessation counseling referral, if a smoker
• Test of kidney function (blood draw)	• Exercise recommendation/facilitation
• Cardiovascular checkup	• Weight loss recommendation, if obese
• Influenza vaccine	• Nutritionist referral (or diet recommendations/facilitation)
• Pneumonia vaccine	

physical disabilities, or mortality. Consequently, persons with diabetes should be taught how to examine their feet carefully for wounds or cuts on a daily basis.

A person with schizophrenia and diabetes should be encouraged continually to adhere to his or her follow-up schedule and self-management regimens. If the person does not follow through with screening or blood draws, it is important to address potential underlying fears or misunderstandings. Follow-up is always a good strategy to ensure that medical visits have occurred. It may also be helpful to accompany someone with schizophrenia to medical appointments.

Very high and very low blood sugar levels are dangerous and potentially life threatening. Consequently, it is important to learn to recognize symptoms of low blood sugar (e.g., cold sweating, shaking, and concentration difficulties) and high blood sugar (e.g., tiredness, increased thirst, hunger, and urination). If these conditions cannot be quickly resolved, then immediate medical attention is urgently needed. The self-management strategies and the choice of medication optimally should limit the frequency of these events. The patient should be encouraged to discuss promptly any such event (even if resolved without medical attention) with his or her medical provider.

Caring for Hypertension and Heart Disease in Persons with Schizophrenia

Hypertension, or high blood pressure, is referred to as *essential hypertension*, or *primary hypertension* when no underlying cause for the high blood pressure is identified. When an underlying condition is the cause, the hypertension is referred to as *secondary hypertension*. Most frequently, a person with high blood pressure does not experience any symptoms. Nevertheless, long-standing high blood pressure can cause damage to many organs and substantially increase the risk of heart attack and stroke. Given the lack of symptoms, it can be difficult to motivate people with hypertension to manage their silent illness with lifestyle changes and medication. This may be especially challenging for persons with schizophrenia, who have numerous challenges in managing serious psychiatric symptoms and may not consider a "silent" medical disorder a priority. For this reason, it is important to provide ongoing education, reminders, and support in addressing the serious long-term risks of hypertension through appropriate preventive and treatment strategies.

Lifestyle changes are important in hypertension, because many lifestyle-related factors themselves represent risk factors for heart disease, such as smoking and obesity. For a summary of relevant lifestyle changes, see Table 41.3. Because hypertension increases the risk for heart disease, it is important to address all risk factors that are amenable to change. For persons with family history of heart disease, it is particularly important to encourage lifestyle changes and appropriate medical management. This group of individuals is at especially high risk of serious complications of hypertension due to an underlying genetic vulnerability.

Regular physical exercise is an important part of achieving and maintaining a healthy blood pressure. Continuous prompting and encouragement are important in helping patients begin and sustain an exercise program. The medical provider should be consulted regarding a suitable level of exercise. In addition, if a person with hypertension is overweight, then it is important to identify a strategy for sustainable weight loss. A nutritionist is an important resource for educating a person with schizophrenia about appropriate dietary changes. Dietary education should be practical and easy to understand, and include basic information on portion size, healthy food items, and easy-to-prepare healthy menus. Additional practical information includes where to find nutritious food items in the grocery store; how to read nutrition labels for important information about salt, fat, and cholesterol content; and how to prepare low-fat meals.

Preferably a person with hypertension should reduce the intake of food items that are high in salt (e.g., salted chips and canned soups) or high in saturated fats (e.g., many meat and dairy products). Diets that focus on fruits, vegetables, whole grains, and low-fat dairy products are generally good, such as the Dietary Approaches to Stop Hypertension (DASH) eating plan. Excessive amounts of alcohol can increase a person's blood pressure. Addressing alcohol and substance use problems is important for effective hypertension management.

When lifestyle measures alone do not reduce the blood pressure to a normal range, medications for hypertension are necessary. For some persons, medication and lifestyle changes may be started concurrently. Many antihypertensive medications exist, including diuretics, beta-blockers, angiotensin-converting enzyme (ACE) inhibitors, and angiotensin receptor blockers. Certain antihypertensive medications, such as some diuretics and beta-blockers, should be avoided by patients on antipsychotic medications because of the risk of heart-related complications. Consequently, to meet both medical and psychiatric needs, and to minimize the risk of drug interactions, a team-based approach of both psychiatric and medical providers is desirable.

Because hypertension usually is not associated with symptoms, it is sometimes hard to motivate patients to take their medications. For the same reason, persons with schizophrenia are likely more aware of the consequences of not taking psychiatric medications than of not taking antihypertensive medications. However, the same medication adherence strategies apply to both psychiatric and medical medications. For example, medication adherence may be improved by placing the medicine container close to one's toothbrush or using written reminders.

When blood pressure is not in the normal range, or when the person experiences antihypertensive medication side effects (e.g., weakness, dizziness, dry mouth, persistent cough, or sexual dysfunction), a change of medications should be considered. A person with schizophrenia and hypertension who experiences side effects should be encouraged to report symptoms promptly to the medical provider. An alternative medication regimen that is more tolerable may improve medication adherence.

TABLE 41.3. Hypertension Lifestyle Changes

• Diet modification (e.g., low-fat, low-salt)	• Weight loss, if obese
• Smoking cessation	• Alcohol screening or counseling
• Exercise	

Caring for Heart Disease in Persons with Schizophrenia

A person with heart disease should generally work toward the same lifestyle goals as persons with hypertension or diabetes. However, physical exercise should be carefully discussed in collaboration with the medical provider. Dietary changes are crucial, and a medical nutritionist should be consulted.

The broad term *heart disease* includes conditions such as *heart failure* (a weakened heart muscle that fails to pump blood adequately to the body), *angina* (chest pain caused by an inadequate blood supply to the heart muscle due to blocked arteries), and *arrhythmias* (irregular heart beats often caused by damage to the heart's natural pacemaker). Many forms of heart disease are caused by a gradual buildup of plaques on the inside of arteries, a process also known as *atherosclerosis*. The buildup slowly makes the arteries narrower and harder, and this makes it more difficult to pump blood to the heart. Furthermore, there is a risk of plaques contributing to blood clot formations. Blood clots can cause a heart attack.

In heart failure, the heart is unable to pump blood adequately; as a consequence, fluid frequently accumulates in the lungs or in the legs. To continually assess the degree of heart failure, persons with heart failure should weigh themselves at the same time every day and check for swelling in the legs, feet, or hands. Any sudden increase in weight is a warning sign of serious problems, and the medical provider should immediately be contacted. Other warning signs are increased swelling, shortness of breath, or tiredness. People with heart failure must be well informed about when and how to contact the medical provider, and those with schizophrenia may need extra support in knowing how to contact their provider and how to describe clearly these important symptoms.

A person with angina (chest pain) must always carry medication and, similarly, needs to be well informed about when and how to seek care. Typically, angina is characterized by a crushing feeling of chest pressure with shortness of breath. Sometimes this is accompanied by pain that moves to the jaw or arm. These and other, related symptoms that do not very quickly resolve upon rest and a tablet of nitroglycerin warrant immediate medical attention. If chest pain associated with angina does not stop promptly (within 5 minutes at the most), then it is of utmost importance that the person get emergency medical attention quickly because he or she may be having a heart attack. Even if the pain goes away, the medical provider should be informed. It is important to keep track of any episodes of angina and, especially, to look for changes in frequency, duration, or intensity. Any observed changes should be reported immediately to the medical provider.

Persons with schizophrenia are at increased risk of ventricular arrhythmias. Antipsychotic medications may be a contributing factor. In selecting antipsychotic medications, it is important to be aware of the risk for arrhythmia and to select a medication that is suitable given overall patient characteristics and risk profile. Communication and consultation between the treating psychiatrist and medical provider are important features of care coordination aimed at identifying unanticipated risk factors and improving quality of care. Medical providers and psychiatrists must similarly consider potential interactions between heart disease and psychiatric medications.

Caring for COPD in Persons with Schizophrenia

COPD is a long-term, irreversible decrease in airflow and lung function due to damage of the airways and lung tissue. Symptoms include persistent cough, sputum production, and breathing difficulties. Smoking is strongly related to COPD. A history of smoking, in combination with a confirmed reduced airflow using a simple test that measures airflow (spirometry), suggests that a person has COPD, which includes a group of related and overlapping chronic respiratory diseases, such as chronic bronchitis chronic obstructive bronchitis, and emphysema.

COPD frequently is diagnosed late in the disease process. No cure exists, but effective management may help to prevent complications and improve quality of life. It is absolutely essential to quit smoking. This may require referral to a specialized smoking cessation program for persons with serious mental illness. Regular flu and pneumonia immunizations help the person to avoid chest infections. Inhaled medications, such as bronchodilators and steroids, can help to control symptoms. In advanced stages of the disease, long-term oxygen therapy and even surgery may become necessary. Individualized rehabilitation programs can teach essential skills and provide education and psychosocial support.

It is important for persons with COPD to know about the factors that trigger episodes of acute exacerbations of the illness, including increased shortness of breath, wheezing, and coughing. Persons with advanced COPD must monitor their pulmonary function with spirometry and carefully watch for worsening of symptoms. Managing symptoms may include increasing or changing medications and knowing when acute medical attention is required. Given the complex challenges associated with smoking cessation and self-management of COPD, persons with schizophrenia require extra support and ongoing monitoring. Collaboration between primary care medical providers and mental health providers (including regular input from pulmonology specialists) is important in identifying and individually tailoring these necessary supports and self-management strategies.

Caring for HIV and Hepatitis in Persons with Schizophrenia

Individuals with serious mental illness are at increased risk for blood-borne infections due to a variety of factors, including high rates of substance abuse, unsafe behaviors, and lack of knowledge about how these infections are transmitted. The prevalence of HBV infection among persons with serious mental illness is approximately five times higher than that in the general population, and the prevalence of HCV infection is more than 10 times higher. Many people are infected with both HCV and HIV, which may worsen the prognosis for both conditions.

Mental health and primary care providers should screen for risk behaviors. This may be a sensitive issue, because some risk behaviors are illegal and most are socially stigmatized. It is important to be aware of the tendency to underreport. Table 41.4 provides examples of risk behaviors. Inquiries about at-risk behaviors should occur in a supportive, nonjudgmental, and confidential manner. Of note, researchers have found that use of computer-based health screening for risky behaviors sometimes overcome barriers to accurate reporting. All persons with schizophrenia and an identified risk factor should be quickly screened to ensure that appropriate treatment is started promptly and to prevent further transmission. Vaccination against hepatitis A and B should also be provided. No vaccinations have yet been developed for HCV and HIV infection.

TABLE 41.4. Risk Behaviors for HBV/HCV/HIV

Current or past use of . . .

• Intravenous drugs	• Multiple or high-risk sexual partners
• Shared needles	• Sexual activity under the influence of drugs
• Unprotected sex	• Commercial sexual activity

Counseling regarding risk reduction is an essential component in reducing the likelihood of becoming infected or of transmitting viral infections. Several risk reduction programs use 8–12 sessions of group and individual cognitive-behavioral therapy. However, brief, individually tailored counseling may be more feasible and still be effective. In three sessions, the newly developed STIRR model (Screen, Test, Immunize, Reduce Risk, and Refer) intervention developed by Rosenberg and colleagues (2004) provides education, risk assessment, risk reduction counseling, screening, pre- and posttest counseling, vaccination against hepatitis A and B, treatment referrals, and follow-up.

Individuals infected with HIV, HBV, or HCV should be referred promptly to specialist medical care. Although no cure is available, appropriate medical care can slow disease progression. Chronic infections with either type of hepatitis can cause cirrhosis or cancer of the liver (this is particularly common in hepatitis C). Because HCV infection often causes no symptoms for the first two decades, it is frequently diagnosed and referred to medical care late in the disease process. Therefore, liver damage is typically present when symptoms appear. When diagnosed with hepatitis, it is vital to stop consuming alcohol and other substances that can be toxic to the liver, including certain medications.

Given the complexity of HIV and hepatitis treatments, efforts to support persons with schizophrenia continually in managing their illness and to follow treatment regimens are particularly helpful.

Smoking

Smoking cessation is an important goal for all persons with schizophrenia. For those who also have diabetes, hypertension, heart disease, or COPD, it is absolutely essential to quit smoking. Although smoking has decreased in the general population, it is still common among persons with serious mental illnesses, including schizophrenia. Research on nicotine receptors of the brain suggests that individuals with schizophrenia may have an increased biological risk for tobacco use and nicotine dependence. Lifestyle, social, and environmental factors also contribute to high rates of tobacco use. For sustainable smoking cessation, it is important to address how the "void" of a cigarette habit may be filled with other useful activities.

Formal smoking cessation programs designed for persons with schizophrenia may be necessary in achieving successful and sustained recovery from nicotine dependence. Along with cognitive-behavioral treatment, smoking cessation programs for schizophrenia generally include bupropion and/or nicotine replacement therapy. Long-term replacement with nicotine may be useful to prevent relapse. It is important to be aware that the process of quitting can affect psychiatric symptoms and increase the risk for relapse. In addition, plasma levels of antipsychotic medications sometimes increase when smoking is discontinued.

Antipsychotic Medications

Antipsychotic medications are associated with a wide range of potential physical side effects and health risks. The newer (atypical), or "second-generation," antipsychotics have fewer nervous system side effects and have been promoted as being potentially more effective than the older "conventional," or "first-generation," antipsychotic medications, such as Haldol and Prolixin. However, as a group, it is not clear that atypical antipsychotics are more effective than first-generation antipsychotics. Furthermore, these medications carry a new and different set of potential health risks that have raised concern among consumers and providers (e.g., weight gain and elevated blood sugar). Atypical antipsychotics have been associated with an increased risk of developing *metabolic syndrome,* characterized by a combination of metabolic risk factors, including abdominal

TABLE 41.5. ADA/APA Consensus on Antipsychotic Drugs: Monitoring Protocol for Patients on Second-Generation Antipsychotics

	Baseline	4 weeks	8 weeks	12 weeks	Quarterly	Annually	Every 5 years
Personal/family history	×					×	
Weight (BMI)	×	×	×	×	×		
Waist circumference	×					×	
Blood pressure	×			×		×	
Fasting plasma glucose	×			×		×	
Fasting lipid profile	×			×			×

Note. More frequent assessments may be warranted based on clinical status. From American Diabetes Association, American Psychiatric Association, American Association of Clinical Endocrinologists, and North American Association for the Study of Obesity (2004). Copyright 2004 by the American Diabetes Association. Reprinted by permission.

obesity, increased blood triglycerides (fats), elevated blood pressure, and insulin resistance. Due to the increased risk of persons with schizophrenia developing metabolic syndrome when taking atypical antipsychotics, close health monitoring is important. It is recommended that body mass index (BMI), waist circumference, plasma glucose level, and blood lipids be evaluated regularly. Before initiating or changing antipsychotic medications, BMI should be recorded and a fasting blood glucose should be obtained. Table 41.5 summarizes the monitoring protocol for antipsychotic medications developed by a consensus workgroup from the American Diabetic Association (ADA) and the American Psychiatric Association (APA). For a detailed description of health monitoring for adults on antipsychotic medications, please refer to the Marder and colleagues (2004) consensus statement (see References and Recommended Readings).

KEY POINTS

- Chronic medical conditions are common among persons with schizophrenia, and contribute to early mortality and poorer quality of life.
- Effective management of medical conditions in persons with schizophrenia requires ongoing collaboration and communication between mental health providers and primary care providers.
- Education and training in self-management of chronic medical conditions are important factors in improving health outcomes.
- Lifestyle factors (e.g., poor diet, overweight, lack of exercise, and smoking) are associated with a number of medical conditions that commonly affect persons with schizophrenia.
- Focusing on improvements in lifestyle-related factors is essential to manage medical conditions effectively in persons with schizophrenia.
- Compared to the general population, persons with schizophrenia need additional encouragement, coaching, and monitoring to achieve a healthy lifestyle.
- Persons with schizophrenia need individually tailored education about their medical condition(s) and associated health risks, signs of serious problems, medication regimens, and nutritional needs.
- Regular contact with medical providers is important to ensure that regular screening tests are on schedule and that optimal treatment is provided.
- Medication adherence is vital for effective chronic disease management, and adherence strategies are similar for both psychiatric and medical medication, including reminders and medication organizers.
- It is critical for persons with serious mental illness and medical comorbidity to acquire the skills and knowledge necessary to effectively access both routine and emergency health services.

REFERENCES AND RECOMMENDED READINGS

Altman, E. (2004). Update on COPD—today's strategies improve quality of life. *Advance for Nurse Practitioners, 12*(3), 49–54.

American Diabetes Association, American Psychiatric Association, American Association of Clinical Endocrinologists, & North American Association for the Study of Obesity. (2004). Consensus Development Conference on Antipsychotic Drugs and Obesity and Diabetes. *Diabetes Care, 27,*(2), 596–601.

Bartels, S. J. (2004). Caring for the whole person. *Journal of the American Geriatric Society, 52*(12), 249–257.

Brunette, M., Drake, R. E., Marsh, B., Torrey, W., Rosenberg, S., & the Five-Site Health and Risk Study Research Committee. (2003). Responding to blood-borne infections among persons with severe mental illness. *Psychiatric Services, 54*(6), 860–865.

Chafetz, L., White, M., Collins-Bride, G., Nickens, J., & Cooper, B. (2006). Predictors of physical functioning among adults with severe mental illness. *Psychiatric Services, 57*(2), 225–231.

Desai, M., Rosenheck, R., Druss, B., & Perlin, J. (2002). Mental disorders and quality of diabetes care in the Veterans Health Administration. *American Journal of Psychiatry, 159*(9), 1584–1590.

Dickerson, F., Goldberg, R., Brown, C., Kreyenbuhl, J., Wohlheiter, J., Fang, L., et al. (2005). Diabetes knowledge among persons with serious mental illness and type 2 diabetes. *Psychosomatics, 46*(5), 418–424.

Dixon, L., Weiden, P., Delahanty, J., Goldberg, R., Postrado, L., Lucksted, A. (2000). Prevalence and correlates of diabetes in national schizophrenia samples. *Schizophrenia Bulletin, 26*(4), 903–912.

Druss, B. G., Bradford, W. D., Rosenheck, R. A., Radford, M. J., & Krumholz, H. M. (2001). Quality of medical care and excess mortality in older patients with mental disorders. *Archives of General Psychiatry, 58*(6), 565–572.

Essock, S., Dowden, S., Constantine, N., Katz, L., Swartz, M., Meador, K., et al. (2003). Risk factors for HIV, hepatitis B and hepatitis C among persons with severe mental illness. *Psychiatric Services, 54*(6), 836–841.

Frayne, S., Halanych, J., Miller, D., Wang, F., Lin, H., Pogach, L., et al. (2005). Disparities in diabetes care: Impact of mental Illness. *Archives of Internal Medicine, 165*, 2631–2638.

Himmelhoch, S., Lehman, A., Kreyenbuhl, J., Daumit, G., Brown, C., & Dixon, L. (2004). Prevalence of chronic obstructive pulmonary disease among those with serious mental illness. *American Journal of Psychiatry, 161*(12), 2317–2319.

Jones, D., Macias, C., Barriera, P., Fisher, W., Hargreaves, W., & Harding, C. (2004). Prevalence, severity, and co-occurrence of chronic physical health problems of persons with serious mental illness. *Psychiatric Services, 55*(11), 1250–1257.

Lawrence, D., Holman, C. D. J., & Jablensky, A. V. (2001). *Preventable physical illness in people with mental illness*. Perth: University of Western Australia.

Lieberman, J., Stroup, S., McEvoy, J., Swartz, M., Rosenheck, R., Perkins, D., et al. (2005). Effectiveness of antipsychotic drugs in patients with chronic schizophrenia. *New England Journal of Medicine, 353*(12), 1209–1223.

Marder, S., Essock, S., Miller, A., Buchanan, R., Casey, D., Davis, J., et al. (2004). Physical health monitoring of patients with schizophrenia. *American Journal of Psychiatry, 161*(8), 1334–1349.

Meadows, G., Strasser, K., Moeller-Saxone, K., Hocking, B., Stanton, J., & Kee, P. (2001). Smoking and schizophrenia: The development of collaborative management guidelines. *Australasian Psychiatry, 9*(4), 340–344.

O'Day, B., Killeen, M., Sutton, J., & Iezzoni, L. (2005). Primary care experiences of people with psychiatric disabilities: Barriers to care and potential solutions. *Psychiatric Rehabilitation Journal, 28*(4), 339–345.

Rosenberg, S., Brunette, M., Oxman, T., Marsh, B., Dietrich, A., Mueser, K., et al. (2004). The STIRR model of best practices for blood-borne diseases among clients with serious mental illness. *Psychiatric Services, 55*(6), 660–664.

Rosenberg, S., Swanson, J., Wolford, G., Osher, F., Swartz, M., Essock, S., et al. (2003). The Five-Site Health and Risk Study of blood-borne infections among persons with severe mental illness. *Psychiatric Services, 54*(6), 827–835.

Rosenberg, S., Trumbetta, S., Mueser, K., Goodman, L., Osher, F., Vidaver, R., et al. (2001). Determinants of risk behavior for human immunodeficiency virus/acquired immunodeficiency syndrome in people with severe mental illness. *Comprehensive Psychiatry, 42*(4) 263–271.

U.S. Department of Health and Human Services/National Institutes of Health/National Heart, Lung and Blood Institute. (2003). *Facts about the DASH eating plan* (NIH Publication No. 03-4082). Rockville, MD: Author.

CHAPTER 42

INTELLECTUAL DISABILITY AND OTHER NEUROPSYCHIATRIC POPULATIONS

RICHARD B. FERRELL
THOMAS W. McALLISTER

Conditions or disorders that alter the motor, sensory, or mental functions of the central nervous system (CNS) may also alter the likelihood of CNS-based disorders or illnesses. These conditions or disorders may also change the symptomatic presentation of psychiatric illnesses, such as schizophrenia. They may also affect response to psychopharmacological, psychotherapeutic, and behavioral treatments. CNS disorders that result in intellectual disability (ID) are a category of such conditions. We think that these ideas are important to the proper understanding and treatment of persons with schizophrenia who also have ID or other neuropsychiatric illnesses. Conditions such as Alzheimer's disease, Parkinson's disease, Huntington's disease, multiple sclerosis, epilepsy, cerebrovascular disease, and traumatic brain injury are often associated with psychotic symptoms or may directly cause psychosis. In this chapter we use ID as a paradigm or example of a neuropsychiatric disorder that can occur concomitantly with schizophrenia. ID is not, however, a single disease or even a disease-state, as are the disorders we named earlier. Its causes are often multiple, obscure, speculative, or unknown. Demonstration of anatomical pathology or of CNS pathophysiology, if it exists, is frequently still beyond the reach of current science.

Although some evidence points to the increased susceptibility to schizophrenia of persons with ID, it is possible that individuals with ID may also develop schizophrenic illness for reasons not related to ID. Our ignorance of the causes of both ID and schizophrenia still greatly exceeds our knowledge. Our purpose is to survey important neuropsychiatric issues and recent findings with respect to the evaluation and treatment of schizophrenia in intellectually disabled people.

OVERVIEW AND EPIDEMIOLOGY OF ID

Intellectual disability (ID) is the current term used to describe individuals who have cognitive impairments present at birth, or early in life, that result in functional life skills deficits. Mental retardation (MR) and developmental disability (DD) are former terms. We use the term ID in this chapter. We sometimes include the terms MR and DD to maintain clarity when reviewing earlier literature.

The *Diagnostic and Statistical Manual of Mental Disorders* (DSM-IV-TR; American Psychiatric Association, 2000) uses the term *mental retardation* to refer to individuals who have below-average intellectual functioning accompanied by deficits in adaptive functioning, with onset in childhood or adolescence. Measures of general intellectual function, such as IQ or some equivalent, are often used as benchmarks for subaverage intellectual functioning. Individuals with an IQ that is two or more standard deviations below the mean, that is, IQ < 70, are generally regarded as having MR if they also have problems in adaptive functioning. In DSM-IV-TR, *adaptive functioning* refers to an individual's ability to cope with problems of everyday life when viewed in the context of social and age-related norms. Adaptive functioning is closely tied to an individual's capacity for age-appropriate independent function.

For the diagnosis of MR, DSM-IV-TR requires that an individual be impaired in at least two of the following domains: communication, self-care, home living, social and interpersonal skills, use of community resources, self-direction, functional academic skills, work, leisure, health, and safety. Because virtually all measures of intellectual functioning have an inherent measurement error; one could possibly make a diagnosis of ID (or MR) in the presence of "low-normal IQ" if the person can be shown clearly to have impairments in adaptive functioning. Conversely, an individual with an IQ that is more than two standard deviations below the mean, but with no clear deficits in adaptive impairment, might not meet diagnostic criteria for MR.

Most classification schemes classify intellectual impairment into four groups: mild (IQ ~ 50–70), moderate (IQ ~ 35–50), severe (IQ ~ 20–35), and profound (IQ < 20). In practice, describing an individual's cognitive and functional strengths and weaknesses instead of applying an arbitrary numerical determination is usually more helpful. This approach gives a more accurate expectation with respect to what an individual can and cannot do.

Using the above-mentioned broad definitions, about 1–3% of the general population probably meet criteria for ID (American Psychiatric Association, 2000). Approximately 85% of these individuals are in the mildly disabled range. Adults with mild ID often live successfully in the community. Depending on their profile of cognitive strengths and weaknesses, they may need residential, vocational, or "life skills" support or supervision. During critical life phase transitions or periods of increased psychosocial stress, they may need extra help.

An additional 10% of persons with ID can be described as moderately impaired. They need much more support in many areas of life function. The remaining ~5% fall into the severe or profound categories and need maximum supports in all areas.

ID, and DD and MR, are minimally helpful, clinical, descriptive terms that give no information about the cause of the intellectual impairment. Estimates are that 250 known causes of ID exist. The number of known causes is likely to increase as understanding of the human genome grows. The major etiological categories include chromosomal or genetic causes, for example, Down's syndrome or trisomy 21, and pre- or perinatal insults (e.g., viral infections, high fever, fetal distress, anoxia, and fetal alcohol exposure).

Schizophrenia remains an illness of unknown cause. Current thinking about this severe illness postulates an etiological hypothesis in which neurodevelopmental or genetic vulnerability, or both, interact with stressful life events of a social, psychological, or possibly physiological nature to produce pathology. Three percent is an often-quoted figure for persons with ID who also have schizophrenia (Turner, 1989), but this number is imprecise and might be low. Some clinical and research interest has focused on whether there might be specific genetic abnormalities that could both cause disabling syndromes and increase risk of schizophrenia and other psychiatric disorders. For example, there appears to be increased risk of developing psychiatric disorders, especially schizophrenia, for persons with velocardiofacial syndrome (VCFS) (Karayiorgou et al., 1995; Murphy, Jones, & Owens, 1999). VCFS is associated with small interstitial deletions on chromosome 22q11. Murphy and colleagues (1999) reported that 12 of 50 persons with VCFS met DSM-IV criteria for schizophrenia.

Another developmental disorder associated with risk of psychosis is Prader–Willi syndrome (Vogels et al., 2004). Characteristic features are neonatal hypotonia and developmental delay, hypogonadism, cognitive abnormalities, and dysmorphia of the face, body, and extremities. Hyperphagia and obesity begin later in childhood. Behavioral problems also begin in childhood, and psychosis emerges in young adulthood in approximately 5–10% of patients (Cassidy, 1997). The onset of psychotic symptoms in persons with Prader–Willi syndrome is typically before age 21 and often follows a period of psychosocial stress. Delusions, hallucinations, anxiety and agitation, bizarre behavior, affective disturbance, and mental anguish are among the described symptoms (Vogels et al., 2004).

Persons with schizophrenia and those with ID might also share other nongenetic risk factors, for example, obstetrical complications (O'Dwyer, 1997) or acquired brain disease of other types.

Brain injury in childhood from trauma also causes cognitive disability. Traumatic brain injury has also been implicated as a synergistic risk factor for development of schizophrenia-like psychosis in individuals whose family pedigrees carry elevated risk for schizophrenia (Malaspina et al., 2001). Nutritional deficiencies, lead poisoning, and sociocultural factors, such as severe neglect or abuse, are additional causes of brain dysfunction in children. ID occurs 1.5 times more frequently in males than in females. Currently, biological causes can be determined for only about one-fourth of individuals. Most cases are of idiopathic etiology.

UNDERSTANDING PSYCHIATRIC ILLNESS IN PERSONS WITH ID

ID and psychiatric illness are not mutually exclusive. Instead, the opposite is true. In 1990, the American Psychiatric Association Committee on Psychiatric Services for Persons with Mental Retardation and Developmental Disabilities estimated that 40–70% of individuals with MR have psychiatric disorders that meet established diagnostic criteria.

More recent studies suggest that the prevalence of psychiatric disorders in the ID population is three to five times higher than that in the non-ID population (Linna et al., 1999). Attention deficit disorder, affective disorders, and pervasive developmental disorder are most commonly seen. The presentation of these disorders, however, can be altered in an individual with ID. Our experience is that depression is underdiagnosed, and that atypical features, especially in more severely impaired groups, often confound the presentation.

Schizophrenia and schizophrenia-like syndromes occur in 2–5% of individuals with ID, but these disorders may account for a much higher percentage of persons with ID who are admitted to psychiatric hospitals. Signs and symptoms of schizophrenia may be more intense in persons with ID than in persons without ID. This may be especially true for negative symptoms and functional decline (Bouras et al., 2004).

When evaluating and treating individuals with ID and behavioral or psychiatric disorders, some important historical sociopolitical factors should be considered. Separate systems of care have often existed for persons with intellectual disabilities and for those with psychiatric disabilities. Lack of collaboration and cooperation between these care systems precludes good care.

Different ideas about the causes of psychiatric illness have played a role in this history. When unconscious psychological conflicts about repressed sexual urges were widely regarded as the cause of most psychiatric illness, many believed that individuals with ID could not develop psychiatric illness, because they lacked the necessary intellectual substrate to develop such psychological conflicts. In this view, all challenging behaviors were characterized as "behavioral" phenomena. These behavioral disturbances were directly attributed to MR. The idea that some of the behaviors might be driven by psychiatric illness had no credibility.

At the other end of the spectrum, the deterioration involved in warehousing and institutionalizing massive numbers of persons with ID in asylums, training schools, and other state facilities with substandard care led to a backlash against the perceived "medical model." A belief evolved that these individuals were not ill. They were not disabled; rather, they were "differently-abled."

The focus of care then turned to community-based models incorporating the principles of normalization, inclusion, and personal choice. Great effort in this care model is devoted to developing a psychosocial environment for the individual that enhances successful adaptation to the world.

Community-based systems have often gone to great lengths to avoid "labeling" individuals with psychiatric diagnoses. They have correspondingly discounted the contribution that rational psychopharmacological management might make in reducing the frequency and intensity of behavioral symptoms. We strongly hold that a combination of community-based models of support and informed neuropsychiatric intervention is a potent therapeutic force. We also recognize that the evaluation, accurate diagnosis, and effective treatment of psychiatric disorders, such as schizophrenia, in persons with ID can be difficult.

Understanding factors that contribute to this difficulty is helpful. Some behavior clusters are so common that they are considered "normal" in many individuals with ID. Diagnostic problems then arise. In some persons with ID, complicating factors include a baseline of psychosis-like behaviors, such as audible self-talk, imaginary friends, and obsessively overvalued ideas.

Where, for example, along a clinical continuum does fondness for routine become obsessive–compulsive disorder (Bodfish et al., 1995)? When does talking to oneself or to imaginary friends become an indicator of psychotic illness? When do overvalued ideas become delusions? We find several indicators helpful in predicting a response to antipsychotic medications: a recognized change in the frequency or intensity of these otherwise possibly normal behaviors; an increase in the frequency or intensity of unpredictable aggression related to these behaviors; or consistent, paranoia-like misinterpretation of events in the immediate environment. Faced with similar challenges, Sovner (1986; Lowry & Sovner, 1991) suggested that four underlying issues common to persons with ID should be considered when formulating a differential diagnosis of psychiatric illness.

- *Intellectual distortion.* This term refers to difficulty in describing emotional symptoms by some persons with ID because of cognitive limitations and insufficient vocabulary or comprehension.

- *Psychosocial masking.* This term refers to how experience affects the pathological meaning of a symptom. For example, for an individual with moderate ID, a belief that he or she can drive a car might represent a grandiose delusion.
- *Cognitive disintegration.* This term refers to a phenomenon in which limited coping skills result in significant behavioral decompensation or symptom emergence in response to relatively minor stress. Such decompensation might not result in symptoms that rise to the level of an Axis I diagnosis.
- *Baseline exaggeration.* This term refers to a tendency to observe an increase in the frequency and severity of chronic symptoms in association with a comorbid psychiatric disorder. The diagnosis may be missed, unless one asks whether the frequency and intensity of these behaviors are new or long-standing.

We consider several additional factors to be important.

- *Mixed and fluctuating symptom pictures.* In our experience, some individuals have a mixed and fluctuating symptom picture that requires a longer observational time to clarify baseline primary behaviors, and their link to psychiatric and environmental triggers.
- *Mixed cognitive deficits.* The presence of deficits in memory, attention, speech and language, and executive functions can make obtaining an accurate history difficult. Placing events and symptoms in proper time sequence, or determining the consistency and intensity of symptoms over time, may be a challenge. This issue highlights the importance of involving family caregivers and other providers or knowledgeable individuals in obtaining a history. Problems in speech and language function can involve both propositional components (i.e., content, and prosodic components such as melody, amplitude, and voice pitch). Such speech and language deficits can make matching affect and content a challenge. Depending also on the degree of intellectual impairment present, perseverative thinking or speech, or a limited repertoire of responses, can create problems of understanding. Persons with this problem may be limited to a few "play loops," which they repeat over and over again, so that the examiner must learn to interpret the meaning of subtle changes in tone, pitch, and amplitude.
- *Filter effects of CNS injury.* Many individuals with ID have other neurological deficits in sensory or motor domains, or in other domains, through which the psychopathology must be expressed, and by which the presentation will be variably altered. For example, consider how depression presents in someone who is nonverbal, how manic hyperactivity presents in someone with quadriplegia, or how hallucinations and delusions present in someone with minimal speech and language function. As a general rule, the milder the cognitive impairment, the more classic the DSM-IV-TR symptom profile, apropos of a particular psychiatric diagnosis. The more severe the cognitive impairment, the more one must rely on the existence of putative risk factors for a given illness, such as schizophrenia, or on other indicators, such as disturbances in sleep, appetite, or overall activity level.

ASSESSMENT OF PSYCHOSIS IN PERSONS WITH ID

When the question is whether a person with ID has a psychosis, circumspect clinical evaluation is essential. Careful assessment begins with obtaining as much historical information as possible. This history includes family history, especially concerning any family members who have neurological or psychiatric illness. Obstetrical and perinatal histories are important, as is an account of success or failure in meeting developmental milestones at appropriate ages. Behavioral problems that emerged during childhood development need close attention. Social and educational histories help to complete the developmental picture. The evaluator should inquire specifically about any history of previous psychiatric symptoms.

Physical examination, with an emphasis on the neurological exam and a careful mental status exam, complement and enhance the understanding gained from the comprehensive history. The initial evaluation of most individuals should include a general laboratory screen, such as complete blood count (CBC), urinalysis, and a metabolic panel. Genetic tests may be indicated depending on the history and on recognized signs and symptoms. We strongly emphasize attention to general medical health, especially for persons with severe disability who are not able to orally communicate symptoms or distress effectively. Medical illness can cause CNS dysfunction that results in delirium with psychotic symptoms. Signs and symptoms of medical illness can also mimic psychosis. One patient, who was incapable of speech, was referred to our care and was thought to have a psychosis that resulted in physical agitation, nonstop yelling, and obvious emotional distress. The etiology of this syndrome proved to be a severe deglutition disorder that resulted in most of his oral intake going into his lungs. The entire syndrome was cured by an appropriate surgical procedure.

A psychologically informed analysis of behavioral function, combined with neuropsychological assessment, almost always yields important data. For individuals with acute psychotic illness, this specialized neuropsychological testing can be deferred until after initial treatment and stabilization.

Electroencephalography (EEG) can give useful information about cerebral function but does not usually open an avenue to treatment of schizophrenia unless epileptic dysrhythmia is present. Brain imaging is indicated for many individuals, especially those having their initial assessment. We generally favor magnetic resonance imaging (MRI) over computed tomography (CT) because of the larger amount of anatomical information obtained.

TREATMENT OF SCHIZOPHRENIA IN PERSONS WITH ID

There are few evidence-based reports in the form of controlled, randomized drug trials concerning pharmacotherapy for schizophrenia in the context of ID. In 1999, Duggan and Brylewski conducted an extensive computer literature search for evidence of efficacy for any antipsychotic drug in treatment of people with a dual diagnosis of schizophrenia and ID. They found "no trial evidence to guide the use of antipsychotic medication for those with both intellectual disability and schizophrenia" (p. 94).

Our MEDLINE search found one other study, which compared risperidone and placebo in a study involving 118 children with ID and severe behavioral disturbance. The risperidone group showed significantly greater improvement than did the placebo group (Aman, DeSmedt, Derivan, Lyons, & Findling, 2002). This report pertained only to children, not to adults.

How do we treat schizophrenia in persons with ID? We use a combination of pharmacotherapy and psychosocial therapy, which represents the two main lines of thinking about the causes and treatment of psychiatric illness over the past 200 years. Neither approach can or should be neglected in 2008. Both aspects of treatment will continue to be needed for the foreseeable future. We do not yet have a cure for schizophrenia.

Pharmacotherapy for schizophrenia in persons with ID does not fundamentally differ from treatment of schizophrenia in nondisabled persons. Except in emergencies, we usually proceed in a manner that is initially cautious and conservative. This is similar in principle to an approach one would use in geriatric psychiatry. The main point is to start with single agents in low doses, followed by slow up-titration of dosage, with sufficient time between dose changes to observe both positive and negative effects. We recommend beginning with single agents and using augmentation strategies, or adding more drugs only when monotherapy clearly has failed.

We usually begin with a low dose of one of the currently available "atypical" antipsychotic drugs, advancing the daily dose in an "as tolerated" manner, depending on positive or negative aspects of the clinical response. We normally increase the dose about once a week. Measuring drug levels may be helpful if there is a question of compliance, or of suspected unusual absorption or metabolism of the drug.

If a positive clinical response is absent or insufficient after about 4–5 weeks, we usually consider a similar trial of another "atypical" antipsychotic. If this second trial does not meet clinical expectations, we might consider trying either two "atypicals" in combination or adding a "typical" drug, such as haloperidol or perphenazine, to the most recent "atypical." We usually pursue a particular regimen for about 1 month before changing or adding a drug.

After two or three unsuccessful drug treatment trials, we consider clozapine. Some case report data suggest that clozapine is a reasonably safe and efficacious drug for persons with ID and symptoms of schizophrenia or schizoaffective disorder (Thalayasingam, Alexander, & Singh, 2004). We also begin with a low dosage of this drug, usually 12.5 mg per day. We usually cross-taper clozapine with the previous drug. One should be aware that selective serotonin reuptake inhibitors (SSRIs), especially fluvoxamine, increase clozapine serum levels.

Long-acting "depot" antipsychotic drug formulations, such as long-acting risperidone, may be considered if there is a significant compliance problem. This has seldom been an issue in our practice, probably because most of our patients have caregivers who can administer oral drugs.

Because a straightforward diagnosis of schizophrenia is frequently not possible in persons with more severe forms of ID, empirical treatment is sometimes necessary. In these more obscure situations, empirical pharmacotherapy based on a dominant symptom or symptom complex should be considered. Our experience and opinion is that the more severe, disruptive, and dangerous the behavior, the stronger the indication for empirical drug treatment trials. Careful analysis of likely risks and benefits is important, but it makes little sense to withhold a trial of rational pharmacotherapy in the face of persistent dangerous or severely disruptive behavior. Most modern antipsychotic drugs have favorable risk–benefit profiles, so their careful use is ethical in these situations.

Although polypharmacy should be avoided in favor of treatment with a single drug whenever possible, complicated neuropsychiatric disorders, including schizophrenia, sometimes require use of combinations of drugs. Tracking target signs and symptoms, so that improvement or worsening can be recognized, is an important treatment tool. Keen awareness of possible drug interactions and adverse drug effects is essential for rational and successful pharmacotherapy. We advise and attempt to use the least number of drugs in the lowest doses necessary to achieve the desired therapeutic result.

Discontinuing drugs that are causing either dangerous or distressing side effects is important. Also, once it is clear that a drug is ineffective, it should also be stopped, even if there is no evident toxicity. Doing so helps to avoid *creeping polypharmacy*, an insidious process in which individuals accrete ever-increasing numbers of unnecessary drugs. This process typically occurs when recurrent behavioral disturbances lead to new prescriptions, while the previous regimen is uncritically maintained.

Indefinitely continuing an initially beneficial drug regimen might not always be a good idea. Our experience is that beneficial drug effects do not necessarily persist over time. Sometimes the good effects appear to "wear off" for unclear reasons. In such instances, prudence suggests trying another antipsychotic drug in the same class, but if this fails, trying a less similar drug would be indicated. Augmentation with mood-stabilizing drugs can also help in some cases, especially if the illness has a strong affective component. Anytime treatment is not working well is a good time to reconsider the accuracy of the working diagnosis.

Another point is that neurobehavioral syndromes, which are etiologically multifactorial, can change for the better over time. Reasons for such change can be hard to identify. With careful consideration of individual cases, gradual tapering and discontinuation of drugs, one at a time, should be considered when a particular regimen has existed for many years. This is especially true if signs and symptoms also have been in substantial remission for many years. When this is the case, we recommend careful consideration of the risks and benefits of continuing antipsychotic drug treatment with fully informed consent of the individual patient, or the guardian or other surrogate medical decision maker, or both. Such a review should occur at least annually.

Literature about use of electroconvulsive therapy (ECT) in the treatment of psychiatric disorders in persons with ID is not extensive. Concerns about ECT for treatment of persons with ID and severe comorbid psychiatric illness include the fear that ECT will cause additional cognitive impairment plus quite legitimate concern about ethical treatment of persons with impaired capacity for medical decision making.

A modest case report literature describes the use of ECT in persons with ID and severe psychiatric illness, including those with psychotic signs and symptoms such as schizophrenia and schizoaffective disorder (Thuppal & Fink, 1999). The consensus of this case report literature is that ECT is a safe and effective treatment for persons with ID and psychiatric illnesses or syndromes for which ECT is indicated. Clinicians should bear in mind that there is not a comparable series of reported negative results of ECT use in persons with ID, but this does not mean that inefficacy or adverse results have not occurred.

Our view is that ECT should be considered for individuals with ID and psychiatric disorders, including signs and symptoms of schizophrenia, that are very severe and very refractory to vigorous pharmacotherapy. Affective syndromes may be more responsive. A careful analysis of likely benefits and risks is essential. Beneficent family members or guardians must provide effective advocacy and surrogate decision making in most instances. The exact extent and form of this help depends on the degree of ID, legal requirements in the relevant jurisdiction, and the clinical situation.

Psychosocial support and treatment are important for persons with schizophrenia and for their families. This is no less true when the ill person also has ID or a neuropsychiatric disorder. Treatment of this type should be tailored to the abilities and needs of the individual, and to his or her overall progress in recovery. Helpful treatment might take the form of individual or group supportive psychotherapy; recreational, occupational, art, or music therapy; or vocational training or supported employment.

WORKING WITH GUARDIANS

Caring for persons with ID and other neuropsychiatric disorders often involves working with a guardian. Guardians may be family members, public guardians, or other individuals. Our overall experience in working with guardians has been positive. Most guardians take their work on behalf of their ward seriously and have a strong moral commitment to his or her welfare. Ethical principles for the practitioner caring for individuals with neuropsychiatric disorders who have guardians are with fundamentally the same as those for any person. Fully informing guardians of possible risks and benefits of proposed treatments enables guardians to do their work well.

Many persons who are judged to be incapacitated and have guardians appointed by a court still possess a degree of clinical capacity; that is, they can understand significant information about their condition and about proposed treatment. They should also be informed about treatment choices or proposals on a level consonant with their ability to comprehend, and when possible, their agreement with planned treatment or tests should also be sought.

KEY POINTS

- Schizophrenia occurs in conjunction with ID.
- Psychosis with schizophrenia-like features also occurs in association with other neuropsychiatric disorders such as Alzheimer's disease, Parkinson's disease, Huntington's disease, epilepsy, and traumatic brain injury.
- Recognition of signs and symptoms, and therefore diagnosis, may be difficult in persons with neuropsychiatric disorders or ID, because signs and symptoms may appear in atypical fashion, or be obscured or altered by impaired cognition or impaired speech and language function.
- Even so, careful attention to accurate diagnosis matters. Not diagnosing schizophrenia when it exists results in dangerous undertreatment. Overdiagnosis and overtreatment are also harmful, for example, by causing long-term exposure to antipsychotic medicines and their possible hazards without commensurate benefit.
- The pharmacological treatment of schizophrenia in persons with ID or other neuropsychiatric disorders is similar to treatment of persons without such conditions, except that extra care is required.
- The long-term prognosis of schizophrenia in persons with concomitant neuropsychiatric disorders is unknown. Lifelong treatment may be needed, but prudence indicates a treatment review at least annually, using clinical judgment to confirm efficacy and a positive benefit-to-risk assessment.

REFERENCES AND RECOMMENDED READINGS

Aman, M., DeSmedt, G., Derivan, A., Lyons, B., & Findling, R. (2002). Double-blind, placebo-controlled study of risperidone for the treatment of disruptive behaviors in children with subaverage intelligence. *American Journal of Psychiatry, 159*(8), 1337–1346.

American Psychiatric Association. (2000). *Diagnostic and statistical manual of mental disorders* (4th ed., text rev.). Washington, DC: Author.

American Psychiatric Association Committee. (1990). *APA Committee on Psychiatric Services for Persons with Mental Retardation and Developmental Disabilities: Task force report: Psychiatric disorders in the developmentally disabled.* Washington, DC: Author.

Bodfish, J., Crawford, T., Powell, S., Parker, D., Golden, R., & Lewis, M. (1995). Compulsions in adults with mental retardation: Prevalence, phenomenology, and comorbidity with stereotypy and self-injury. *American Journal of Mental Retardation, 100*(2), 183–192.

Bouras, N., Martin, G., Leese, M., Vanstraelen, M., Holt, G., Thomas, C., et al. (2004). Schizophrenia-spectrum psychoses in people with and without intellectual disability. *Journal of Intellectual Disability Research, 48*(6), 548–555.

Cassidy, S. B. (1997). Prader–Willi syndrome. *Journal of Medical Genetics, 34*, 917–923.

Duggan, L., & Brylewski, J. (1999). Effectiveness of antipsychotic medication in people with intellectual disability and schizophrenia: A systematic review. *Journal of Intellectual Disability Research, 43*(2), 94–104.

Karayiorgou, M., Morris, M. A., Morrow, B., Shprintzer, R. J., Goldberg, R., Borrow, J., et al. (1995). Schizophrenia susceptibility associated with interstitial deletions of chromosome 22q11. *Proceedings of the National Academy of Sciences, USA, 92,* 7612–7616.

Linna, S. L., Moilanen, I., Ebeling, H., Piha, J., Kumpulamen, K., Tamminen, T., et al. (1999). Psychiatric symptoms in children with intellectual disability. *European Child and Adolescent Psychiatry, 8*(Suppl. 4), 77–82.

Lowry, M., & Sovner, R. (1991). The functional existence of problem behavior: A key to effective treatment. *Habilitative Mental Health Care Newsletter, 10,* 59–63.

Malaspina, D., Goetz, R. R., Friedman, J. H., Kaufmann, C. A., Faraone, S. V., Tsuang, M., et al. (2001). Traumatic brain injury and schizophrenia in members of schizophrenia and bipolar disorder pedigrees. *American Journal of Psychiatry, 158*(3), 440–446.

Murphy, K. C., Jones, L. A., & Owen, M. J. (1999). High rates of schizophrenia in adults with velo-cardio-facial syndrome. *Archives of General Psychiatry, 56*(10), 940–945.

O'Dwyer, J. M. (1997). Schizophrenia in people with intellectual disability: The role of pregnancy and birth complications. *Journal of Intellectual Disability Research, 41*(3), 238–251.

Sovner, R. (1986). Limiting factors in the use of DSM-III criteria with mentally ill/mentally retarded persons. *Psychopharmacology Bulletin, 22*(4), 1055–1059.

Thalayasingam, S., Alexander, R. T., & Singh, I. (2004). The use of clozapine in adults with intellectual disability. *Journal of Intellectual Disability Research, 48*(6), 572–579.

Thuppal, M., & Fink, M. (1999). Electroconvulsive therapy and mental retardation. *Journal of ECT, 15*(2), 140–149.

Turner, T. (1989). Schizophrenia and mental handicap: An historical review, with implications for further research. *Psychological Medicine, 19*(2), 301–314.

Vogels, A., De Hert, M., Descheemaeker, M. J., Govers, V., Devriendt, K., Legius, E., et al. (2004). Psychotic disorders in Prader–Willi syndrome. *American Journal of Medical Genetics, 127*(3), 238–243.

CHAPTER 43

TRAUMA AND POSTTRAUMATIC STRESS SYNDROMES

STANLEY D. ROSENBERG
KIM T. MUESER

NATURE OF THE SPECIAL POPULATION

In the wake of 9/11 and Hurricane Katrina, mental health providers and the general public have become increasingly aware of the emotional and psychiatric consequences of exposure to traumatic events—consequences that can persist for many years after the trauma. It is important that providers who work with clients with schizophrenia also be aware of the presentation of posttraumatic stress syndromes and their treatment. What we have discovered in recent years is that trauma exposure is close to universal in clients with schizophrenia and other severe mental illnesses, and multiple traumatization over the lifespan is the rule rather than the exception in this population. For example, studies of the prevalence of interpersonal trauma in women with severe mental illness indicate especially high exposure to violent victimization (a particularly toxic form of trauma), with rates ranging as high as 77–97% for episodically homeless women.

Approximately one-third of all clients with schizophrenia spectrum disorders enrolled in treatment services also meet diagnostic criteria for current posttraumatic stress disorder (PTSD), making it perhaps the most common psychiatric comorbidity in this group. Moreover, trauma exposure and PTSD in clients with schizophrenia spectrum diagnoses are associated with more severe symptoms, substance abuse, higher service utilization (including medical and psychiatric hospitalizations), increased medical problems, overall distress, and increased high-risk behaviors.

Why do we see so much trauma and trauma-related impairment in clients with schizophrenia and other severe mental illnesses? Several models have been put forth to account for these relationships. First, because there is abundant evidence that stress can precipitate psychotic episodes, negative life events have long been thought to act as stressors that contribute to an underlying vulnerability to psychotic symptoms. Second, schizophrenia and severe mental illness generally may increase the likelihood of trauma exposure through associated correlates such as homelessness and substance abuse. Third, a preexisting psychiatric disorder may increase vulnerability to the emergence or chronicity of posttraumatic symptoms following exposure. Research to date supports the likely contribution of these, and other possible mechanisms, linking trauma exposure, schizophrenia, and PTSD.

Several other contributory factors have also been hypothesized. For example, psychosis and associated treatment experiences (e.g., involuntary commitment) may themselves represent DSM-IV-TR Criterion A traumas. The potential symptom overlap between schizophrenia and PTSD (e.g., flashbacks being misinterpreted as hallucinations; extreme avoidance and anhedonia interpreted as negative symptoms), may conflate the apparent rates of PTSD in those diagnostic groups. Alternatively, PTSD associated with psychotic symptoms may be misdiagnosed as a primary psychotic disorder.

Clients and advocacy groups often point to posttraumatic symptoms as among the most troubling of these individuals' life problems, and many U.S. states have prioritized the development of "trauma-sensitive services" as a key reform to mental health and substance abuse service systems. Major elements of trauma-sensitive services include (1) increased awareness by providers about trauma history and sequelae among clients; (2) better understanding of special requirements of survivors; and (3) knowledge of trauma-specific interventions for persons requiring such services. We discuss these three topics in this chapter, and provide tools and useful references to increase mental health providers' knowledge and competence in regard to trauma-related issues. Posttraumatic stress disorders are among the most treatable of psychiatric syndromes, and it is important to recognize and treat PTSD symptoms in clients with schizophrenia.

DEFINITIONS

Psychological *trauma* refers to the experience of an uncontrollable event perceived to threaten a person's sense of integrity or survival. A *traumatic event* is defined by DSM-IV-TR as an event involving direct threat of death, severe bodily harm, or psychological injury, which the person at the time finds intensely distressing (i.e., the person experiences intense fear, helplessness, or horror). Common traumatic experiences include sexual and physical assault, combat exposure, and the unexpected death of a loved one. Negative psychiatric and health outcomes are associated with the total number of exposures to traumatic events and with their intensity. Sexual assault and other forms of interpersonal violence in which the victim suffers actual physical harm, along with childhood sexual abuse, represent the forms of trauma most likely to lead to persistent psychiatric disorders, including PTSD. PTSD is defined by three types of symptoms: (1) *reexperiencing the trauma*; (2) *avoidance of trauma-related stimuli*; and (3) *overarousal*. These symptoms must be related to the index trauma and persist, or develop at least 1 month after exposure to that trauma. Examples of reexperiencing include intrusive, unwanted memories of the event, nightmares, flashbacks, and distress when exposed to reminders of the traumatic event (e.g., being in the vicinity of the traumatic event, meeting someone with similarities to the perpetrator). Avoidance symptoms include efforts to avoid thoughts, feelings, or activities related to the trauma; inability to recall important aspects of the traumatic event; diminished interest in significant activities; detachment; restricted affect; and a foreshortened sense of one's own future. Overarousal symptoms include hypervigilance, exaggerated startle response, difficulty falling or staying asleep, difficulty concentrating, and irritability or angry outbursts. DSM-IV-TR criteria require that a person must have at least one intrusive, three avoidant, and two arousal symptoms to be diagnosed with PTSD.

How do clients with both schizophrenia and PTSD present differently from those with schizophrenia alone? First, it is important to recognize that most of these clients do not spontaneously talk about their trauma experiences and related symptoms. Clinicians generally believe that they know their client well enough to be aware when a particular client has experienced a very adverse event. Thus, providers are often surprised when they systematically inquire about trauma history in clients they have know for years, and learn for the first time about traumatic events clients have experienced. The reality is that a central feature of PTSD is avoidance. The last thing that most trauma survivors are likely to do is to discuss spontaneously or describe past traumatic events, or associated problems such as nightmares and avoidance (e.g., fear of going back to a setting where a sexual assault occurred). Because clients with PTSD tend to appear more fearful, avoidant, and distrustful of others, they are more difficult to engage. On average, they are more likely to abuse substances (often to avoid memories of their traumatic experiences), to experience revictimization, and to be assaultive toward others, including providers. In general, clients with PTSD tend to be more impaired, low function, and symptomatic than individuals without PTSD.

For example, one client reported believing that others could see into his mind, and he frequently heard persecutory voices when he was out in public, which made him very wary of leaving his house. Only when he was assessed for PTSD symptoms did his providers become aware that the voices referred both to childhood incidents of being sexually abused and his own subsequent abuse of other, younger children. He believed that people on the street knew about his past actions and were highly critical of him. The voices were a form of expressing guilt and shame (common among abuse survivors), and of reexperiencing the trauma. What was somewhat unusual in terms of PTSD (although not unknown in severe cases) was that this client utilized psychotic mechanisms to express these symptoms and associated distorted cognitions. However, once he was treated for PTSD, the voices essentially disappeared, and the client became less psychotic. Another client frequently relapsed into substance abuse when exposed to reminders of her past trauma (so-called "triggers"). These slips also tended to lead to more general decreases in her ability to function independently, including unstable housing, inability to hold a job, and frequent rehospitalizations. Treatment for PTSD helped this client develop alternative strategies to alcohol use in response to trauma-related stressors, and a period of relative stability followed. The trauma-related problems described in these clients represent either the primary or associated symptoms of PTSD. An understanding of this disorder is crucial to clinicians' ability to recognize the behaviors, attitudes, and symptoms that people with schizophrenia and PTSD present.

POSTTRAUMATIC STRESS SYNDROMES: THE EVOLUTION OF THE CONCEPT

Recognition of the psychiatric complications associated with extreme forms of trauma exposure has a long history, dating back at least to the U.S. Civil War. In the last half of the 19th century, the concept of Da Costa syndrome, or irritable heart, appeared in the medical literature. Seen first in combat veterans, it was characterized by anxiety (fearfulness, chest pain mimicking heart attack), extreme fatigue, and arousal symptoms (palpitations, sweating). By the end of the 19th century, Breuer and Freud had recognized and described the role of trauma in various neurotic disorders, particularly so-called "hysteria," and Freud continued for many years to theorize about the role of traumatic events in personality formation and disruption of functioning. Throughout the 20th century, posttraumatic reactions were recognized in psychiatry and military medicine, and generally conceptualized under various labels that suggested organic etiologies (e.g., "shell shock" in World War I, and "combat fatigue" in World War II). Psychiatry has also long recognized that civilian traumas (e.g., dramatic changes in life circumstances; car accidents) can produce similar emotional reactions.

In more recent years, the psychological and psychophysiological components of posttraumatic disorders have been better characterized through empirical studies, and the affective, cognitive, and interpersonal alterations associated with trauma exposure have been extensively researched and described in the literature. Neuroimaging techniques have more recently allowed the field to examine the neurobiological alterations in persons who develop PTSD, including hippocampal changes (atrophy) and alterations in amygdala function. Both lines of research have been associated with advances in treating PTSD. A variety of psychotherapeutic interventions (primarily based on cognitive-behavioral techniques) have become well established through multiple clinical trials, and effective treatments are available for a variety of trauma populations, including children, combat veterans, sexual assault survivors, and women who experienced abuse in childhood. Biological treatments, which build on the similarities between the neurobiology of PTSD and depression, have also shown utility in reducing symptoms. Systematic reviews of these treatments and their relative efficacy are available (see References and Recommended Readings). However, until very recently, no proven treatments for clients with both schizophrenia spectrum disorders and PTSD have been available. Several clinical research groups are now actively addressing this gap in services, and promising treatment models are described below.

TRAUMA, SCHIZOPHRENIA, AND PTSD

Unfortunately, until the last decade, theory and practice regarding severe mental illnesses, such as schizophrenia, and posttraumatic stress syndromes were quite separate and distinct. Much of the seminal work on trauma-related psychiatric disorders focused on combat-related stress responses, and scant research—and almost no treatment models in the field—explicitly considered the intersection of trauma-related disorders with other major DSM Axis I disorders. Following the inclusion of PTSD as a diagnosis in DSM-III, research on trauma-related disorders accelerated. The field became increasingly aware that many forms of civilian trauma exposure, including childhood physical and sexual abuse, are not only common events but also are frequently comorbid and possible contributory factors in a variety of other psychiatric disorders. Exposure to traumatic events in general population studies is associated with increased psychiatric morbidity, substance abuse, increased medical utilization, and generally poor health and functional outcomes. These relationships are often mediated by PTSD.

TRAUMA EXPOSURE AND SCHIZOPHRENIA

Limited systematic research has investigated trauma exposure in clients with schizophrenia spectrum disorders. Most studies have looked at the broader category of *severe mental illness* (typically including both schizophrenia spectrum and bipolar disorders, and chronic and disabling major depression). These studies have reported overwhelmingly high levels of trauma exposure, both prior to illness onset and throughout the course of illness. In those few studies looking specifically at clients with schizophrenia, the same relationships are evident. For example, in a recently completed study of adverse childhood events in a large sample of clients with schizophrenia receiving public mental health services (Rosenberg, Lu, Mueser, Jankowski, & Cournos, 2007), rates of childhood physical abuse were much higher than those found in the National Comorbidity Study: 56.4% abused versus 3.3% in the general population. Sexual abuse in childhood (33.6 versus 10.1%) was also elevated in the schizophrenia sample.

These rates are consistent with the larger set of studies looking at the combined group of people with severe mental illness. These studies report almost universal (e.g., 98%) exposure to any or all types of trauma over the lifetime. Although there are many types of civilian trauma, the most common of which is the sudden, unexpected death of a loved one, 87% of clients report more severe and less common traumas, including either physical or sexual assault in childhood, in adulthood, or in both. Indeed, more than one-third of clients living in the community report either physical or sexual assault in the last year alone. By all accounts, being a person with schizophrenia or other severe mental illness is generally a frightening and dangerous way to live, at least in the United States. Often confined to low-income urban areas, likely to be intermittently homeless and incarcerated, sometimes forced by circumstance into sex trading, and disproportionately likely to abuse drugs in unsafe places such as crack houses, clients live in the most dangerous spaces in a society where violence is rather common. In addition, it seems likely that these clients' common isolation and vulnerability make them likely targets of opportunity for predators in such environments.

CORRELATES OF TRAUMA EXPOSURE

What happens to people following exposure to extreme, life-threatening events? For many people, the hours and days following exposure are filled with anxiety, agitation, and distress. Clients may feel emotionally numb, lose focus on the immediate environment, and feel as if they or events are "unreal" or "in a daze." They may be unable to stop thinking about the events, even though thinking about them is highly distressing. People in the United States as a whole had at least an indirect experience of these symptoms following 9/11, when, for example, people were horrified by the television footage of the Twin Towers but could not help ruminating about the event. People found themselves unable to concentrate on work or school. Some reported watching the news replays over and over; others tried to avoid any news or mention of the attack. When these reactions become clinically significant and last for more than 2 days, they are called *acute stress disorder*. For an unfortunately high percentage of trauma survivors, acute stress disorder persists beyond 30 days, and progresses to PTSD. Other people exposed to trauma may not meet criteria for acute stress disorder, but have instead delayed response to the events and develop symptoms later. In either sequence, PTSD is the most common and directly attributable psychiatric disorder to develop following trauma exposure, although depression and substance use disorders may also ensue, with or without diagnosable PTSD symptoms.

The steps by which PTSD develops after a trauma exposure have been well documented. During and immediately following the event, the survivor experiences an intense emotional response, including fear, anxiety, grief, helplessness, and often a complex mixture of all of these. Memories of the event are associated with reexperiencing all of these emotions and, subsequently, elaborated emotions and ideas (e.g., guilt, sense of loss) as the person continues to process the implications of the trauma. Because these recollections are so emotionally charged and distressing, the person attempts to avoid memories or situations that are reminders of the trauma, which leads to further vigilance and avoidant behavior. In addition, some traumatic events are so overwhelming that survivors' assumptions about the world (e.g., "People are mostly OK") and themselves ("I know how to look out for danger as well as the next person") can be shattered. They may construct new cognitive frames or internal scripts that keep them locked in aspects of the traumatic moment (e.g., "I could be attacked at any moment" or "No one can be trusted").

The severity of the trauma, the number of traumas to which persons have been exposed in their lifetime, the nature of available social supports, and the quality known as psychological hardiness, or resilience, all influence the likelihood of developing PTSD following exposure, as well as the severity and chronicity of this disorder. All these factors seem to conspire to make people with schizophrenia highly vulnerable to developing chronic PTSD.

Recent estimates of lifetime prevalence of PTSD in the general population range between 8 and 12%, and the few available, community-based studies reporting point prevalence of PTSD (the number of people who meet diagnostic criteria on any given day) suggest rates of approximately 2%: 2.7% for women and 1.2% for men. Studies of clients with severe mental illness suggest much higher rates of PTSD. Seven studies have reported *current* rates of PTSD ranging between 29 and 43% (Mueser, Rosenberg, Goodman, & Trumbetta, 2002), yet PTSD, as discussed earlier, was rarely documented in clients' charts. In the few studies with samples large enough to assess PTSD in clients by diagnosis, clients with schizophrenia spectrum diagnoses had slightly lower rates (33%) than clients with mood disorders (45%), but rates in both groups were nevertheless much higher than those in the general population. Another study reported that among persons hospitalized for a first episode of psychosis, 17% met criteria for current PTSD. This study, in combination with the others, suggests that childhood trauma exposure and PTSD not only occur more often in persons who develop schizophrenia and other forms of severe mental illness, but that having severe mental illness also increases subsequent risk for trauma and PTSD. As in the general population, PTSD severity in clients with severe mental illness is related to severity of trauma exposure, and the high rates of PTSD in this population are consistent with clients' increased exposure to trauma. These rates also suggest an elevated risk for developing PTSD given exposure to a traumatic event. For example, in a sample of clients drawn from a large health maintenance organization, Breslau, Davis, Andreski, and Peterson (1991) reported that the prevalence of PTSD among those exposed to trauma was 24%. This rate of PTSD following trauma exposure is approximately half the rate (47%) found in studies of trauma and PTSD in persons with severe mental illness. The high PTSD rate in this population and its correlation with worse functioning suggests that PTSD may interact with the course of co-occurring severe mental illnesses, such as schizophrenia and major mood disorders, worsening the outcome of both disorders. We developed a model to help us understand how trauma and PTSD may interact with schizophrenia and other severe mental illnesses (see Figure 43.1).

TRAUMA, PTSD, AND THE COURSE OF SCHIZOPHRENIA

This model describes how PTSD directly and indirectly mediates the relationships among trauma, more severe psychiatric symptoms, and greater utilization of acute care services in clients with schizophrenia (Mueser et al., 2002). Specifically, we suggest that the symptoms of PTSD may *directly* worsen the severity of schizophrenia due to clients' *avoidance of trauma-related stimuli* (resulting in social isolation), *reexperiencing the trauma* (resulting

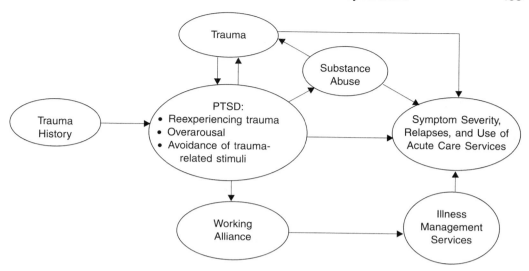

FIGURE 43.1. Heuristic model of how trauma and PTSD interact with schizophrenia to worsen the course of illness. From Mueser, Rosenberg, Goodman, and Trumbetta (2002). Copyright 2002 by Elsevier. Reprinted by permission.

in chronic stress), and *hyperarousal* (resulting in increased vulnerability to stress-induced relapses). In addition, the model suggests that common clinical correlates of PTSD might *indirectly* worsen schizophrenia, including increased *substance abuse* (leading to substance-induced relapses), *retraumatization* (leading to stress-induced relapses), and *poor working alliance* with case managers. It is important to treat PTSD in clients with schizophrenia to reduce the suffering related to the disorder, *and* because PTSD may exacerbate the course of schizophrenia, contributing to worse outcomes and greater utilization of costly services through a number of mechanisms.

PTSD AND SCHIZOPHRENIA

PTSD is frequently chronic, often ebbs and wanes in intensity, and is characterized by both clear biological changes and psychological symptoms. PTSD is also complicated by the fact that it frequently occurs in conjunction with related disorders, such as depression, substance abuse, problems of memory and cognition, and other physical and mental health problems. The disorder is also associated with impairment of the person's ability to function in social or family life, including occupational instability, marital problems and divorces, family discord, and difficulties in parenting. Given this cluster of primary and secondary symptoms, it is readily apparent how some PTSD symptoms might be overlooked in clients with schizophrenia, who frequently have problems in these life spheres. Possible symptom overlap may lead to masking of PTSD in clients with a primary psychotic disorder. For example, concentration and memory problems are common in schizophrenia, as are restricted or blunted affect and sleep difficulties associated either with the primary illness or with medication side effects. As with a client described earlier in this chapter, PTSD may be expressed in psychotic terms, or in psychotic distortion of actual traumatic events by clients with schizophrenia diagnoses. A client who was sexually abused in childhood might, for example, allude to this experience as being assaulted by the devil, expressing both confusion about the event and the common desire of children to protect the actual perpetrator, who might even be a primary caretaker. Whatever the sources of diagnostic ambiguity, including lack of provider awareness of trauma-related disorders and lack of standardized screening for clients, multiple studies have now reported that only about 5% of clients with severe mental illness and PTSD have the latter diagnosis even listed in their charts, and almost none currently receive trauma-specific treatment.

ASSESSMENT OF TRAUMA AND PTSD

Providers should be aware that there are simple, straightforward techniques for assessing trauma history and PTSD in clients with schizophrenia and other severe mental illnesses. Several studies, and much recent clinical experience, have now shown that clients respond reliably and coherently to straightforward questions about trauma exposure (both early and more recent), and can be assessed for PTSD symptoms with brief symptom inventories. These tests have been used successfully in paper-and-pencil format, as interviews, and in computerized formats. They generally take about 10 minutes to complete. Despite earlier concerns, these assessments rarely lead to increased distress (even in acutely ill clients), and are often appreciated by clients as indicators of provider concern about the issues that really trouble them, yet have not been a focus of traditional mental health care. One note of caution is worthy of mention: Providers who ask clients to participate in these assessments, or who conduct them, may be uncomfortable themselves with some of the topics covered (e.g., childhood sexual abuse or recent sexual assault experiences). When this is the case, the providers may need some information and supervision on how to conduct these assessments in a neutral, matter-of-fact, supportive way to ensure client comfort and accurate, open reporting.

We have discussed how clients with both schizophrenia and PTSD may differ from clients with schizophrenia alone. It is also important to observe that clients with both disorders tend to present with many of the same issues as people with so-called "complex PTSD," as described by Herman (1992) and others. Complex PTSD has been observed in people exposed to early or extreme stress, to neglect or abuse, and to multiple trauma experiences. In addition to the core symptoms of PTSD, which may be expressed in very intense form, complex PTSD involves dissociation, relationship difficulties, somatization, revictimization, affect dysregulation, and disruptions in sense of self. Experts have argued that people with complex PTSD are often diagnosed as having borderline personality disorder, and this sometimes appears as a secondary diagnosis in clients with schizophrenia who have extremely adverse life histories.

CURRENT TREATMENT APPROACHES

At this point in time, no published studies exist of treatment for clients with both schizophrenia and posttraumatic stress syndromes. To our knowledge, none of the drug trials for PTSD have included clients with schizophrenia or other psychotic disorders, so we do not discuss pharmacological treatments in this chapter. Instead, we describe several psychotherapeutic treatment models designed for the broader category of people with severe mental illness. The list is not comprehensive, but it is representative of what is being developed, assessed, and implemented in the field. Developmental work with these treatment models has included some (but not necessarily a majority) of clients with schizophrenia. Assessment of the treatment models has involved either open or randomized clinical trials of varying levels of rigor (e.g., uniform implementation; good characterization of clients served; use of well-validated, standard outcome measures).

Like trauma and PTSD treatments designed for the general population, these interventions have relied on a relatively small set of therapeutic ingredients, often combining with or employing somewhat different mixes and emphases. Common therapeutic elements include psychoeducation, stress management techniques, teaching strategies and resources to enhance personal safety, prolonged exposure to trauma-related stimuli (e.g., memories, safe but fear-eliciting situations), cognitive restructuring, group support, skills training, and empowerment. Of these elements, the empirical literature on PTSD treatment in the general population has shown that prolonged exposure and cognitive restructuring are the most effective treatments. Interventions designed for more vulnerable populations, including those with psychotic disorders, have used both group and individual formats (with some models combining the two), and intervention length has ranged from 12 weeks to 1 year or more. Some models have been developed specifically for women, particularly women survivors of sexual abuse, whereas other, more general models are for all types of trauma exposure (in either childhood or adulthood) leading to PTSD. Several models focus on PTSD per se, whereas others attempt to address a broader array of problems associated with chronic victimization. These models, and the level of evidence supporting them, are summarized in Table 43.1.

TREATMENT GUIDELINES

1. All clients with schizophrenia spectrum disorders should be assessed with standardized instruments for trauma exposure and for PTSD.

2. Providers working with these clients should be trained to understand posttraumatic stress syndromes, and to recognize their symptom presentation in schizophrenia.

3. Services for such clients should be trauma-aware (e.g., housing recommendations; gender of providers; guidelines for use of restraints for abused clients that factor in trauma-related issues).

4. Clients should receive psychoeducation about trauma and posttraumatic stress syndromes, including how to recognize PTSD symptoms, how PTSD might exacerbate psychotic illness, and what treatments might be available.

5. Trauma-specific treatments (with different levels of empirical support) are available and well described in the literature. Service systems that provide care for clients with schizophrenia should choose trauma interventions best suited for their clients and settings, and train staff in providing these treatments.

6. Providers should learn who in their area is able to provide trauma-specific treatments for clients with both schizophrenia and PTSD symptoms.

7. Given the high level of ongoing trauma in clients with schizophrenia, periodic reassessment for trauma exposure and PTSD should be part of standard care.

8. PTSD symptoms can persist over many years, and symptoms ebb and wane, often in response to external stressors. Providers should be aware that clients' PTSD may reemerge, and follow-up treatments or "booster" sessions may be required when clients undergo stress.

TABLE 43.1. Treatment Approaches for PTSD and Other Posttraumatic Syndromes in Persons with Schizophrenia and Other Severe Mental Illnesses

Intervention name (developer)	Target population	Format and length	Therapeutic elements	Level of evidence	Reference
Beyond Trauma (Covington)	Women abuse survivors	Both group (11 sessions) and individual and group (16–28 sessions)	Strengths-based approach; empowerment oriented	Pre–post trial under way (150 participants)	*Beyond Trauma Manual* (S. Covington; 858-454-8528)
Seeking Safety (Najavits)	Clients with substance abuse and PTSD or partial PTSD	25 topics (variable length); group and individual	Establish safety. Teaches 80 safe coping skills for relationships, substances, self-harm, etc.	Several RCTs; multiple open trials (none with identified SMI clients)	Najavits (2002)
Target (Ford)	Multiple-trauma-exposed populations	Group and individual versions; variable length, 3–26 sessions	Strengths-based; teaches symptom monitoring and self-regulatory skills, experiential exercises	Multiple open trials (none for SMI); one RCT completed for substance abuse population	*www.ptsdfreedom.org* for updates
Trauma Recovery and Empowerment (TREM; Harris)	Women trauma survivors	Group format, 24–33 sessions	Skills training, psychoeducation, peer support, elements of CBT	Multiple open trials, RCT under way (women with SMI)	Harris (1998)
CBT for PTSD among Public Sector Consumers (Frueh)	People with SMI and PTSD	Group (10–14) and individual (6–12) sessions	Anxiety management, exposure, coping and skills enhancement	Treatment development phase (open trial under way)	Frueh et al. (2004)
CBT for PTSD in SMI (Mueser, Rosenberg)	Clients with SMI and PTSD	Individual (12–16) sessions	Psychoeducation, relaxation	One open trial and one RCT completed	Mueser et al. (2004); Rosenberg et al. (2004)
Atrium (Miller & Guidry)	Abuse survivors with related problems (substance abuse, self-injury, violence, severe psychiatric disorders)	12-session individual, group, or peer-led program	Psychoeducation, relaxation, mindfulness, expressive modalities, elements of CBT	Participated in multisite, open trial (women and violence study)	*www.dustymiller.org*
Syndrome-Specific Group Therapy for Complex PTSD (Shelley & Munzenmeier)	People with complex PTSD and SMI	12 sessions, group intervention	Psychoeducation, skills training, and social support	Pilot data only	Syndrome-Specific Treatment Program for SMI Manual (Vols. I–VI) (*shelleybpc @aol.com*)

Note. CBT, cognitive-behavioral therapy; RCT, randomized controlled trial; SMI, severe mental illness.

KEY POINTS

- Trauma exposure is ubiquitous in clients with schizophrenia, as is PTSD, but trauma history and posttraumatic syndromes are rarely assessed and treated in this population.
- Trauma history and PTSD are associated with more severe symptoms (especially depression, anxiety, and psychosis), worse functioning, and a more severe course of illness in clients with schizophrenia.
- Reliable and valid evaluations of trauma exposure and PTSD can be obtained in clients with schizophrenia through the use of standardized assessment instruments, including interview, self-report, and computer-administered formats.
- The assessment of traumatic experiences and PTSD in schizophrenia rarely leads to symptom exacerbations or other untoward clinical effects.
- Treatment programs for trauma and PTSD in schizophrenia, based on effective interventions for posttraumatic syndromes in the general population, have recently been developed and are being evaluated.
- Preliminary experience with these treatment programs suggests that people with schizophrenia can be engaged and retained in treatment, and experience benefits from their participation.

REFERENCES AND RECOMMENDED READINGS

Blanchard, E. P., Jones-Alexander, J., Buckley, T. C., & Forneris, C. A. (1996). Psychometric properties of the PTSD Checklist. *Behavior Therapy, 34,* 669–673.

Breslau, N., Davis, G. C., Andreski, P., & Peterson, E. (1991). Traumatic events and posttraumatic stress disorder in an urban population of young adults. *Archives of General Psychiatry, 48,* 216–222.

Cusack, K. J., Frueh, B. C., & Brady, K. T. (2004). Trauma history screening in a community mental health center. *Psychiatric Services, 55,* 157–162.

Da Costa, J. M. (1871). On irritable heart: A clinical study of a form of functional cardiac disorder and its consequences. *American Journal of the Medical Sciences, 61,* 17–52.

Frueh, B. C., Buckley, T. C., Cusack, K. J., Kimble, M. O., Grubaugh, A. L., Turner, S. M., et al. (2004). Cognitive-behavioral treatment for PTSD among people with severe mental illness: A proposed treatment model. *Journal of Psychiatric Practice, 10,* 26–38.

Harris, M. (1998). *Trauma Recovery and Empowerment: A clinician's guide for working with women in groups.* New York: Free Press.

Harris, M., & Fallot, R. (Eds.). (2001). *New directions for mental health services: Using trauma theory to design service systems.* San Francisco: Jossey-Bass.

Herman, J. L. (1992). *Trauma and recovery.* New York: Basic Books.

Janoff-Bulman, R. (1992). *Shattered assumptions: Towards a new psychology of trauma.* New York: Free Press.

Mueser, K. T., Bolton, E. E., Carty, P. C., Bradley, M. J., Ahlgren, K. F., DiStaso, D. R., et al. (2007). The Trauma Recovery Group: A cognitive-behavioral program for PTSD in persons with severe mental illness. *Community Mental Health Journal, 43*(3), 281–304.

Mueser, K. T., Rosenberg, S. D., Goodman, L. A., & Trumbetta, S. L. (2002). Trauma, PTSD, and the course of schizophrenia: An interactive model. *Schizophrenia Research, 53,* 123–143.

Mueser, K. T., Rosenberg, S. D., Jankowski, M. K., Hamblen, J., & Descamps, M. (2004). A cognitive-behavioral treatment program for posttraumatic stress disorder in severe mental illness. *American Journal of Psychiatric Rehabilitation, 7,* 107–146.

Mueser, K. T., Salyers, M. P., Rosenberg, S. D., Ford, J. D., Fox, L., & Carty, P. (2001). A psychometric evaluation of trauma and PTSD assessments in persons with severe mental illness. *Psychological Assessment, 13,* 110–117.

Myers, A. B. R. (1870). *On the etiology and prevalence of diseases of the heart among soldiers.* London: Churchill.

Najavits, L. M. (2002). *Seeking safety: A treatment manual for PTSD and substance abuse.* New York: Guilford Press.

Pratt, S. I., Rosenberg, S. D., Mueser, K. T., Brancato, J., Salyers, M. P., Jankowski, M. K., et al. (2005). Evaluation of a PTSD psychoeducational program for psychiatric inpatients. *Journal of Mental Health, 14,* 121–127.

Rosenberg, S. D., Lu, W., Mueser, K. T., Jankowski, M. K., & Cournos, F. (2007). Correlates of adverse childhood events in adults with schizophrenia spectrum disorders. *Psychiatric Services, 58,* 245–253.

Rosenberg, S. D., Mueser, K. T., Friedman, M. J., Gorman, P. G., Drake, R. E., Vidaver, R. M., et al. (2001). Developing effective treatments for post-traumatic disorders: A review and proposal. *Psychiatric Services, 52,* 1453–1461.

Rosenberg, S. D., Mueser, K. T., Jankowski, M. K., Salyers, M. P., & Acker, K. (2004). Cognitive-behavioral treatment of posttraumatic stress disorder in severe mental illness: Results of a pilot study. *American Journal of Psychiatric Rehabilitation, 7,* 171–186.

Salyers, M. P., Evans, L. J., Bond, G. R., & Meyer, P. S. (2004). Barriers to assessment and treatment of posttraumatic stress disorder and other trauma-related problems in people with severe mental illness: Clinician perspectives. *Community Mental Health Journal, 40,* 17–31.

CHAPTER 44

MANAGEMENT OF CO-OCCURRING SUBSTANCE USE DISORDERS

DAVID J. KAVANAGH

NATURE OF THE ISSUES IN COMORBID POPULATIONS

In recent years there has been increasing interest in effective ways to manage people with both psychoses and co-occurring substance use disorders (SUDs). Despite the importance of these problems, treatment research in this area remains at a relatively early stage, with few well-controlled trials and outcomes that are often quite weak. However, we now have a substantial body of research on the nature, incidence, and correlates of SUDs in psychoses, and on the nature and perceived limitations of existing services. This research has clear implications for interventions.

SUDs Are Very Frequent in People with Psychoses

About half of people with schizophrenia spectrum disorders have an SUD at some time in their lives. In treatment settings, rates can be even higher—especially in acute or crisis services, or in services for people with high needs for ongoing support, because the combination of problems increases problem severity and risk of relapse.

There are important implications for clinical practice that arise from this observation. First, because comorbidity is so common, screening for substance use should be universal and routine in initial assessments and status reviews of people with psychosis. Second, routinely offering more intensive or prolonged treatment than that available at present to everyone with schizophrenia and an SUD would have substantial resource implications. Unless budgets and staffing receive a substantial boost, or other consumers receive less intervention, there will be severe limitations on the extent to which such additional treatment can be contemplated. Exporting the problem to another service (e.g., an alcohol and other drug service) just shifts rather than solves the resource problem.

Three potential strategies present themselves. One would be to embed most treatment for comorbidity within standard treatment sessions. A second would ensure that all affected patients received at least a brief intervention. A third would restrict substantial amounts of additional treatment to the patients most likely to benefit from it. This chapter takes the view that a combination of all three ideas should be considered (Table 44.1).

Risk Factors and Selected Substances Are Similar to the Rest of the Population

Rates of co-occurring SUDs typically follow community patterns, so that young people and men are at increased relative risk, as are people from groups with higher consumption (e.g., single or divorced people, the unemployed, members of alienated indigenous communities or of cultural groups with heavy substance use). Substance use is also more common in time periods or in geographical areas where substances are readily obtained at low cost.

The substances selected by people with psychoses also follow the pattern in the general community. Typically, surveys in Western countries over the last 20 years have found that the recreational drugs most commonly used by people with psychoses (other than caffeine) are nicotine, alcohol, and cannabis, usually in that order. However, drug selection can vary dramatically across time and locality, with changes in production, law enforcement, and fashion or acceptance. In the last 10 years, amphetamine, cocaine, and heroin consumption have each demonstrated this phenomenon. There is also evidence that the pattern of demographic correlates may differ across particular drugs—for example, that age may be a weaker predictor for alcohol than for cannabis, because alcohol has been less subject to cohort effects over the last 50 years. The predominant drug and the demographic correlates can also vary across treatment services, according to local characteristics and the nature of the service.

Together, these observations suggest that we need to design and offer treatments that are appropriate for high-volume groups, such as young men, and for the substances currently in most common use. At the same time, the needs of other groups (e.g., women, older people, users of less common drugs) should not be ignored.

SUDs Have a Substantial Impact on People with Psychoses

The high frequency of comorbidity would not be such a major issue if it did not have substantial impact. Unfortunately, comorbidity has severe individual and collective effects that encompass patients, their families and friends, a wide range of health and social services, and the community at large. SUDs contribute to costs by exacerbating symptoms, producing functional deficits and triggering impulsive behaviors (including self-harm, aggression, and high-risk sexual activity). The impact is not just financial, as large as that is; it also includes emotional and psychological impacts, and both objective and subjective quality of life. Mental health services are not immune to the increased costs. Untreated, this group is overrepresented by those who repeatedly relapse or have chronic, severe functional deficits. They are particularly common in users of high-cost services, such as crisis and emergency care, high-support community housing, and inpatient facilities. Unless service capacity is high, this means that other consumers miss out on the level of services they need. Despite the difficulties in addressing comorbidity in a proactive fashion, there is an imperative to do so.

The complexity of comorbid problems is usually compounded by multiple substance use. An obvious implication is that treatment focusing on only one drug may have limited

TABLE 44.1. Treatment Recommendations on Co-Occurring Mental Disorders and SUDs

Recommendations from epidemiological research

1. Universally screen for SUDs in people with psychosis.
2. To maximize access and restrict cost:
   - Integrate comorbidity work in standard treatment.
   - Routinely apply brief interventions.
   - Restrict high-cost interventions to those who will benefit only from those treatments.
3. Have treatments that are suitable for the following, while ensuring that less common groups are also addressed:
   - High-risk groups (e.g., young men).
   - Substances currently in common use among the service's consumers (e.g., nicotine, alcohol, cannabis, cocaine/amphetamines).
   - Use of multiple substances.
4. Ensure that treatments can deal with initial instability in substance control, and that optimism about recovery is expressed. Even in low-intensity treatments, some ongoing, assertive contact may be required.
5. Intervene early to help preserve prospects of functional recovery.
6. Present comorbidity interventions in the context of maintaining optimal physical and mental health to reduce stigma and maximize engagement. Nicotine smoking should be an important focus.
7. Any problematic responses by others should be addressed (e.g., in family intervention) and highly confrontational approaches to clients should be avoided.
8. Any responses by the service to substance-related infractions should be proportional and expected, and minimize threats to engagement or relapse.
9. Treatments should offer more opportunities for pleasure and mood enhancement than are taken away.
10. Treatments for complex problems should sequentially focus on the single behavioral change with the greatest potential impact on the current problems.

Recommendations based on treatment outcome research

1. Mental health and SUD treatments for people with serious mental disorders should be fully integrated and routinely offered by the mental health service, with consultative support from alcohol or other drug services where required.
2. People with serious mental disorders and severe substance dependence may require input from multiple services.
3. Current trials do not offer strong support for any specific treatment component or set of components. Approaches used with each disorder have some effect.
4. A staged approach to treatment intensity should be considered, with higher intensity treatments reserved for consumers who do not respond to lower intensity treatments.

impact or leave people at risk of relapse, if it ignores potential relationships with other substances. Examples are people's difficulties resisting consumption when intoxicated with another drug; ongoing contact with suppliers, users, or usage contexts for other drugs; use of the same mode of administration, such as smoking or injection for multiple drugs; and strategic consumption to deal with effects of other drugs. Both clients and treatments may productively target one substance at a particular time, but this focus should not become myopic and miss cross-substance influences.

The high levels of service contact and poor response to previous treatment commonly seen in this group lead many therapeutic staff to be doubtful of success or to lack self-efficacy about being able to provide effective treatment. It is important to remind ourselves that recovery from a substance-related problem often requires several attempts,

and that we have sometimes found it hard to maintain attempts to change our own behaviors in the past. People with comorbid mental health problems may find it particularly
difficult to initiate and maintain behavior change, especially if they have deficits in problem solving or prospective memory, experience severe negative symptoms, or are depressed—
as so many are. If their practitioners do not model persistence and optimism, it is difficult
for consumers to maintain optimism and persistence themselves.

There is an upside. Although SUDs have a very negative impact on outcomes, people
who develop a co-occurring SUD often have levels of premorbid functioning that are as
good as or better than those of patients without an SUD. One possible reason for this observation is that people with higher premorbid social functioning may be at greater risk
of exposure to substance use. To the extent that premorbid abilities are preserved, treating the SUD may offer a relatively good prognosis. This effect is most evident in consumers whose psychosis is truly secondary to their substance use, and who typically recover
rapidly once they stop consuming the drugs, but it may also be true of persons with truly
independent disorders. There may, however, be some urgency in addressing the problem
before it is too late. Use of cannabis and other substances triggers an earlier average trajectory of psychosis, interfering with both education and social development, and with
the final stages of brain maturation. It is imperative that we help consumers address
SUDs and maximize their potential, before windows of opportunity for socialization and
career development are lost. Ideally, we need to prevent the brain insult that underlies the
first episode of psychosis. If we cannot do that, we need to try to ensure that consumers'
initial episode is also their last, and that their ultimate functioning is maximized.

Small Amounts of Drugs Can Have Large Effects

As a group, people with psychosis and an SUD are very different from the majority of
people in the general population who request treatment for SUDs. On average their consumption is lower, and they are less likely to show a severe substance dependence syndrome. This is partly because they can rarely afford large amounts, and partly because
many people with severe mental disorders are exquisitely vulnerable to negative impacts
from small quantities of drugs. The vulnerability does not extend only to symptoms and
interactions with prescribed drugs. Because this population usually already has significant
functional deficits, these individuals are very susceptible to additional impact. Given that
most have a very low income, smoking and other substance use have an early effect on
other spending, in many cases, affecting not only discretionary spending (e.g., movies,
outings, or small indulgences) and narrowing sources of pleasure but also impacting essential purchases, such as food, clothing, and shelter.

The same amount of a drug may have very different effects on the same person, depending on the situation at the time. So, a person within a more vulnerable period for
psychotic symptoms, or with temporarily less disposable money, may have more negative
effects than usual. There is also substantial individual variation. In some people, any use
of particular substances creates havoc for their mental state and functioning. This can be
difficult for consumers to acknowledge if they are using considerably less of the drugs
than their peers. As in other addiction contexts, highly vulnerable consumers often adopt
an initial goal of harm reduction or moderation before they appreciate that abstinence offers the best outcome. Respecting their decision and assisting them in the attempt does
not imply agreement that the goal is appropriate; it acknowledges their positive motivation and maintains an alliance that can ultimately result in more complete success.

Not all effects of substances are direct. Some problems arise from negative responses
of other people. Intoxication is more salient in people who are displaying odd behavior. It

is also tempting for friends and relatives to blame substance users with serious mental disorders for their own symptoms. These reactions substantially increase the risk of subsequent psychotic relapse. In fact, this indirect influence can sometimes be stronger than direct effects of the drug. Exclusion and rejection are seen in a number of contexts, unfortunately, including health services and assisted accommodation. Effects of such exclusion can be catastrophic.

There are at least two implications for treatment. First, interventions assisting families and friends to cope with the person's co-occurring psychosis and SUD may be very important. Second, we should ensure that our reactions to these people do not worsen their prognosis or lead to their permanent exclusion. Although there are good reasons to ban substance use within specific contexts (e.g., on treatment or accommodation sites, or before sessions), avenues for support and treatment of those who do use must remain open. Any consequences should be proportional, temporary, demonstrably fair (e.g., abbreviation and rescheduling of the session), and protective of the health and welfare of all parties. It is no more appropriate to exclude lapsing substance users from service than to exclude people with symptomatic exacerbation from appropriate service responses.

The large impact that typically follows relatively low consumption of recreational drugs means that the majority of people with serious mental disorder and an SUD who are seen in most mental health services do not show high levels of physical dependence or need assisted withdrawal. This is not to say that attention to physical risk is unimportant: Both the psychosis and the substance use increase the risk of physical exposure, impaired self-care, injury, and infection (including infection with HIV). Self-harm, suicide, and either committing assault or being the victim of it are more likely in people with an SUD than in those without an SUD, and assessment of these risks is essential. Given the heightened risk of serious physical disorder in this population, and the risk of misdiagnosis or inadequate treatment, mental health and SUD services have an obligation to provide relevant consultation and training to ensure that general medical staff are able to meet the significant challenges this population may pose. Services are also needed for people with both a severe mental disorder and severe substance dependence, who often need a high level of ongoing treatment and support, and input from a range of specialist services.

Often There Is Little Else in the User's Life

Substance use in people with psychosis is usually in the context of a very impoverished existence, with drug users constituting their primary or only friends, and with few alternative recreational activities. These individuals rarely use substances to address psychotic symptoms, but they often cite relief of dysphoria or boredom as key reasons for consumption. Corollaries are that motivation enhancement and relief of dysphoria may be important components of successful treatment. Because dysphoria lowers self-efficacy, strategies that boost confidence and address responses to perceived failures may often be required. Interventions need to provide more social advantages and opportunities for mood enhancement than they take away.

This Group Usually Has Complex, Intertwined Issues

The term *dual diagnosis* comes nowhere near an accurate description of the complexity of problems typically seen in this population. Most people with psychosis and co-occurring SUD use more than one substance, and many have additional mental health problems (e.g., depression, social anxiety, and personality disorders). As already noted, often they also have physical disorders and a complex web of social, financial, legal, housing, and occupational issues. It is time that we recognize this complexity by using a different term.

Significant practical issues are raised by this complexity. Which problem should be addressed first? Which ones are critical to overall recovery?

In some cases, the mental disorder may be secondary to the substance use, and treating the latter can resolve the former. However, this is not strictly a group with independent, co-occurring disorders. For most people with both psychosis and an SUD, the problems are linked by threads of mutual influence. For example, symptom exacerbation is more likely after greater cannabis use, but higher cannabis use is also more likely when symptoms are worse.

A more complex or multifaceted treatment is not necessarily the answer—especially if treatment strategies simultaneously impose high memory or performance demands on participants. Focusing on one current treatment target that is likely to produce the most impact on the total set of problems may be a better approach. An example of a potential target with multiple impacts is increasing positive, nondrug activities: This potentially affects not only the time spent on substance use and total amount consumed but also addresses dysphoria and perhaps social contact. Another example, employment, offers multiple opportunities for pleasure and increased functioning, provides a strong reason for substance control, and is inconsistent with substance use over most of the week. Multi-impact treatment targets need to be identified for each individual and tailored to his or her current status and valued goals.

Priority Setting Requires a Balance of Frequency, Severity, and Acceptability

The most commonly used drugs are not necessarily the ones with greatest impact on psychotic symptoms, physical health, or social functioning. Injected or smoked drugs and illegal drugs of unknown content or potency, of course, pose particular risks. Hallucinogens and amphetamines have particularly strong effects on symptoms, as can cannabis, but as I already noted, nicotine and alcohol are by far the most commonly used substances. As a result, the latter drugs have the greatest impact in the population with severe mental disorders, just as they do in the general population. There are sometimes difficult priority issues relative to substances: Should we focus on the substances that most commonly affect clients, or on those that have the greatest impact on individual users?

Clearly, there is not a single answer to this question, but initial work with individual clients is usually more productive if it focuses on substances about which they are already concerned. One substance that scores high on both frequency and risk is also a common focus of client concern. Nicotine is not only the most common substance used by people with psychoses (up to 80% smoke cigarettes according to surveys) but it is also the greatest single contributor after suicide to excess mortality and morbidity in psychosis. Nicotine use is often neglected as a treatment target—perhaps because of high rates of smoking by staff, because of its use in the past to calm or reward clients, or because there is little evidence that it exacerbates psychotic symptoms. In fact, nicotine moderates negative symptoms, improving cognitive performance in particular. However, the additional dopamine release and faster drug metabolism seen in smokers mean that up to 50% more of the older antipsychotics is needed for effective symptom control. Cigarette smoking is a noncontentious target for many consumers, because of exposure to public campaigns on the dangers of smoking, and because it is not subject to the same opprobrium as illegal substance use. Nicotine should not be neglected in assessment and intervention for comorbidity.

DESCRIPTION OF TREATMENT APPROACHES, AND EVIDENCE FOR THEM

There are three main approaches to multiple disorders. One is to address them *sequentially*. This may be especially useful when clearly there is one primary problem, and other problems simply flow from it. A second approach is to treat the disorders *in parallel*. This implies that they are independent disorders that co-occur by chance, and also that treatments for the disorders will not interfere with each other. A third approach is *integrated treatment* for both disorders by a single treatment agent. Each aspect of the treatment takes the full set of issues into account and is tailored to have maximum impact on multiple areas. A single, coherent treatment plan attempts to address the disorders and the associations between them. This does not, of course, require that all treatment components are applied simultaneously—just that all elements take account of the total context.

A body of research has attempted to determine which of these models is best for people with psychosis and SUDs. Although there are few randomized controlled trials and significant methodological limitations to the current research, the current evidence is more in favor of an integrated treatment by a single agent than treatment with other models. There are several possible reasons for this observation: Integrated treatment, by definition, ensures some treatment for both conditions, and communication is ensured. There is more likely to be consistency in advice and objectives, and each aspect is more likely to be tailored and timed to take into account other comorbid conditions. Consistency is also present in the therapeutic relationship. Each of these features could conceivably be obtained in a model involving more than one treatment agent, and with parallel or sequential aspects, but it would be much more difficult.

In many countries, services for mental health problems and SUDs are offered by separate agencies, with a very different mix of professional backgrounds, inclusion criteria, treatment foci and objectives, methods, and degree of assertive follow-up. Frequently they are in separate locations, and intersectoral communication is often problematic. Gaps are commonly reported in perceived ability to manage problems that are seen as the province of the companion sector. These structural features create significant difficulties for individuals with multiple, complex problems. Historically, often they have been excluded from one or both services altogether, or left to negotiate treatments with multiple agencies themselves. This has sometimes meant that only the most motivated and resourceful consumers and families have been able to obtain an acceptable standard of treatment for comorbidity. Sequential treatments often become sequential culs-de-sac; parallel treatments may take diverging or conflicting paths, and integrated treatment may be extremely difficult if not impossible.

How then do we resolve this problem? Even if services are combined, attitudes, practices and professional specialities may still carry over. Should specialist comorbidity teams be established? Such teams can be very useful in promoting cross-sectoral training and offering supervision or specialist consultation, but a risk is that other staff members may attempt to slough off all relevant consumers to that team, so that it is soon overwhelmed by the caseload. A set of service criteria and priorities would inevitably have to be established, and there would be a new basis for service exclusion.

There is a practical alternative. If the regular treatment staff from each service takes responsibility for the assessment and management of the kinds of comorbidity that routinely present in its service, an integrated model of treatment can be delivered. Consumers with serious mental disorders could be assured of treatment by the mental health service for a comorbid SUD. Conversely, individuals presenting to a specialist SUD service could expect to have comorbid anxiety or depression treated. Some services already run on this model, although some others remain stuck in a less flexible or encompassing role. A corollary of the recommended approach is that staff members acquire competence in managing the commonly presenting comorbidities in their service, and that quality control and accreditation encompass management of comorbidity as a core function. Comanagement of comorbid disorders across services, or management by specialist comorbidity trainers or consultants, could then be limited to individuals with particularly severe or apparently intractable problems.

EVIDENCE ON TREATMENT EFFECTS

Current evidence suggests that some atypical antipsychotic medications may reduce other substance use, and that most medications for substance misuse may (with some provisos) be safely applied in people with serious mental disorders. However, there are few data as yet on the specific efficacy of the latter drugs for people with psychosis.

There are still very few randomized controlled trials on psychological interventions for comorbidity in the literature. They often obtain relatively weak, short-lived, or patchy results across different substances, and many positive results are not subsequently replicated. This is the case even when the intervention is much more substantial and intensive than would be practical in a standard service. On the one hand, in common with the general literature on the treatment of SUDs, initial changes by individual participants are often unstable, and multiple attempts at control are often needed. Extended treatment may often be required.

On the other hand, evidence on interventions for risky alcohol consumption in the general population suggests that opportunistic brief interventions can be remarkably effective. These interventions typically involve feedback of results from screening and assessment, and advice to stop or reduce substance use, sometimes with specific suggestions on how to do it. The number and duration of treatment sessions differ widely, but single-session interventions of 5 minutes or less still have significantly better effects than no treatment, and brief interventions give the same average impact as longer ones.

Motivation enhancement, or *motivational interviewing* (Miller & Rollnick, 2002), is a style of intervention that can be used in either a brief format or as the precursor to longer treatment. It encourages clients to express ambivalence about their current substance use, and how it fits with their self-concept and goals. There is no attempt to persuade or argue with clients—instead, they are encouraged to develop awareness of their own motivations for change. Both brief interventions in general and motivation enhancement have particularly strong supportive evidence for change in alcohol consumption (Miller & Wilbourne, 2002), but they have also been applied to other behavior targets.

There is some evidence that motivation enhancement can be effectively adapted to comorbid populations, generating engagement in subsequent extended treatment, and serving as a relatively brief, stand-alone intervention. However, as in the case of longer treatments, evidence on substance-related changes is inconsistent. At least some of the difficulty that is experienced in controlled trials may reflect the fact that some clients successfully make significant and sustained changes in their substance use after having an inpatient admission, with little or no specific intervention. Perhaps their reaction to an admission and their awareness (whether preexisting, or triggered by staff comments) that substances may have triggered it is as much intervention as this group needs. Or it may be just a matter of regression to the mean: Their substance use before admission was more than usual, triggering an episode, but they then returned to more usual consumption. We need to find out more about natural recovery processes in this population to understand how we can increase the proportion of people who fall into this group.

Up to now, there has been little success in a priori identification of consumers who will benefit from brief comorbidity interventions. Those with less severe or less chronic problems, for example, do not necessarily show better outcomes. This observation, together with cost considerations, suggests that a staged model of intervention may be indicated, in which all affected consumers receive a brief intervention, with some repetition in individuals with fragile motivation. Motivated consumers who have difficulty maintaining an attempt may need additional support and targeted skills training, or adjunctive pharmacotherapy. A small group that is at acute physical and psychiatric risk and is unable to respond to skills training may need more intensive environmental support (e.g., supervised living environments). Such a staged approach to treatment delivery would need to ensure that consumers not see stage progression as a reflection of their own failure (perhaps by drawing an analogy to particular medications being more effective with some people than others).

GUIDELINES FOR PSYCHOLOGICAL TREATMENT

Where does this leave us as practitioners? Given the current state of the evidence, any recommendations must be tentative. When the epidemiological and treatment outcome research are considered, some specific guidance is given. Table 44.1 summarizes the implications for treatment relative to the issues already discussed in preceding sections. But what components of psychological intervention should be considered?

Development of Rapport

It is critical that clients trust that the information they divulge will not result in negative outcomes (exclusion from service, legal consequences, or disapproval); otherwise, they will withhold information about substance use (and other potentially sensitive issues). One the one hand, at least "denial" of problems may also be more accurately described as nondisclosure. On the other hand, provided that rapport and trust are well established, reports of consumption can be as accurate as assays (or more so, if a report extends beyond the detection period of the assay). Trust is established by the therapist demonstrating empathy and positive regard in response to other personal information, and by providing specific reassurance about lack of consequences for disclosure. General conversations about the person's interests, usual activities, and goals are especially useful in later motivational interviewing.

Brief Intervention or Advice

If there is insufficient opportunity for anything more, people with comorbidity should be provided nonjudgmental feedback on outcomes of screening and assessment. Brief advice from an expert may be persuasive in some cases, particularly if the person is already concerned about the issue. However, highly confrontational interactions should be avoided in this population, because of their potentially detrimental symptomatic impact. Furthermore, some people are likely to react defensively to direct suggestions about either their substance use or concurrent mental disorder. Motivational interviewing (Miller & Rollnick, 2002) minimizes defensive reactions and often elicits motivation for change, even when the person was not initially contemplating it. Adjustments for people with serious mental disorder may include splitting the process into several short sessions, revising the process on each occasion, and including more summaries than usual. We have found that the approach can even be used during a psychotic episode, as long as clients are not acutely distressed, and can maintain attention to a single topic of conversation over a 5- to 10-minute period (with prompting, if necessary).

Planning behavior change should initially focus on preparations that specify when and how action will occur, and strategies to support the person through the initial days. Potential challenges in the first 7 days are identified, and ideas on how to address them are generated, rehearsed, and practiced. Our version of this intervention (Start Over and Survive [SOS]) totals 3 hours, including rapport development, motivational interviewing, and planning, and leaves participants with a series of pocket-sized personalized leaflets to remind them about their own situations and plans. In the case of participants who are living at home, we also deliver a single session to relatives, to generate empathy and encourage their continued support, while setting appropriate limits. If there is a delay in appointing case managers after discharge, we make brief, weekly telephone calls to clients over the first month to acknowledge progress, to review their reasons for change, and to cue problem solving.

Our research group uses individual sessions, because this provides maximum flexibility in delivering coherent, integrated, and individualized treatment over the course of short inpatient stays (often 3–5 days), when consumers are acutely psychotic and thought disordered. Within longer admissions or ongoing outpatient contact, group sessions may be used to consolidate motivation and to model success. Obviously, care needs to be taken that negative modeling, supplying drugs to other members, and conflict are avoided.

Skills Training and Ongoing Group Support

Some clients need training in problem solving, substance refusal, management of dysphoria, medication adherence, or other specific skills, before they are on track for recovery. Many also need ongoing encouragement, reengagement after lapses or symptom exacerbations, or additional support when external stressors or dysphoria are higher than usual. Development of pleasant activities, social relationships, and social roles that are unrelated to substance use (including employment) may be particularly important for overall recovery. Ongoing peer groups can be a cost-effective way to provide social rewards, to alternate activities, and to assist with problem solving over a substantial period. One way to provide group support for abstinence has been through adaptations of 12-step approaches, although that is not the only model and may not be the best for all clients.

Family members potentially offer extremely valuable support for substance use and symptom management. However, comorbidity presents difficult challenges for them. Even in our brief SOS intervention, we routinely ask relatives to a single session to elicit empathy and help them to find ways to continue providing appropriate assistance. A psychoeducational group workshop may provide similar benefits, if material is readily applied to each family's situation. More extended support and training through relatives groups or single-family interventions may improve the whole family's quality of life and reduce relapse risks for an affected family member.

Environmental Structure

When people with very high disability pose a significant risk to themselves or others (e.g., recurrent personal neglect or dangerous behavior), environmental support, such as assistance with finances, shopping and cooking, or a staffed home environment, should be considered. More intrusive forms of care should, of course, be restricted to those with pressing current needs. Although some clients may require indefinite support, everyone should, of course, be offered opportunities to develop the maximum degree of culturally appropriate adult functioning.

KEY POINTS

- Comorbidity of SUDs and serious mental disorders should be core business for mental health services, because of its frequency and impact.
- Current evidence favors integration of treatments for SUDs and serious mental disorder, provided by a single practitioner.
- It is time to stop talking about dual diagnosis, and to recognize the complexity of comorbidities.
- Relatively low levels of substance use can have substantial negative effects in people with serious mental disorders, and most people with this comorbidity do not have severe substance dependence.
- Complex disorders do not necessarily imply more complex treatments: Clients and practitioners may benefit maximally from strategies that have impact on multiple problems.
- Although the evidence on effective treatments is still in its infancy, some potentially useful treatments may be readily implemented by practitioners without substantial additional training.
- As in other populations with substance use problems, people with serious mental health disorder may need several attempts to achieve sustained success in controlling substance use. We need to maintain our belief in ultimate success and help clients maintain their own optimism.

REFERENCES AND RECOMMENDED READINGS

General reviews of comorbidity and its management are given by Donald, Dower, and Kavanagh (2005); Drake, Mercer-McFadden, Mueser, McHugo, and Bond (1998); Graham, Copello, Birchwood, and Mueser (2003); Kavanagh, Mueser, and Baker (2003); and Kavanagh and Mueser (2007). Castle and Murray (2004) offer an overview of the effects of *cannabis*, the use of cannabis by people with psychosis, and the management of comorbidity with psychosis. Reviews of *pharmacological management* of comorbidity are provided in Kavanagh, McGrath, Saunders, Dore, and Clark (2001) and Mueser, Noordsy, Drake, and Fox (2003). Reviews on effectiveness of *brief interventions* in general populations with alcohol abuse or dependence are offered by Moyer, Finney, Swearingen, and Vergun (2002) and Wilk, Jensen, and Havighurst (1997). *Motivational interviewing* is described and relevant evidence is reviewed by Miller and Rollnick (2002). Methods to adapt motivational interviewing to serious mental disorder are in Martino, Carroll, Kostas, Perkins, and Rounsaville (2002). *Start Over and Survive* (SOS) is guided by a manual that is available on a link from *http://www.uq.edu.au/coh*. Select Online Psych.

Castle, D., & Murray, R. (Eds.). (2004). *Marijuana and madness.* Cambridge, UK: Cambridge University Press.

Donald, M., Dower, J., & Kavanagh, D. J. (2005). Integrated versus non-integrated management and care for clients with co-occurring mental health and substance use disorders: A qualitative systematic review of randomised controlled trials. *Social Science and Medicine, 60,* 1371–1383.

Drake, R. E., Mercer-McFadden, C., Mueser, K. T., McHugo, G. J., & Bond, G. R. (1998). Review of integrated mental health and substance abuse treatment for patients with dual disorders. *Schizophrenia Bulletin, 24,* 589–608.

Graham, H., Copello, A., Birchwood, M., & Mueser, K. T. (Eds.). (2003). *Substance misuse in psychosis: Approaches to treatment and service delivery.* Chichester, UK: Wiley.

Kavanagh, D. J., McGrath, J., Saunders, J. B., Dore, G., & Clark, D. (2001). Substance abuse in patients with schizophrenia: Epidemiology and management. *Drugs, 62,* 743–755.

Kavanagh, D. J., & Mueser, K. T. (2007). Current evidence on integrated treatment for serious mental disorder and substance misuse. *Journal of the Norwegian Psychological Association, 5,* 618–637.

Kavanagh, D. J., Mueser, K., & Baker, A. (2003). Management of comorbidity. In M. Teesson & H. Proudfoot (Eds.), *Comorbid mental disorders and substance use disorders: Epidemiology, prevention and treatment* (pp. 78–120). Sydney: National Drug and Alcohol Research Centre.

Martino, S., Carroll, K. M., Kostas, D., Perkins, J., & Rounsaville, B. J. (2002). Dual diagnosis interviewing: A modification of motivational interviewing for substance-abusing patients with psychotic disorders. *Journal of Substance Abuse Treatment, 23,* 297–308.

Miller, W. R., & Rollnick, S. (2002). *Motivational interviewing: Preparing people for change* (2nd ed.). New York: Guilford Press.

Miller, W. R., & Wilbourne, P. L. (2002). Mesa Grande: A methodological analysis of clinical trials for alcohol use disorders. *Addiction, 97,* 265–277.

Moyer, A., Finney, J. W., Swearingen, C. E., & Vergun, P. (2002). Brief interventions for alcohol problems: A meta-analytic review of controlled investigations in treatment-seeking and non-treatment-seeking populations. *Addiction, 97,* 279–292.

Mueser, K. T., Noordsy, D. L., Drake, R. E., & Fox, L. (2003). *Integrated treatment for dual disorders: A guide to effective practice.* New York: Guilford Press.

Wilk, A. I., Jensen, N. M., & Havighurst, T. C. (1997). Meta-analysis of randomized control trials addressing brief interventions in heavy alcohol drinkers. *Journal of General Internal Medicine, 12,* 274–283.

CHAPTER 45

PARENTING

JOANNE NICHOLSON
LAURA MILLER

EPIDEMIOLOGY AND SOCIAL CONTEXT

Parenthood is a desired life goal and meaningful role for many adults with schizophrenia. An analysis of national prevalence data indicated that 62% of women and 55% of men with schizophrenia spectrum disorders are parents. Parents with schizophrenia spectrum disorders have their first children, on average, at about age 20, with up to 35% experiencing their first episode of psychosis before becoming parents.

Systematic data on the parenting experiences of individuals with schizophrenia are sparse, and most studies to date do not fully take into account the influence of gender, onset and course of illness, extent and domain of disability, family and community resources and supports, and access to effective treatment and rehabilitation on parents' experiences. Some studies have shown that individuals with schizophrenia who become parents tend to have had better premorbid social adjustment. Women with mental illness who become mothers are more likely to have been married than are women with mental illness who do not become mothers. However, women with schizophrenia, compared with women without mental illness, are less likely to have a current partner and have a higher number of lifetime sexual partners.

Fathers with serious mental illness (SMI) are significantly more likely than mothers with SMI to be younger and to abuse substances. Fathers with schizophrenia tend to be socially isolated. In one study, for example, fewer than 20% of fathers with schizophrenia were married, and fewer than 30% lived with their children.

Many parents with SMI lack material and emotional supports. They report that their mental illnesses limit their social networks and contribute to poverty, joblessness, homelessness, and lack of transportation. They may have limited ability to supply children's necessities. Whereas relationships with adult family members can be an important source of support in some cases, they can undermine parents' abilities and efforts, and contribute to their stress in other cases.

Comorbid substance abuse may contribute to poor overall functioning and impaired parenting. Medical comorbidity, including higher rates of hypertension, diabetes, and sexually transmitted diseases, may decrease energy for parenting and is especially difficult when limited child care alternatives allow ill parents no respite.

For many parents with schizophrenia, intermittent parenting is the norm. Their children may live with others in informal caregiving arrangements or in legal custody situations. The relationship between a parent with schizophrenia and other child caregivers is a key factor in the well-being of the ill parent and the children. In the worst case scenario, custody may be awarded to relatives who were abusive to the parent; the resultant anxiety about the children's safety and well-being may undermine the parent's treatment and recovery. In the best case scenario, alternative caregivers are supportive coparents, possibly living close by or in the same home. Coparents provide respite, support the parent–child relationship, provide guidance and advice, and serve as role models of effective parenting behavior for the parent with SMI.

THE IMPACT OF SCHIZOPHRENIA ON PARENTING

Parenting capability in individuals with schizophrenia can range from highly attuned and competent to adequate, to abusive and/or neglectful. Mental illnesses, including schizophrenia, are more prevalent in samples of parents who are known to abuse their children; however, there are no systematic data on prevalence of child abuse by parents with schizophrenia. Some studies have demonstrated that when schizophrenia *does* impair parenting capability, it can do so in specific ways. Understanding these disease-linked functional impairments can help clinicians plan parenting rehabilitation interventions.

Negative Symptoms

Parent–infant interactions that are synchronous and contingent promote healthy development. Difficulty in reading nonverbal cues especially limits parenting of babies and toddlers. Blunted affect, apathy, and withdrawal can reduce a parent's capacity to convey moods clearly and to respond appropriately to children. Prolonged lack of stimulation can impair children's cognitive and social development. Compromised executive functioning can impair day-to-day family functioning (e.g., meal planning and preparation) and child behavior management.

Positive Symptoms

Thought disorder can interfere with a parent's ability to recognize antecedents and to anticipate consequences of children's behavior. Parents with schizophrenia may have delusional fears regarding potential harm to their children, may misinterpret their children's behavior, or may erroneously believe their children are causing problems or have problems. Hallucinations involving children, particularly command hallucinations, may contribute to a parent injuring a child. However, although command hallucinations have been linked to violence, there are no systematic data on the likelihood that parents with schizophrenia will act upon command hallucinations to harm their children.

Impaired Insight

A parent's level of insight into his or her illness has been found to correlate with responsive parenting behavior, and to be inversely correlated with risk of child maltreatment in parents with SMI.

THE IMPACT OF PARENTAL SCHIZOPHRENIA ON CHILDREN

Offspring of mothers with schizophrenia are more likely to have developmental, emotional, social, behavioral, and cognitive problems. This is due in part to genetics and in part to adverse childhood experiences, perhaps exacerbated by common correlates of serious mental illness (e.g., unemployment, poverty, family conflict and disruption, and homelessness). Children born to women with schizophrenia spectrum disorders are at higher risk for emotional symptoms during early childhood than children born to women without psychiatric illness, and are more prone to social inhibition during their school years. Children with unmet special needs or those who pose behavior management difficulties may contribute to greater stress for parents with schizophrenia, and provide additional challenges to their parenting capabilities. Screening during early childhood can lead to timely implementation of prevention and intervention strategies for children.

Children whose parents have schizophrenia may be pressed into service as caretakers of ill parents, or of siblings. Some children whose parents have schizophrenia suggest that this role reversal enhanced their coping and caregiving skills; others report having suffered from age-inappropriate family burdens.

Children whose parents have schizophrenia may be at greater risk of family disruption, through the increased likelihood of parental divorce and/or being removed from their parental home. Although children's safety is a priority, the disruption of family relationships has costs. Children may be extremely loyal to the most disturbed of parents and have difficulty forming what they view as competing attachments. They may worry that their parents will suffer if they are separated from them. Children placed in different foster homes may lose contact with siblings. Multiple placements over time may seriously impair children's capacity to form healthy relationships.

THE EXPERIENCES OF PARENTS WITH SCHIZOPHRENIA

Many mothers with SMI describe motherhood as rewarding and central to their lives, and feel pride in fulfilling the maternal role. Mothers with schizophrenia, like many mothers, may also be stressed by the demands of parenting, particularly if supports are insufficient; such stress may precipitate illness relapse. Hospitalizations and resultant separations from children can also be stressful, particularly if mothers are forced to place children with strangers in foster care. Mothers may prioritize their children's needs, jeopardizing their own health and well-being by not keeping treatment appointments or not taking medications if these conflict with parenting responsibilities. Many mothers with SMI fear that their children will be adversely affected by their illnesses, and may become overly concerned when their children express normal, age-appropriate, though "difficult" behavior (e.g., temper tantrums in a 2-year-old).

INCREASED VULNERABILITY TO LOSS

Parenthood is somewhat less prevalent among women with nonaffective psychoses than among women with other mental illnesses. Women with SMI have more unplanned and unwanted pregnancies than do women without psychiatric disorders. This relative lack of planning may decrease the chance for successful parenting. Other women with schizophrenia may not define motherhood as an option; consequently, they may need to grieve the loss of this life role.

The major reason for loss of the parenting role among adults with schizophrenia appears to be loss of custody of children. Although there are no nationally representative data on the prevalence of parents' ultimate loss of custody or contact with children, researchers conducting smaller, treatment-setting-based studies find rates of custody loss from 30 to 70% or higher for women with SMI. Whereas maintaining custody or relationships with children can motivate some mothers to participate in treatment, other mothers may avoid treatment, or avoid disclosing parenting difficulties, if they fear this may result in custody loss. Parents may also have difficulty visiting children who live with others, because they anticipate the painful feelings of loss that recur each time a visit ends.

PREGNANCY AND PARENTHOOD
IN THE TREATMENT OF SCHIZOPHRENIA

Treatment interventions can directly support parental functioning, via psychosocial rehabilitation and support strategies, or indirectly, via incorporating consideration of the effects on parenting into all aspects of treatment. Because antipsychotic medication is the cornerstone of treatment for schizophrenia, it is important to consider the effects of these medications on parental functioning.

Pharmacotherapy for Parents with Schizophrenia

Optimal pharmacotherapy can support effective parenting for women with schizophrenia, beginning even before pregnancy. Effective antipsychotic medications, especially those that alleviate both positive and negative symptoms, can improve overall functioning, strengthen social networks, and promote capacity for committed, intimate relationships, paving the way for better parenting support. By contrast, antipsychotic medications that elevate prolactin, most notably risperidone and haloperidol, can impair fertility and cause menstrual unpredictability, making it more difficult to plan a pregnancy.

During pregnancy, withholding or underdosing antipsychotic medication may reduce prenatal care and increase the risk of obstetric complications. The postpartum period, a high-risk time for developing an exacerbation of schizophrenia, may contribute to parenting difficulties. Additionally, discontinuing and then resuming antipsychotics can increase the risk of tardive dyskinesia and adversely affect long-term morbidity from schizophrenia.

While no antipsychotic medications to date are approved by the U.S. Food and Drug Administration (FDA) for use during pregnancy, understanding pregnancy-related advantages and disadvantages of commonly used antipsychotic medications allows for optimal prescribing. Relevant data are summarized below and may also be found in Table 45.1.

First-generation antipsychotic agents (FGAs) have been relatively well studied during pregnancy due to decades of use. Haloperidol used to be a common treatment for excessive nausea and vomiting during pregnancy in nonpsychotic women. Studies have shown no increased risk of congenital anomalies in offspring after *in utero* haloperidol exposure. Other high-potency FGAs, such as trifluoperazine and fluphenazine, have been less systematically studied, but available data do not show increased risk of physical anomalies in exposed offspring. By contrast, low-potency FGAs such as chlorpromazine have been found to increase the risk of physical anomalies nonspecifically after *in utero* exposure. This may result from decreased placental perfusion due to the orthostatic hypotension that is a relatively common side effect of these agents.

Haloperidol does not appear to increase the risk of cognitive or neurodevelopmental problems in children exposed *in utero*. However, some data show that children exposed

TABLE 45.1. Antipsychotic Medications in Pregnancy

Medication	Advantages	Disadvantages	Metabolic change
Aripiprazole	• No weight gain • No diabetes risk • Less sedation	• Lack of systematic study	CYP450 3A4, CYP450 2D6 increased; may need dose increase
Clozapine	• Highly effective	• Risk of weight gain • Risk of diabetes • Risk of sedation • Lower seizure threshold • Risk of agranulocytosis • Accumulates in fetus • Accumulates in breast-feeding baby	Variable, but CYP450 1A2 (predominant enzyme) decreased; may need dose decrease
Haloperidol	• Relatively well studied • No increased risk of physical anomalies • No adverse effects on neurodevelopment	• Elevated prolactin can decrease fertility	CYP450 3A4 increased; may need dose increase
Olanzapine	• No increased risk of physical anomalies	• Risk of weight gain • Risk of diabetes • Risk of sedation	CYP450 1A2 decreased; may need dose decrease
Risperidone	• No increased risk of physical anomalies • Less sedation	• Elevated prolactin can decrease fertility	CYP450 2D6 increased; may need dose increase
Quetiapine	• No morphological teratogenicity	• Risk of sedation	CYP450 3A4 increased; may need dose increase
Ziprasidone	• No weight gain • diabetes risk • Less sedation		CYP450 3A4 increased; may need dose increase

to haloperidol *in utero* are taller and/or heavier than comparable nonexposed children. This suggests that haloperidol may have an enduring effect on fetal dopaminergic systems that affect growth hormone and/or appetite.

FGAs may cause extrapyramidal side effects (EPS). Relatively low calcium may increase the risk of EPS, perhaps due to effects at the neuromuscular junction. Pregnancy is a time of relatively high calcium need, and women whose diets do not contain enough calcium may be at heightened risk of EPS during pregnancy.

Rarely, newborns can also experience a form of EPS after prolonged exposure to FGAs during pregnancy. This is posited to be withdrawal dyskinesia. Signs can include tremor, hand posturing, jerky eye movements, a shrill cry, arched back, tongue thrusting, increased tone, and hyperreflexia. These effects begin within hours to days after birth and resolve gradually over several months, with no lasting abnormalities.

Pregnant women and newborns can have side effects related to the anticholinergic properties of FGAs. Constipation can be exacerbated by intestinal slowing during pregnancy. Rarely, intestinal slowing from anticholinergic effects can result in functional intestinal obstruction in newborns. The likelihood of this side effect is increased if the mother also took an anticholinergic agent to treat EPS during the pregnancy.

Haloperidol has not been associated with side effects from exposure during breast feeding. By contrast, more sedating, low-potency FGAs such as chlorpromazine have been observed to cause somnolence in some breast-feeding babies.

As newer agents, *second-generation antipsychotic agents* (SGAs) are less well studied during pregnancy than FGAs. One prospective study compared pregnancy and neonatal outcomes for women taking the SGAs olanzapine, risperidone, quetiapine, and clozapine, and for demographically comparable women who were taking medications known not to be teratogenic. There was no significant difference in rates of malformations, reported labor complications, or mean gestational age between exposed and comparison infants.

The SGA side effects posing the highest risk during pregnancy are obesity and diabetes. Obesity during pregnancy increases the risk of hypertension, preeclampsia, neural tube defects, and need for caesarean section. Infants born to mothers with obesity have a higher risk of macrosomia or low birthweight. Gestational diabetes doubles the rate of spontaneous abortion and increases the rate of birth defects by three- to fourfold. Weight gain and increased risk of diabetes are particularly pronounced for clozapine and olanzapine. Weight gain can also occur with risperidone and quetiapine; data about whether these agents increase diabetes risk are equivocal. Ziprasidone and aripiprazole are usually weight-neutral and do not appear to increase the risk of diabetes.

A prospective, comparative study of SGAs in human pregnancy indicated that women taking quetiapine during pregnancy had significantly higher body mass indices (BMIs) than pregnant women not taking psychotropic medication. No significant differences in BMI were found between pregnant women taking olanzapine and comparison pregnant women taking no psychotropic medication. Although there are case reports of new-onset or worsening gestational diabetes in women taking clozapine during pregnancy, a prospective study indicated no significant difference in rates of diabetes, hypertension, or caesarean section between pregnant women taking SGAs and pregnant women taking no psychotropic agents.

Postpartum, sedation is an especially problematic medication side effect. Some women report being unable to awaken to their babies' cries due to altered sleep quality from antipsychotic medication. Others report that medication-induced sedation saps the energy they need for parenting. Clozapine, quetiapine, and olanzapine have higher reported rates of sedation than risperidone, ziprasidone, and aripiprazole.

Few data are available regarding exposure of breast-feeding infants to SGAs. Some breast-feeding babies whose mothers were taking olanzapine were noted to have sedation, poor suck reflex, jaundice, shaking, diarrhea, sleep problems, tongue protrusion, cardiomegaly, and heart murmur. However, no causal connection was established. Clozapine, which is highly lipophilic, is found in relatively high concentrations in breast milk and can accumulate in breast-feeding babies.

Dosing Strategies during Pregnancy

Pregnancy affects medication absorption, distribution, and metabolism. The most significant change appears to be effects on hepatic cytochrome P450 (CYP450) systems. Pregnancy increases the activity of CYP450 3A4 and 2D6. Most antipsychotic agents are predominantly metabolized by CYP450 3A4 (aripiprazole, haloperidol, quetiapine, and ziprasidone) and/or CYP450 2D6 (aripiprazole and risperidone). Pregnancy may therefore lower the levels of each of these medications at a given dose. Breakthrough symptoms may necessitate a dose increase. By contrast, pregnancy decreases the activity of CYP450 1A2, the primary metabolizer of olanzapine and clozapine. At a given dose, these medications may have higher levels in the pregnant than in the nonpregnant state, resulting in additional side effects.

Guidelines for Prescribing Antipsychotic Medication before, during, and after Pregnancy

Preconception

- Incorporate discussions of family planning into discussions about pharmacotherapy.
- For patients attempting to become pregnant:
  - Consider medications that do not elevate prolactin levels.
  - Choose a medication regimen with an optimal benefit–risk ratio during pregnancy.

During Pregnancy

- When possible, choose medications that have been studied in human pregnancy and have not been found to increase risk of congenital anomalies in offspring.
- Adjust doses as needed when pharmacokinetic changes lead to altered reactions (e.g., less therapeutic effect and/or more side effects) at a given dose.
- Encourage use of prenatal vitamins with calcium; this may decrease risk for EPS.
- Do not use routine anticholinergic medication prophylaxis for EPS.
- Communicate with the patient's obstetrician about careful blood sugar monitoring and glucose tolerance tests when prescribing agents that increase the risk of diabetes.

Postpartum

- Inquire about sedative effects and effects on sleep depth, including the mother's ability to awaken to her baby's cries.
- Readjust doses as needed as pharmacokinetics return to the prepregnancy state.
- If a breast-feeding infant shows possible side effects, confer with the pediatrician and check infant serum levels of the medication and any active metabolites.

Psychosocial Rehabilitation and Other Supports for Parents

Along with medication, the other cornerstone of effective treatment for schizophrenia is psychosocial rehabilitation. For mothers with schizophrenia, this can encompass interventions to enhance parenting capability. Assessing parenting strengths, challenges, resources, and goals can identify targets for intervention.

Comprehensive *parenting assessment* includes the following elements: (1) parent interview that includes specific questions to elicit effects of symptoms on parenting perceptions and behaviors, and parental report of strengths, challenges, resources, and goals; (2) direct observation of the parent with the child, either informally or using systematic assessments, such as the Crittenden Index; (3) an assessment of the parent's insight into the psychiatric disorder; (4) assessment of the parent's understanding of her or his child's capabilities at different stages of development (e.g., the Parent Opinion Questionnaire); and (5) assessment of available social support and resources, informal and formal.

There are no evidence-based parenting interventions specifically for adults with schizophrenia. However, interpersonal skills-building interventions with demonstrated efficacy have been adapted for use in parents with schizophrenia. Additional guidance for useful intervention comes from studies of parents themselves, in which they identify peer supports, parent skills training, respite services, and supports for children as especially helpful.

A U.S. survey identified approximately 20 programs specifically developed for parents with mental illness (Hinden, Biebel, Nicholson, Henry, & Katz-Leavy, 2006), repesenting a variety of theoretical frameworks and treatment approaches, from a residential rehabilitation model with on-site family services and supports, to a therapeutic nursery program with support services for parents, to hospital-based inpatient and clinic services, to community-based comprehensive case management services. Interventions offered by these programs may include:

- *Parenting classes.* These are didactic sessions in which parents can learn basic knowledge about parenting (e.g., child nutrition, sleep patterns, behavior shaping, and developmental norms).
- *Parenting coaching.* In this form of dyadic or family therapy, a therapist, or coach, teaches parenting skills directly to parents. Techniques can include the coach "speaking" for a nonverbal child to help train parents to understand nonverbal cues, role modeling effective parenting behaviors with the parent practicing them, or praising effective behaviors that parents exhibit naturally, so as to encourage and further develop those strengths.
- *Parent support groups.* Parents may be encouraged to give each other parenting tips, to role-model effective behaviors for one another, and to problem-solve together to overcome obstacles to effective parenting.
- *Coparenting support.* A relative or friend may serve as a coparent, with specific delineation of roles for the parent and the coparent with respect to the child and to each other. Such arrangements may include plans for progressive assumption of the parenting role by the parent as rehabilitation proceeds.

Using Existing Treatment Resources to Support Parents

Adults who do not have access to specific programs for parents with SMI can benefit from the adaptation of existing resources to support parental functioning. Evidence-based psychosocial interventions for adults with mental illness, though not specifically tested with parents with schizophrenia, suggest strategies that may prove effective. For example, assertive community treatment (ACT) services can address parenting as a role domain, and help to build skills and access resources. Family psychoeducation programs can address the education and communication needs of parents with schizophrenia and their children. Skills training interventions for adults with mental illness can be adapted to include parent skills training. Symptom self-management strategies can be modified to take the sometimes competing demands of parenting into consideration.

Barriers to Treatment for Parents with Schizophrenia and Their Families

Parenting responsibilities may compromise treatment adherence by either interfering with appointments with providers or thwarting compliance with treatment recommendations (e.g., medications and hospitalization). For example, parents may not take medications that make them lethargic in the morning if they must prepare breakfast and get children ready for school. Mothers with SMI may delay hospitalizations if they have no child care. Consequently, parents may be labeled "treatment resistant" or "noncompliant" by providers or family members when they are in fact choosing to prioritize what they perceive as the demands of parenthood.

Many treatment settings are not designed to encourage or support family contact. Clinic reception areas may not be child-friendly; treatment settings may not be able to provide safe space for children to wait while parents are receiving treatment. Inpatient settings are not likely to have appropriate space or resources (e.g., toys or games for children to use while visiting with hospitalized parents).

The impact of stigma is pervasive; providers themselves may have negative perceptions of parents with schizophrenia. They may not ask adult clients about reproductive goals, status, or responsibilities as parents. Clients who are parents may be sensitive to providers' disapproval and withhold information about their children.

KEY POINTS

- Incorporate questions about goals, strengths, and needs related to parenting and family life within comprehensive assessments of adults with schizophrenia (e.g., whether they are thinking about becoming parents, actively caring for children, or living apart from children).
- Conduct a parenting assessment and use the findings to guide an intervention strategy to promote parenting capability and to minimize the risk of emotional, social, and behavioral problems in the children. Interventions may range from simple suggestions (e.g., advice to parents about how to communicate with their children about their illness) to formal parenting rehabilitation strategies.
- Assess parents' medication regimens in terms of their effects on pregnancy and parenting, and modify medication to support parenting goals optimally.
- Assess the need for concrete material supports for parents with schizophrenia, including access to benefits and entitlements, and so forth, and refer to family-centered case management services, if available.
- Identify ways to expand the formal and informal support networks of parents with schizophrenia and their children when needed.
- Identify and eliminate barriers to treatment for parents with schizophrenia.
- Help families plan prospectively for meeting the needs of children in case of relapse of parental illness, and identify alternative caregivers and supports.

REFERENCES AND RECOMMENDED READINGS

Professional References

Bosanac, P., Buist, A., & Burrows, G. (2003). Motherhood and schizophrenic illnesses: A review of the literature. *Australian and New Zealand Journal of Psychiatry, 37,* 24–30.

Caton, C. L. M., Cournos, R., & Boanerges, D. (1999). Parenting and adjustment in schizophrenia. *Psychiatric Services, 50,* 239–243.

Cowling, V. (Ed.). (1999). *Children of parents with mental illness.* Melbourne: Australian Council for Educional Research Press.

Cowling, V. (Ed.). (2004) *Children of parents with mental illness: Personal and clinical perspectives* (Vol. 2). Melbourne: Australian Council for Educational Research Press.

Craig, T., & Bromet, E. J. (2004). Parents with psychosis. *Annals of Clinical Psychiatry, 16,* 35–39.

Dickerson, F. B., Brown, C. H., Kreyenbuhl, J., Goldberg, R. W., Fang, L. J., & Dixon, L. B. (2004). Sexual and reproductive behaviors among persons with mental illness. *Psychiatric Services, 55,* 1299–1301.

Gentile, S. (2004). Clinical utilization of atypical antipsychotics in pregnancy and lactation. *Annals of Pharmacotherapy, 38,* 1266–1271.

Gopfert, M., Webster, J., & Seeman, M. V. (Eds.). (2004). *Parental psychiatric disorder: Distressed parents and their families* (2nd ed.). Cambridge, UK: Cambridge University Press.

Hinden, B., Biebel, K., Nicholson, J., Henry, A., & Katz-Leavy, J. (2006). A. survey of programs for parents with mental illness and their families: Identifying common elements to build the evidence base. *Journal of Behavioral Health Services and Research, 33,* 21–38.

Jablensky, A. V., Morgan, V., Zubrick, S. R., Bower, C., & Yellachich, A. (2005). Pregnancy, delivery, and neonatal complications in a population cohort of women with schizophrenia and major affective disorders. *American Journal of Psychiatry, 162,* 79–91.

McKenna, K., Koren, G., Tetelbaum, M., Wilton, L., Shakir, S., Diav-Citrin, O., et al. (2005). Pregnancy outcome of women using atypical antipsychotic drugs: a prospective comparative study. *Journal of Clinical Psychiatry, 66,* 444–449.

Miller, L. J. (1997). Sexuality, reproduction, and family planning in women with schizophrenia. *Schizophrenia Bulletin, 23,* 623–635.

Nicholson, J., Biebel, K., Katz-Leavy, J., & Williams, V. (2004). The prevalence of parenthood in adults with mental illness: Implications for state and federal policymakers, programs, and providers. In M. J. Henderson & R. W. Manderscheid (Eds.), *Mental health, United States, 2002.* Rockville, MD: U.S. Department of Health and Human Services, Substance Abuse and Mental Health Services Administration, Center for Mental Health Services.

Nicholson, J., & Henry, A. D. (2003). Achieving the goal of evidence-based psychiatric rehabilitation practices for mothers with mental illnesses. *Psychiatric Rehabilitation Journal, 27*(2), 122–130.

Resources for Families

Australian Infant, Child, Adolescent and Family Mental Health Association, Ltd. (2004). *Family talk: Tips and information for families where a parent has a mental health problem or disorder* and *The best for me and my baby: Managing mental health during pregnancy and early parenthood.* Available on AICAFMHA website for Children of Parents with a Mental Illness, an Australian Government initiative. Retrieved September 14, 2007, at *http://www.copmi.net.au/files/Family Talk_final.pdf*

Chovil, N. (2004). *Understanding mental illness in your family: For children who have a parent with schizophrenia.* (Available from the British Columbia Schizophrenia Society, 201-6011 Westminster Hwy., Richmond, BC V7C 4V4)

Internet Resources

Children of Parents with a Mental Illness National Resource Centre: *www.copmi.net.au*
National Alliance on Mental Illness: *www.nami.org*
National Mental Health Association: *www.nhma.org*
Parenting Well: *www.parentingwell.info*

CHAPTER 46

CHILDREN AND ADOLESCENTS

JOHN G. COTTONE
SANJIV KUMRA

Schizophrenia is considered to be a major contributor to the "global burden of disease," particularly for adolescents and young adults. Perhaps not surprising, some data suggest that functional outcome may be worse when the onset of the disorder occurs during childhood and adolescence. There is increasing evidence that a number of adverse environmental exposures may increase risk for the development of schizophrenia in genetically vulnerable adolescents, and that the origins of schizophrenia may be detected in early childhood. It has now become well established that schizophrenia can be diagnosed in children with the same criteria as those described in DSM-IV-TR (American Psychiatric Association, 2000) for adults. Also, though autism and schizophrenia are separate disorders, they share symptom overlap of disturbances in social-cognitive development.

This chapter is divided into two parts. The first part focuses on the clinical and neurobiological aspects of early-onset psychotic disorders, and the second part focuses on the general principles of treatment, with special attention to the latest developments in research since the publication of "Schizophrenia and Other Psychotic Disorders" (Tsai & Champine, 2004). The reader is referred to this chapter and to other sources (see References and Recommended Readings) for additional information regarding the care of children and adolescents with psychotic disorders.

CLINICAL AND NEUROBIOLOGICAL ASPECTS OF EARLY-ONSET PSYCHOTIC DISORDERS

Onset of schizophrenia before age 12, which is exceedingly rare, has usually been referred to as childhood-onset schizophrenia (COS). In contrast, the incidence of the disorder sharply increases after puberty, and when schizophrenia occurs before age 18 it is referred to as early-onset schizophrenia (EOS). The assessment of a child or adolescent with possible psychosis involves obtaining a careful history and assessment of mental status over multiple sessions.

Prior to the onset of psychotic symptoms, children may present with nonspecific symptoms suggestive of pervasive development disorder, learning disabilities, oppositional behavior/violent aggression, and attentional dysfunction. Regarding the latter, because high doses of stimulant medications have been shown to induce psychotic symptoms in normal individuals, and low doses can induce psychotogenic symptoms in individuals susceptible to psychosis, physicians should be extremely cautious when prescribing these medications for children with attentional deficits who may also be vulnerable to psychosis. Premorbid abnormalities, similar to those noted earlier, have been observed in patients with adult-onset schizophrenia. However, the rate of language impairments and transient, autistic-like symptoms appears higher in children and adolescents with schizophrenia relative to their adult counterparts, potentially suggesting that a more disturbed neurodevelopmental course is associated with an earlier onset of schizophrenia.

The few studies to examine the phenomenology of COS using DSM-III (American Psychiatric Association, 1980) criteria have supported a hypothesis of phenomenological continuity with later-onset schizophrenia. Schizophrenia in children is frequently insidious rather than acute in onset, and the most common psychotic features reported by patients are developmentally appropriate auditory hallucinations and delusions. The presence of formal thought disorder, however, is more variable and depends on the sample, and there is little agreement on how to describe the disorganized speech patterns of children with schizophrenia, because terms such as *illogicality*, *loose associations*, *tangentiality*, and *speech poverty* have been used very differently by different clinicians. Medication status at time of assessment is important to note, because both psychotic and affective symptoms may be masked by the administration of psychotropic medications, and patients may not experience a relapse of their symptomatology immediately after discontinuation of their medications. Additionally, collateral data, such as reports from other specialists consulted (e.g., school reports, previous neuropsychological test data, speech and language evaluations, and neurological and genetics consultations), should be obtained. To prevent misdiagnosis, each child or adolescent with a diagnosis of schizophrenia should be followed closely for several years, and a medication-free period, if feasible, should be considered to help clarify diagnosis.

There is a requirement in DSM-IV-TR that the signs of a psychotic disturbance must be present for at least 6 months, with at least 1 month of active-phase psychotic symptoms (fewer, if successfully treated). The 6-month duration may include periods of prodromal or residual symptoms. In community settings there is typically a lag of approximately 2 years from the time that psychotic symptoms first manifest to the time that children and adolescents with schizophrenia first present for psychiatric treatment. Objective evidence of deterioration in function for a child might include a need for psychiatric hospitalization or day treatment, as well as worsening grades in school and/or placement in special education classes due to behavior problems.

In terms of differential diagnosis, it should be stressed that hallucinations and delusions are commonly observed in patients with affective psychoses and pervasive developmental disorders, and the prevalence of these disorders is far more common than COS from an epidemiological perspective. A number of children with pervasive developmental disorders report psychotic symptoms; however, this group typically does not exhibit marked deterioration in social or school functioning for a sufficient amount of time coincident with the onset of psychotic symptoms to warrant an additional diagnosis of schizophrenia. Psychosis due to a general medical condition, medication, or illicit drug use should always be ruled out with a careful history, physical examination, and appropriate laboratory testing. There has been increasing awareness that cannabis use prior to the age of 15 may be associated with early onset of schizophrenia, but whether this usage is involved in the etiopathogenesis of the disorder remains a topic of future research. In such cases, it may be very important to clarify whether the usage of cannabis preceded the onset of psychotic symptoms, because many adolescents may attempt to self-medicate with cannabis.

Also, for a diagnosis of schizophrenia, a careful assessment of affective symptoms is necessary to rule out mood disorders and schizoaffective disorder, because adolescents with bipolar disorder frequently present with psychotic symptoms, and many young children with severe affective disturbances and transient psychotic symptoms develop classic symptoms of bipolar disorder as they mature into adulthood.

Last, isolated "psychotic-like" symptoms may be elicited from children with conduct disorder, posttraumatic stress disorder, and obsessive–compulsive disorder in the context of intact reality testing and preservation of social relatedness.

Children with Psychotic Disorder Not Otherwise Specified

A considerably large group of children with complex developmental disorders and brief "psychotic" symptoms fall outside of current syndrome boundaries, and these children have provisionally been labeled as having borderline or schizoid personality disorder, multiplex developmental disorder (MDD), and multidimensional impairment syndrome to emphasize the developmental nature of their difficulties and phenomenological similarities to children with schizophrenia.

As a group these children are characterized as having brief psychotic symptoms that do not meet the psychotic symptom severity or duration criteria for a diagnosis of schizophrenia. Typically, it is their prominent attention and impulse control difficulties that trigger a request for psychiatric assessment and services. These children are typically males and frequently have comorbid language and learning disabilities, poor interpersonal skills, and increased rates of schizophrenia spectrum disorders in first-degree relatives and sex chromosome aneuploidies compared to children in both the general population and the population with mild mental retardation.

Neurocognitive Function

Neuropsychological assessment cannot be used for diagnostic purposes at present, but it may assist in treatment planning and school placement after a child has been clinically stabilized with antipsychotic medications following an acute episode of psychosis. Adolescents with EOS have been found to have generalized neurocognitive deficits between 1.5 and 2.0 standard deviations below those of healthy children. These cognitive deficits most likely lead to academic impairments and social dysfunction, which may manifest as early as first grade. Although a generalized pattern of neurocognitive deficits has typically been reported in most studies of children and adolescents with schizophrenia, deficits in attention, executive function, and motor skills appear relatively more pronounced compared to other neurocognitive domains, such as language.

Within the realm of executive functioning, decision making may represent an area of specific disability for adolescents with EOS. Similar to adults with substance use disorders, adolescents with EOS have been shown to be hypersensitive to rewards and relatively insensitive to future consequences on tasks assessing complex decision-making skills. Executive function impairments may also play a role in the verbal learning and memory deficits reported for this clinical group. Adolescents with EOS show similar dysfunction to that of their adult-onset schizophrenia (AOS) counterparts in verbal learning and memory skills, and more widespread dysfunction than adolescents with bipolar disorder. In healthy adolescents there is a developmental transition from the use of less efficient strategies to facilitate verbal encoding (i.e., rote rehearsal) in early adolescence to the use of more efficient strategies (i.e., semantic organization) by late adolescence, and there is evidence that this transition may not occur as robustly in adolescents with EOS. Overall, these data suggest a pattern of abnormal frontal lobe development in adolescents with schizophrenia.

In adolescents with schizophrenia, there is some evidence for a steep decline in IQ around the time of onset of psychosis, with relative stabilization in cognitive function thereafter. From a clinical point of view, it should be reiterated that none of the currently described neurobiological or neuropsychological deficits in children and adolescents with schizophrenia are diagnostic at this point. Thus, the primary role for laboratory tests and neuroimaging studies in the assessment and diagnosis of children and adolescents with schizophrenia is to rule out other medical disorders.

Neurobiological Features

In the absence of a specific indication based on history or physical examination, most clinical magnetic resonance imaging (MRI) scans for children and adolescents with schizophrenia are typically read as "normal" by radiologists. However, several lines of evidence suggest that ongoing changes in cortical gray and white matter in healthy adolescents may provide the basis for ongoing cognitive development during this time period. Because genetic studies of schizophrenia have identified disruptions in genes involved in myelin formation, development, and repair—all of which may be disrupted in the pathogenesis of schizophrenia—new research protocols using MRI techniques (i.e., diffusion tensor imaging [DTI]), have provided an opportunity to study white matter development *in vivo* in adolescents with schizophrenia. Using both a region-of-interest and voxel-based methodologies, abnormalities in white matter integrity have been identified in adolescents with schizophrenia. Additional studies are needed to describe the stability and functional importance of these structural abnormalities.

Family Studies and Cytogenetic Abnormalities

Neuropsychological data indicate that healthy first-degree relatives of COS probands perform more poorly than controls on measures of oculomotor–psychomotor speed, working memory, and executive function. Similarly, smooth pursuit eye-tracking dysfunction (ETD), one of the most well-replicated biological markers of schizophrenia, is significantly more common in parents of COS and AOS probands. Together, these findings suggest that neuropsychological and neurobiological assessments of first-degree relatives can shed light on markers that may be part of the endophenotypic profile of children at risk for COS/EOS.

There appears to be a high rate (5.3%) of cytogenetic abnormalities in children and adolescents with schizophrenia, particularly for 22q11 deletion or velocardiofacial syndrome, compared to what is found in the community and the 0.46% rate found in adults with schizophrenia. The role of 22q11 in the etiopathogenesis of schizophrenia remains unclear, because a high-density mapping of the 22q11 region did not indicate that one or more important genes implicated in schizophrenia lie within this deleted region.

TREATMENT PRINCIPLES

In adult patients with schizophrenia, psychoeducational interventions aimed at improving awareness of the illness and the need for medication, family function, problem solving, and communication skills have been shown to decrease relapse rates in conjunction with good pharmacological treatment. In adolescents with early prodromal features of the illness, some experts have argued that psychosocial and educational interventions should be the first line of treatment, because the natural history and diagnostic stability of these prodromal symptoms in adolescents has not been established.

Similar to adults, children and adolescents with schizophrenia and related psychotic disorders also appear to benefit from a combined treatment approach, including medication and psychosocial interventions. The development of a treatment plan requires the consideration of many issues, including current clinical status, cognitive level, developmental stage, and severity of illness. Individual educational plans need to be developed for each child in accordance with his or her specific needs, as assessed by a multidisciplinary team. The general principles of the care of children and adolescents with psychotic disorders include (1) establishing a supportive therapeutic relationship with the patient and family; (2) providing education to the patient and family as to the nature of the child's illness, prognosis, and treatment, as well as how to recognize changes in mood, behavior, or thought processes that may be indicative of clinical deterioration, so that adequate treatment can be provided quickly; and (3) increasing understanding of and adaptation to the disorder by helping patients cope with their environments by improving family relationships and communication skills, teaching personal safety, reviewing educational plans, advocating for special rehabilitative services, accessing appropriate medical care, and securing disability income support when appropriate.

Pharmacological Treatments

Since 1996, there has been a substantial increase in the number of prescriptions for antipsychotic medications, predominantly for children with severe emotional disturbances. Although substantial, well-designed clinical trial data support the use of antipsychotics in adult patients with schizophrenia, few studies have included pediatric patients (under age 18). Thus, most of the currently available evidence to support the use of these medications in children has been based on open-label studies in small groups of patients and case reports, and should be considered preliminary. Therefore, the general lack of controlled clinical trials and outcome data in children with schizophrenia spectrum disorders has precluded the development of evidence-based treatment guidelines. However, several multisite, industry-sponsored and National Institute of Mental Health (NIMH)–funded controlled trials of antipsychotic medications are currently under way, and the results should be available shortly. Nevertheless, apart from differences in side effects and dosing, treatment efficacy appears to be similar in both adult and pediatric patients. Short-term efficacy has generally been measured by reductions in positive or negative symptoms among treated patients during 4- to 8-week medication trials. An advantage is that these studies clearly demonstrate how well a medication can reduce target symptoms; however, what remains less clear is whether short-term symptomatic improvement will lead to improvements in functional outcome and prevention of future relapse.

In assessing treatment effects and outcomes, there has been an increased push for clinicians to incorporate standardized symptom and behavior rating scales with proven reliability and validity to measure the severity and frequency of target symptoms before treatments are initiated, at regular intervals during treatment, and during acute episodes and when treatments are changed or discontinued. All antipsychotic drugs are indicated for the acute and preventive treatment of psychotic episodes, but no curative treatment for psychotic disorders is currently available. Because the onset of clinically meaningful therapeutic effects of neuroleptics may take several weeks, high-dose trials and antipsychotic polypharmacy should be avoided except in unusual cases in which clear documentation of symptom ratings demonstrates the need for such practices. In this regard, before switching, augmenting, combining, or discontinuing antipsychotic medications because of lack of response or partial response, physicians should ensure that patients have received adequate trials of medication, as well as psychosocial intervention.

Pretreatment Screening

For all new cases, clinicians should review the results of, or conduct, a comprehensive psychiatric diagnostic interview with the patients and parent(s)/guardian(s) before prescribing, changing, or discontinuing medication. In addition, a detailed medical workup that includes the following measures and tests should be considered: (1) measurement of height and weight to allow for calculation of body mass index; (2) neurological examination for tics, stereotypies, extrapyramidal disorders, and tardive dyskinesia; (3) baseline laboratory evaluations (e.g., thyroid function tests, screen for toxic substances, pregnancy test, serum ceruloplasmin, erythrocyte sedimentation rate, antinuclear factor, complete blood count, urinalysis, renal function tests, and liver function tests); (4) MRI scan of the brain; (5) electroencephalogram; (6) karyotype and molecular fragile X analysis; (7) cerebrospinal fluid analysis (as clinically indicated, especially for acute-onset cases); and (8) genetics examinations (necessary to exclude known medical causes of psychotic disorders in childhood).

Conventional Antipsychotic Medications

Though psychiatrists have been prescribing typical neuroleptics (e.g., haloperidol, thiothixene, and loxapine) with less frequency, they are still considered to be acceptable first-line treatments for children with psychotic disorders under certain circumstances. The selection of an antipsychotic medication is frequently guided by past response, family history of response, cost, and the patient's tolerance of side effects. Two controlled trials support the use of typical neuroleptics in children and adolescents with schizophrenia. The major limitations of conventional antipsychotic drugs in patients with COS include inadequate treatment response, lack of efficacy against negative symptoms, galactorrhea, gynecomastia, excessive weight gain, sedation, and neurological side effects, particularly treatment-emergent dyskinesias.

Second-Generation Antipsychotics

As a class, second-generation antipsychotics (e.g., clozapine, risperidone, olanzapine, ziprasidone, quetiapine) are linked by characteristic binding profiles to dopamine and serotonin receptors that differentiate these drugs from conventional antipsychotics. Because of their lesser propensity to induce extrapyramidal side effects as a class, there was initially considerable enthusiasm about the introduction of second-generation antipsychotics; however, a recent large-scale study found that intolerable metabolic side effects, severe weight gain, and other adverse effects resulted in treatment discontinuation within the first 18 months in 74% of adult patients who were prescribed these medications.

Also, the therapeutic benefits of the second-generation medications relative to conventional antipsychotics appeared much smaller than what would have been assumed from the initial industry-sponsored studies.

To date, most of the clinical data to support the use of second-generation antipsychotics in children and adolescents with schizophrenia have been derived from studies of clozapine, olanzapine, and risperidone. In comparison, no systematically collected data regarding the use of ziprasidone, aripiprazole, and quetiapine in children and adolescents with schizophrenia spectrum disorders have demonstrated either the safety or efficacy of these medications in this population.

The best of the available published data supporting the use of second-generation antipsychotics are for clozapine, the first drug with convincing data that show it is superior to other conventional (e.g., haloperidol) and second-generation antipsychotics (e.g., high-dose olanzapine) in the treatment of adolescents with treatment-refractory schizophrenia. In accord with these data, naturalistic studies have found that clozapine is effective in reducing the frequency of aggressive behaviors in youth with schizophrenia, and that the rate of serious hematological disturbances, such as agranulocytosis, does not appear to be higher in children and adolescents compared to adults.

In addition to clozapine, risperidone and olanzapine have demonstrated efficacy comparable to, if not exceeding, that of haloperidol in a recent randomized, double-blind trial with adolescents. Unfortunately, recent evidence suggests that weight gain and extrapyramidal side effects may be more prevalent and severe for youth than for adults treated with risperidone and olanzapine.

Despite the lack of evidence supporting the use of the other second-generation antipsychotic agents, based on expert opinion and current community standards, aripiprazole, olanzapine, quetiapine, and risperidone are all considered acceptable first-line agents for pediatric patients with psychoses. If patients fail to respond to an adequate trial (dose and duration) of an initial atypical antipsychotic, physicians should first reassess the diagnosis to rule out the presence of a comorbid condition that may be contributing to the poor clinical response. For example, after the resolution of psychotic symptoms, underlying affective symptoms and/or attentional impairments that may become evident might be effectively treated with a mood stabilizer or antidepressant. If failure to respond to an initial treatment does not appear to be due to a secondary or comorbid condition, monotherapy with a different atypical antipsychotic should be tried (Pappadopulos et al., 2003); however, a clozapine trial should be attempted only after two adequate antipsychotic drug trials. Due to the comparative lack of published safety data, limited use of clozapine in pediatric populations, and risk for agranulocytosis, clozapine should be considered as a second-line agent at the present time.

Polypharmacy in young children, particularly in those who are poor treatment responders, has become a major problem. It has been suggested that if patients have not shown meaningful responses to multiple psychotropic medications administered in combination, then physicians should reexamine the diagnoses and consider tapering and discontinuing one or more medications.

Weight gain has emerged as the major adverse side effect associated with second-generation antipsychotics in adolescents, particularly for clozapine, olanzapine, and risperidone. Although diet, exercise, and behavioral treatments are the most commonly recommended strategies for preventing and treating atypical antipsychotic–induced weight gain in adults with schizophrenia, the use of these strategies has not been systematically examined in controlled studies of youth with schizophrenia, and such strategies may not be feasible during the acute phase of treatment, when a substantial portion of weight gain is likely to occur. Also, there has been increasing recognition that both olanzapine and clozapine treatment may be associated with hyperglycemia, hyperlipidemia, and diabetes among youth. Isolated reports have described hepatic side effects associated with long-term risperidone treatment secondary to excessive weight gain, suggesting the need for baseline liver function tests, careful monitoring of weight, and periodic monitoring of liver function tests during the maintenance phase of therapy.

At relatively higher doses (> 4 mg/day) extrapyramidal side effects may be problematic for some youth treated with risperidone. The risk of tardive dyskinesia with use of second-generation antipsychotics in children and adolescents is presently unknown, but it is probably less than the rates associated with traditional neuroleptics. Other problematic side effects associated with second-generation antipsychotics, particularly risperidone, include increased prolactin secretion and galactorrhea.

Although there are some safety data regarding QTc prolongation in exposing children with tic disorders to ziprasidone, these data did not include patients exposed to typical doses used for children with schizophrenia (i.e., 120–160 mg/day). To date, no reported cases of torsade de pointes have been associated with ziprasidone usage, and the clinical significance of its electrocardiographic (ECG) changes remains unclear. Thus, the side effects of ziprasidone in youth need further investigation.

Maintenance Phase of Treatment

There are no available systematic data to guide the long-term treatment of adolescents with schizophrenia. In general, the goals of the maintenance phase are to minimize stress on the patient, to provide support to minimize the likelihood of relapse, to empower parents to be strong advocates for their children, and to integrate the children back into their environments. It is important to leave no gaps in service delivery, because many patients are vulnerable to relapse and need support in readjusting to their home communities. In addition, because relapses are part of the expected course of the illness, provision should be made for respite and wraparound services. With this extra support, patients can often be cared for effectively and safely in a less restrictive setting.

After completion of an 8-week antipsychotic treatment trial, many patients remain symptomatic; thus, slow titration of their medication upward to find their optimal dose and/or the addition of adjunctive agents for symptom control (e.g., valproic acid, lithium carbonate, and lorazepam) may be required. After the resolution of an acute psychotic episode, both depressive symptoms and/or persistent negative symptoms may be problematic.

In adult patients with schizophrenia it has been suggested that medication discontinuation can be considered for individuals with multiple prior episodes of schizophrenia who have no positive symptoms and who have been stable for 5 years and are compliant with treatment. If discontinuation of antipsychotic medication is attempted, additional precautions—such as gradual dose reduction over several months, more frequent visits, and rapid resumption of medication when schizophrenic symptoms appear—should be instituted.

The clinical utility of measuring plasma concentrations of antipsychotic drugs in children and adolescents remains uncertain. As in adults, pharmacokinetic processes in children and adolescents vary from individual to individual and may be variable within the same individual. The half-life of psychotropic drugs in children and adolescents is often unknown. Plasma drug levels can identify patients with low plasma levels who are noncompliant, nonresponders, or rapid metabolizers, or aid in the differential diagnosis of patients with high plasma levels and drug toxicity.

KEY POINTS

- Functional outcome in schizophrenia may be worse when the onset of the disorder occurs during childhood and adolescence.
- Prior to the onset of psychotic symptoms, children may present with nonspecific symptoms suggestive of pervasive development disorder, learning disabilities, oppositional behavior/violent aggression, and attentional dysfunction.
- Generalized neurocognitive performance for children–adolescents with schizophrenia is between 1.5 and 2.0 standard deviations below that of healthy children, and may be manifest as early as the first grade.
- Some data suggest a steep decline in IQ around the time of onset of psychosis, with relative stabilization in cognitive function thereafter.
- Before switching, augmenting, combining, or discontinuing antipsychotic medications, physicians should ensure that patients have received adequate trials.
- If patients fail to respond to an adequate trial of an initial atypical antipsychotic, then their diagnosis should be reassessed to rule out a comorbid condition.
- Clozapine has shown superior efficacy over conventional and second-generation antipsychotics in adolescents with treatment-refractory schizophrenia.
- Weight gain has emerged as a major side effect of second-generation antipsychotics in adolescents, particularly for clozapine, olanzapine, and risperidone.
- Very few data are available regarding the potential long-term side effects of all atypical antipsychotics in children.

REFERENCES AND RECOMMENDED READINGS

American Psychiatric Association. (2000). *Diagnostic and statistical manual of mental disorders* (4th ed., rev. text). Washington, DC: Author.

Barnea-Goraly, N., Menon, V., Eckert, M., Tamm, L., Bammer, R., Karchemskiy, A., et al. (2005). White matter development during childhood and adolescence: A cross-sectional diffusion tensor imaging study. *Cerebral Cortex, 15,* 848–1854.

Bilder, R. M., Goldman, R. S., Robinson, D. E., Reiter, G., Bell, L., Bates, J. A., et al. (2000). Neuropsychology of first-episode schizophrenia: Initial characterization and clinical correlates. *American Journal of Psychiatry, 157,* 549–559.

Gerbino-Rosen, G., Roofeh, D., Tompkins, A., Feryo, D., Nusser, L., Kranzeler, H., et al. (2005). Hemotological adverse events in clozapine-treated children and adolescents. *Journal of the American Academy of Child and Adolescent Psychiatry, 44,* 1024–1031.

Kranzler, H., Roofeh, D., Gerbino-Rosen, G., Dombrowski, C., McMeniman, M., DeThomas, C., et al. (2005). Clozapine: Its impact on aggressive behavior among children and adolescents with schizophrenia. *Journal of the American Academy of Child and Adolescent Psychiatry, 44,* 55–63.

Kumra, S., Ashtari, M., Cervellione, K. L., Henderson, I., Kester, H., Roofeh, D., Wu, J., et al. (2005). White matter abnormalities in early-onset schizophrenia: A voxel-based diffusion tensor imaging study. *Journal of the American Academy of Child and Adolescent Psychiatry, 44,* 934–941.

Kumra, S., Ashtari, M., McMeniman, M., Vogel, J., Augustin, R., Becker, D. E., et al. (2004). Reduced frontal white matter integrity in early-onset schizophrenia: A preliminary study. *Biological Psychiatry, 55,* 1138–1145.

Kumra, S., Frazier, J., Jacobson, L. K., McKenna, K., Gordon, C. T., Lenane, M. C., et al. (1996). Childhood-onset schizophrenia: A double-blind clozapine–haloperidol comparison. *Archives of General Psychiatry, 53,* 1090–1097.

Pappadopulos, E., MacIntyre, J. C., II, Crismon, M. L., Findling, R. L., Malone, R. P., Derivan, A., et al. (2003). Treatment recommendations for use of antipsychotics for aggressive youth (TRAAY): Part II. *Journal of the American Academy of Child and Adolescent Psychiatry, 42,* 145–161.

Reichenberg, A., Weiser, M., Rapp, M., Rabinowitz, J., Caspi, A., Schneidler, J., et al. (2005). Elaboration on premorbid intellectual performance in schizophrenia: Premorbid intellectual decline and risk for schizophrenia. *Archives of General Psychiatry, 62,* 1297–1304.

Rhinewine, J. P., Lencz, T., Thaden, E. P., Cervellione, K. L., Burdick, K. E., Henderson, I., et al. (2005). Neurocognitive profile in adolescents with early-onset schizophrenia: Clinical correlates. *Biological Psychiatry, 58,* 705–712.

Sikich, L., Hamer, R. M., Bashford, R. A., Sheitman, B. B., & Lieberman, J. A. (2004). A pilot study of risperidone, olanzapine, and haloperidol in psychotic youth: A double-blind, randomized, 8-week trial. *Neuropsychopharmacology, 29,* 133–145.

Schaeffer, J. L., & Ross, R. G. (2002). Childhood-onset schizophrenia: Premorbid and prodromal diagnostic and treatment histories. *Journal of the American Academy of Child and Adolescent Psychiatry, 41,* 538–545.

Sporn, A. L., Addington, A. M., Gogtay, N., Ordonez, A. E., Gornick, M., Clasen, L., et al. (2004). Pervasive developmental disorder and childhood-onset schizophrenia: Comorbid disorder of a phenotypic variant of a very early onset illness. *Biological Psychiatry, 55,* 989–994.

Tsai, L. Y., & Champine, D. J. (2004). Schizophrenia and other psychotic disorders. In J. M. Wiener & M. K. Dulcan (Eds.), *The American Psychiatric Publishing textbook of child and adolescent psychiatry* (3rd ed.). Washington, DC: American Psychiatric Publishing.

CHAPTER 47

SUICIDE

MARNIN J. HEISEL

Suicide, a leading cause of preventable morbidity and mortality worldwide, accounts for as many as 1 million deaths annually, exceeding the number of fatalities due to homicide and war combined. Suicide leaves in its wake tremendous confusion, pain, and suffering for suicidal individuals and for their families, friends, and care providers. Thus, prevention of suicide is a critical public health imperative. Suicide prevention spans universal, selected, and indicated strategies. *Universal strategies* include population-level initiatives such as national strategies for suicide prevention and programs of means restriction. *Selected strategies* target groups at elevated risk for suicide with mental health promotion efforts such as public health education and community outreach. *Indicated strategies* target individuals imminently at risk for suicide with clinical assessment and intervention initiatives. This chapter provides a brief overview of the epidemiology of suicide in schizophrenia, associated risk and resiliency factors, and mental health assessment and treatment strategies, and concludes with key considerations for clinical care with individuals at elevated risk for suicide.

EPIDEMIOLOGY

Over 30,000 Americans die by suicide annually, accounting for more deaths than homicide and HIV combined. Suicide was the 11th leading cause of death in the United States in 2004, and accounted for more than 1.25 million years of potential life lost before age 85. Mental illness has been implicated in over 90% of suicides in rigorous research studies. A review article assessing suicide risk factors covering a 40-plus-year period reported the presence of mental illness in over 99% of psychiatric inpatients who died by suicide, and in 88% in the general population who died by suicide. Mood disorders (30.2%), substance misuse disorders (17.6%), schizophrenia (14.1%), and personality disorders (13.0%) were the leading forms of mental illness associated with death by suicide; schizophrenia was more prevalent in psychiatric inpatient suicide (19.9%), second in prevalence only to mood disorders (20.8%).

Individuals with schizophrenia are at excess risk for suicidal behavior and for death by suicide. Suicide may be the most common cause of death associated with schizophrenia; between 20 and 40% engage in self-harm behavior, and the estimated lifetime risk for suicide is approximately 9–13%. Estimated rates of suicide in schizophrenia vary widely, ranging from 147 to 750 deaths per 100,000 persons per year (Heilä et al., 1997), greatly exceeding the U.S. national rate of approximately 11 deaths per 100,000 persons per year. The reported proportion of suicides by individuals with schizophrenia ranges from 3 to 10% overall and may be as high as one-third of psychiatric patients who die by suicide, necessitating clinician assessment of suicide risk and resiliency in the routine care of patients with schizophrenia.

RISK AND RESILIENCY FACTORS FOR SUICIDE IN SCHIZOPHRENIA

Despite the high rates of suicide in schizophrenia, suicide is a low base-rate occurrence limiting research and hindering risk detection. Epidemiological data typically derive from national mortality data or population polls. Risk factor research necessitates alternative methodologies; prospective studies are indispensable in determining risk and resiliency; however, they require immense sample sizes and lengthy follow-up, raising feasibility constraints. Retrospective research typically uses the so-called "psychological autopsy" methodology, involving collection of all-source information from medical and mental health records, coroner and/or police reports, and interviews with family, caregivers, and acquaintances of those who died by suicide. Psychological autopsy studies have revealed nonmodifiable risk factors (including age, gender, ethnicity, and historical variables), and potentially modifiable factors (including presence and severity of psychological and physical symptoms, access to care, psychosocial factors, and potential resiliency factors that decrease risk for suicide). Risk and resiliency factors for suicide in schizophrenia are summarized below (also see Table 47.1).

Demographic Factors

Demographic risk factors are typically nonmodifiable; however, awareness of groups at elevated risk for suicide can help in identifying individuals who might benefit from targeted interventions. Sex, ethnicity, and age are common demographic variables associated with risk for suicide. Men account for approximately 60–75% of suicides in schizophrenia. Women with schizophrenia have higher suicide rates than do those without the disorder. In the general population, men more commonly die by suicide, yet women more commonly engage in suicidal behavior. Among individuals with schizophrenia, men more commonly die by suicide, yet rates of suicidal behavior may be equivalent between the sexes (Harkavy-Friedman & Nelson, 1997).

Whites or Caucasians are at elevated risk for suicide compared with other ethnic groups in the United States. Relatively few researchers have explored the effect of ethnicity on risk for suicide in schizophrenia. In one study, 87% (13/15) of individuals with schizophrenia who died by suicide were white, compared with 51% (42/82) of those who died by other causes (Kelly et al., 2004).

Risk for suicide in schizophrenia increases over time since onset of illness; nonetheless, young men with schizophrenia are at elevated risk compared with the general population in the initial months to years following diagnosis, especially those with high premorbid intelligence (Hawton, Sutton, Haw, Sinclair, & Deeks, 2005; Heilä et al.,

TABLE 47.1. Selected Risk Factors for Suicide in Schizophrenia

Domain	Risk factor	Comment
Demographics	Younger age	Older age confers risk for suicide in the general population and can increase risk for suicide in schizophrenia. However, younger adults with schizophrenia have high risk for suicide, especially in the context of high premorbid intelligence.
	Male sex	Men have higher suicide rates than women; women with schizophrenia have higher suicide rates than do women without the disorder. Although women typically attempt suicide more frequently than men in the general population, there may be no sex difference in rates of suicide attempts in schizophrenia.
	Caucasian ethnicity	Whites/Caucasians generally have higher rates of suicide than non-whites.
Suicide symptoms	Death ideation	The wish or desire for death is a strong risk factor for suicide in schizophrenia.
	Suicide ideation	Suicidal thoughts and wishes greatly increase risk for suicide in schizophrenia. Reports of suicidal thoughts are to be taken extremely seriously; however, absence of suicide ideation should not be interpreted as absence of risk.
	History of suicide attempt	Lifetime and recent history of suicidal behavior is among the strongest risk factors for suicide. One study found a history of previous suicide attempt in nearly three-fourths of individuals with schizophrenia who died by suicide. Family history of suicide also increases risk.
Clinical course and symptoms of schizophrenia	Diagnostic subtype	Paranoid and undifferentiated subtypes may confer greater risk for suicide than the other diagnostic subtypes of schizophrenia.
	Time since onset of illness	A majority of individuals with schizophrenia who die by suicide do so within the first 6–10 years following onset of illness; however, individuals recently diagnosed with schizophrenia may be at elevated risk for suicide. Schizophrenia confers excess risk for suicide throughout the course of the disorder, even decades after initial onset.
	Positive and negative symptoms	Individuals with schizophrenia may be at risk for suicide in the context of positive and/or negative symptoms. Psychotic symptoms greatly increase risk for suicide; suicidal command hallucinations can also increase risk. Paranoid ideation, suspiciousness, delusions about thought control, flight of ideas, and loose associations may also increase risk for suicide, as may fear of mental disintegration. Active illness and acute exacerbations both increase risk for suicide.
	Recency of hospitalization	Risk for suicide increases with recent hospital admission. Risk remains high within 6 or more months following discharge from the hospital, and can continue for years following discharge from mental health hospitalization. An increasing number of mental health admissions confers greater risk for suicide.
	Recency of health care	As with the general population, individuals with schizophrenia often present for health care days to months prior to suicide.

(continued)

TABLE 47.1. (*continued*)

Domain	Risk factor	Comment
Mental health symptoms	Depression	A majority of individuals with schizophrenia die by suicide in the context of depression, hopelessness, and despair. Risk for suicide is especially high among those with schizoaffective disorder.
	Impulsivity, anxiety, and agitation	Behavioral impulsivity, increased agitation, and motor restlessness may increase risk for suicide in schizophrenia. Concurrent depression and anxiety may be a potent risk factor for suicide.
	Alcohol misuse	Misuse of alcohol may increase risk for suicide, alone or in the context of depression and/or other mental health symptoms.
	Misuse of other substances	Abuse of drugs and/or reliance on nicotine may increase risk for suicide in schizophrenia.
Psychosocial factors	Stressors and losses	Negative life events, psychosocial stressors, and losses all may increase risk for suicide in schizophrenia.
	Marital status	Being single, widowed, divorced, or separated can increase risk for suicide in the general population. Marital status has not yet been shown to increase risk for suicide in schizophrenia, perhaps due to a greater likelihood of individuals with schizophrenia being unmarried. Loneliness and isolation may increase risk.

Note. This table lists selected variables shown in the literature to be associated with potentially heightened risk for suicide. It is not comprehensive and should not be taken as a checklist. It is intended to provide information to consider when conducting a suicide risk assessment. It is not intended to replace clinical judgment.

1997; Kelly, Shim, Feldman, Yu, & Conley, 2004). Hopelessness and impulsivity may confer suicide risk for this group, along with negative attitudes toward treatment, psychosis, and recent major loss. Conversely, community care, involvement in daily activities, and being asymptomatic may reduce risk for suicide (De Hert, McKenzie, & Peuskens, 2001). Clinicians are advised to be vigilant to increased risk for suicide in individuals newly diagnosed with schizophrenia, especially young males with high premorbid intelligence.

Suicidal Ideation and Behavior

History of suicidal behavior is perhaps the strongest risk factor for death by suicide across age groups and clinical populations, including among individuals with schizophrenia (Harkavy-Friedman & Nelson, 1997; Kallert, Leisse, & Winiecki, 2004). A rigorous, controlled psychological autopsy study in Finland found that 71% of individuals with schizophrenia who died by suicide had previously engaged in suicidal behavior (Heilä et al., 1997). Elevated suicide risk is not restricted to those who have previously engaged in suicidal behavior; presence of the wish to die, thoughts of suicide, presence and lethality of a suicide plan, and associated intent to die all confer excess risk for suicide in schizophrenia and in other populations. Fifty-two percent of the individuals with schizophrenia who died by suicide in the Finnish study had expressed suicide ideation to a health provider, family member, or friend; those with schizophrenia who died by suicide were more likely than those without the disorder to have ever expressed suicide ideation and/or engaged in suicidal behavior (84 vs. 70%), necessitating clinical vigilance to expressions of suicide ideation and to related signs of clinical distress.

Clinical Course and Symptoms of Schizophrenia

Suicide risk factors specific to schizophrenia include diagnostic subtype, time since onset of illness, presence of positive and negative symptoms, and recency of mental health hospitalization. Paranoid and undifferentiated subtypes may be the most common diagnostic subtypes associated with suicide in schizophrenia. As many as 60% of individuals with schizophrenia who die by suicide do so within the initial 6–10 years of being diagnosed; however, suicide risk remains high throughout the course of the disorder, even decades after the onset of illness (Harkavy-Friedman & Nelson, 1997; Heilä et al., 1997). Suicide risk may be especially high after acute psychotic exacerbations, especially for women.

Conflicting evidence has been reported regarding suicide risk associated with both positive and negative symptoms of schizophrenia, due in part to limited available data (Hawton et al., 2005). Researchers in Finland reported that 78% of individuals with schizophrenia who died by suicide had active psychotic symptoms at the time of death; approximately 10% experienced suicidal command hallucinations (Heilä et al., 1997). Individuals with schizophrenia who were actively ill more frequently expressed suicide ideation or engaged in suicidal behavior in the 3 months prior to suicide than did nonpsychotic individuals (56 vs. 41%). Other positive symptoms associated with elevated suicide risk include paranoid ideation, suspiciousness, delusions of thought control, flight of ideas, and loose associations. Fear of mental disintegration may further increase risk for suicide, as may loss of interest.

As with the general adult population, risk for suicide in schizophrenia increases with recent hospital admission, whether voluntary or involuntary, necessitating vigilance to suicide risk during discharge planning and follow-up in the community. Risk is especially high within 6 months of discharge from hospital. Heilä and colleagues (1997) reported that approximately 33% of individuals with schizophrenia who died by suicide did so within 3 months of hospital discharge, more than 25% were mental health inpatients at the time of death, more than 50% were outpatients at the time, and only 3% had never been hospitalized. Those who died by suicide had an overall mean of eight lifetime mental health hospitalizations (standard deviation [SD] = 8, range: 0–49); women had a higher number of mean admissions than men (11.5 vs. 6.6). Individuals with schizophrenia who die by suicide are more likely to be recipients of mental health care; those without schizophrenia who die by suicide are more likely to receive treatment in general medical practices. Presentation to a health care provider is quite common prior to suicide; in the Finnish study, over 50% of individuals with schizophrenia who died by suicide saw a health care provider within 4 days of death, and over 95% did so in the prior 3 months, necessitating clinician vigilance to patient distress and other mental health symptoms.

Depression, Substance Misuse, and Other Mental Health Symptoms

There are high rates of comorbidity of depression and substance misuse in individuals with schizophrenia. Those who harm themselves often do so in the context of extreme depression, despair, hopelessness, and feelings of worthlessness. A review of psychological autopsy studies of suicide in schizophrenia reported that depression, but not physical illness, increases risk for suicide (Hawton et al., 2005). Heilä and colleagues (1997) reported that 64% of individuals with schizophrenia experienced depressive symptoms at the time of suicide; depression was quite common among middle-aged women with schizophrenia who died by suicide. Clinicians often did not detect these symptoms. It is critical that clinicians attend to mood symptoms and hopelessness in people with schizophrenia and not focus exclusively on treating diagnosis-specific symptoms.

Alcoholism may be common among middle-aged men with schizophrenia who die by suicide (Heilä et al., 1997). Although Hawton and colleagues (2005) did not find a clear risk for suicide among individuals with schizophrenia and alcoholism, they reported elevated risk associated with drug abuse. Behavioral impulsivity, increased agitation, and motor restlessness have been implicated in elevated risk for suicide in schizophrenia; however, no clear association was found linking violence with elevated risk for suicide in this population (Hawton et al., 2005). Thus, clinicians should attend to mood symptoms, possible substance abuse, and impulsivity and agitation in individuals with schizophrenia, because these factors can increase risk for suicide.

Psychosocial Factors

Stressful life events, transitions, and impaired general and social functioning may all increase risk for suicide. Negative life events are prevalent in individuals with schizophrenia who die by suicide but may be even more common among those without schizophrenia who die by suicide, possibly due to the more restricted lifestyles of individuals with schizophrenia, affording them fewer social and occupational contacts. Negative life events are generally more common among outpatients than among inpatients who die by suicide, and among those with a greater abundance of social contacts. Problems with finances and imprisonment are more common among those with schizophrenia and comorbid alcoholism who die by suicide. Losses, disappointments, frustrations, living alone, and social isolation increase risk for suicide in schizophrenia (Hawton et al., 2005). Clinicians are advised to monitor the reactions of individuals with schizophrenia to negative life events, stressors, and losses, which can increase risk for suicide. No clear effect of marital status on suicide risk is apparent in people with schizophrenia, unlike the general population, which may be due partly to the fact that individuals with schizophrenia are more likely to be unmarried (Harkavy-Friedman & Nelson, 1997). A study of suicide in men in Montréal, Canada, indicated that most men with schizophrenia died during the winter/fall seasons, possibly reflecting effects of seasonal biological changes and/or restriction of social activity, which suggests the potential value of enhancing community outreach to at-risk populations, especially during high-risk periods.

Resiliency Factors

There is a paucity of research on resiliency factors that protect against suicide among individuals with schizophrenia. Research generally suggests that degree of religious commitment and/or religious activities help to decrease suicide risk; this issue is complicated among individuals with delusions of good versus evil, or with suicidal command hallucinations. Clinical research findings indicated less suicide ideation in patients with greater life satisfaction, perceived social support, future orientation, and perceived meaning and purpose in life (Heisel & Flett, 2004). Research exploring risk and resiliency to suicide in schizophrenia is needed.

RISK FACTORS FOR SUICIDAL BEHAVIOR IN SCHIZOPHRENIA AND/OR SCHIZOAFFECTIVE DISORDER

Research supports elevated suicide risk among all patients with psychotic symptoms (Busch, Fawcett, & Jacobs, 2003; Radomsky, Haas, Mann, & Sweeney, 1999); however, there is evidence of differing risk factors in patients with schizophrenia compared to those with schizoaffective disorder. Modai, Kuperman, Goldberg, Goldish, and Mendel (2004) constructed computerized models of risk factors for medically serious suicide attempts, and reported different patterns of risk factors for individuals with schizophrenia compared to those with schizoaffective disorder. Elevated risk for suicidal behavior in schizophrenia was associated with method of last suicide attempt, being over 18 years of age, having paranoid delusions, time elapsed since the last suicide attempt, experiencing stress, unemployment, poor overall functioning, number of previous suicide attempts, having command hallucinations, and rarely being in contact with others.

Researchers have reported that elevated risk for suicidal behavior among individuals with schizophrenia or schizoaffective disorder is associated with history of suicidal behavior, severity of suicide ideation and fewer reasons for living, presence and severity of depression, longer duration of untreated psychosis (≥ 1 year), number of hospitalizations in the prior 36 months, more frequent prescription of typical (vs. atypical) antipsychotic agents, and history of abuse or dependence on nicotine or other substances.

ASSESSMENT

Assessment of Suicide Risk

Clinician knowledge of risk and resiliency factors can aid suicide risk assessment and influence care. Clinicians should actively assess for suicide risk and resiliency factors among individuals with schizophrenia, and provide enhanced care for those with multiple risk factors and/or without sufficient social supports or other protective factors, in collaboration with patients' families, supports, and other health care providers. Efforts to predict individual deaths by suicide based on a risk factor approach have not yet proven successful, because prediction of statistically rare occurrences, such as suicide, is considered to be impossible. Risk factors for suicide are derived from aggregated information and typically do not reflect variation in risk over time. Demographic and historical variables may confer lifelong risk for suicide but be insufficient for determining a particular patient's imminent risk for suicide at a specific moment in time, thus necessitating attention to clinical warning signs associated with risk for suicide.

Assessing Suicide Warning Signs

An expert panel of the American Association of Suicidology recently proposed the mnemonic "ISPATHWARM," which reflects a set of suicide warning signs for use in community and clinical contexts. Associated warning signs include *I*deation (conceptualized as thoughts of death or of suicide, wish to die or to hurt or kill one's self, giving away prized possessions or putting one's affairs in order, and writing about death or writing a suicide note), *S*ubstance (alcohol or drug misuse), *P*urposelessness (or absence of reasons for living or perceived meaning in life), *A*nxiety (or agitation), *T*rapped (feeling like there is no way out), *H*opelessness (anticipating no improvement in the future or being unable to conceptualize the future), *W*ithdrawal (from friends, family, and/or care providers), *A*nger (rage or wish for revenge), *R*ecklessness (risk-taking or behavioral impulsivity), and *M*ood (dramatic mood swings or affective lability). Many of these characterisitics are chronically present in schizophrenia, so clinicians and family members are advised to be especially vigilant to increases in these warning signs, because they might be associated with elevated imminent risk for suicide. Research is needed to assess the effectiveness of suicide warning signs in helping to identify individuals at elevated suicide risk and to prevent suicidal behavior.

Suicide Assessment Measures

Monitoring of suicide risk can be enhanced by thoughtful use of standardized measures with acceptable reliability and validity for individuals with schizophrenia. Research supports the assessment of suicide ideation among psychotic patients; however, a paucity of clinical measures exists assessing suicide risk specifically in schizophrenia. Rating scales for assessing suicide risk in schizophrenia include the Schizophrenia Suicide Risk Scale (SSRS; Taiminen et al., 2001) and the InterSePT Scale for Suicidal Thinking (ISST; Lindenmayer et al., 2003). The 25-item SSRS, developed as a semistructured tool for estimating short-term risk for suicide, includes 13 "History items" assessing demographic and clinical variables derived from a psychological autopsy study of suicide in schizophrenia, items assessing clinical severity, and items derived from the Calgary Depression Scale, given the high risk for suicide among depressed individuals with schizophrenia. The Interview items have acceptable interrater reliability among living respondents (kappa = .79, SD = 0.30) but poor reliability when completed using all-source data, including collateral records and interviews with informants of individuals who died by suicide (kappa = .31, SD = 0.45). The History items also had unacceptably low internal consistency for both the living (Cronbach's alpha = .54) and the deceased groups (Cronbach's alpha = .38). SSRS total scores, and History and Interview subscales significantly differentiated living respondents with schizophrenia from those who died by suicide. Acceptable sensitivity and specificity could not be demonstrated for any SSRS cut score in predicting risk for suicide; however, scores above 36 out of a total possible 90 points yielded poor sensitivity (32%) and only a marginal negative predictive value (59%), despite strong specificity (97%) and a strong positive predictive value (92%). The scale's authors concluded that "the SSRS seems not to be a practical screening instrument for suicide risk in schizophrenia, and it is probably impossible to construct a suicide risk scale with both high sensitivity and high specificity in this disorder" (Taiminen et al., 2001; p. 199).

The ISST was developed for use as a primary outcome measure in the International Suicide Prevention Trial (InterSePT; Meltzer et al., 2003). The ISST is a 12-item version of the 19-item Scale for Suicide Ideation, developed by deleting items with low item–total correlations or redundancy, or judged to be difficult to interpret based on the findings of a factor analysis, and adding an item assessing delusions or hallucinations of self-harm. An initial investigation of the interrater reliability of the ISST with 22 patients yielded a strong intraclass correlation coefficient (ICC = .90) and a mean weighted kappa of .77 (SD = 1.0). A subsequent validation study with 980 study patients yielded strong internal consistency for the ISST items for the principal investigator (range: alpha = .86–.89) and for a blinded rater (range: alpha = .88–.90), with a total scale alpha of .88. A factor analysis yielded a three-factor model, representing "Current Suicidal Thinking," "Volitional Suicidal Thinking," and "Cause of Suicidal Thinking," together explaining 55.2% of the total variance in ISST scores. Criterion validity was demonstrated by significant associations between ISST scores and measures of suicide ideation and depression; convergent validity, by associations with measures of symptom severity and substance misuse; and discriminant validity, by differentiating between study patients with higher versus lower levels of suicidality. Research is needed to assess the predictive validity of the ISST and other measures of suicide risk in schizophrenia with respect to future suicidal ideation and behavior, and as a treatment outcome measure.

Clinicians wishing to use standardized psychological assessment instruments should have appropriate training and clinical experience in the selection, administration, scoring, and interpretation of such measures. Unsophisticated or otherwise ineffective use of assessment tools can compromise therapeutic rapport and/or yield incorrect findings. Some individuals at excess risk for suicide do not admit to suicidal thoughts and plans when asked directly. Busch and colleagues (2003) explored the characteristics of 76 patients who died by suicide while in the hospital or immediately after discharge, over half of whom had evidence of psychosis. Of the 50 patients for whom information on suicide ideation was present in the hospital chart, 78% were reported to have denied suicidal thoughts and intent in their final communication before suicide. Clinical experience in working with individuals with schizophrenia is especially warranted when using assessment scales given the potential impact of cognitive and psychotic symptoms on response characteristics.

TREATMENT

Early Intervention Programs

The high rate of suicide among individuals with schizophrenia early in the course of the disorder supports the importance of mental health promotion, prevention, and early intervention programs. Melle and colleagues (2006) compared patients with "nonorganic" and "nonaffective psychosis" who sought treatment in hospital catchment areas, with or without early detection of psychosis programs, and reported higher rates of suicidal ideation, plans, and attempts in communities without such programs. Results from the OPUS Study demonstrated effectiveness for an integrated treatment regimen, including assertive community treatment, antipsychotic medication, family treatment, and social skills training, in reducing hopelessness among individuals with first-episode psychosis. Research is needed to investigate the efficacy of early intervention programs in reducing risk for suicidal ideation and behavior. Clinicians should exercise caution and sensitivity when communicating to patients the diagnosis of schizophrenia and associated prognosis to minimize the likelihood of hopelessness and despair.

Medication

Research findings support so-called "antisuicidal" properties of certain medications, such as lithium for patients with bipolar affective disorder, antidepressants for patients with major depressive disorder, and antipsychotics for patients with schizophrenia and schizoaffective disorder. Evidence of efficacy in reducing suicide risk among patients with schizophrenia and schizoaffective disorder derives primarily from the InterSePT trial, one of the largest randomized controlled treatment studies to date on prevention of suicidal behavior (Meltzer et al., 2003). Investigators compared 980 patients, recruited from 67 medical centers worldwide, who were treated with clozapine ($n = 490$) or olanzapine ($n = 490$), on 2-year outcomes of suicide attempts or hospitalizations to prevent suicide attempts and worsening of suicide ideation. Study patients were 18–65 years of age, diagnosed with schizophrenia or schizoaffective disorder, and had a history of suicide attempts, or hospitalizations to prevent a suicide attempt, in the previous 3-year period, and/or moderate-to-severe current suicide ideation and depressive symptoms, and/or command hallucinations for self-harm within the previous week. Findings indicated that patients receiving clozapine treatment had significantly fewer "significant suicide attempts" (6.9 vs. 11.2%, $p = .03$), hospitalizations to prevent suicide attempts (16.7 vs. 21.8%, $p = .05$), and fewer episodes of "much worsening" suicide ideation (24.5 vs. 32.9%, $p = .005$) than patients treated with olanzapine. Patients receiving clozapine were additionally less frequently prescribed antidepressants (49.1 vs. 55.1%, $p = .01$) and anxiolytics/

soporifics (60.2 vs. 69.4%, *p* = .05) than those treated with olanzapine. Overall, there were no significant between-group differences in number of adverse events or reasons for study discontinuation, except for "unsatisfactory therapeutic effect for lowering suicide risk," which favored the clozapine over the olanzapine group (0 vs. 1.2%; *p* = .03). There was a higher frequency of deaths by suicide in the clozapine (*n* = 5, 1.0%) compared with the olanzapine group (*n* = 3, 0.6%); however, this difference did not reach statistical significance (*p* = .73). This trial suggests benefit to clozapine treatment for at-risk patients with schizophrenia; replication studies are warranted.

Heilä and colleagues (1999) reported inadequate active-phase treatment or nonadherence in 57% of individuals with schizophrenia who died by suicide, with low rates of antidepressants prescribed (13%) and no use of electroconvulsive therapy (ECT). Clinicians are advised to consider appropriate antidepressant and anxiolytic medications for individuals with comorbid mood and/or anxiety disorders given the high prevalence of mood disorders among suicidal individuals with schizophrenia and research implicating serotonergic dysfunction in elevated risk for suicide (Radomsky et al., 1999). Clinicians must carefully consider patient medical history prior to prescription of any medication, as well as response to past medications and potential medication interaction effects, side effects, withdrawal effects, toxicity of overdose, and potential for abuse and nonadherence.

Poor adherence to treatment has been associated with elevated suicide risk among individuals with schizophrenia (De Hert et al., 2001; Hawton et al., 2005); Heilä and colleagues (1997) found that a majority of those who died by suicide during an active phase of illness were being inadequately treated or were nonadherent to treatment. One study reported a fourfold increased risk for suicidal behavior among nonadherent individuals with schizophrenia. Partial medication adherence or nonadherence may increase the likelihood of relapse or resurgence of psychotic symptoms, necessitating involuntary hospitalization and hospitalizations of longer duration, and contribute to suicide risk (Leucht & Heres, 2006). Patients are nonadherent for a variety of reasons, including fear of taking medication, familiarity with certain auditory hallucinations (i.e., "supportive" voices), amotivation, cognitive impairment, comorbid substance abuse, and presence of nonsupportive or overly emotional and/or demanding caregivers. Given that physicians tend to overestimate patients' medication adherence, they are encouraged to ask patients explicitly about their adherence to treatment; to provide clear instructions to patients on when and how to take their medications, and reminders to refill prescriptions; and to be clear and supportive in educating patients on the importance and value of taking medications, unpleasant side effects notwithstanding. Psychosocial interventions, including psychoeducation for the patient and/or his or her family and social support providers, and provision of literature and resources, peer-support, family-to-family support, compliance therapy, and shared patient–physician decision making may increase treatment adherence (Leucht & Heres, 2006). One psychoeducational trial did not show a reduction in relapse rates for individuals with schizophrenia, and demonstrated a paradoxical increase in suicide ideation in the treatment arm (Cunningham Owens et al., 2001). Notably, insight has not been found to be a risk factor for suicide in schizophrenia (Hawton et al., 2005).

Psychotherapy and Other Psychosocial Interventions

Suicidal individuals are typically excluded from clinical trials, severely limiting available evidence for psychotherapeutic and psychosocial interventions with those at-risk for suicide. There is a growing body of evidence that specific psychotherapies help to reduce risk for suicide, including cognitive approaches, such as problem-solving therapy, cognitive therapy, and dialectical behavior therapy, and more interpersonal approaches, such as psychodynamic and interpersonal psychotherapy. Clinical psychotherapy trials have not yet focused on suicide risk reduction in schizophrenia; however, efficacious psychotherapies that reduce depression, hopelessness, impulsivity, agitation, and other mental health symptoms may help reduce risk for suicide in schizophrenia. Research is critically needed in this area.

Additional Clinical Care Issues

Clinicians are strongly advised to be ever-cautious for signs and symptoms of mounting clinical distress and suicide warning signs among individuals with schizophrenia given their high risk for suicidal behavior and for suicide throughout the course of the disorder. Clinicians should initially collect a thorough medical and mental health history, and assess for suicide risk factors, including personal and familial history of suicidal behavior and of suicide, and presence of suicidal command hallucinations. Vigilance is needed for signs of increasing suicide risk, such as depressed mood, hopelessness, agitated depression, suicidal expressions and communications expressing a longing for death, or vague references regarding not being around much longer. A patient who has been depressed and suddenly appears much brighter or energetic, even in the context of medication changes, should be watched very carefully, because that patient may have decided to end his or her life. Additionally, it is advisable to assess for homicidal ideation and/or plans to harm or kill others. This is especially important in individuals with paranoid schizophrenia, who may be at risk of harming others in what they perceive to be preemptive self-defense. Clinicians should additionally assess for the presence of guilt and shame, and misuse of substances, including nicotine, alcohol, and both illicit and prescribed medication. Assessment of social supports and social support deficits, negative life events, perceived burdensomeness, and other sources of stress or emotional pain, is essential for assessing increased risk for suicide. Other telltale signs of increased suicide risk include getting one's affairs in order, as if planning for a lengthy vacation; writing a will or suicide note; giving away prized possessions or pets, stockpiling lethal implements; and withdrawing from social networks and/or discontinuing clinical care.

When providing pharmacological care to persons judged to be at-risk for suicide, clinicians are advised to prescribe only small doses of medications that may be potentially lethal on overdose, and to consider eliciting assistance from family members or other care providers in administering medications. Increasing the frequency of health care visits and/or psychotherapy sessions may be advisable in the face of mounting distress and risk for suicide. ECT may have beneficial short-term effects in reducing suicide risk in individuals with mood disorders; however, there is a paucity of evidence from the literature exploring randomized controlled trials of suicide risk and ECT in individuals with schizophrenia (see McClintock, Ranginwala, & Husain, Chapter 20, this volume, for a discussion of ECT as a treatment for individuals with schizophrenia).

Hospitalization may be needed for individuals with schizophrenia at excess risk for suicide. Hospitalization can be an important safeguard for a person at risk for suicide and should be considered when an individual is judged to be at risk for harming self and/or others, when risk for suicide and/or medical complications is high during periods of starting, stopping, augmenting, or switching medications, and/or for medical or psychological stabilization. Removal from stressful life circumstances can provide the suicidal individual with respite, and a structured hospital milieu, close supervision, and access to medical and psychosocial interventions can all prove therapeutic. Absolute safety is not ensured with hospitalization; people have died by suicide while on 24-hour in-hospital suicide watch (Busch et al., 2003), and suicide risk is high immediately following hospital discharge. Clinicians must weigh the potential benefits and risks of hospitalization to the therapeutic relationship, while recognizing that patient safety must always take precedence. Clinicians should consider discussing hospitalization with their patients as a viable treatment option early in the course of treatment, and agreeing upon voluntary hospitalization during times of elevated risk. In less ideal circumstances, involuntary hospitalization might be necessary. When permitted, it may be advisable for clinicians to discuss the possible range of treatment options and elicit cooperation from at-risk clients, their families, and other social supports as early as possible. Following hospitalization, clinicians should promote outpatient aftercare, including day hospitalization and other step-down care programs, recognizing that suicide risk is high for individuals with schizophrenia in the immediate period following hospital discharge.

When a patient is judged to be at imminent risk for suicide, he or she should not be left alone. Clinical work with individuals at risk for suicide should never be a solitary endeavor; clinicians should work to build a collaborative network of care providers to ensure the highest quality of care for individuals at risk for suicide, and to provide support for one another, because working with at-risk populations can be highly stressful, and loss of a patient to suicide devastating. Clinicians are further advised to develop a safety plan with the patient, listing explicit resources and supports to be accessed when risk is high, including support groups, distress lines and crisis centers, emergency access phone numbers (e.g., 911), and use of emergency services and hospital emergency departments. There is little, if any, evidentiary support for use of so-called "no suicide contracts"; however, developing a safety plan to be enacted when a patient is suicidal can be helpful. Clinicians should endeavor to restrict access to potentially lethal means. Detailed note keeping is essential, and consultation is strongly encouraged. It is crucial that clinicians be empathic and supportive of the patient's needs, and attentive to the therapeutic alliance. Mindfulness to suicide risk factors and warning signs, and provision of sensitive clinical care, may help to reduce risk for suicide in individuals with schizophrenia.

KEY POINTS

- Assess for potentially modifiable suicide risk factors and provide enhanced care for those who have multiple risk factors and/or lack sufficient resiliency factors.
- Be vigilant to increased risk for suicide during high-risk periods: following initial diagnosis and hospital discharge; and when starting, stopping, augmenting, or switching medications.
- Attend to suicide warning signs on an ongoing basis (e.g., ISPATHWARM).
- Clinicians employing standardized psychological measures to assess suicide risk should have appropriate training and experience in selecting, administering, scoring, and interpreting these measures in individuals with schizophrenia.
- Consider prescribing antipsychotics, antidepressants, and anxiolytics to help reduce symptoms associated with schizophrenia and comorbid mood and/or anxiety disorders, carefully considering patient medical history, past response to medications, and potential interaction effects, side effects, withdrawal effects, toxicity of overdose, potential for abuse, and likelihood of medication nonadherence.
- Attend to the client's potential for treatment nonadherence by providing clear instructions and education about medication use and anticipated side effects.
- Consider using psychotherapeutic and psychosocial interventions to help reduce the clients' symptoms, increase treatment adherence, and enhance social functioning and psychological well-being.
- Discuss the range of treatment options, including hospitalization, and elicit cooperation from at-risk individuals, and their personal and professional supports, at the earliest possible point.
- Develop a safety plan with clients, listing explicit resources and supports to be accessed when risk is high, including support groups, distress lines and crisis centers, emergency access numbers (e.g., 911), and emergency services (including hospital emergency rooms).

ACKNOWLEDGMENTS

I gratefully acknowledge the very helpful comments and editorial feedback of Drs. Paul S. Links, Ross M.G. Norman, Abraham Rudnick, and the book's editors. Thank you as well to Megan Nichols, MSc, for assistance in editing an earlier draft of this chapter.

REFERENCES AND RECOMMENDED READINGS

American Psychiatric Association. (2003). *Practice guidelines for the assessment and treatment of patients with suicidal behaviors.* Arlington, VA: Author.

Busch, K. A., Fawcett, J., & Jacobs, D. G. (2003). Clinical correlates of inpatient suicide. *Journal of Clinical Psychiatry, 64,* 14–19.

Cunningham Owens, D. G., Carroll, A., Fattah, S., Clyde, Z., Coffey, I., & Johnstone, E. C. (2001). A randomized, controlled trial of a brief interventional package for schizophrenic out-patients. *Acta Psychiatrica Scandinavica, 103,* 362–369.

De Hert, M., McKenzie, K., & Peuskens, J. (2001). Risk factors for suicide in young people suffering from schizophrenia: A long-term follow-up study. *Schizophrenia Research, 47,* 127–134.

Harkavy-Friedman, J. M., & Nelson, E. A. (1997). Assessment and intervention for the suicidal patient with schizophrenia. *Psychiatric Quarterly, 68,* 361–375.

Hawton, K., Sutton, L., Haw, C., Sinclair, J., & Deeks, J. J. (2005). Schizophrenia and suicide: Systematic review of risk factors. *British Journal of Psychiatry, 187,* 9–20.

Heilä, H., Isometsä, E. T., Henriksson, M. M., Heikkinen, M. E., Marttunen, M. J., & Lönnqvist, J. K. (1997). Suicide and schizophrenia: A nationwide psychological autopsy study on age- and sex-specific clinical characteristics of 92 suicide victims with schizophrenia. *American Journal of Psychiatry, 154,* 1235–1242.

Heilä, H., Isometsä, E. T., Henriksson, M. M., Heikkinen, M. E., Marttunen, M. J., & Lönnqvist, J. K. (1999). Suicide victims with schizophrenia in different treatment phases and adequacy of antipsychotic medication. *Journal of Clinical Psychiatry, 60,* 200–208.

Heisel, M. J., & Flett, G. L. (2004). Purpose in life, satisfaction with life and suicide ideation in a clinical sample. *Journal of Psychopathology and Behavioral Assessment, 26,* 127–135.

Kallert, T. W., Leisse, M., & Winiecki, P. (2004). Suicidality of chronic schizophrenic patients in long-term community care. *Crisis, 25,* 54–64.

Kelly, D. L., Shim, J.-C., Feldman, S. M., Yu, Y., & Conley, R. R. (2004). Lifetime psychiatric symptoms in persons with schizophrenia who died by suicide compared to other means of death. *Journal of Psychiatric Research, 38,* 531–536.

Leucht, S., & Heres, S. (2006). Epidemiology, clinical consequences, and psychosocial treatment of nonadherence in schizophrenia. *Journal of Clinical Psychiatry, 67*(Suppl. 5), 3–8.

Lindenmayer, J. P., Czobor, P., Alphs, L., Nathan, A.-M., Anand, R., Islam, Z., et al. (2003). The InterSePT Scale for suicidal thinking reliability and validity. *Schizophrenia Research, 63,* 161–170.

Maris, R. W., Berman, A. L., & Silverman, M. M. (2000). *Comprehensive textbook of suicidology.* New York: Guilford Press.

Melle, I., Johannesen, J. O., Friis, S., Haahr, U., Joa, I., Larsen, T. K., et al. (2006). Early detection of first episode of schizophrenia and suicidal behavior. *American Journal of Psychiatry, 163,* 800–804.

Meltzer, H. Y., Alphs, L., Green, A. I., Altamura, C., Anand, R., Bertoldi, A., et al. (2003). Clozapine treatment for suicidality in schizophrenia: International Suicide Prevention Trial (InterSePT). *Archives of General Psychiatry, 60,* 82–91.

Modai, I., Kuperman, J., Goldberg, I., Goldish, M., & Mendel, S. (2004). Suicide risk factors and suicide vulnerability in various major psychiatric disorders. *Medical Informatics, 29,* 65–74.

Radomsky, E. D., Haas, G. L., Mann, J. J., & Sweeney, J. A. (1999). Suicidal behavior in patients with schizophrenia and other psychotic disorders. *American Journal of Psychiatry, 156,* 1590–1595.

Simon, R. I., & Hales, R. E. (Eds). (2006). *American psychiatric textbook of suicide assessment and management.* Arlington, VA: American Psychiatric Publishing.

Taiminen, T., Huttunen, J., Heilä, H., Henriksson, M., Isometsä, E., Kähkönen, J., et al. (2001). The Schizophrenia Suicide Risk Scale (SSRS): Development and initial validation. *Schizophrenia Research, 47,* 199–213.

SELECTED RESOURCES AND REFERENCES ON SUICIDE PREVENTION

Website

American Association of Suicidology: *www.suicidology.org*
American Foundation for Suicide Prevention: *www.afsp.org*
Canadian Association for Suicide Prevention: *www.suicideprevention.ca*
Centre for Research and Intervention on Suicide and Euthanasia: *www.crise.ca*
Centre for Suicide Prevention: *www.suicideinfo.ca*
International Academy of Suicide Research: *www.iasronline.org*
International Association for Suicide Prevention: *www.med.uio.no/iasp*
NIMH: Suicide Prevention Resources: *www.nimh.nih.gov/suicideprevention/index.cfm*
Suicide Prevention Resource Center: *www.sprc.org*
Suicide Prevention Action Network USA: *www.spanusa.org*
U.S. National Strategy for Suicide Prevention: *mentalhealth.samhsa.gov/suicideprevention/strategy.asp*
Web-Based Injury Statistics Query and Reporting System (WISQARS). Centers for Disease Control and Prevention: *cdc.gov/ncipc/wisqars*
WHO: Suicide Prevention (SUPRE): *www.who.int/mental_health/prevention/suicide*

Journals Focusing on Suicide

Archives of Suicide Research
Crisis: The Journal of Crisis Intervention and Suicide Prevention
Omega: The Journal of Death and Dying
Suicide and Life-Threatening Behavior

PART VII

POLICY, LEGAL, AND SOCIAL ISSUES

CHAPTER 48

THE ECONOMICS
OF SCHIZOPHRENIA

MIHAIL SAMNALIEV
ROBIN E. CLARK

Although schizophrenia is a relatively rare condition, it has a broad-ranging economic impact on individuals, families, and societies. Disability associated with schizophrenia impairs earning power for individuals with the illness, and often places increased costs and caregiving demands on family members. Treatment is expensive, and lifetime costs exceed those of many other chronic conditions. Private insurance coverage is often inadequate, and a high proportion of care is covered by publicly financed programs. Health care financing has a profound impact on access to effective treatment. Over the past decade, increasing attention has been given to studying the cost-effectiveness of various treatments in an attempt to use scarce health care dollars most efficiently and effectively.

In this chapter, we address the economic aspects of schizophrenia. We begin by discussing prevalence and costs at the societal level, then how those costs are distributed to various payers. Next, we review current knowledge about the cost and effectiveness of treatment. How health care financing affects the accessibility and efficiency of treatment is the final topic in our discussion.

COSTS OF THE ILLNESS

Prevalence and Burden

Schizophrenia affects at least 24 million people worldwide and 2.5 million, or about 1% of the population, in the United States. The global burden of the illness is disproportionately high compared to other mental disorders, because it affects people in the most productive period of their lives, may cause lifetime disability, and requires expensive treatment and long-term involvement of caregivers. Schizophrenia is listed by the World Health Organization (WHO) among the top 10 leading causes of disability worldwide and the second largest contributor to the overall burden of disease, after cardiovascular diseases. The substantial economic burden of schizophrenia stems from direct costs incurred for its treatment in the health care system, and a wide range of indirect costs, including nontreatment expenditures and intangible costs associated with emotional and physical burden. Direct treatment expenditures have been well documented and are of particular concern to public payers, such as the Medicaid program, states, and counties. Indirect costs have received much less attention but are equally important; they allow for calculations of the full cost of schizophrenia, thus providing information about the true societal value of public health care programs targeting people with severe mental disorders.

Direct Costs

Spending for mental care treatment in the United States was more than $85 billion in 2001, accounting for 6.2% of all health care spending. Outpatient care accounted for the largest share of expenditures (52%), followed by inpatient (22%) and residential care (19%). About one-fourth of all expenditures were for services provided in hospitals, including specialty hospitals (11%), specialty units in general hospitals (7%), and in nonspecialty care in general hospitals (9%). Treatment of schizophrenia alone accounted for 2.5% of all health care spending and almost one-third of all mental health care spending, roughly approximating $34 billion (Mark, Coffey, Vandivort-Warren, Harwood, & King, 2005).

Trends in Spending

Spending for mental health services in the last 15 years is characterized by the increasing shares of outpatient and general care and declining use of inpatient and specialty care. Between 1991 and 2001 there was a 12% decrease in the relative share of expenditures for specialty hospitals, no change for general hospitals, and a 6% decrease in the share for nursing homes and home health services. At the same time, there was a 4% increase in expenditures for multiservice mental health organizations (e.g., community mental health centers and psychosocial treatment programs) and a 14% increase for retail drugs (Mark et al., 2005).

Spending on Drugs

The rising expenditures for atypical antipsychotic drugs are particularly prominent. Most notably, between 1996 and 2001, an increase of 5.5 million people using atypical antipsychotic drugs was paralleled by a 77% annual increase in prices, mostly attributable to introduction of new medications. These two trends have been the major factors in the escalating costs of mental health care: As of 2004, drug expenditures accounted for $20 billion, or 21% of all mental health spending. During the same period, spending for older antipsychotics remained almost unchanged.

Geographic Variation

Mental health spending varies significantly by state. For example, the $16 billion distributed by the 50 State Mental Health Agencies in 1997 varied fivefold across states, from $23 to 112 per capita. New England, Mid-Atlantic, and Far West regions had the highest per capita expenditures, mostly driven by community-based programs, whereas the Southeast and the South Central regions had the lowest per capita spending.

Indirect Costs

Direct expenditures for treatment reflect only part, likely less than half, of the resources utilized for people with schizophrenia. They do not capture a range of additional resources associated with schizophrenia morbidity and mortality, including informal care and financial help by family members and forgone opportunities to work by both individuals with schizophrenia and their caregivers (opportunity costs). These costs are often estimated by the *human capital approach*, which is based on the productivity, or output, of the individual in the economy, as determined by the prevailing labor wages.

The main criticisms of the human capital approach are its often unrealistic assumption that wages reflect one's true economic "worth"; that it does not capture the costs of physical and emotional distress caused by a disease; and that lost wages do not reflect how much people actually value their health. These issues are addressed by a more recent method based on *willingness to pay*, that deduces how much people value their health. The main criticism of this approach is that estimates are often elicited with hypothetical questions—for example, about the purchase of a hypothetical drug that will increase numbers of symptom-free days—and do not necessarily correspond to actual purchasing behavior.

Using these two methods, studies have found that a significant indirect cost of schizophrenia arises from mortality, increased morbidity, unemployment, family caregiving, and physical and emotional distress associated with the illness. In addition, schizophrenia is associated with increased financial assistance by family members and criminal justice costs.

Mortality and Morbidity

Opportunity costs to people with schizophrenia are driven by the high rates of mortality, mainly because of increased risk of suicide. The WHO reports an average reduced life expectancy of 10 years among people with the disease. Among patients with schizophrenia, 30–60% attempt suicide at least once in a lifetime, and an estimated 10% die from suicide. Opportunity costs also stem from impaired social functioning. People with severe mental disorders have high rates of coexisting medical conditions that can severely impair social functioning and quality of life. For example, 80% of older adults with mental disorders have at least one comorbid, chronic physical condition; one-half of people with schizophrenia also have a substance use disorder at some point in their lifetimes. Costs of schizophrenia mortality and morbidity according to the human capital approach (lost productivity) were estimated to be $1.3 billion, and $10.7 billion, respectively, in 1990 (Rice & Miller, 1996).

Family Caregiving

The value of all informal health care in the United States was conservatively estimated to be $200 billion in 1999, almost twice as much as the formal spending for nursing homes and home health care (Arno, Levin, & Memmott, 1999). Informal caregiving by family members, however, has been largely unacknowledged in health care policy. Caregivers spend a significant amount of time with their ill relatives, and to be able to do so, many of them either reduce their work time or stop working. The value of informal family care for people with schizophrenia, based on market wages for caregivers, was estimated to be $2.5 billion in 1990 (Rice & Miller, 1996), or $11,500 a year per family. In addition, family members provide direct financial assistance to people with schizophrenia. For example, one study reported that parent financial assistance for people with schizophrenia and co-occurring substance use disorders was two times higher than that for children without chronic conditions (Clark, 1994). Family expenditures for members with schizophrenia were more often for daily maintenance needs and less likely to involve investments such as support for education or assistance in purchasing a home. Because informal family care appears to be linked with use of formal mental health care, reductions in public spending may shift costs to family members.

Costs of Physical and Emotional Suffering

Estimating the monetary value of physical suffering and emotional distress, also referred to as *intangible costs*, is a very new area of health economics research. One study has argued that people with schizophrenia can distinguish, assess, and place utility rankings or willingness to pay amounts for improved health status (Voruganti et al., 2000). This study suggested that the cost of physical and emotional burden of schizophrenia is considerable: Willingness to pay to maintain current health status was more than $2,000 (Canadian) per year.

Criminal Justice Costs

The deinstitutionalization and transition to community-based care has led to a well-documented rise in encounters of people with severe mental illnesses with the criminal justice system. Individuals with schizophrenia are much more likely to be arrested and charged with a crime, and prevalence of severe mental illness in prisons is two to three times higher than that in the general population. Criminal justice costs are incurred for law enforcement, legal defense, and incarceration. Updated estimates of these costs are unavailable, but an older study reported a total cost of $464 million in 1990 (Rice & Miller, 1996). Legal system encounters among people with severe mental illnesses are uneven, with a small group of people incurring the majority of encounters and related law enforcement costs.

The costs of schizophrenia in the United States are summarized in Table 48.1.

COST-EFFECTIVENESS

The value of specific pharmacological or psychosocial interventions is grounded in their evidence-based ability to improve symptoms, social functioning, or quality of life. Cost-effec-

TABLE 48.1. The Cost of Schizophrenia in the United States

Cost	$, billion	Diagnostic group	Study (year)
Direct	85 in 2001	All mental disorders	Mark et al. (2005)
Drugs	18 in 2001		
Other outpatient	45 in 2001		
Inpatient	19 in 2001		
Residential	17 in 2001		
Indirect		Schizophrenia	Rice (1999)
Morbidity	10.7 in 1990		
Mortality	1.3 in 1990		
Informal caregiving	2.5 in 1990		
Criminal justice	0.46 in 1990		
Intangible costs	National estimates not available		

tiveness analyses of interventions allow consumers to compare their efficiency (ability to achieve effects at the least cost) whenever financial resources are limited. Cost-effective interventions do not necessarily mean cost savings. Expensive technologies that have large benefits may increase overall costs of treatment but be more effective, and more cost-effective.

Pharmacological Treatment

Evidence of the cost-effectiveness of pharmacological interventions is only recently emerging and for the most part is still contradictory. Research in the United States has focused mostly on the relative cost-effectiveness of newer antipsychotics, such as clozapine, risperidone, olanzapine, and quetiapine, compared to haloperidol, a popular traditional antipsychotic. Pharmacological cost-effectiveness studies need to be viewed with caution, because they often omit important components of costs such as the side effects of medications, or societal benefits such as reduced encounters with the criminal justice system after switching to atypical antipsychotics.

Clozapine

Clozapine appears to be the most cost-effective antipsychotic drug compared to both atypical and typical antipsychotics. It is the most cost-effective medication used among treatment-resistant patients and has proven clinical benefits, resulting in reduced hospitalization and a shift to outpatient treatment. Clozapine is also associated with fewer relapses and higher patient satisfaction, although its effect on global/social functioning is ambiguous. The benefits of clozapine seem to offset its higher acquisition costs compared to typical antipsychotics. However, use of clozapine has been limited because of rare but potentially lethal side effects.

New Atypical versus Traditional Antipsychotics

There is still a lack of consensus about whether new atypical antipsychotics are cost-effective compared to traditional antipsychotics. Acquisition prices of atypical antipsychotics are much higher than those for typical antipsychotics. For example, the federally negotiated price for a 30-day supply of olanzapine or risperidone exceeds $400, whereas a 30-day supply of haloperidol may cost as little as $20. This difference in prices makes a case against the use of atypical antipsychotics from an economic point of view, unless they have a clear clinical advantage. Some studies suggest that risperidone, olanzapine, and quetiapine enjoy greater acceptance by patients and can offset higher acquisition costs by improving clinical outcomes. However, as mentioned, most studies typically have not included side effects and indirect benefits in their calculations. Furthermore, the majority of trials comparing new atypical antipsychotics to haloperidol may be biased, because patients taking haloperidol in these trials were not given prophylactic medications that would alleviate side effects (Rosenheck, 2005).

Cost-Effectiveness of New Antipsychotics

The comparative value of atypical antipsychotics is still unclear. Each drug has a different side effect profile, which makes it difficult to assess cost-effectiveness. Research in this area is contradictory and should be viewed with caution. The net effect of years of research can probably be summarized by the findings of a recent study published in the *New England Journal of Medicine*, suggesting that olanzapine has the advantage of lower dropout rates compared to risperidone, quetiapine, and perphenazine (Lieberman et al., 2005), but it is also associated with greater risk for side effects. There is not yet sufficient evidence to conclude whether the higher acquisition cost of olanzapine can be offset by clinical and/or social functioning benefits in the long run.

Psychosocial Interventions

Several psychosocial programs are now considered evidence based and are recommended to individuals with schizophrenia. Assertive community treatment (ACT), supported employment, and integrated treatment for patients with co-occurring substance use disorder have received considerable research attention and are consistently found to be effective. Cognitive-behavioral therapy has demonstrated promising results among people with schizophrenia. Cost-effectiveness of psychosocial treatment is a relatively new area of research, and most studies have focused on its short-run effects. In addition, costs of psychosocial treatment are often borne by states, whereas benefits accrue to individuals. In such cases, tight state budgets can become a limiting force, even if interventions are beneficial and cost-effective from a broader societal perspective.

Assertive Community Treatment

ACT has proven effective in reducing hospital admissions and length of stay (ranging from 10 to 85% across studies), improving housing stability (likelihood and duration of independent accommodation), and leads to patient and family caregivers' satisfaction with ACT services. ACT is expensive and in most situations is unlikely to be cost-effective, at least in the short run. ACT has been found to be cost-effective among high service users, for example, among consumers with a history of substance use disorders, and among homeless people with severe mental illness. Cost savings of ACT arise mainly because of reduced hospitalizations, and recent downward trends in hospitalization may make ACT less cost-effective.

Integrated Treatment

For individuals with co-occurring severe mental and substance use disorders, integrated treatment of both disorders is considered the "gold standard." In integrated care, psychiatric and substance abuse treatment is typically provided by a team that includes clinicians with skills in both areas. The benefits of the integrated treatment approach have been clearly demonstrated in experimental settings but have not been widely implemented in clinical practice yet due to organizational, policy, and financial barriers. Clinical guidelines for implementation of integrated treatment have only recently been published. Whether integrated treatment is more cost-effective than separate care is still a largely unanswered question. One study found that the integration of individual and family psychosocial intervention, along with pharmacological treatment, was more cost-effective, mainly due to reduced inpatient expenditures, fewer symptoms, and improved functioning. However, the small number of patients in this study affected the statistical robustness of its findings (Haddock et al., 2003).

Supported Employment

Most people with schizophrenia want to work, but employment rates are as low as 10%. Supported employment (SE) is the most effective vocational model for people with severe mental disorders, leading to a rate of almost 40% employment among those who enroll in SE programs. Earlier vocational rehabilitation approaches (e.g., sheltered employment and prevocational training) have not been as effective. A form of SE, the *individual placement model*, is specifically adapted for people with severe mental illness. Some of the distinguishing characteristics of this approach are ongoing, onsite, individualized support in a competitive employment environment and integration with mental health services. Because, earnings among people with schizophrenia are typically not high, the cost-effectiveness of SE is largely dependent on how the program is implemented. For example replacing SE to existing vocational programs or day treatment can be cost-effective. SE has not been found to translate into reduced utilization rates and costs of treatment.

Cognitive-Behavioral Therapy

Cognitive-behavioral therapy (CBT) among people with schizophrenia is a relatively recent practice that shows promising results. Randomized clinical trials consistently indicate that compared to conventional pharmacological treatment or other psychosocial interventions, CBT reduces or stabilizes psychotic symptoms, although it is unclear whether CBT improves relapse or hospitalization rates in the long run. The cost-effectiveness of CBT among schizophrenia patients has barely been addressed. Among people with co-occurring schizophrenia and substance misuse, CBT (in combination with motivational and family therapy), along with routine pharmacological treatment, has been found to be more effective and of comparable cost to pharmacological treatment alone (Haddock et al., 2003).

FINANCING OF MENTAL HEALTH CARE

Public Payers

Compared with treatment in other chronic illnesses, a greater proportion of schizophrenia treatment costs tend to be paid by government. Almost two-thirds of mental health treatment in the United States is paid by local, state, or Federal government. Between 1991 and 2001, the percentage of mental health care coverage by public payers increased from 58 to 65%. Less than one-half of all other health care is paid by public sources.

The largest government payers for mental health treatment in the United States are Medicaid, a joint state–Federal insurance program for people with low income, and direct appropriations by state or local government. Each of these sources pays slightly more than 25% of the costs. An additional 13% is paid by Federal programs such as Medicare, which covered about 7% of all mental health care in 2001.

Private Payers

Low rates of employment among people with schizophrenia prevent many individuals from accessing private health insurance. Most private insurance policies also have lifetime coverage caps that effectively end reimbursement after a beneficiary reaches a preset utilization or spending limit. Insurers often limit mental health coverage more stringently than care for other conditions in an effort to discourage *adverse selection*, enrollment of persons with schizophrenia or other severe and persistent psychiatric disorders whom they see as poor financial risks. Legislative attempts to achieve parity between coverage for physical and mental disorders have had limited success.

Managed Care

Enrollment of people with schizophrenia in managed care plans, which have incentives to reduce costs, has lagged behind that of other diagnostic groups, largely because of the perceived risk of catastrophic costs. However, special "carveout" managed care plans have been created in a growing number of states (15 states as of 2005, according to the National Alliance on Mental Illness [NAMI]). These plans usually include higher payments for persons with severe mental illness and often offer special protections from financial risk, such as *reinsurance*, which insures managed care organizations against substantial financial losses or outlier payments that cover some or all additional payments for beneficiaries with unusually high costs.

Managed care for persons with severe mental illness has been hotly contested in the United States over the past two decades. Many questions remain about its impact on the health of individuals and cost to payers. However, dire predictions of greatly restricted access to needed service and adverse health effects have not been borne out by research to date. It is likely that managed care will play an increasing role in coverage for people with schizophrenia in coming years.

KEY POINTS

- Schizophrenia imposes a disproportionately high cost on society compared to other mental disorders.
- Treatment of schizophrenia consumes almost one-third of all mental health expenses in the United States.
- The indirect costs associated with the illness are also considerable and at least as high as the direct cost of treatment.
- With continuing reliance on drug treatment, there is concern about the sharply escalating cost of atypical antipsychotic drugs.
- With the exception of clozapine, which emerges as the most efficacious and cost-effective drug for patients with treatment-resistant schizophrenia, evidence has failed to clearly establish clinical or cost-effectiveness advantage of new atypical antipsychotics.
- Several evidence-based psychosocial interventions, including ACT, SE, and integrated treatment of people with co-occurring severe mental and substance use disorders can be cost-effective compared to standard care, mainly among high health service users.
- Treatment of mental disorders in the United States is predominantly and increasingly paid for by government, because private insurers and market forces fail to meet the need of people with persistent psychiatric disorders.
- Evidence of the impact of managed care on quality of care for individuals with severe mental disorders is ambiguous; however, managed care for people with schizophrenia has not expanded as much as for the remainder of the U.S. health sector.

REFERENCES AND RECOMMENDED READINGS

Arno, P., Levine, C., & Memmott, M. (1999). The economic value of informal caregiving. *Health Affairs, 18*(2), 182–188.

Center for Mental Health Services. (2000). *Mental health, United States, 2000 (Sections 3 and 4)* (DHHS Publication No. (SMA) 01-3537). Washington, DC: Author.

Clark, R. (1994). Family costs associated with severe mental illness and substance use. *Hospital and Community Psychiatry, 45*(8), 808–813.

Clark, R., & Samnaliev, M. (2005). Psychosocial treatment in the 21st century. *International Journal of Law and Psychiatry, 28*, 532–544.

Haddock, G., Barrowclough, C., Tarrier, N., Moring, J., O'Brien, R., Schofield, N., et al. (2003). Cognitive-behavioral therapy and motivational intervention for schizophrenia and substance misuse: 18-month outcomes of a randomised controlled trial. *British Journal of Psychiatry, 183,* 418–426.

Knapp, M., Mangalore, R., & Simon, J. (2004). The global costs of schizophrenia. *Schizophrenia Bulletin, 30*(2), 279–293.

Lieberman, J. A., Stroup, T. S., McEvoy, J. P., Swartz, M. S., Rosenheck, R. A., Perkins, D. O., et al. (2005). Effectiveness of antipsychotic drugs in patients with chronic schizophrenia. *New England Journal of Medicine, 353*(12), 1209–1223.

Mark, T., Coffey, R., Vandivort-Warren, R., Harwood, H., & King, E. (2005, January–June). U.S. spending for mental health and substance abuse treatment, 1991–2001. *Health Affairs,* pp. W5-133–W5-142.

National Institute for Health Care Management Research and Educational Foundation. (2002). *Prescription drug expenditures in 2001: Another year of escalating costs.* Washington, DC: Author.

Rice, D. (1999). The economic impact of schizophrenia. *Journal of Clinical Psychiatry, 60*(Suppl. 1), 4–6.

Rice, D., & Miller, L. (1996). The economic burden of schizophrenia: Conceptual and methodological issues, and cost estimates. In M. Moscarelli, A. Ruff, & N. Sartorius (Eds.), *Handbook of mental health economics and health policy* (Vol. 1, pp. 321–334). Chichester, UK: Wiley.

Rosenheck, R. (2005). The growth of psychopharmacology in the 1990s: Evidence-based practice or irrational exuberance. *International Journal of Law and Psychiatry, 28,* 467–483.

Voruganti, L. N., Awad, A. G., Oyewumi, L. K., Cortese L., Zirul, S., & Dhawan, R. (2000). Assessing health utilities in schizophrenia. *Pharmacoeconomics, 17*(3), 273–286.

CHAPTER 49

INVOLUNTARY COMMITMENT

JONATHAN BINDMAN
GRAHAM THORNICROFT

BACKGROUND

Involuntary Commitment and Coercive Treatment

Involuntary commitment is a term used in North America for the use of legal measures to compel patients to accept psychiatric treatment. This may include treatment in a hospital or in the community (involuntary outpatient commitment [IOC]). The use of the law to compel treatment is only one aspect of a more general issue, coercion, by which patients who decline treatment may be persuaded, pressured, or threatened by professionals or others before, or as an alternative to, legal commitment.

The use of coercion as a routine part of care fundamentally distinguishes psychiatry from other areas of medicine, in which the autonomy of the competent patient to refuse treatment is more usually assumed. The association of physical restraint with mental health care has historic roots, certainly established before the English law of 1714, which permitted Justices of the Peace to secure the arrest of any person "furiously mad and dangerous" and to lock them up securely for as long as "such lunacy and madness shall continue."

Involuntary Commitment in the Hospital and in the Community

Involuntary commitment has historically been taken to mean detention in a hospital, though this was commonly associated with restrictions that could be applied after discharge to the community, using the threat of readmission (conditional discharge). As community care has developed in economically developed countries in the last 40 years, the association between coercion and hospital admission has increasingly been questioned. It has been successfully argued that as the locus of treatment moves to the community, coercive powers that can be applied outside a hospital are needed. The spread of IOC through a number of jurisdictions in recent decades as a result has also aroused controversy and calls for restrictions on its use. The extent to which evidence supports and contests IOC is considered further below.

Commitment in Different Jurisdictions

The legal structures that govern the use of involuntary commitment vary in their detailed application between jurisdictions, resulting in differences between countries and states; however, broad themes are common to all jurisdictions.

First, it is commonly the case that a specific law regulates the commitment of mentally ill persons. Therefore, from a legal point of view they are distinguishable from other people who may require medical treatment but are unable to consent to treatment due to temporary or permanent mental incapacity, such as dementia or learning disability. However, as the core concept of mental illness has changed over time, so lawmakers must decide whether to leave the definition entirely to clinical judgment or to circumscribe it in some way. This might involve inclusion criteria, such as a diagnosis included in a formal classification system, or exclusion criteria, such as substance abuse problems or unusual sexual behaviors.

Second, the law must state the criteria for commitment. The criteria that are usually included are considered further below. A distinction is usually made also between the stringency of the criteria applied in an emergency or to detain someone for a short period of assessment, and those applied for longer term treatments, and additional safeguards may be required for controversial or irreversible treatments, such as electroconvulsive therapy (ECT) and psychosurgery.

Third, the law must describe the way in which compulsion will be exercised, the roles assigned to police, doctors, other professionals (e.g., social workers or nurses), and the role of the courts. In different jurisdictions, the courts may have the primary role in authorizing detention, or this may be left to mental health professionals, who have varying degrees of police powers to exercise physical restraint. However, even in systems in which mental health professionals are given wide discretion to manage commitment, they are likely to rely on the police to support them in physically removing patients to hospital.

Fourth, the law will include mechanisms of appeal whereby a committed patient, or an authorized representative, can challenge professional decisions, and relatives or caregivers are also likely to have specified rights either to seek commitment or to oppose it.

Fifth, a distinction is usually made between the application of mental health legislation to people with mental disorders who have committed criminal offenses, with compulsory psychiatric treatment being one of the "disposal" options available to the courts, and to those who have not committed offenses and are therefore subject to civil commitment measures.

Criteria for Commitment

Criteria for commitment, although they do vary in different jurisdictions, also have common themes. It is usual for them to include the presence of mental illness, a consequent risk to the patient or to others, and the likelihood of treatment having a positive effect. The *least restrictive principle*, that treatment should be given with the least restriction of liberty possible, may be stated.

A useful version of these criteria is that prepared by the World Health Organization (WHO) in its *Resource Book on Mental Health, Human Rights and Legislation*, which recommends minimum standards to be applied in all jurisdictions (see Table 49.1).

Although these are desirable criteria, and most appear in some form in jurisdictions in which mental health legislation is well developed, there is room for debate. For example, WHO criteria include both the concept of mental illness as judged by an expert prac-

TABLE 49.1. WHO Criteria for Involuntary Committment

1. A person may be admitted involuntarily to a mental health facility . . . if . . . a qualified mental health practitioner authorized by law determines . . . that the person has a mental illness and considers
   a. that because of that mental illness, there is a serious likelihood of immediate or imminent harm to that person or other persons; or
   b. that in the case of a person whose mental illness is severe and whose judgment is impaired, failure to admit . . . is likely to lead to serious deterioration . . . or will prevent the giving of appropriate treatment that can only be given by admission.
2. In the case referred to in subparagraph (b) above, a second such mental health practitioner, independent of the first, should be consulted where possible.
3. A mental health facility may receive involuntarily admitted patients only if the facility has been designated to do so by a competent authority prescribed by domestic law.

Note. From World Health Organization (2005). Copyright 2005 by the World Health Organization. Adapted by permission.

titioner and the concept of impaired judgment (also known as *impaired capacity* to make decisions). It has been argued that if impaired judgment (assessed by a doctor or by another legal process) is present, then the criterion of diagnosed mental illness is redundant. By this argument, people with mental illness, but without impaired judgment, should be allowed to determine their own treatment, whereas people with impaired judgment may be treated involuntarily, in their own best interests, regardless of diagnosis.

The criteria allow wide latitude for clinical judgment, about not only the presence of mental illness but also the seriousness or imminence of risk (notoriously hard to assess accurately), the likelihood of deterioration without treatment, or what treatment is appropriate. Legal criteria provide a framework for clinical decisions but do not determine them.

NATURE AND IMPORTANCE OF INVOLUNTARY COMMITMENT

Involuntary commitment is widely used, with an estimated 2 million uses in the United States per year (0.8%, 800 per 100,000 population), somewhat higher than the total incarceration rate in the criminal justice system (500 per 100,000 per year). In England, 26,000 people were committed to hospital in 2004, and a further 3,000 were detained after entering a hospital voluntarily (a total of 58 per 100,000 per year), somewhat less than the total incarcerated by the criminal justice system (220 per 100,000 in 2002).

These numbers, although they demonstrate the scale of involuntary commitment, do not convey the importance of the issue to consumers of mental health care, for many of whom the use of forced treatment is a key issue in determining their attitude toward treatment and the professionals who provide it. They also cannot convey the extent to which the perceived threat of involuntary treatment may affect people receiving treatment voluntarily, even when compulsion is not actually threatened, or even considered, by the psychiatrist.

Studies of this perception that psychiatric treatment is coercive by researchers in the United States and Europe have shown that it is indeed widespread, and that although involuntary commitment is, as expected, an important factor in determining perceived coercion, patients who are treated "voluntarily" in the strict legal sense may perceive coercive pressures to take treatment from a number of sources, including family, housing organizations or the welfare system, as well as mental health professionals.

It has been suggested that coercion can helpfully be understood as forming part of a spectrum of "treatment pressures" placed on people. Szmukler and Applebaum (2001) have conceptualized a hierarchy of "treatment pressures" (Table 49.2) that may assist in understanding and making decisions to treat an individual involuntarily.

Persuasion, Leverage, and Inducement

These may be described as "positive pressures" to take treatment—the "carrots" rather than the "sticks." The lowest level of treatment pressure is *persuasion*, in which the professional sets out for the client the benefits of a particular course of action and attempts to counter objections. The patient is free to reject advice. The next level of pressure, *leverage*, assumes an interpersonal relationship between the client and professional that has an element of emotional dependence. This gives the professional power to pressure the client by demonstrating approval of one course of action or disapproval of another. Greater pressure may be exerted by *inducement*, in which acceptance of treatment is linked to material help, such as support in accessing charitable or welfare funds over and above any basic entitlement.

Threats and Compulsion

These "negative pressures" are overtly coercive. A threat could be made to withdraw services on which the client normally relies (which is more coercive than simply failing to offer inducements over and above normal services), or to detain the client in the hospital. Finally, involuntary commitment, at the highest level of the hierarchy of pressure, carries with it the power to use physical force to overcome resistance to treatment.

PERTINENT RESEARCH FINDINGS

The act of detaining a patient is a legal intervention, though one with clinical consequences. Depending on the research question being addressed, legal analysis, the principally qualitative methods of the social sciences, or the epidemiological and statistical methods of the medical sciences may be required.

An example of a question requiring legal analysis arose when the United Kingdom passed the Human Rights Act (2000), which introduced into domestic law the rights afforded by the European Convention on Human Rights (ECHR). It was suggested that this might lead to widespread challenges to psychiatric practice in the United Kingdom as articles of ECHR protecting the liberty and privacy of the subject were invoked, and some commentators predicted a "flood" of cases. An analysis of decisions of the Euro-

---

TABLE 49.2. Hierarchy of Treatment Pressures

- Persuasion
- Leverage
- Inducements
- Threats
- Compulsion (including the use of physical force)

Note. From Szmukler and Applebaum (2001). Copyright 2001 by Oxford University Press. Adapted by permission.

pean Court over many years, combined with a review of cases arising in the first year of the new Act, suggested that in fact courts, both European and UK, have historically been deferential to medical expertise and very unlikely to regard the current routine practice of commitment as breaching the human rights protected by the ECHR. This appears to be correct, and no flood of cases has resulted, though the low level of evidence presented for doctors' assertions about the level of risk posed by many committed patients would appear to leave their decisions vulnerable to legal challenge.

In an example of the application of qualitative methods, Peay (2003) sought to understand the reasoning underlying professionals' decisions to detain and to discharge patients using the English Mental Health Act. She did this by developing "case vignettes," videotaped interviews of "typical" patients, that were shown to professional pairs, a psychiatrist and a social worker, who were then asked to discuss the cases together, replicating the process by which actual commitment decisions are arrived at. It became apparent that a majority of psychiatrists made an initial assessment favoring compulsion. The social workers were much less likely to start from this position, and once dialogue between the professionals began, the eventual joint decision was more likely to reflect the social workers' initial assessment, with a joint recommendation of fewer commitments than the psychiatrists initially had suggested would be necessary. It was possible to distinguish three distinct approaches to the decision: *Clinical* decision makers formed their own view of the best interests of the patient and the wider society, and looked to interpret the legal criteria in such a way as to serve those interests. *Legal* decision makers had a detailed awareness of the legal criteria and attempted to use these to guide their decision. *Ethical* decision makers attempted to assess patients' capacity for judgment and take account of the patients' own views of their best interests. A general finding of the research was that the same vignette resulted in widely differing decisions, with different professional pairs assessing the various admission criteria relative to risk or the appropriateness of noncompulsory treatment as either justifying or not requiring involuntary commitment.

Though legislation in different jurisdictions may have elements in common, the actual rate of involuntary commitment that results is highly variable between cultures and nations. Evidence for this comes from survey data and analysis of routine statistics; for example, a recent review of psychiatric detention across Europe found that comparable estimates of rates of detention could be obtained from 12 states (Salize & Dressing, 2004). They varied enormously, from 6 per 100,000 population per year in Portugal and 11 per 100,000 in France, to 175 per 100,000 in Austria and Germany and 218 in 100,000 in Finland. England had a fairly high rate, 93 per 100,000 (in 1998). Generally countries with high detention rates also had high rates of informal admission, but Sweden and the United Kingdom had only moderate levels of overall admissions, a high proportion of which were involuntary (25–30%, including those detained after informal admission). The rate of detention appeared to have risen during the 1990s in many countries, but this seemed to be due to more frequent, but shorter, admissions rather than an absolute increase in compulsion. Though there are considerable differences between countries' criteria for detention, legal processes, and the use of detention for dementia or substance abuse, none of these account for the difference in rates. However, there tend to be lower levels of detention in countries that require involvement of a legal representative for all detained patients.

The results of epidemiological studies also suggest that individual clinicians' interpretation of criteria for commitment vary. An ecological study of rates of detention in hospitals in 34 catchment areas in England showed that rates varied widely, and that although the level of socioeconomic deprivation was a strong predictor of the rate, there was a high level of unexplained variation, likely due to differing approaches by clinical teams or individual clinicians.

POLICY AND SOCIAL IMPLICATIONS

Evidence for and Justification of IOC

An important and controversial policy issue in many jurisdictions has been the extent to which involuntary treatment should be extended into the community.

Two randomized controlled studies have compared the effectiveness of IOC in reducing hospital admission. The first, carried out in New York, randomly assigned 78 people discharged from Bellevue Hospital to compulsory community treatment and compared them with 64 people treated voluntarily by the same intensive treatment team (Steadman et al., 2001). Over the following 11 months, no difference was observed in the rate of admission, symptoms, or quality of life, and no patient in either group was charged with a violent offense.

The second study, in North Carolina, randomly assigned 129 people to compulsory treatment and 135 to voluntary treatment of varying intensity and by four different teams (Swartz et al., 2001). In this study, the compulsorily treated group had 57% fewer admissions and spent 20 days more in the community over the 1-year follow-up. However, the reduction in admissions occurred only when compulsory orders were associated with more intensive treatment. It may be that it is the availability of intensive treatment that matters, and if this is available to everyone, as in New York, compulsion adds nothing. A 2000 review published by the RAND Corporation also concluded that the evidence gathered across the United States did not support the use of IOC, and a database study in Australia had similar negative conclusions (Kisely, Xiao, & Preston, 2004). Although research evidence is only one of a number of factors that should be taken into account in formulating policy, it has had very little impact on the spread of IOC legislation introduced in many jurisdictions in recent decades. However, the question of whether IOC "works" remains an important one for future research.

Ethical Basis of Detention

As described earlier, legislation usually requires that commitment be justified on the grounds that failure to accept psychiatric treatment involve risks to the health or safety of the patient or of others, though these risks are often rather poorly defined and rarely quantifiable. Deciding what level of treatment pressure is commensurate with the risk is not straightforward, but it may be helpful to try to apply an ethical framework commonly used to assist decision making in general medicine. This requires consideration of the person's capacity to take treatment decisions that are in his or her best interests. *Capacity* is usually defined as the ability to understand and retain information about the proposed treatment, and to weigh in the balance the consequences of alternative decisions about it. People with capacity can determine what treatment is in their own best interests, even where their views are not in accord with those of clinicians, and minimal pressure, perhaps limited to persuasion, is all that can be justified. If capacity is lacking, the treatment that is in the person's best interest may need to be determined by clinicians, though taking account, if possible, of the past and present wishes of the patient, and the views of significant others. Advance statements about treatment preferences, made with capacity in anticipation of a future loss of capacity, such as might occur in psychotic relapse, carries weight in the assessment of what is in someone's best interests. Once the treatment that is in the best interests of the patient is established, the minimal level of pressure necessary to achieve the objectives of this treatment can then be exerted.

Although the application of this framework is helpful in clarifying the decision to be made, mental health professionals are often faced with situations in which a simple judgment of capacity is not easy to make. A client may, apparently through choice, live in squalor or on the streets. Does such an apparently irrational choice necessarily imply a lack of capacity, or must delusional reasoning be established? Even if capacity seems to be absent, what minimum standard of living is in the best interests of a patient who expresses no desire for material comforts?

Faced with such complex issues, it is tempting to resort to the traditional medical approach of assuming that best interests are best determined by a beneficent doctor. However, attempting to apply a capacity-based approach clarifies that the client's reasoning about his or her situation is the starting point for the decision, and makes it less likely that the values, anxieties, or prejudices of others will prevail over the client's expressed views. Sharing difficult decisions with multidisciplinary teams, caregivers and advocates similarly reduces the risk of poor or hasty judgments.

Though the law may allow compulsion on the grounds of risk to others, and mental health services are exposed to strong societal expectations that they should prevent violence by their patients, attempting to take an ethical approach to treatment pressure on these grounds presents considerable difficulties. There are very few circumstances in which citizens without mental disorder can be detained preventively on the grounds of risk, and it is hard to justify taking a different approach to clients with capacity. The challenge for professionals is to avoid being pressured into applying an ethical double standard, in which behavior that would not justify significant sanction in the absence of mental disorder is used to justify loss of liberty, or in which levels of treatment pressure are not commensurate with the actual level of risk.

KEY POINTS

- Involuntary commitment has historically been seen as a central aspect of the treatment of schizophrenia.
- Criteria for commitment vary between jurisdictions but typically include the presence of a mental disorder, risk to the patient, risk to others, and an expectation of therapeutic benefit (or the prevention of deterioration).
- These criteria are seldom capable of rigid definition, and their interpretation varies among clinicians and jurisdictions, resulting in highly variable proportions of those diagnosed with schizophrenia being assumed to require commitment in different mental health systems.
- The ethical basis of this is not always made explicit in law; therefore, clinicians must combine an understanding of the legal criteria for commitment with an ethical understanding of the basis for clinical involvement in state-sanctioned detention.
- Good clinical practice requires the use of the least restrictive form of treatment.

REFERENCES AND RECOMMENDED READINGS

Allen, M., & Smith, V. F. (2001). Opening Pandora's box: The practical and legal dangers of involuntary outpatient commitment. *Psychiatric Services, 52,* 343–346.

Applebaum, P. (2001). Thinking carefully about outpatient commitment. *Psychiatric Services, 52,* 347–350.

Bindman, J., Tighe, J., Thornicroft, G., & Leese, M. (2002). Poverty, poor services, and compulsory psychiatric admission in England. *Social Psychiatry and Psychiatric Epidemiology, 37,* 341–345.

Holloway, F., Szmukler, G., & Sullivan, D. (2000). Involuntary outpatient treatment. *Current Opinion in Psychiatry, 13,* 689—692.

Kisely, S., Campbell, L., & Preston, N. (2005). Compulsory community and involuntary outpatient treatment for people with severe mental disorders. *Cochrane Database Systematic Reviews, 3,* CD004408.

Kisely, S. R., Xiao, J., & Preston, N. J. (2004). Impact of compulsory community treatment on admission rates: Survival analysis using linked mental health and offender databases. *British Journal of Psychiatry, 184,* 432–438.

Monahan, J., Bonnie, R. J., Applebaum, P. S., Hyde, P. S., Steadman, H. J., & Swartz, M. S. (2001). Mandated community treatment: Beyond outpatient commitment. *Psychiatric Services, 52,* 1198—1205.

Peay, J. (2003). *Decisions and dilemmas working with mental health law.* Oxford, UK: Hart.

Rand Corporation. (2000). *Does involuntary outpatient treatment work?* (Law & Health Research Brief No. RB-4537), Santa Monica, CA: Author. Retrieved from *http://www.rand.org/pubs/research_briefs/RB4537/index1.html*

Salize, H. J., & Dressing, H. (2004). Epidemiology of involuntary placement of mentally ill people across the European Union. *British Journal of Psychiatry, 184,* 163–168.

Steadman, H. J., Gounis, K. L., Dennis, D., Hopper, K., Roche, B., Swartz, M., et al. (2001). Assessing the New York City involuntary outpatient commitment pilot program. *Psychiatric Services, 52* 330–336.

Swartz, M. S., Swanson, J. W., Hiday, V. A., Wagner, H. R., Burns, B. J., & Borum, R. (2001). A randomized controlled trial of outpatient commitment in North Carolina. *Psychiatric Services, 52,* 325–329.

Szmukler, G., & Appelbaum, P. (2001). Treatment pressures, coercion and compulsion. In G. Thornicroft & G. Szmukler (Eds.), *Textbook of community psychiatry* (pp. 529–544). Oxford, UK: Oxford University Press.

Torrey, E. F., & Zdanowicz, M. (2001). Outpatient commitment: What, why, and for whom. *Psychiatric Services, 52,* 337—341.

World Health Organization. (2005). *Resource book on mental health, human rights and legislation.* Geneva: Author.

CHAPTER 50

JAIL DIVERSION

JOSEPH P. MORRISSEY
GARY S. CUDDEBACK

Currently, more people with severe mental illness are admitted to jails in the United States each year than are admitted to psychiatric hospitals. The numbers are truly staggering. In 2000, there were more than 1 million jail admissions of persons with severe mental illness and only about 645,000 hospitalizations. That means the relative risk of jail detention for a person with severe mental illness is about 150% *greater* than the risk of hospitalization. The phrase often bandied about is that "jails have become the new mental hospitals," but jails provide mental health services only as a last resort to meet obligations concerning the conditions of safe confinement mandated by the U.S. Constitution. Most have very inadequate mental health staffing even for assessment and immediate crisis intervention, which together, at a minimum, should be the limited goals for any in-jail mental health service program.

Many mental health experts would agree that any in-jail mental health services should focus on assessment, crisis stabilization, and diversion—*not* on long-term treatment. Given this goal, any needs for ongoing treatment and rehabilitation are more efficiently and effectively met in community-based settings. This principle underlies the many attempts to use jail diversion to deal with this problem in communities across the country. This chapter reviews the basic types of jail diversion programs, their common features, the available research evidence about their successes and failures, and some directions for more effective approaches in the future.

NATURE AND IMPORTANCE OF JAIL DIVERSION

Jails and Prisons

There are about 3,365 jails in the United States. Jails are local detention facilities, usually operated by county sheriffs. In some large cities a municipal jail is operated by the police department separate from the county jail that serves multiple cities and towns. Some municipal or county jails are operated by civilian correctional administrations, independent of law enforcement. Jails range in size from 10-cell facilities in rural counties to the megajails in large cities, such as Chicago, New York, and Los Angeles, that accommodate 8,000–10,000 detainees in single or multiple complexes. Jails serve as adjuncts to the courts, detaining individuals awaiting trial, those convicted and sentenced for 1 year or less, and those on hold pending transfer to other state or Federal authorities. Jails are designed as short-term facilities, so they are not equipped or staffed to provide a lot of services for their detainees. Most individuals admitted to jails are released within 48 hours.

In 2000, there were 1,320 adult state prisons, 84 Federal prisons, and 264 private prisons that operated under contract with government (mostly Federal) agencies. Prisons house *convicted felons*, persons who have committed serious crimes and are sentenced by the courts for a few years to life imprisonment. These facilities are operated by state or Federal departments of corrections, which are staffed separately from law enforcement. As long-stay facilities, they are equipped and staffed to provide recreational, vocational, and health care services for their inmates. All persons serving time in prison have spent some time in jail as part of their criminal justice processing.

On June 30, 2004, there were 713,990 persons in jails and another 1,494,216 in prisons. Although prisons house twice as many inmates as jails on any given day, more people pass through jails than through prisons over the course of a year, because jails are short-stay, quick-turnaround facilities, whereas prisons are long-stay facilities. In 2004, jails had about 13.5 million admissions, whereas state and Federal prisons combined had only 28,000 admissions.

The fates of persons with mental illness have always been intertwined with the shifting boundaries between the criminal justice and mental health systems. The presence of persons with mental illness in jails is not new; the problem has been around for 200 years, since the very beginnings of organized efforts to improve the care of persons with mental disorders in the United States. What is new is the volume of cases involving persons with severe mental illness now processed through jails. Just as state mental hospitals once served as the institutions of last resort for the care and confinement of persons with mental illness, jails have become the last secure environment in most communities for the control of difficult-to-manage and noncompliant behavior. So, to a large extent, jails have now taken on the social custody and time-out role once reserved for state mental hospitals, but on a short-term, revolving-door basis.

The primary locus of diversion for persons with mental illness is law enforcement and jails, not prisons. With determinant sentencing, by the time a person with a severe mental illness is convicted of a serious crime and gets sentenced to prison, it is too late to divert him or her to a community-based treatment program. The opportunity for diversion, if there is one, occurs during the initial, pretrial detention period in the jail or, for less serious offenders, during their sentenced time in jail. The more serious the offense, however, the less the likelihood that criminal justice authorities will consent to diversion of a person with mental illness. As a consequence, diversion of most people at the point of jail detention is for misdemeanor, nonviolent charges.

There is growing concern about the large numbers of people with severe mental illness being released either through parole, when a substantial portion of a sentence has been served, or at completion of a full sentence. For prisons, effective reentry into the community requires arrangements for housing, restoration of entitlements, and participation in appropriate treatment to ease reintegration of prisoners whose ties to family and the community have been strained or severed as a result of several years of incarceration. Although it is correct to view these reentry programs as efforts to avoid future incarcerations, they are better thought of as *prevention* programs rather than true diversion programs that avoid arrest or secure early release of persons from criminal justice sanctions.

In this chapter, then, the term *diversion* is used only with reference to law enforcement and jail-based programs.

What Is Jail Diversion?

The goal of jail diversion is to eliminate or reduce the time a person with severe mental illness is detained or incarcerated as a result of potential or pending criminal charges. Diversion has two key components: (1) eliminating/reducing jail time and (2) linking diverted individuals to community-based treatment. Beginning in the 1990s, a variety of jail diversion programs began to crop up in various locales around the country, funded primarily by Federal and state demonstration programs. By 2005, according to GAINS Center estimates, there were 294 operational jail diversion programs.

Who Benefits from Jail Diversion?

The prime beneficiary of jail diversion is the person with severe mental illness. There is evidence that persons with mental illness will often be charged, convicted, and sentenced more severely than other people arrested for similar behavior. Moreover, it has been reported that persons with mental illness spend two to five times longer in jail than persons without mental illness. While in jail, they may spend more time in segregated housing and isolation cells, and have more restricted privileges than other detainees. So diversion to community-based mental health treatment can make a significant difference in quality of life and functioning.

It is also important to recognize that there are other beneficiaries in jail diversion. Mental health clinicians and police/jail authorities can find common ground in diverting people with severe mental illness from the criminal justice system. Clinicians seek to help people with severe mental illness stay out of hospitals and jails by facilitating access to and use of treatment and support services that improve their functioning and quality of life. Police officers want to keep the peace, to avoid any escalation of violence when called to a disturbance, and to secure arrangements that help persons with mental illness who are repeatedly involved in disturbances or behaviors that warrant arrest. Jail correctional personnel want to maintain conditions that promote detainee and correctional officer safety while holding people with criminal charges pending their adjudication. Jail authorities are also motivated to reduce the administrative burden that detainees with severe mental illness often place on the jail by exacerbating jail overcrowding and requiring specialized in-jail housing, extra staffing, and special precautions, such as suicide watch.

The common ground here is that recognizing someone has a severe mental illness and engaging that person in mental health treatment minimizes or averts untoward situations that would otherwise compromise the public health and public safety goals of all parties. Finally, families and consumer advocates share a common ground with mental health clinicians and police/jail authorities in that all parties desire the most appropriate treatment in the least restrictive settings for persons with mental illness who are involved with the criminal justice system.

When Does Diversion Occur?

Pathways into, through, and out of criminal justice processing involve a series of steps through which any criminal defendant passes, regardless of his or her mental health status. The GAINS Center has conceptualized criminal justice processing as a pathway with several distinct points at which a defendant with severe mental illness might be intercepted and diverted to community-based mental health treatment (Munetz & Griffin, 2006; see Figure 50.1). For a mental health clinician the significance of this "sequential intercept model" is that the different intercept points identify the main criminal justice partners that must be engaged if diversion is to work, as well as the legal constraints with which he or she must deal in developing a diversion plan, as discussed below.

Basically, there are two types of jail diversion programs: prebooking and postbooking diversion. *Prebooking diversions* occur before arrest and before charges are filed. Here, the partnership is between mental health clinicians and police officers. The goal is to avoid charging a person with a crime when there is evidence of severe mental illness and the behavior or offense is a nonviolent misdemeanor (low-level offense). This is diversion at the "front door" of the criminal justice system, because the individual never enters the system via arrest and detention.

Several models of police–mental health clinician collaboration have been developed, including the traditional *referral approach*, whereby police officers bring persons with mental illness to a community mental health center for evaluation and treatment, and the *colocation approach*, in which civilian mental health clinicians are employed by the law enforcement agency to work alongside police officers. But the most effective current form of police-based diversion is the crisis intervention team (CIT), whose members are sworn officers trained to act as liaisons to the mental health system and to learn about basic concepts of mental illness, special management techniques for diffusing disturbances involving persons with mental illness, and procedures for transporting persons with mental illness to a no-refusal psychiatric emergency service rather than jail. With the endorsement and support of the National Alliance on Mental Illness (NAMI), CITs have diffused rapidly since the prototype program was developed in Memphis, Tennessee, in the early 1990s. Now CITs can be found in police departments in many large and mid-size cities across the country.

Postbooking diversions occur at one of several points after the filing of formal charges by a police officer. Here, the police officer exits the diversion scene, and several

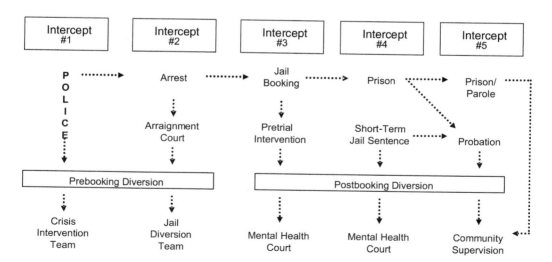

FIGURE 50.1. GAINS Center sequential intercept model. This diagram is a modification of the *Sequential Intercepts for Change: CJ-MH Participation* model, which can be found at *www.gainscenter. samhsa.gov.*

new partners come on stage—judges, district attorneys, jail administrators, public defenders, and possibly probation officers. Postbooking diversion can occur at first arraignment court; during pretrial detention in the jail; at adjudication by a regular or mental health court; or following conviction and sentencing to prison, jail, or probation (community supervision). All of these options represent "backdoor" diversions, in that the person already has been booked into the jail, and the effort shifts to reducing the length of time under criminal justice supervision. This is accomplished by negotiating with the criminal justice partners to secure alternative sentencing, conditional release, or dropped charges given the rationale that the person will enter into well-supervised mental health treatment. These arrangements are mandated or ordered by a criminal court or a specialty mental health court, with stipulations that create continuing obligations to the court for both the offender and the treatment provider. If probation is the intercept point, then probation officers become important partners in the postbooking diversion process as well.

How Does Postbook Diversion Work?

There are times when an informal or ad hoc approach might work for diverting a person with severe mental illness from jail, but a formal, well-planned, programmatic approach is much more effective. The APIC model (Assess, Plan, Identify, and Coordinate) offers a best practice approach to managing the early release and reentry of jail detainees (Osher, Steadman, & Barr, 2003; see Table 50.1). This model provides guidance for mental health and criminal justice partners, and proposes a set of critical elements that, if implemented, is likely to improve outcomes for persons with mental illness who are being released from jail. The four stages of the APIC model are described below.

Assess

In this initial stage, a detainee's psychosocial, medical, and behavioral needs and strengths are carefully evaluated. Information is compiled from law enforcement, court, corrections, correctional health, families, and community providers, with the goal of creating a plan for transitioning the person to community care. Consistent with empowerment principles, efforts are made to engage the detainee in an assessment of his or her own needs. Also, logistical issues around access to and means to pay for community-based treatment and services must be explored. It is self-defeating to refer a detainee to a community service that only takes insured persons, for example, without first checking to see that the individual has Medicaid, Veterans Administration entitlements, or other third-party coverage.

TABLE 50.1. The APIC Model for Postbook Diversion

Item	Description
Assess	Assess the inmate's clinical and social needs, and public safety risks.
Plan	Plan for the treatment and services required to address the inmate's needs.
Identify	Identify required community and correctional programs responsible for postrelease services.
Coordinate	Coordinate the transition plan to ensure implementation and avoid gaps in care with community-based services.

Note. From Osher, Steadman, and Barr (2003). Copyright 2003 by Sage Publications, Inc. Reprinted by permission.

Plan

The goal of transition planning is to address both the detainee's short- and long-term needs. To this end, special consideration must be given to the critical period immediately following release to the community—the first hour, day, and week after leaving jail. How will the person's basic needs for food, shelter, and clothing be met outside the jail? In addition, a major problem that can arise when a person is released from jail is disruption in the supply of psychotropic medications started in jail. Good practice calls for providing a sufficient amount of medication to last at least until the person can be seen for a follow-up appointment in the community.

Identify

At this stage, the challenge is to identify specific community referrals that are appropriate to each releasee based on the underlying clinical diagnosis, cultural and demographic factors, financial arrangements, geographic location, and the person's legal circumstances. The goal is to ensure that treatment and supportive services match the person's level of disability, motivation for change, and availability of community resources. It is also important to negotiate with the court and probation officer, so that the conditions of release and community supervision match the severity of the person's criminal behavior. Another important consideration is to address the community treatment provider's role (with regard to limits of confidentiality) vis-à-vis other social service, parole, and probation agencies, and the court system.

Coordinate

The APIC model sensitizes clinicians to the complex, multiple needs that detainees with severe mental illness often have, and to the use of case managers who coordinate multiple sources of community care and help the detainee span the jail–community boundary following release. Other considerations at this stage are confirming that the releasee knows the details about follow-up appointments and has identified contact persons in the community for tracking purposes if aftercare appointments are not kept.

PERTINENT RESEARCH FINDINGS

Is jail diversion effective? The answer to this question depends upon whether criminal justice or mental health outcomes are used as the standard of evidence. Current research suggests that for people with severe mental illness compared to nondiverted individuals, jail diversion does lead to more time in the community (i.e., fewer days in jail). However, individuals who are diverted do not have more favorable mental health outcomes (reduced symptoms, improved functioning, etc.) than those who are not diverted. The most comprehensive effort to address these issues was the 5-year (1997–2002) multisite demonstration study funded by the Substance Abuse and Mental Health Services Administration (SAMHSA), as described below.

The SAMHSA study used a quasi-experimental, nonequivalent comparison group design to examine the public health and public safety outcomes of three prebooking diversion programs in Oregon, Pennsylvania, and Tennessee, and three postbooking diversion programs in Arizona, Connecticut, and Oregon (Broner, Lattimore, Cowell, & Schlenger, 2004). Research staff interviewed participants at baseline, at 3 months, and at

12 months using a common interview protocol. A total of 1,966 participants (971 diverted and 995 nondiverted) were enrolled, with 76% retention at 3 months and 69% at 12 months.

The main findings (based on 1,185 participants who completed 12-month interviews) indicated the following:

1. Diverted participants spent an average of 2 months less time in jail (i.e., more time in the community) than did the nondiverted participants (303 vs. 245 days, respectively).
2. Despite more days in the community, diverted and nondiverted participants had comparable rearrest rates (1.03 vs. 1.2, respectively) during the 12-month follow-up period, so diversion did not appear to increase public safety risk.
3. Diverted participants were linked to community-based services at a higher rate (+6 to +13% across several services) than were nondiverted participants, but whether participants actually received appropriate evidence-based services consistent with their needs could not be determined.
4. Although diverted participants received significantly more mental health treatment than nondiverted participants, the outcomes on mental health symptoms at 12 months did not significantly differ between the two groups.
5. Service use costs were examined at four sites. Overall, jail diversion resulted in lower criminal justice costs and greater community mental health treatment costs, because diverted participants received more community mental health treatment than did nondiverted participants. And, at least in the short run, the additional community mental health treatment costs were higher than criminal justice agency savings.

These findings suggest that diversion works from a criminal justice perspective, in that it reduces time spent in jail and does not increase public safety risks (Steadman & Naples, 2005). However, diversion to routine community mental health treatment does not seem to improve mental health outcomes (e.g., symptom reduction, improved quality of life). Would diversion to evidence-based, intensive services make more of a difference in mental health outcomes? Further research is needed to determine whether diversion to intensive evidence-based services such as assertive community treatment or dual-diagnosis treatment teams would significantly improve mental health and criminal justice outcomes.

POLICY AND SOCIAL IMPLICATIONS

Diversion programs for persons with severe mental illness who come in contact with local law enforcement and jails have emerged over the last 30 years as one strategy to keep persons with severe mental illness out of our jails and in the community, where they can receive the best possible treatments in the least restrictive settings. There are a number of social and policy implications to developing and providing jail diversion services. Some of these issues are discussed below.

Access to Evidence-Based Treatments

Although access to evidence-based practice for persons with mental illness is generally poor, the gulf is especially wide in the criminal justice area. Current evidence clearly indicates that jail diversion programs can successfully divert people from criminal justice processing. What is less clear is the programs' ability to link diverted individuals to appropriate, evidence-based treatment for severe mental illness, co-occurring substance abuse disorders, and a host of other medical and social problems. The continuing challenge for mental health clinicians and policymakers is to mobilize sufficient and effective interventions for this population. The goal of providing care in the least restrictive setting is elusive and often does not provide effective treatments. A number of treatments with known effectiveness have not yet been made available in sufficient quantity or duration to help people with severe mental illness stay out of jail. This remains one of the greatest challenges in community mental health.

Parallel Systems of Care

Current mental health and criminal justice policies have created parallel systems of care for treating persons with severe mental illness in both community and correctional settings. For many communities, allocating more dollars to mental health services in correctional settings often means there are fewer dollars available to support community-based treatment. This creates a situation in which scarce resources for mental health care are stretched between two inadequate systems of care. If inmates are to be confined against their will in detention settings, the U.S. Constitution requires that their health care needs be met. The implications seem clear enough. As many persons with severe mental illness as possible should be diverted from the criminal justice system to community care. Until community care is adequately funded, however, persons with mental illness will continue to pass through the revolving door of jails and prisons.

Who Benefits, Who Pays?

Jail diversion programs are precarious efforts that try to link two systems that, left to their own separate priorities, usually have competing philosophies and objectives. With distressed mental health and corrections budgets at all levels of government, diversion programs often fall between the cracks, with neither system feeling ownership or responsibility to fully fund these diversion programs. Typically, jail diversion programs, both pre- and postbooking, are started with Federal or state seed money. Unfortunately, once these Federal or state demonstration dollars stop, most jail diversion programs either cease operations altogether or convert to a more generic and less effective service modality. Current evidence points to a mismatch between who benefits and who pays for jail diversion programs, with local mental health authorities shouldering more of the costs and correctional programs realizing more of the benefits. One goal, then, is to strive for partnership and collaboration among mental health and criminal justice stakeholders, such that the costs and benefits of jail diversion can be shared by both.

Here is where services research can come to the aid of clinical practice. Research aimed at establishing the cost-effectiveness of calibrated interventions—those designed to meet the varying needs of people with mental illness in the criminal justice system—can go a long way toward sustaining jail diversion efforts. The challenge here is that current evidence suggests that diversion is not cost-effective, but no long-term studies that examine the balance of up-front costs and downstream savings have been conducted. To the extent that research could address the value-added nature of diversion, then there would be a stronger evidence base for insisting upon adequate funding for programs that improve community living opportunities for the thousands of persons with mental illness now caught up in the criminal justice system.

KEY POINTS

- Diversion of detainees with severe mental illness is essential given that the goal of in-jail mental health services is to focus on assessment, crisis stabilization, and diversion—*not* on long-term treatment.
- Jail diversion can occur at the front door (prebooking) or the back door (postbooking) of the jail, and there are a number of sequential intercept points in both areas where persons with severe mental illness can be diverted from criminal justice processing.
- Partnerships between mental health clinicians and criminal justice authorities are essential for a workable diversion program.
- Current research evidence suggests that jail diversion is more successful in reducing jail time and lowering criminal justice system costs; however, jail diversion may increase mental health treatment costs, and these increases appear higher than the criminal justice savings associated with jail diversion.
- Many jail detainees with severe mental illness also have co-occurring substance abuse disorders, poor functioning, and long histories of repeated incarcerations and hospitalizations; the intensity of the services provided to these individuals must be calibrated to their needs.
- Further research is needed to determine whether diversion to intensive, evidence-based services such as assertive community treatment or dual-diagnosis treatment teams would significantly improve both mental health and criminal justice system outcomes for jail detainees with severe mental illness.
- Further research aimed at establishing the cost-effectiveness of calibrated interventions can go a long way toward sustaining diversion efforts and improving community living opportunities for thousands of persons with mental illness who cycle in and out of the criminal justice system.

REFERENCES AND RECOMMENDED READINGS

Borum, R., Deane, M., Steadman, H., & Morrissey, J. (1998). Police perspective on responding to mentally ill people in crisis: Perceptions of program effectiveness. *Behavioral Sciences and the Law, 16*, 393–405.

Broner, N., Lattimore, P. K., Cowell, A. J., & Schlenger, W. (2004). Effects of diversion on adults with co-occuring mental illness and substance use: Outcomes from a national multi-site study. *Behavioral Sciences and the Law, 22*, 1–23.

Harrison, P., & Beck, A. (2005). *Prison and jail inmates at midyear 2004.* Washington, DC: Bureau of Justice Statistics, U.S. Department of Justice Office of Justice Programs.

Massaro, J. (2004). *Working with people with mental illness involved in the criminal justice system: What mental health service providers need to know.* Delmar, NY: National GAINS Technical Assistance and Policy Analysis Center for Jail Diversion.

Munetz, M. R., & Griffin, P. A. (2006). Use of the sequential intercept model as an approach to decriminalization of people with serious mental illness. *Psychiatric Services, 57*(4), 544–549.

Osher, F., Steadman, H. J., & Barr, H. (2003). A best practice approach to community reentry from jails for inmates with co-occurring disorders: The APIC model. *Crime and Delinquency, 49*(1), 79–96.

Reuland, M., & Cheney, J. (2005). Enhancing success of police-based diversion programs for people with mental illness. Delmar, NY: GAINS Technical Assistance and Policy Analysis Center for Jail Diversion.

Steadman, H. J., Deane, M. W., Morrissey, J. P., Westcott, M. L., Salasin, S., & Shapiro, S. (1999). A SAMHSA research initiative assessing the effectiveness of jail diversion programs for mentally ill persons. *Psychiatric Services, 50*(12), 1620–1623.

Steadman, H. J., McCarty, D. W., & Morrissey, J. P. (1989). *The mentally ill in jail: Planning for essential services.* New York: Guilford Press.

Steadman, H. J., & Naples, M. (2005). Assessing the effectiveness of jail diversion programs for persons with serious mental illness and co-occurring substance use disorders. *Behavioral Sciences and the Law, 23*, 163–170.

CHAPTER 51

STIGMA

PATRICK W. CORRIGAN
JONATHON E. LARSON

Mental illness presents a complex phenomenon that cuts into human lives like a double-edged sword. On the one hand, illness and medication side effects negatively impact emotions, cognitive abilities, memory, problem-solving skills, decision-making abilities, social skills, communication skills, and other domains. On the other, stigma leads to discrimination, which removes people's opportunities to reach and maintain life goals. Complete intervention requires addressing both problems. This chapter focuses on the latter: the stigma of mental illness. Several processes initiate the stigma of mental illness. We review the impact of stigma by first discussing the mental illness label.

PROCESSES AND STRUCTURES THAT LEAD TO STIGMA

Mental Illness Label

Individuals *labeled* with mental illness often fall victim to the corresponding stigma. These labels arise through different mechanisms. Health care professionals label individuals with mental illness through diagnostic processes. Professionals intend to help rather than to harm people with mental illness; despite the intent, diagnoses produce labels that orient the public to be prejudicial. Similarly, people may receive the label through association; for example, individuals observed leaving a support group held at a mental health center might be labeled "mentally ill." Labels lead to stigmatizing public reactions against individuals so labeled. The negative social reactions exacerbate the course of psychiatric disorders. Individuals with mental illness may also label themselves and internalize the label, which can result in self-stigma.

Common responses to the labels of mental illness include fear and disgust. People experiencing these reactions tend to minimize contact and distance themselves socially from individuals with the label. Avoidance negatively impacts individuals with mental illness, because they lose opportunities to interact with people and to pursue life goals. These kinds of experiences facilitate the process of becoming a "mental patient" rather than becoming a human being with hopes, dreams, and life goals. Labels produce stigmatizing reactions that cause harm in the lives of individuals experiencing mental illness.

Public Stigma

The general population primarily demonstrates public stigma through negative reactions and behaviors toward people with severe mental illness. Public stigma describes society's negative beliefs, reactions, and behaviors toward individuals with mental illness. As outlined in Figure 51.1, public stigma consists of stereotypes, prejudice, and discrimination. First, stereotypes provide cognitive structures that categorize information about social groups: "Those crazy people are incompetent, commit dangerous acts, and possess weak characters." Second, prejudice includes the endorsement of a stereotype and in turn an emotional response: "Yes, those crazy people commit dangerous acts and that scares me." Third, discrimination contains a behavioral reaction to the prejudice: "I will not employ or rent to people with mental illness, because they commit dangerous acts that scare me."

Public stigma negatively impacts the lives of individuals with mental illness. First, stigma may rob individuals of important life opportunities, including gainful employment, safe and comfortable housing, relationships, community functions, and educational opportunities. Specifically, individuals labeled with mental illness find it difficult to obtain these important life goals because of discriminating practices endorsed by employers, landlords, neighbors, friends, family, community members, and education professionals. Second, stigma negatively interacts with the criminal justice system; mental illness becomes criminalized rather than being treated as a mental health problem. Individuals with psychiatric symptoms more often face the likelihood of being arrested than do members of the general public; this leads others to treat individuals with mental illness as criminals rather than to provide mental health treatment for psychiatric symptoms. Third, health care systems withhold appropriate medical services from individuals due to stigma. Specifically, individuals with mental illness receive fewer insurance benefits and medical services than do members of the general public, and insurance plans provide fewer mental health benefits than physical health services. Moreover, when individuals with mental illness present with physical symptoms, health care providers may be more likely to attribute any health concerns to psychiatric symptoms, such as delusions or paranoia, rather than to actual physical ailments.

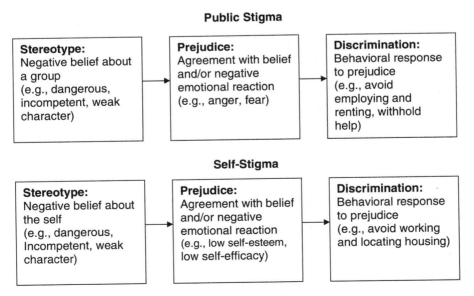

FIGURE 51.1. The cognitive components of stigma that influence public stigma and self-stigma.

Label Avoidance

Label avoidance refers to individuals' concealment of their mental illness to avoid being labeled "mentally ill"; this may then cause significant harm in their lives. They may decide to avoid the harm of stigma by hiding their mental illness and "staying in the closet." Coming out of the closet may have negative impacts on personal relationships, housing, career opportunities, and other life goals. Alternatively, individuals may opt to bypass the stigma altogether by denying their group status and avoiding recovery support of community mental health centers that tag them with labels. In label avoidance, individuals decide that hiding their mental illness causes less harm than obtaining the recovery support that typically leads to the label of mental illness. This type of label avoidance is the most significant way that stigma impedes mental health care–seeking behaviors.

Many individuals avoid disclosure of their mental illness to coworkers, friends, family, and community members to escape negative statements that lead to decreased self-esteem, minimized self-efficacy, and increased shame upon themselves and family members. Within this type of label avoidance, protecting the self and one's social image from harm outweighs benefits from receiving support that leads to the mental illness label.

Self-Stigma

Individuals with mental illness may endorse and demonstrate self-stigma through harmful self-thoughts and turning negative behaviors inward. As outlined in Figure 51.1, self-stigma includes the same components as public stigma, although the components interact differently. First, individuals may hear and believe mental illness stereotypes: "People say I am incompetent because of my illness, and I believe it." Second, prejudiced individuals agree with and internalize stereotypes: "Because I am incompetent, I believe that I can't accomplish anything." Third, discrimination includes individuals reacting to prejudice with a behavioral response: "I am incompetent, so I'm not going to apply for that job."

Just like public stigma, self-stigma negatively impacts many aspects of individuals' lives. Specifically, individuals who engage in self-prejudice and self-discrimination avoid trying to achieve employment, housing, political, educational, relationship, and health care goals. By being continually bombarded publicly with stigmatizing images and behaviors, individuals who endorse these notions may have minimal self-esteem, self-efficacy, and confidence, which may lead to a lack of drive to pursue life goals. Moreover, by internalizing stigma, individuals may believe they are less valued in society.

Structural Stigma

At the social level, political, economic, and historical forces create stigmatizing social barriers that restrict life opportunities for individuals with mental illness. Structural stigma comprises two levels: institutional policies and social structures. Examples of institutional policies, based on prejudice of leaders, include laws and regulations that discriminate against individuals with mental illness. For example, some states maintain laws and administrative rules that restrict the rights of individuals with mental illness in the areas of jury service, voting, holding public office, marriage, parenting, gun ownership, and professional licensure. Government entities develop these laws and rules based on the label of mental illness rather than on the severity of disability resulting from the impact of psychiatric symptoms on functioning.

Structural stigma developed historically through economic and political injustices wrought by prejudice and discrimination. The essential aspect of structural stigma is not the intent to stigmatize, but rather the effect of keeping individuals with mental illness in subordinate positions. There is not a specific prejudicial group in power maintaining structural stigma; rather, it is the product of discriminatory historical trends relative to mental illness. For example, current structural stigma maintains a political and economic environment that promotes the inability to achieve parity between mental and physical health insurance coverage. For several decades, insurance benefits for physical illness have continued to surpass benefits for mental illness; this leads to the assumption that greater benefits for mental health decrease the benefits available for physical health. In another example of structural stigma, mental illness research receives minimal Federal dollars compared to other health care research. Because agencies fund physical health research at a much higher rate, knowledge that reduces mental illness stigma and enlightens mental health policies cannot be gained at the same rate as knowledge in physical health fields. Overall, structural stigma manifests itself as either institutional policies or social structures that negatively impact the lives of individuals with mental illness.

Social Justice

From a clinical perspective, symptoms may appear to be the main cause of stigma. Individuals with manifest psychotic and bizarre behavior experience greater stigma than individuals with symptoms under control. This type of assertion exemplifies the "kernel of truth" perspective. Stigmatization and prejudice relative to any group is based on a kernel of truth, or separate evidence about that group. For example, the public views Irishmen as drunken sots, because the Irish, as a culture, imbibe more than most other cultural groups. The public discriminates and fears people with mental illness because of the kernel of truth in the belief that they may be more violent than the rest of the population.

This "kernel of truth" perspective suggests that one way to decrease stigma is to diminish the social belief. Widespread programs that foster recovery provide one mechanism to decrease the kernel of truth and erase the stigma of mental illness. Note, however, that dealing with stigma is not a clinical agenda. New generations of medication and psychosocial treatment will not bring about its demise, because stigma is a problem of social justice. Stigma is not the natural result of symptoms; rather, stereotypes exist as social constructs that lead to stigmatization of the targeted group. Erasing intrinsically stigmatizing social injustices increases opportunities for individuals with mental illness to pursue crucial hopes, dreams, and life goals.

STIGMA CHANGE STRATEGIES

Effective stigma change strategies match the type of stigma they address. Antistigma approaches that counter stereotypes, prejudice, and discrimination address public stigma, and personal strategies address components of self-stigma.

Changing Public Stigma

Research identifies three approaches that diminish the impact of public stigma experienced by people with mental illness: protest, education, and contact. Groups *protest* inaccurate and hostile representations of mental illness to challenge the stigmas they represent. These efforts send two messages. First, to the media to *stop* reporting inaccurate representations of mental illness, and second, to the public to *stop* believing negative reports about mental illness. Largely anecdotal evidence suggests that protest campaigns have been effective in getting stigmatizing images of mental illness withdrawn from the media. Consider, for example, what happened to the ABC show *Wonderland*, in which the first episode depicted a person with mental illness shooting police officers and stabbing a pregnant psychiatrist in the belly with a hypodermic needle. In response to coordinated effort, advocates forced the network to cut the show after only a few episodes. This approach demonstrates that economic protest might have a significant impact on the news and entertainment media.

Protesting against Stigma

Despite the previous example, protest seems to have a limited effect on public prejudice. In fact, research suggests that protest might lead to a rebound effect, which increases stigmatizing attitudes about mental illness. Instructing a group of people to not think bad thoughts about people with mental illness can lead to worse attitudes. There are various explanations for this iatrogenic effect. Perhaps most prominent is the construct of psychological reactance: The public may react to protest by responding, "Don't tell me what to think." Hence, protest is ineffectual if the goal of the antistigma program is, for example, to change landlord attitudes about renting to people with mental illness. Protest as an economic deterrent provides an effective strategy when stigma and discrimination are affected by market influences. Theater owners may be less likely to show a stigmatizing film when they experience the disapproval inherent in protest.

Stigma and Education

Protest attempts to diminish negative attitudes about mental illness but fails to promote more positive attitudes supported by facts. Education may achieve this latter goal. Typically education involves challenging the myths of mental illness (e.g., people with mental illness are incapable of being productive members of the work world) with facts (e.g., most people who receive vocational rehabilitation for psychiatric disability will achieve the goals of his or her work world). One additional benefit of pursuing antistigma goals via education is exportability. Educational materials, including curricula and videotaped testimonials, can be easily dispersed to the public at large. Both government and private advocacy groups continually develop educational programs. The SAMHSA Center for Mental Health Services provides a website with information about educational programs about stigma. Despite these benefits, research suggests the impact of educational programs may be limited. Research on program participation with immediate follow-up measures indicates small, positive effects on changing the stigma of mental illness. However, any positive effects seem to return to baseline when periodic follow-up measures are obtained.

Changing Stigma through Contact

Contact is the final public approach to stigma. Members of the public who interact with people with mental illness are less likely to endorse stigmatizing behaviors and more likely to internalize positive statements about the group. In addition, change in attitudes is likely to be maintained over time; follow-up evaluations of a month or more indicate that improvements at baseline remain during subsequent months. NAMI provides In Our Own Voice, a consumer-based, antistigma program in which participants tell their stories about illness and recovery.

Despite its promise, there are limitations to contact, especially in terms of exportability. Videos and other materials that are the foundation of education may be disseminated easily and quickly. Contact requires that individuals have the courage to come out of the closet to tell their stories to one group at a time. Educational materials can be absorbed almost anywhere: school, work, home, and community settings. Within contact, identified and willing individuals must prepare antistigma presentations. Program organizers identify specific situations or settings (e.g., police officer roll call to address the burgeoning concerns about criminal justice). These tasks tend to create labor-intensive barriers that decrease the broad use of contact. One episode of contact yields significant change in stigma. Multiple interventions demonstrate an even better impact on stigma.

To increase massively the effect of contact on stigma, individuals with mental illness may need encouragement and incentives to come out of the closet via disclosure. If one considers the epidemiology of psychiatric disorder, as much as 20% of the adult population could come out of the closet by disclosing serious mental illnesses. Lessons about coming out may be learned from gay men and lesbians. The gay and lesbian community has accrued benefits from coming out, both as a group and as individuals. In like manner, the community of people with mental illness might experience fewer problems by coming out en masse. The impact of this kind of courage might broaden the impact of contact programs. Ultimately, individuals who are deciding whether to come out should be highly attuned to the negative aspects of disclosure.

Diminishing Self-Stigma

As stated earlier, stigma provides a fundamental example of social injustice. Stigma is diminished through specific strategies, which brings us to the heart and soul of this injustice. However, antistigma programs that address self-stigma might give the wrong impression (i.e., that stigma is a product of the person's disease or disability). Stigma is not a clinical problem that resolves itself through medications, psychosocial services, and support. Despite these concerns, people with mental illness may need some immediate strategies to deal with the internal impact of stigma. For people who internalize the stigma experience, personal stigma strategies provide avenues to attenuate the personal impact of stigma. Three specific strategies are useful to combat self-stigma: (1) cognitive reframing of the negative self-statements that result from stigma, (2) disclosure of one's psychiatric history, and (3) programs that enhance the person's sense of empowerment, thereby countering self-stigma.

Cognitive reframing provides a mechanism to change negative self-thoughts related to stigmatizing stereotypes. Self-stigmatizing people internalize self-statements representing the negative stereotype: "All people with mental illness are lazy" is a negative bias; "I must be lazy" is the result of applying the stereotype to oneself. These self-statements may lead to low self-esteem ("I must be a bad person because I am incompetent") and diminished self-efficacy ("A lazy person like me is not capable of finding and keeping a job"). Cognitive reframing teaches the stigmatized person to identify and to challenge these harmful self-statements.

A stigma is a set of belief statements influenced and perpetuated by the attitudes and behaviors of one's community. How might self-stigma of this ilk be diminished? Stigmatization is reduced when people with mental illness survey their community about these beliefs and behaviors. People with self-stigmas, such as "I am a lazy person," may challenge these stigmas by asking friends and acquaintances whether they agree: "Do you think I am lazy or in some other way bad because I have a mental illness?" This process is even more effective if the person with a stigma picks a life mentor and asks him or her about the self-statement. Life mentors may include spiritual leaders and senior family members. Once individuals learn to challenge the internalized stereotype, they may develop a counterperception that diminishes the effects of these stereotypes: "I am not lazy and, despite my disabilities, I am working as much as possible."

Disclosing One's Mental Illness

The stigma of mental illness is largely hidden. The public may not know whether specific individuals meet the criteria for mental illness. Hence, individuals need to decide whether to disclose their illness history. As we suggested earlier, disclosure may result in several disadvantages. People may risk the disapproval of peers, bosses, coworkers, neighbors, and community members. Disapproval may include being fired from one's job, being cut out of opportunities to interact with neighbors, and not being included in community functions. Moreover, people who disclose may become more stressed by worrying about what others think of them.

There are also benefits to disclosure. Avoidance of disclosure may suggest avoidance of shame, although people who come out typically feel better about themselves. This sense of shame disappears with the act of disclosing. Because mental illness is largely hidden, people with stigma may not be able to find (on the job or in the community) peers with mental illness who might provide support as illness issues emerge. Coming out also decreases the general prejudice against the community of people with mental illness. As we described earlier, contact with other individuals with mental illness can greatly diminish stigma.

Stigma is not a categorical experience. Telling some people about mental illness does not necessarily mean that one must disclose to everyone in the community. The various social spheres in which to disclose may include work settings, family situations, and community functions. People may opt to tell peers in one sphere but not in another. Moreover, disclosure is not an unequivocal decision. There are different ways in which people can approach this issue. They may selectively let others know about their experience by approaching individuals who seem open-minded to general issues related to stigma, or they may let everyone know about their mental illness. This does not mean either blatantly proclaiming or hiding one's experience with mental illness. The elements related to disclosure are complex; hence, only the disclosing individuals make these decisions.

Addressing Stigma by Fostering Empowerment

Research suggests that empowerment is at the opposite end of a continuum anchored by self-stigma. Put another way, people who view themselves as having power over their lives are less likely to be tortured by self-stigma. Several treatment decisions enhance empowerment and decrease stigma. State-of-the-art services are collaborative rather than based in adherence frameworks. In collaborative exchanges, individuals and practitioners view each other as peers and work together to understand the illness and develop a treatment plan; this gives people control over an important part of their lives. Another element of treatment that diminishes self-stigma is consumer satisfaction; people with mental illness feel more empowered when program change is the result of their own efforts.

Coaching-based psychosocial services also facilitate empowerment. Coaches provide services and support that help people to be successful in various important areas: work, housing, education, and health settings. This type of success provides an excellent source of empowerment. The impact on empowerment increases exponentially when peers with psychiatric illness provide coaching services. Individuals offering services and overcoming mental illness describe personal success stories that provide significant inspiration. People with mental illness present special experiences and critical viewpoints that enhance the quality of care. People with mental illness gain empowerment when they develop programs and provide services to assist people with recovery goals. Within these settings, people with mental illness provide peer support and grapple with program elements.

KEY POINTS

- Public stigma, self-stigma, structural stigma, and label avoidance rob individuals of important life opportunities, including gainful employment, health care services, safe and comfortable housing, relationships, and educational opportunities.
- Members of society commonly react to the label of mental illness with fear and disgust, which leads to reduced contact with individuals with mental illness and minimizes their opportunities for life growth.
- Public stigma and self-stigma consist of their stereotypes (negative beliefs), prejudice (agreement with beliefs), and discrimination (behavior in response to beliefs).
- Three approaches have been identified that diminish aspects of the public stigma experienced by people with mental illness: protest, education, and contact.
- Three specific strategies have been identified as useful for reducing self-stigma: cognitive reframing, decisions about disclosure, and empowerment programs.

REFERENCES AND RECOMMENDED READINGS

Chamberlin, J. (1978). *On our own: Patient-controlled alternatives to the mental health system.* New York: McGraw-Hill.

Corrigan, P. W. (Ed.). (2005). *On the stigma of mental illness: Implications for research and social change.* Washington, DC: American Psychological Association Press.

Corrigan, P. W., & Lundin, R. K. (2001). *Don't call me nuts: Coping with the stigma of mental illness.* Tinley Park, IL: Recovery Press.

Goffman, E. (1963). *Stigma: Notes on the management of spoiled identity.* Englewood Cliffs, NJ: Prentice-Hall.

Heatherton, T., Kleck, R. E., Hebl, M. R., & Hull, J. G. (Eds.). (2000). *The social psychology of stigma.* New York: Guilford Press.

Jones, E. E., Farina, A., Hastorf, A. H., Markus, H., Miller, D. T., & Scott, R. A. (1984). *Social stigma: The psychology of marked relationships.* New York: Freeman.

Phelan, J. C., Cruz-Rojas, R., & Reiff, M. (2002). Genes and stigma: The connection between perceived genetic etiology and attitudes and beliefs about mental illness. *Psychiatric Rehabilitation Skills, 6,* 159–185.

Link, B. G., & Phelan, J. C. (2001). Conceptualizing stigma. *Annual Review of Sociology, 27,* 363–385.

Link, B. G., Yang, L. H., Phelan, J. C., & Collins, P. Y. (2004). Measuring mental illness stigma. *Schizophrenia Bulletin, 30,* 511–541.

Pescosolido, B. A., Monahan, J., Link, B. G., Stueve, A., & Kikuzawa, S. (1999). The public's view of competence, dangerousness, and need for legal coercion of persons with mental health problems. *American Journal of Public Health, 89,* 1339–1345.

Stangor, C. (Ed.). (2000). *Stereotypes and prejudice essential readings.* Philadelphia: Psychology Press.

Wahl, O. (1997). *Media madness: Public images of mental illness.* New Brunswick, NJ: Rutgers University Press.

Wahl, O. (1999). *Telling is risky business: Mental health consumers confront stigma.* New Brunswick, NJ: Rutgers University Press.

CHAPTER 52

EVIDENCE-BASED PRACTICES

MATTHEW R. MERRENS
ROBERT E. DRAKE

The desire to improve outcomes by promoting evidence-based health care has recently led to a proliferation of practice recommendations, guidelines, and algorithms throughout medicine. Research indicates, however, that the distribution of information regarding effective treatments has been largely insufficient to transform the health care system. Implementing and sustaining new approaches to health care are difficult, notwithstanding the evidence of benefits to patients.

In a parallel fashion, the mental health field has been attempting to facilitate the widespread adoption of evidence-based practices in routine mental health care settings, so that persons with mental illnesses can benefit from interventions that have been shown to work. Yet implementing and sustaining major changes in mental health care has also proven to be difficult.

THEORY

Several models of organizational change have gained attention (Everett M. Rogers's *Diffusion of Innovations* [2002] is a scholarly presentation, whereas Malcolm Gladwell's *The Tipping Point* [2002] is a popular best seller). Theorists agree that behavior changes when intention to change is combined with the necessary skills and the absence of environmental constraint.

Theorists also agree that promotion of organizational change has at least three phases:

1. *Predisposing* or disseminating strategies include building information, enthusiasm, and planning, often through educational events or written material.
2. *Enabling* methods refer to processes of putting a new intervention or method of practice into place, and include training and supervision based on practice guidelines and decision supports.
3. *Sustaining* strategies are mechanisms to reinforce continuation of a new practice, and include information technology, financing, and outcomes-based contracting.

Many researchers do not believe that a simple theory of any kind can ever explain successful implementation of a new practice. Health care systems, or even individual practices, are complex microsystems governed by their own unique constraints and facilitators, and successful implementation probably requires several large-scale system changes, as well as local strategies.

RESEARCH

Several research findings are clear. No single model of practice change or implementation is strongly supported by empirical evidence. Research shows that education alone does not strongly influence the practice behaviors of health care providers. Additional efforts, such as increasing consumer demand for services, changing financial incentives and penalties, using administrative rules and regulations, and providing clinicians with ongoing supervision and feedback on practices, are also necessary. In general, greater intensity of effort produces greater change. The more elements of the system of care that can be brought to bear to support change and reduce resistance, the more likely practice improvements will occur. As a corollary, complex changes, such as modifying the practice of an entire clinical team, require a greater intensity of effort or supports than is needed to effect a relatively simple change, such as shifting a single prescription pattern. Guidelines are not self-implementing and must be adapted to the actual processes of services used in a specific center. Sustained change requires a restructuring of daily workflow and incentives, often based in information technology, so that routine procedures make it easy rather than difficult for the clinician to provide services in the new way.

EVIDENCE-BASED MENTAL HEALTH INTERVENTIONS

Research on public mental health systems strongly supports the use of several evidence-based practices for persons with severe mental illness. These interventions improve clients' outcomes in recovery-oriented domains such as independent living, employment, avoidance of hospitalization and incarceration, family relationships, and subjective quality of life. Research also indicates that when mental health programs attempt to implement evidence-based practices, the quality of the implementation strongly influences client outcomes. For example, when two programs offer a practice of care that is known to be effective, the program with higher fidelity to the defined practice tends to produce superior clinical results. This finding suggests that efforts to promote evidence-based practice must include fidelity measures and self-correcting feedback mechanisms. Implementation efforts are most effective when they address the specific needs, values, and concerns of the persons whose behavior the implementation aims to change. Specifically, administrative features of an implementation plan must be tailored for mental health administrators, providing clinical training elements for clinicians, and consumer and family education to those groups.

Evidence-based mental health practices include the following:

- Illness management and recovery services, which help clients learn to manage their own illnesses.
- Systematic medication management services, which enable practitioners and clients to use evidence-based guidelines, to engage in shared decision making, and to use medications effectively.

- Supported employment services, which help the 70–80% of clients whose goal is competitive employment.
- Family psychoeducation services, which enable families and their member with mental illness to acquire knowledge, coping skills, and supports.
- Integrated dual-disorder services, which help the 50% of clients who have co-occurring substance use disorders to achieve abstinence.
- Assertive community treatment services, which provide intensive in-community interventions to the 15–20% of clients who have difficulty maintaining housing and avoiding hospitalizations and homelessness.

Other mental health practices have research support as well, but the aforementioned practices have been the focus of several large-scale studies of implementation.

Although these evidence-based practices could improve many lives, they are not routinely available to people in mental health settings. In the most extensive demonstration of this issue, the Schizophrenia Patient Outcome Research Team (PORT; Lehman, Steinwachs, & Survey Coinvestigators of the PORT Project, 1998) showed that people with a diagnosis of schizophrenia in two state mental health systems were highly unlikely to receive effective services. Even simple medication practices only met standards of effectiveness about half or less than half of the time. Only 10% or fewer people received psychosocial interventions supported by effectiveness research.

IMPLEMENTATION PROJECTS

Research on implementation is accumulating rapidly as a result of several large, multisite projects. Key examples are the Johnson & Johnson–Dartmouth Community Mental Health Program, the National Evidence-Based Practices Project, the Texas Medication Algorithm Project, and the Social Security Administration's Mental Health Treatment Project. In each of these projects, one or more of the evidence-based practices we mentioned have been implemented in multiple sites with careful monitoring and evaluation. We next outline several lessons from these large implementation studies.

Starting with "Early Adopters"

One common strategy for large-scale systems change involves comprehensive top-down change. Frequently, this has been accomplished in single-payer systems, such as those used in European countries or by the federal Veterans Administration health system in the United States. These systems are characterized by centralized control of policies and procedures. Comprehensive change is sometimes feasible in such systems. For example, every health practitioner in Veterans Administration hospitals is required to use the same medical record, so that specific decision supports and requirements can be inserted into the medical record within this system. There are also many examples within single-payer systems of resistance to top-down change efforts, especially when the interventions are complex and not easily enforced or monitored by electronic medical records.

Efforts at comprehensive change have generally failed in state mental health systems, where there is much less centralized authority. For example, state mental health programs that have attempted to implement a new practice, such as integrated dual-disorders treatment, on a uniform and simultaneous statewide basis have not been successful.

An alternative strategy is to start with early adopters and plan for the gradual spread of a new practice. This approach recognizes that some states, organizations, and practitioners—the "early adopters"—are more interested than others in adopting new practices. It also assumes that the others will be more likely to follow suit once change has proven successful among the early adopters, and once enthusiasm, expertise, and trained staff have spread to other organizations. Many of the demonstrations listed earlier have used the early-adopter strategy with success.

Implementing New Practices in Stages

A common misconception is the belief that training is a sufficient step for implementation. In practice, considerable work must precede training. Health policy personnel, such as state-level administrators, need to address financing, regulations, contracts, credentialing, data collection, and other procedures that allow delivery of a new practice without impediments. Administrators in local sites must address mission, leadership, service organization, medical records, personnel policies, training, supervision, and other procedures that facilitate implementation. In addition, other stakeholders, such as clients, family members, and clinicians, need to be involved in the process of building consensus, planning for change, and solving local problems.

Once the setting is prepared for change, training can begin. The need to solve local problems must continue, because unanticipated reactions and consequences occur. Data collection, outcomes-based supervision, and quality improvement procedures must be in place to ensure continuous movement toward effective practice. Changing the culture of treatment, attaining clinical competence, and overcoming local barriers generally occur over about 1 year.

Once a new practice is in place, staff turnover, inattention, and natural tendencies encourage drift back to traditional forms of care, unless the structural elements of the practice setting have been thoroughly changed to reinforce the new practice. Supervision, records, billing, and other procedures must be aligned properly. For example, although delivering services in the community is more effective, clinicians drift back to office-based practice if organizational incentives are not properly directed toward in-community care.

Involving All Stakeholders

As described earlier, all stakeholders have roles to play in practice change. They need to be involved from the beginning, and at each stage, or they are likely to become barriers themselves, whether by resistance, resentment, or misunderstanding. Furthermore, particular tasks at each level can only be addressed by relevant stakeholders. Of particular importance, local leaders must coalesce to form an implementation planning team.

Toolkits and Training Centers

Two strategies used in the National Evidence-Based Practices Project (Substance Abuse and Mental Health Services Administration [SAMHSA], 2006) were to produce comprehensive and multimodal training materials for all stakeholders on each evidence-based practice and to establish local training centers within each participating state. The training materials (also called *toolkits*) were intended to be used in conjunction with a longitudinal process of training and supervision, not as stand-alone manuals.

The data regarding toolkits are still being analyzed, but preliminary findings indicate that the toolkits were only partially successful. They tended to be used extensively by state trainers, team leaders, and clinical supervisors (who found them useful in the process of overseeing implementations), but not by other stakeholder groups. Policymakers felt that they needed more specific and detailed guidelines for facilitating implementation. Clinicians generally did not read the materials instead relying on their team leaders and supervisors to understand and to help them apply the principles of evidence-based practice to their current activities. For a variety of reasons, the materials rarely got to clients and family members.

In 2006, the toolkits were redesigned, based on the qualitative and quantitative feedback from the Implementing Evidence-Based Practices Project. The format for the re-edited toolkits is found in Table 52.1. As is evident, the aim was to break down the toolkit materials into smaller units in booklet form rather than a large binder format. Table 52.1 also describes each toolkit component and how best to use it in implementing the practice.

State training centers, often established in conjunction with academic partners, were almost uniformly successful. Trainers needed to be experienced and skilled in the practices, of course, and to have skills as trainers, but nearly all training centers were able to hire staff with these qualities. Uniform training across large systems was appreciated by clinical programs and state administrators, and trainers successfully reduced their roles in individual centers as local supervisors and team leaders acquired the expertise to take over supervisory responsibilities. Trainers were then able to move on to work with other centers as enthusiasm for the evidence-based practices spread.

Care Coordinators

A number of implementation studies, particularly those related to the Texas Medication Alogrithm studies, have shown that use of care coordinators to collect data and to provide longitudinal information regarding symptoms, side effects, and algorithms to practitioners at the time of contact with clients can improve the quality of implementation. For example, medication prescribers improve their adherence to guidelines from approximately 50–90% based on helpful information from care coordinators.

Information Technology

Experiences across medicine, and particularly in the Veterans Administration health care system, make it clear that standards, guidelines, monitoring, quality improvement, and safety can be enhanced by attaching electronic decision support systems to electronic medical records. These vehicles can be used to ensure that clinicians and clients attend to important information when they are making decisions about care. Thus far, few behavioral health systems have clinically oriented electronic medical records, but we anticipate that this will change over the coming decade, in part because of the positive experience within the Veterans Administration system.

Behavioral health guidelines and algorithms need to be computerized for these changes to occur. Information technology is rapidly developing in many sectors, and electronic monitoring of evidence-based practices is a central feature of quality improvement and quality assurance in the Social Security Administration Mental Health Treatment Study.

Advocacy

Advocacy can help systems move toward evidence-based practices. For example, the National Alliance on Mental Illness (NAMI) has had success in promoting assertive community treatment. By focusing on the replication of assertive community treatment as a

TABLE 52.1. A Description and Suggested Usage Guide for Revised Toolkit Components

Toolkit component	Description of toolkit component	How to use toolkit component
Quick Reference Guide	The guide describes all the components of the toolkit and presents a plan for using materials most effectively.	To provide a quick summary of all toolkit materials for all stakeholders.
Booklet 1	This booklet provides a more detailed description of all toolkit components and how to use them. A discussion of evidence-based practice philosophy and values, an introduction to the concept of fidelity, the General Organizational Index, the assessment of client outcomes, and a discussion of the importance of cultural competency are included. In addition, reference, resource materials, and articles are presented.	To provide a more detailed presentation of all toolkit materials for all stakeholders.
Booklet 2	This booklet provides an introduction to the practice. The concept of quality assurance is addressed by describing the quality improvement measures employed in the evidence-based practice. These measures include the Evidence-Based Practice Fidelity Scale, the General Organizational Index (GOI), and Client Outcome Measures. In addition, articles on evidence-based practices and reference and resource material are presented. An appendix on special populations is included.	To provide an orientation to the practice, as well as resources for ensuring the quality of the implementation. References, resource materials, and information on special populations provide additional information to stakeholders.
Booklet 3	This booklet includes information and implementation materials for both mental health administrators and mental health authorities.	Assists stakeholders in facilitating the implementation of the practice.
Booklet 4: *Integrated Treatment for Co-Occurring Disorders Workbook for Practitioners*	Describes the practice principles and the practice skills. Employs vignettes for illustration. The workbook is the major practitioner tool for learning and implementing the practice.	The workbook presents the essential practice skills necessary for practice implementation. It is divided into modules to enhance the process of learning the practice.
Introductory video in DVD format	A short video based on consumer and family experiences. Describes principles of the practice and how it has been helpful for consumers and families. Spanish and English versions are available.	Excellent to show at the beginning of the training process, and to community organizations and civic groups.
Practice demonstration video in DVD format	An illustration of the practice skills described in the workbook.	Coordinates with workbook and provides skills development training for all those wishing to acquire practice skills.
Trifold brochure	A brief overview of the principles of the practice and its goals.	Display this brochure prominently in a wide variety of community agencies, so that people can become familiar with the practice.
Introductory PowerPoint presentation	A short PowerPoint presentation that describes the principles of the practice and how it has been designed to help consumers and families.	Excellent to show at the beginning of the training process and to community organizations and civic groups.
Booklet 5: *Forms and Handouts*	A collection of forms and handouts from the toolkit.	Facilitates copying and distribution of evidence-based practice materials.

national priority, packaging the practice for implementation, engaging the media, coordinating state advocacy efforts, and communicating progress, NAMI has created a grassroots demand for assertive community treatment. In fact, active NAMI assertive community treatment steering committees are working with providers to establish the practice in several states.

Policy

Ultimately, extensive policy changes are needed to support the full implementation of evidence-based practices. States and local mental health care systems cannot create integrated, continuous systems of behavioral health care without Medicaid, Medicare, Social Security, managed care, and other organizations shifting their attention to quality. For example, current Social Security Administration and Medicaid policies encourage people to claim lifetime disability status rather than to participate in evidence-based supported employment. These policies need to be significantly realigned. Researchers, administrators, advocates, clinicians, and others need to speak out for science- and values-based health care systems.

KEY POINTS

- Distribution of information regarding effective treatments does not change practice.
- Implementing and sustaining major practice changes are difficult tasks.
- Promoting organizational change has three phases: predisposing, enabling, and sustaining.
- Successful implementation requires large-scale systems changes, as well as local strategies.
- Generally, the greater the intensity of effort, the greater the change.
- Research supports evidence-based practices for persons with severe mental illness, although they are not routinely available.
- Implementation is facilitated when systems start with "early adopters."
- New practices are implemented in stages.
- All stakeholders are involved in the implementation process.
- Implementation works best when toolkits are combined with training and supervision.
- Information technology is a valuable asset that benefits treatment.
- Advocacy (e.g., NAMI) can help systems move to evidence-based practices.
- It is ultimately necessary for Federal and state mental health authorities to establish policy to facilitate the full implementation of evidence-based practices.

REFERENCES AND RECOMMENDED READINGS

Becker, D. R., Torrey, W. C., Toscano, R., Wyzik, P. F., & Fox, T. S. (1998). Building recovery-oriented services: Lessons from implementing IPS in community mental health centers. *Psychiatric Rehabilitation Journal, 22,* 51–54.

Center for Mental Health Services. (1999). *Mental health: A report of the surgeon general.* Rockville, MD: Author.

Drake, R. E., Goldman, H. H., Leff, S. H., Lehman, A. F., Dixon, L., Mueser, K. T., et al. (2002). Implementing evidence-based practices in routine mental health settings. *Compendium on Psychosis and Schizophrenia, 2,* 18–19.

Drake, R. E., Merrens, M. R., & Lynde, D. (2005). *Evidence-based mental health practice: A textbook.* New York: Norton.

Drake, R. E., Torrey, W. C., & McHugo, G. J. (2003). Strategies for implementing evidence-based practices in routine mental health settings. *Evidence-Based Mental Health, 6,* 6–7.

Fishbein, M. (1995). Developing effective behavioral change interventions: Some lessons learned from behavioral research. In T. E. Backer, S. L. David, & G. Soucy (Eds.), *Reviewing the behavioral science knowledge base on technology transfer* (NIDA Research Monograph 155). Rockville MD: National Institute of Mental Health.

Gladwell, M. (2002). *The tipping point: How little things can make a big difference.* New York: Little, Brown.

Jerrel, J. M., & Ridgely, M. S. (1999). Impact of robustness of program implementation on outcomes of clients in dual diagnosis programs. *Psychiatric Services, 50,* 109–112.

Lehman, A. F., Steinwachs, D. M., & the Survey Coinvestigators of the PORT Project. (1998). Translating research into practice: The Schizophrenia Patient Outcomes Research Team (PORT) treatment recommendations. *Schizophrenia Bulletin, 24,* 1–10.

McDonnell, J., Nofs, D., & Hardman, M. (1989). An analysis of the procedural components of supported employment programs associated with employment outcomes. *Journal of Applied Behavioral Analysis, 22,* 417–428.

Mueser, K. T., Torrey, W. C., Lynde, D., Singer, P., & Drake, R. E. (2003). Implementing evidence-based practices for people with severe mental illness. *Behavior Modification, 27,* 387–411.

Rogers, E. M. (1995). The challenge: Lessons for guidelines from the diffusion of innovations. *Journal on Quality Improvement, 21,* 324–328.

Rogers, E. M. (2003). *Diffusion of innovations* (5th ed.). New York: Simon & Shuster.

Substance Abuse and Mental Health Services Administration (2006). *SAMHSA implementation resource kits for assertive community treatment, family psychoeducation, illness management and recovery, integrated treatment for co-occurring disorders, and supported employment—Revised.* Rockville, MD: Author. Available online at *www.samhsa.gov*

CHAPTER 53

SCHIZOPHRENIA IN DEVELOPING COUNTRIES

VIHANG N. VAHIA
IPSIT V. VAHIA

Demographic projections in the year 2000 indicated that approximately 24.4 million individuals with schizophrenia live in undeveloped nations. Since the late 1960s, the issue of schizophrenia in the developing world has been a source of much study and debate. In the developing world, there is an intricate interplay among the biological illness, its phenomenological manifestations, cultural interpretation of this illness, its contextualization within society, and systems of care involved in its management. Moreover, research findings consistently indicate this affects outcome, and studies have consistently shown better outcome in the developing world. We aim to highlight this complex issue and its implications for the understanding and management of schizophrenia.

THE NATURE OF SCHIZOPHRENIA ACROSS CULTURES

The Cross-Cultural Conflict in Systems of Care

Globalization of health care policies mandates that all member countries of the World Health Organization (WHO) conform to a standardized pattern of curative, preventive, and epidemiological strategies. Health care guidelines are formulated along the theories of the allopathic or European system of care. Developing countries refer to this system of medicine as modern medicine, thus indicating that the "developing" countries have a parallel system of traditional medicine.

Developing countries in India and South Asia, China and Far Eastern Asia, the Middle East, Latin and South America, and the Caribbean and Africa each have had a parallel stream of traditional health care that has retained its popularity despite the dominance of allopathy in health education and policies. The traditional healers are the customary practitioners of curative and preventive care. They continue to influence several treatment-related variables, such as acceptance of care and outcome of the illness. The importance of emotional and mental well-being is a part of the illness constructs and the healing process in these systems of medicine.

Allopathy has its strength in a strong "scientific" evidence base, created through laboratory data and collective strength of documented individual case studies. Teachings of traditional medicine are based on documents that conceptualize physical and mental illness in general terms. The texts do not abound in descriptive pathology or psychopathology. They describe physical ailments, thinking, feeling and actions, personality traits, and syndromes of mental illness (including insanity) in general terms. The metaphors correspond to the current descriptions of schizophrenia and bipolar disorder. Such similes correspond to similar descriptions in Greek medicine.

The task of studying schizophrenia across cultures therefore poses formidable challenges in terms of how to explain and to standardize findings within cross-cultural contexts. Although a substantial body of literature now addresses this topic, a frequent criticism is that using evidence-based techniques for this purpose may not be the most valid standard for assessment of the issue.

"Traditional Care"

Treatments in the system of traditional health care tend to be a mixture of religion, mysticism, and rational healing. Treatment methods include rituals, use of somatic treatments, and drugs that have to be inhaled, ingested, or massaged into the head, hair, or skin. A common principle used in traditional care involves identification of a causal entity, and a reversal of the identified cause is believed to induce cure. This is the basis for exorcism in cultures where possession by an external entity is believed to be the cause of psychosis. A subgroup of traditional healers subscribe to the thought that strong fear or severe loss induces insanity. They believe that the dysfunction caused by exposure to such fear can be reversed by a second exposure to an identical stimulus. Hence, exposure to wild animals or inducing pain in other forms is believed to be a cure for insanity. Popular past practices of confinement to a cellar, solitary confinement in a room without sanitation or ventilation, whipping the patient, or blood letting from the skull at a point near the temporal region have now been abandoned.

Leaders, or the hierarchically higher class of society, often counsel individuals and the public at large on religious norms and social customs, and provide psychosocial counseling. In several cultures, religious and faith healers have helped people with psychological and psychosocial problems. Faith healers differ from practitioners of traditional medicine in that they claim to cure the illness through occult and magical practices. A common factor in such healing practices is a strong and unchallenged mutual belief and social approval of healers, who have strong personalities and usually deliver the services without seeking monetary compensation. Anecdotal reports of physical or sexual abuse by such healers have not been verified.

The literature documents that, in some cultures, the socially conscientious and the rich provided food and medicine to the sick and the needy. However, the seriously mentally ill were viewed inauspiciously, and the society was often encouraged to renounce them. Violent and unreasonably aggressive patients were considered unworthy of treatment. The theorists often blamed the family or the celestial influences as factors causing the illnesses.

It is of note that the practice of contemporary psychiatry does not differ in different cultures across the globe, but in the developing world, psychiatrists are constantly faced with the issue of educating persons with mental illness about the nature of the illness, and the notion of the illness being a biological entity with phenomenological manifestations that are related to cultural norms. Practitioners of Western medicine in developing countries are required to spend long hours dispelling the myths and misconceptions about mental illness being a curse or punishment for wrongdoings in a past life, past deeds, bad parenting, or a form of divine punishment. Issues related to the stigma of mental illness have far-reaching social consequences and necessitate persuasive skills of psychiatrists to soothe the suffering families, whose children may not find spouses or business partners.

RESEARCH

The Importance of Studying Schizophrenia across the Globe

Historically, science initially needed to substantiate the notion that schizophrenia was indeed a biological entity, and that this could be accomplished by establishing the prevalence of schizophrenia across cultures and nations. Additionally, for the purpose of strengthening the reliability and validity of psychiatric diagnosis, it was important to test prevailing taxonomic systems globally. In addition, schizophrenia was, and remains, a source of significant burden on individuals with the ailment, and their families and communities. It was a large enough problem to merit investigation to facilitate a better understanding of the illness.

There remains a need for localized research studies within communities, especially within the developing world, by researchers from the same culture/geographical region, who can more reliably seek to explain the interplay between illness, socioeconomics, and culture. The application of this information into a broader global perspective will be the next major step in enhancing our knowledge of this enigmatic universal condition.

International Collaborative Studies

Over the years, the WHO organized two trend-setting studies—the International Pilot Study of Schizophrenia (IPSS) and the Determinants of Outcome of Severe Mental Disorder (DOSMD). The IPSS, a groundbreaking study initiated jointly by the WHO and the National Institute of Mental Health (NIMH) in 1967, brought together researchers from nine countries across the "developed" and the "developing" world. The research teams studied progress of schizophrenia across multiple cultures, and compared outcomes in the nine centers for the study. This pioneering study was considered a model for successful international cross-cultural collaboration.

The IPSS revealed multiple highly consequential and even controversial findings. It showed almost universally better outcomes in all outcome measures in the developing world. IPSS findings have led to much investigation worldwide to establish this pattern, and several scholars have proposed hypotheses in an attempt to explain this pattern. Initially, this finding was considered by many to be counterintuitive given the more sophisticated health care available in the developed world. The WHO has reviewed the IPSS data at intervals to study whether this "developed" versus "developing" divide persists. It also launched the DOSMD, a 10-center international study that confirmed IPSS findings and offered culture-based explanations. The WHO has also launched the more recent International Study of Schizophrenia (IsoS), which used many of the patients studied in the DOSMD.

Proposed Explanations for Better Outcomes in the Developing World

This remains a controversial topic, with no universally accepted explanation. Early death of the more seriously ill, genetic heterogeneity, social tolerance, better family support, less competitive society, and several such psychosocial factors are considered to contribute this apparently superior outcome. Culture-based explanations have not been extensively studied, but it is accepted that cultural norms often provide explanations and promote more optimistic stances. Supernatural causes (possession, "evil eye"), alternative explanation for behavioral changes (isolation as a way to avoid being cursed), and more socially tolerant stances based on these explanations often play critical roles in destigmatizing mental illness, which may be a key factor in these outcomes.

A body of literature contests the existence of the "developing" versus "developed" world divide in schizophrenia outcomes, citing methodological flaws in the IPSS study design as potential sources of bias, but there is not enough evidence either to revalidate this finding soundly or, indeed, to disprove it.

The Need for More Local Studies

It is important to note that no evidence currently links the etiology of schizophrenia to cultural or social factors. In light of this, the fact that culture affects outcome suggests that there is much to learn about the role of specific cultures in schizophrenia. These cultural factors have intricate links to schizophrenia, and it may not be possible to examine this in a broad, global study. It has often been pointed out that the aforementioned IPSS, DOSMD, and IsoS all aimed at studying schizophrenia from a "Western" perspective, and this may not be the ideal perspective to identify the interplay of culture and schizophrenia.

Several small studies in Africa, India, and South America have looked at this, but more literature is necessary. Indeed, there may be valuable lessons in this form of activity for the entire global community.

TREATING SCHIZOPHRENIA IN THE DEVELOPING WORLD

In addition to sociocultural attitudes influencing perception of both psychiatry and schizophrenia, there are unique challenges to overcome in addressing the issue of mental health in the developing world. Two major factors tend to be shortage of adequately trained staff (especially in rural areas) and poor access to available services. The treatment gap for schizophrenia tends to be exaggerated in rural areas in developing nations. Given the socioeconomic diversity in different parts of the world, it has been difficult to create a care model that can be meaningfully generalized.

A strategy that has been employed in multiple areas is a decentralized system of mental health care that involves setting up community-based outreach programs. This remains the most extensively implemented and studied model worldwide, with historical origins in the "barefoot doctor" system of care practiced in China from 1967 to 1981, where specialized training is provided to volunteer outreach workers who are not medical professionals. Identification of illness and referral to appropriate care is done by these workers. They also perform the critical task of educating patients and families about the nature of the illness. This has proven to be an effective tool for identifying untreated schizophrenia and ensuring compliance to medication once care is received. An adaptation of this model has been well studied in India, where "multipurpose health workers" are trained to identify mental illness and to refer patients to primary health centers (PHCs), where they have access to medical professionals and, if necessary, specialized psychiatric care via referral to district health care centers. This model was found to significantly reduce symptoms of psychosis, family burden, and disability. Increased costs of outreach were found to be balanced by reduction in costs of informal care sector visits and family caregiving time, and the model was found to be an effective tool for improving the quality and quantity of care for schizophrenia in rural communities. This model has since been expanded and is currently implemented in several parts of the world. Outreach workers have also assisted in creating customized manuals for care based on prevalent sociocultural beliefs, as well as availability of resources.

It is also important to note the role played by nongovernmental organizations (NGOs) in developing nations. NGOs perform a variety of functions in multiple settings, ranging from performing outreach functions similar to those performed by government workers to provision of medications at subsidized rates—a function that is likely to increase in significance and impact in light of recent economic developments (see the following section). Given the lack of available resources in several parts of the developing world, and overburdening of resources where available, the role of NGOs is likely to take on importance.

The outreach model does have impediments and limitations. In several parts of the world outreach remains a voluntary activity, and this leads to poor continuity of care and observation of patients with schizophrenia. Furthermore, lack of sufficient training, education, and expertise is a problem derived from poor availability of economic and intellectual resources. Accessing updates on health care and health information is a problem commonly faced by both outreach workers and more specialized care providers. There is also an absence of centralized coordination of NGOs worldwide, leading frequently to situations in which multiple NGOs work simultaneously on similar projects in the same region without knowledge of each other's activities, leading to duplicity of effort. Innovative initiatives to facilitate better communication, such as information communication technology (ICT), which aims to uses telecommunication, as well as Internet-based systems to facilitate better long-distance coordination and distance learning/training, need to be implemented and studied systematically.

Also of note is that in most parts of the world, the relationship between practitioners of allopathic medicine and more traditional, faith-based healers tends to be one of distrust and hostility. The need for better integration of traditional and modern health care services was recognized even in the Alma-Ata Declaration of 1978. In most parts of the developing world the traditional healer:patient ratio is far superior to the doctor:patient ratio. As much as 80% of the population of developing countries has been estimated to utilize traditional care. Given this, it is important for all of medicine, but especially psychiatry, to foster better communication with this care community. This may also serve as a means to improve communication between psychiatry and the population it aims to serve.

Finally, it is important to note that many of the problems faced by psychiatry in tackling the issue of schizophrenia in the developing world are similar to those faced by medicine at large in tackling chronic illness such as diabetes mellitus or hypertension. Much may be gained and learned in terms of strategies and ideas by attempting to adapt models used in different parts of the world for dealing with chronic medical illness.

CURRENT SOCIAL AND ECONOMIC ISSUES

The social structure is changing in the developing countries. Industrial globalization, cultural mix and extensive migration, changing social norms, and economy-driven social attitudes have altered the differences between the developing and the developed world. Economy-driven research and progressive restrictions on research have now distorted the ground realities. Ever-increasing numbers of drug makers are now looking at the developing countries to conduct industry-driven studies. Data obtained from developing countries are now applied as the norms for industrialized countries. In general, both brand-name and generic drugs have been readily available to the mentally ill in the developing world. However, the impact of recent trade laws enforcing intellectual patency rights will change the distribution of newer medications across the globe and likely have a profound impact on management of mental illness. Factors such as responsiveness to medications and compliance, which have been overshadowed by larger public health concerns regarding availability of care, are likely to become more important as medications become more expensive. In light of this, a better understanding of the role of culture in illness is likely to become more important in devising creative methods to improve compliance and monitor response. It is possible to postulate that economic and health policy will have to take this into account.

The eventual impact of these changed circumstances on health care delivery and disease outcome will require close study.

KEY POINTS

- Manifestation of schizophrenia varies across cultures and geographical regions of the planet.
- Application of Western concepts of schizophrenia to different cultures and use of evidence-based research methods to study them may lead to conflicts and bias if cultural and economic factors in the developing world are not taken into account.
- Studies have consistently demonstrated better outcomes for patients with schizophrenia in the developing world.
- The outcome difference is broadly attributed to cultural factors, though the precise nature of this complex interplay remains a matter of speculation.
- Access to specialized care for patients with mental illness, and especially schizophrenia, is a major problem in the developing world.
- A closer collaboration with nontraditional systems of care may become important, because such caregivers are often treated with greater trust and have easier access to the community.
- There is a need for closer study of this fascinating phenomenon in light of its implications for our understanding of not only the illness process itself but also economic policy.

REFERENCES AND RECOMMENDED READINGS

Bhugra, D., Gopinath, R., & Patel, V. (2005). *Handbook of psychiatry: A South Asian perspective*. New Delhi: Byword Viva.

Bodeker, G., & Kronenberg, F. (2002). A public health agenda for traditional, complementary and alternative medicine. *American Journal of Public Health, 92*(10), 1582–1591.

Grover, S., Avasthi, A., Chakrabarti, S., Bhansali, A., & Kulhara P. (2005). Cost of care of schizophrenia: A study of Indian out-patient attenders. *Acta Psychiatrica Scandinavica, 112*(1), 54–63

Hugo, C. J., Boshoff, D. E., Traut, A., Zungu-Dirwayi, N., & Stein, D. J. (2003). Community attitudes toward and knowledge of mental illness in South Africa. *Social Psychiatry and Psychiatric Epidemiology, 38*(12), 715–719.

Jablensky, A., Sartorius, N., Emberg G., Anker, M., Korten, A., Cooper, J. E., et al. (1992). Schizophrenia manifestations, incidence, and course in different countries: A WHO ten country study. *Psychological Medicine, 20*(Suppl.), 97.

Mateus, M. D., dos Santos, J. Q., & Mari Jde, J. (2005). Popular conceptions of schizophrenia in Cape Verde, Africa. *Revista Brasileira de Psiquiatria, 27*(2), 101–107.

McConnell, H., Haile-Mariam, T., & Rangarajan, S. (2004). The World Health Channel: An innovation for health and development. *World Hospital Health and Services, 40*(4), 36–39.

Shaikh, B. T., & Hatcher, J. (2005). Complementary and alternative medicine in Pakistan: Prospects and limitations. *Evidence-Based Complementary and Alternative Medicine, 2*(2), 139–142.

Shorvon, S. D., & Farmer, P. J. (1988). Epilepsy in developing countries: A review of epidemiological, sociocultural, and treatment aspects. *Epilepsia, 29*(Suppl. 1), S36–S54.

Srinivasa Murthy, R., Kishore Kumar, K. V., Chisholm, D., Thomas, T., Sekar, K., & Chandrashekari, C. R. (2005). Community outreach for untreated schizophrenia in rural India: A follow-up study of symptoms, disability, family burden and costs. *Psychological Medicine, 35*(3), 341–351.

Wig, N. N. (1977). Schizophrenia in the Indian scene—keynote address. In P. Kulhara, A. Avasthi, & S. Verma (Eds.), *Schizophrenia: The Indian scene.* Chandigarh: Postgraduate Institute of Medical Education and Research.

Williams, C. C. (2003). Re-reading the IPSS research record. *Social Science and Medicine, 56*(3), 501–515.

World Health Organization. (1979). *Schizophrenia: An international follow-up study.* New York: Wiley.

PART VIII

SPECIAL TOPICS

CHAPTER 54

REMISSION

BERNARD A. FISCHER, IV
WILLIAM T. CARPENTER, JR.

Schizophrenia has traditionally been conceptualized as a disease entity defined by psychosis, deterioration, and poor outcome. Emphasis on remission and recovery has been limited by this traditional view. Each aspect of the traditional view is flawed. An alternative paradigm is described, and remission is considered within this framework. Recovery in the medical sense is discussed in this chapter, whereas Chapter 55 deals more extensively with recovery from the vantage point of the care recipient.

A BACKGROUND ON SCHIZOPHRENIA

Schizophrenia is a clinical syndrome that has not been established as a single disease entity. Clinical heterogeneity is evident, and it is probable that subgroups of the syndrome have different etiology and pathophysiology. This being the case, differences in treatment response, course, and outcome are expected. Indeed, concepts of a typical course of schizophrenia are not compatible with research observations. European and North American long-term outcome studies have consistently documented about eight course types. Favorable outcomes are reported in 20–50% of cases, and a progressive course with persistent deterioration is rarely observed (see References and Recommended Readings). To the extent that schizophrenia is associated with progression, this appears to occur early in the psychotic phase, reaching a plateau within the first 5–10 years of illness. There may be a small subgroup of very chronic patients who decline rapidly in late life; however, advancing age is often associated with improvement—perhaps because the psychotic component becomes less intense. In any event, the view that there is a typical course of schizophrenia is simply incorrect, but the influence of this view has impeded research and clinical application relating to remission and recovery.

The "domains of pathology" paradigm is slowly replacing the disease entity paradigm. The domains paradigm is based on observations that various pathological manifestations observed in persons with schizophrenia have little relationship with each other. Symptoms segregate into *domains* representing reality distortion (i.e., hallucinations and delusions), disorganization of thoughts and behaviors, and negative symptoms (e.g., decreased motivation, restricted expression of emotion, and reduced social drive). These symptom domains are relatively independent of each other, have different patterns of onset, and different treatment responses. Negative symptoms appear as trait pathology and do not vary with the severity of psychosis. The impact of some aspects of negative symptoms on outcome appears stronger than that of psychosis. In addition, impaired cognition is almost universal in persons with schizophrenia. This impairment, measured with neuropsychological tests, has low to nil correlation with the symptom domains. Impaired cognition, however, is a primary determinant of poor functional outcome. The implication of this body of data is that schizophrenia can be deconstructed into separable domains of pathology, and that concepts of remission and recovery must be considered for each domain.

Schizophrenia can be fairly viewed as a disorder involving psychosis, but an almost exclusive emphasis on psychosis in diagnosis and treatment has distorted the concept of schizophrenia. The presence of psychosis has been foremost in assessing response in clinical trials and real-world practice. But concepts of remission and recovery based on psychosis runs afoul of observations of continuing negative symptoms, impaired cognition, and poor functioning. Despite the low relationship between a psychotic symptom course and other aspects of pathology and function, the presumption that treating psychosis is key to improved outcomes has persisted. Treatment research, especially clinical trials of pharmacotherapy, has reported outcomes in percentage of improvement in symptom scores, or percentage of patients crossing an improvement threshold. These approaches have no known relationship to remission or recovery, and the field has been criticized for being content with improvement without aggressively pursuing remission.

The impact of overemphasizing psychosis can be illustrated by the influence of antipsychotic drug trials on the concept of remission. During the 1950s and 1960s, effects of drug–placebo differences on measures of time in the hospital, level of psychotic symptoms, and relapse rates were very robust. The differences were direct, and it was easy to understand the implications for treatment. However, other outcome measures were virtually ignored, and it is still unclear how much improvement in long-term outcomes has been achieved (Hegarty, Baldessarini, Tohen, Waternaux, & Oepen, 1995). More recent clinical trials show less robust drug–placebo differences, presumably because more treatment-resistant individuals are participating in clinical trials. The introduction of clozapine, and the documentation of superior efficacy in treatment-resistant individuals, stimulated hope for more favorable outcomes. This hope, carried forward with second-generation antipsychotic drugs, has not been fulfilled. Cochrane Library reviews have failed to find superior efficacy for second-generation antipsychotic drugs other than clozapine, results substantiated in the recent publicly funded Clinical Antipsychotic Trials of Intervention Effectiveness (CATIE; Lieberman et al., 2005) in the United States and Cost Utility of the Latest Antipsychotic Drugs in Schizophrenia (CUtLASS; Jones et al., 2006) trial in the United Kingdom, and in industry-sponsored first-episode studies in which lower doses of first-generation drugs were used. Rather than evaluating treatments with concepts of remission, studies have usually reported percentage of improvement and number of subjects achieving a 20% reduction in a symptom rating scale. It is difficult to tell from such measures whether a clinically meaningful difference is achieved. In fact, it would appear that such changes reflect a very small improvement—which may be barely noticeable clinically (Leucht et al., 2003).

A BACKGROUND ON REMISSION VERSUS RECOVERY

The medical concept of *remission* implies significantly reducing core features of a disease, achieving a certain functional level, and remaining stable. The medical concept of *recov-*

ery generally means complete cessation of signs and symptoms of pathology. This does not imply a cure, because relapse from recovery is possible. The term *cure* implies eradication of the disease. Any apparent recurrence would be a new onset of the disease, not a relapse of existing disease. Recovery from a nonmedical point of view represents a process of optimal adaptation, with certain core values such as autonomy and hope. This is dealt with in Chapter 55. The differences in the concepts are illustrated in Figure 54.1. The narrow, but vitally important, medical goal is to establish a symptomatic response, minimize psychopathology, and achieve clinical stability. Simultaneously, work on the road to recovery should begin. This work can be described within the biopsychosocial medical model, with attention to quality of life and personal goals related to decision making, independent living, attainable self-defined goals, and responsibility for treatment.

RELEVANT RESEARCH

Previous Studies and Defining Remission in Schizophrenia

A number of studies have tracked the outcomes of people diagnosed with schizophrenia, but most of these studies have not focused on remission per se, but have looked at groups of patients and their illness course. *Good outcomes* have been variously defined as lack of symptoms, absence of hospitalizations, decreased or no use of antipsychotics, and so forth. Recognizing that people diagnosed with schizophrenia do not have a uniformly poor prognosis, the next step is to use this information. Being able to define, in measurable terms, what is meant by concepts such as remission will allow researchers to test interventions and make statements about results. Furthermore, having an agreed-upon definition of *remission* will allow comparison of interventions across trials and effective communication in the field.

To this end, a working group of experts in schizophrenia convened to determine practical criteria for establishing remission in schizophrenia. This group examined remis-

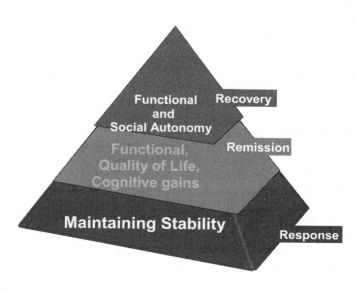

FIGURE 54.1. An illustration of the distinctions between the concepts of response, remission, and recovery in schizophrenia. Note that the concepts build on one another toward the ultimate goal of recovery.

sion criteria in other illnesses—including depression and anxiety. Their deliberation is summarized in the sections below.

Remission in Depression and Anxiety versus Schizophrenia

Experts in both depression and anxiety have defined *remission* as a significant decrease in symptoms. An individual does not have to be completely symptom-free to be in remission. When determining the level of symptom decrease that would merit the qualifier *remission*, the consensus is to examine the patient's functioning. Depression and anxiety are considered to be "in remission" if symptoms are mild and the impact of those symptoms on an individual's functioning is minimal.

However, schizophrenia presents a unique challenge to using identical criteria. Although it is certainly possible to measure symptoms, it is worth noting how the symptoms of schizophrenia differ from those of depression and anxiety. In some sense, the symptoms of depression and anxiety may be experienced—albeit to a lesser degree—by individuals without a diagnosable depression or anxiety disorder. Therefore, someone with generalized anxiety disorder could be recognized as being "in remission" despite experiencing symptoms of anxiety around an important meeting. Could a person with schizophrenia similarly be considered to be "in remission" when he or she still occasionally hears voices?

Another challenge to adopting the same type of remission criteria for schizophrenia is the requirement that symptoms have only a minimal impact on functioning. In a disorder in which the very diagnosis depends on social and/or occupational dysfunction, the requirement that dysfunction be "minimal" may not be useful in defining remission in schizophrenia.

In answer to the first of these challenges, we have seen that negative, indeed even psychotic, symptoms are on a continuum of severity—with low levels of both recognized in persons without mental illness. For that reason, complete cessation of symptoms may not be necessary for remission in schizophrenia. Regarding a person's disability, it has been determined that full neurocognitive and psychosocial functioning should not be a condition of remission in schizophrenia. Rather, symptoms should not interfere with a person's behavior. Improved cognitive, social, and occupational functioning should be goals of treatment, but these goals are long term and best addressed during periods of symptomatic remission. As a practical matter, remission in schizophrenia is defined by absent or mild symptoms, clinical stability, and the absence of a direct and immediate, symptomatic adverse effect on behavior.

Measuring Remission in Schizophrenia

There are no validated biomarkers for remission, and assessment is based on clinical observation of symptoms and function. Reality distortion, disorganization, and disturbed affect are the symptoms with the most temporal fluctuation and are potentially episodic. They are also the symptoms that appear largely treatable. Thus, they are most relevant to the medical definition of *remission*. Negative symptoms not only appear to be more stable over time but are also relevant to the definition of remission. Severe negative symptoms, even in the presence of clinical stability, are not compatible with the definition of *remission*. Cognitive impairment, as measured with neuropsychological test procedures, is not an aspect of the *remission* definition.

The definition of *remission* requires absent or mild symptoms. Clinicians may vary in how they calibrate judgment of remission, but the concept is common in medicine. In research studies, there needs to be a uniform and reliable way of assessing symptom severity. Instruments are already in place that can be applied to a systematic definition of *remission*. These instruments can be used reliably by trained raters and are sensitive to changes in clinical status. The most commonly used instruments are (1) the Scale for Assessment of Positive Symptoms and Scale for Assessment of Negative Symptoms (Andreasen & Olson, 1982), (2) the Brief Psychiatric Rating Scale (Lukoff, Neuchterlein, & Ventura, 1986; Overall & Gorham, 1962), and (3) the Positive and Negative Syndrome Scale (Kay, Fizbein, & Opler, 1987).

To warrant the qualifier "in remission," an individual must rate no higher than "mild" on any of the items on these scales for a period of at least 6 months. Additionally, any symptom, when present, must not interfere with a person's behavior.

TREATMENT IMPLICATIONS

Clinical Criteria for Remission in Schizophrenia

Translating the instrument-based operationalized criteria for remission into clinical practice does not require the administration of these scales. Clinicians schooled in the psychopathology of schizophrenia can implement the concept based on clinical evaluation.

Psychotic symptoms include reality distortion and disorganization. Examples of reality distortion are hallucinations—whether auditory or involving any of the other senses—and delusions. Disorganization can take the form of difficulties with tasks requiring an integration of planning and behavior, such as driving or getting dressed properly. Thoughts (as expressed in speech), too, may be disorganized—jumping to unrelated topics or jumbling incoherently.

Negative symptoms are generally conceptualized as a lack of something in the patient that people without schizophrenia seem to have. Some examples of negative symptoms are alogia (not speaking much), anhedonia (not getting pleasure out of things), blunted or flat affect (not expressing feelings through speech tone or body movements), poor hygiene, and decreased social engagement. Negative symptoms have been further categorized as primary versus secondary.

Secondary negative symptoms are due to causes other than the disorder of schizophrenia. Examples include depression, effects of medication (especially the older antipsychotics; see Chapters 16 and 17 of this volume), and prolonged institutionalization. Primary negative symptoms are those seen as being attributable to the individual's schizophrenia. People who have a significant amount of and problems with primary negative symptoms are said to have the *deficit* form of schizophrenia.

The scales used to measure remission in schizophrenia assess more than just the positive and negative symptoms we reviewed earlier. They also measure preoccupation with physical health, anxiety, motor agitation, depressed mood, guilt, disorientation, attention, and cooperation with the interviewer. Therefore, in a clinical setting, the individual with schizophrenia in remission does not have—or has only mildly—problems with these symptoms.

In summary, the patient who is in remission from schizophrenia will have at least 6 months of no symptoms or mild symptoms, as assessed by a health care professional. The next piece of the definition of remission is that the symptoms, when present in mild form, cannot interfere with a person's behavior.

Clinical Implications of Defining Remission in Schizophrenia

The principal benefit of defining *remission* in schizophrenia is to raise expectations and to maximize therapeutic efforts. There are other benefits as well. Treatment algorithms based on evidence of treatments achieving remission may be more informative than small changes based on symptom rating scales. Available evidence already suggests that integrated treatment that personalizes treatment decisions, and incorporates medication and psychosocial interventions, leads to the most favorable outcome. Finally, work toward remission can be responsive to the recovery/wellness movement of patients, families, and advocates.

KEY POINTS

- Schizophrenia is a syndrome with varied prognosis and does not necessarily entail an inevitable downhill course.
- There is a need for a consensus definition of the medical concept of remission in schizophrenia.
- The proposed definition of *remission* is at least 6 months of no symptoms or mild symptoms that do not interfere with a person's behavior.
- A consistent definition will allow both standardization in research and new ways of measuring treatment.
- Clinicians should integrate medication and psychosocial interventions to maximize outcome of patients.
- Remission should be the clinical goal in treating people with schizophrenia.
- The clinical concept of remission should be integrated with the concept of recovery.

REFERENCES AND RECOMMENDED READINGS

On Remission

Andreason, N. C., Carpenter, Jr., W. T., Kane, J. M., Lasser, R. A., Marder, S. R., & Weinberger, D. R. (2005). Remission in schizophrenia: Proposed criteria and rationale for consensus. *American Journal of Psychiatry, 182*(3), 441–449.

Doyle, A. C., & Pollack, M. H. (2003). Establishment of remission criteria for anxiety disorders. *Journal of Clinical Psychiatry, 64*(Suppl. 15), 40–45.

On Outcomes in Schizophrenia

Carpenter, W. T., Jr. (Ed.). (2005). Recovery [Special issue]. *Schizophrenia Bulletin, 31*(3).

Vaillant, G. E. (Guest Ed.). (1978). Prognosis and the course of schizophrenia [Special issue]. *Schizophrenia Bulletin, 4*(1).

Medication Trials and Their Evaluation

Cochrane Library: Available online at *www.cochrane.org*

Hegarty, J. D., Baldessarini, R. J., Tohen, M., Waternaux, C., & Oepen, G. (1995). One hundred years of schizophrenia: A meta-analysis of the outcome literature. *American Journal of Psychiatry, 152*(11), 1409–1416.

Jones, P. B., Barnes, T. R., Davies, L., Dunn, G., Lloyd, H., Hayhurst, K. P., et al. (2006). Randomized controlled trial of the effect on quality of life of second- vs. first-generation antipsychotic drugs in schizophrenia: Cost Utility of the Latest Antipsychotic Drugs in Schizophrenia Study (CUtLASS 1). *Archives of General Psychiatry, 63*, 1079–1087.

Leucht, S., Barnes, T. R., Kissling, W., Engel, R. R., Corell, C., & Kane, J. M. (2003). Relapse prevention in schizophrenia with new-generation antipsychotics: A systematic review and exploratory meta-analysis of randomized, controlled trials. *American Journal of Psychiatry, 160*(7), 1209–1222.

Lieberman, J. A., Stroup, T. S., McEvoy, J. P., Swartz, M. S., Rosenbeck, R. A., Perkins, D. O., et al. (2005). Effectiveness of antipsychotic drugs in patients with chronic schizophrenia. *New England Journal of Medicine, 353*(12), 1209–1223.

Scales

Andreason, N. C., & Olsen, S. (1982). Negative v positive schizophrenia: Definition and validation. *Archives of General Psychiatry, 39,* 789–794.

Kay, S. R., Fiszbein, A., & Opler, L. A. (1987). The Positive and Negative Syndrome Scale (PANSS) for schizophrenia. *Schizophrenia Bulletin,13,* 261–276.

Lukoff, D., Nuechterlein, K. H., & Ventura, J. (1986). Manual for the expanded Brief Psychiatric Rating Scale (BPRS). *Schizophrenia Bulletin, 12,* 594–602.

Overall, J. E., & Gorham, D. R. (1962). The Brief Psychiatric Rating Scale. *Psychological Reports, 10,* 799–812.

Integrated Treatment

Hogarty, G. E., Flesher, S., Ulrich, R., Carter, M., Greenwald, D., Pogue-Geile, M., et al. (2004). Cognitive enhancement therapy for schizophrenia: Effects of a 2-year randomized trial on cognition and behavior. *Archives of General Psychiatry, 61*(9), 866–876.

Lenroot, R., Bustillo, J. R., Lauriello, J., & Keith, S. J. (2003). Integrated treatment of schizophrenia. *Psychiatric Services, 54*(11), 1499–1507.

CHAPTER 55

RECOVERY

DAVID ROE
LARRY DAVIDSON

For over 20 years, the notion of recovery in schizophrenia was cherished by only a small—but energetic—group on the fringe of the field of mental health. However, recently this concept has taken center stage in major policy documents and initiatives in the United States and around the world. This chapter includes a review of some of the central developments that led to this "era of recovery" for persons with schizophrenia, grapples with some of the complex and confusing elements of the concept, and discusses different theoretical approaches to and definitions of recovery. Finally, a consideration of the main implications of such notions for the treatment and rehabilitation of persons with schizophrenia and related disorders is discussed.

HISTORY AND BACKGROUND OF THE CONCEPT

Toward the end of the 19th century, Émil Kraepelin identified a disease entity that he termed *dementia praecox* and described as having a characteristic downward and deteriorating course beginning in adolescence, leading irreversibly to severe, persistent impairment, and ending in a premature death. Although his observations were based primarily on long-term residents of institutions, his basic idea that *dementia praecox*, later referred to as schizophrenia, inevitably leads to progressive deterioration still reigns dominant today in the field and in society in general, leading to frequent lifelong pessimistic pronouncements about persons with the disorder. This view justified—as well as grew out of—the custodial care of people with schizophrenia, who, as a result, were perceived as chronic and "maintained" for long periods of times in large state hospitals, with little care or hope for a better future. This static, grim picture went on for years. However, toward the middle of the 20th century, a number of developments changed the conceptualization of the course and outcome of schizophrenia. Recovery is central to these new ways of thinking about severe mental illness in general and about schizophrenia in particular. The following sections describe the context, development, and substance of a variety of perspectives on recovery. Specifically, we briefly discuss four different meanings of recovery: (1) recovery as cure, (2) recovery as rehabilitation, (3) recovery from the trauma of mental illness and its aftermath, and (4) recovery as institutional change.

THE MANY MEANINGS OF RECOVERY

Recovery as Cure

In the 1950s, the deterioration of 100-year-old state hospitals and the introduction of effective psychotropic medication encouraged policymakers to consider less restrictive and confining living arrangements for persons with schizophrenia. Once people diagnosed with the disease began to live their lives outside of institutional settings, a tremendous diversity in course and outcome in the illness became apparent. This heterogeneity in outcome has now been confirmed consistently over the past 30 years of clinical research by standardized rating scales for assessing symptoms and functioning, and rigorous longitudinal designs that followed people over time. These studies revealed how some of the people in these studies fell at either of the far ends of the spectrum, with some showing a classic Kraepelinian deterioration in functioning, whereas many others showed no observable signs or symptoms and no residual impairments from the disorder between 11 and 32 years after onset. Given that symptoms are the classic marker of illness, these people could be considered to have recovered. On this basis, *recovery* became a synonym for *cure*, similar to the typical definition of *recovery* from illness, implying that the person has been restored, through whatever means, to the same presumably normal condition that existed prior to the onset of the illness.

In this way, definitions of *recovery* as returning to a normal condition based on explicit criteria of levels of symptoms imply that there is a point at which symptom remission might be said to have occurred. This definition has many advantages, such as being reliable; clear; and relatively easy to define, measure, and link to levels of functioning and well-being in other areas of life. Appearing never to have had a serious mental illness, such persons could be considered to have recovered from their schizophrenia in the same sense that people recover from a severe infection, a broken leg, or asthma.

In addition to discovering this sense of full recovery, the longitudinal outcome research described earlier also painted a multidimensional picture of schizophrenia, identifying several conceptually and empirically distinct domains of functioning. Some people recovered function in one or more of these areas, while remaining impaired or symptomatic in other domains. For example, some could work in challenging jobs and live independently, while continuing to hear voices or to entertain delusions. Others might no longer experience such symptoms at all, but still have moderate functional impairments in social relationships and/or employment. Taking into account only the loosely linked nature of these distinct domains, clinicians used concepts of partial, social, symptomatic, and other definitions of recovery to describe these different outcomes. Thus, it became clear that recovery was a multidimensional concept. Following are a number of conceptualizations of recovery, each of which emphasizes different aspects.

Recovery as Rehabilitation

Recovery as applied to schizophrenia and related disorders has often been interpreted as adapting rehabilitation principles developed in the area of physical disabilities to psychiatric disabilities. Examples drawn from the broader disability field provide a more concrete glimpse into what this concept of recovery adds to current approaches. In the case of paraplegia, for instance, several things need to be in place for persons who have lost their mobility to resume the activities they enjoyed prior to the accident or illness. The most obvious—therefore, the most often overlooked—requirement is that people not wait to regain their mobility before pursuing these and other activities. This is occasionally referred to as *acceptance* of the trauma and disability, but for many people such a notion of acceptance connotes resignation and despair. The same has been true in mental illness, with many people refusing or being reluctant to *accept* the diagnosis of schizophrenia because of the helplessness and hopelessness—as well as the stereotypical pessimistic prognosis—associated with it.

An alternative conceptualization is that people need not wait to regain their mobility to resume their lives. Although it is not preferable, it is nonetheless possible to have a life without use of one's legs. Once people acknowledge that they cannot simply sit around and wait to regain their mobility, a next important step is to be fitted for, and learn to use, prostheses or other compensatory devices, such as a wheelchair. No matter how well they learn to maneuver the wheelchair, however, certain activities remain extremely difficult, if not impossible, to resume unless other environmental accommodations are made. Understanding this crucial point has been a major contribution of the independent living movement led by people with physical disabilities, and a source of inspiration for the consumer/survivor movement in mental health. Beginning with passage of the American Rehabilitation Act of 1973, the independent living movement established that society had an obligation to promote the independence and self-sufficiency of people with disabilities. Fulfilling this obligation involved making public spaces accessible to people who used wheelchairs or other compensatory devices. Without curbs cut into sidewalks and bars installed in bathrooms, for example, the world had remained fairly restricted for people who used wheelchairs. Similarly, without Braille signs posted on doors and elevators, and without the mandate that service dogs be allowed in public spaces, people who had lost their vision had very limited access to the kinds of lives they wanted to lead in the community. The independent living movement successfully established that for people with these and other disabilities, issues of access and accommodation were fundamental to the rights and responsibilities of citizenship. Although they do not restore people's mobility or vision, they can and do restore people's lives as valuable and contributing members of society. The same should be true, according to the mental health recovery movement, for people with psychiatric disabilities.

Recovery from the Trauma of Mental Illness and Its Aftermath

Exploratory qualitative research shifted attention from the more objective, public, and observable domains to the more subjective, private, and personal ones. This research drew attention to complex interactions between the person and the disorder, revealing how the person is both influenced by as well as influences the course of his or her disorder. From this perspective, schizophrenia and many of its common social and personal consequences, such as stigmatization, discrimination, rejection, loss of job and status, loss of social roles and valued identities, unemployment, poverty and isolation, are experienced as traumatic events that generate profound changes. Accordingly, *recovery* is not defined as a return to a previous condition, but rather as an active process of confronting and working through or integrating the trauma, so that it has a less destructive impact, enabling the person to continue to live a personally meaningful life despite the trauma. While striving to overcome the pain of these many losses, people often learn lessons, make gains, and further their development. Recovery, in this sense, is the person's active effort to internalize the faith that change and renewal are still possible, and even to find new meaning in the extreme situation of trauma. According to this approach, the potential for growth implies that recovery can be seen as a developmental process and continuum through and along which new capabilities can emerge. At least one such capacity includes striving beyond personal recovery to the collective recovery of a group that for most of history has been grossly deprived of rights, neglected, and robbed of hope. This form of collective recovery is manifested through advocacy, activism, and striving for institutional change.

Recovery as Institutional Change

In the 1970s, there appeared early advocacy efforts by individuals who have since come to refer to themselves as ex-patients, ex-inmates, psychiatric survivors, or consumers or users of mental health services. Having left or been released from mental hospitals, these advocates became living proof of the research findings described earlier, demonstrating and arguing that people with schizophrenia and other serious mental illnesses can, and should be entitled to, have a life beyond that of a "mental patient." As advocates intent on reforming psychiatric policy and practice, leaders of the consumer movement had little interest in the conceptual or empirical distinctions employed in clinical research, drawing more from their own firsthand experiences of illness, incarceration, and success in recovering their lives. For these people, the categories of abnormal and normal, illness and health, were not nearly as black and white as research and diagnostic practice at times suggested. In fact, the lines between these categories seemed fuzzy and permeable at best, and arbitrary and political at worst. As a result, their agenda was not so much getting better, or getting over a psychiatric disorder such as schizophrenia, as figuring out how to live a safe, dignified, and meaningful life given whatever hand they had been dealt. For guidance in this process, they had to go outside of the mental health service system to find examples in populations that had managed adversity. It was within the context of this agenda and this movement outside of mental health services that another concept of recovery emerged.

Advocates of this approach emphasize that the recovery movement is first and foremost a civil rights movement, but this emphasis is quickly lost or overlooked in clinical settings, where the focus typically remains on disorder, deficit, and disability. Clinicians often focus primarily on minimizing and/or containing pathology. But from the perspective of the person with the psychiatric disability, the focus on deficits and pathology not only is overly narrow and limited in its utility but it also misses the very point of the civil rights argument. It would be pointless for society to accord people with disabilities the rights and responsibilities of citizenship if those rights and responsibilities were contingent on individuals overcoming their disability first. It is in the presence of enduring disability that these rights become most pressing and relevant. Similarly, it is when people with schizophrenia are most disabled by the illness that their civil rights and responsibilities become most pressing and relevant. Recovery speaks primarily to the person's rights for social inclusion and self-determination, irrespective of the nature or severity of his or her psychiatric condition. In this sense, *recovery* refers to the rights to access and to join in those elements of community life the person chooses, and to be in control of his or her own life and destiny, *while remaining disabled*. It also speaks to the need to work toward a redistribution of power in the mental health system in particular and in society in general, so that persons diagnosed with schizophrenia have a meaningful say in the way they are treated both within the mental health system and in society at large.

A RECOVERY REVOLUTION IN MENTAL HEALTH?

The first noticeable step in the direction of institutionalizing recovery in mental health in the United States was the landmark 1999 publication of the *Surgeon General's Report on Mental Health*, which marked the entry of this notion of recovery into mainstream mental health services and education, with its insistence that all mental health services be consumer- and family-oriented, and have as their overarching aim the promotion of recovery (U.S. Department of Health and Human Services, 1999). Expanding on this position, the President's New Freedom Commission on Mental Health—whose report was entitled *Achieving the Promise: Transforming Mental Health Care in America* (U.S. Department of Health and Human Services, 2003)—even more forcefully advocated for "fundamentally reforming how mental health care is delivered in America" (p. 4) to be reoriented to recovery. In the opinion of the New Freedom Commission, even the term *fundamentally reforming* was inadequate for capturing the magnitude of the changes required by a recovery orientation, resulting in their eventually settling on the term *transformation*. Continuing this momentum, the most recent policy statement contained in the *Federal Action Agenda* (U.S. Department of Health and Human Services, 2005) for implementing the New Freedom Commission recommendations takes this rhetoric one step further: "Transformation . . . is nothing short of revolutionary. . . . It implies profound change— not at the margins of a system, but at its very core. In transformation, new sources of power emerge and new competencies develop" (p. 4). Clearly, if holding out hope were the only requirement for clinical improvement of people with schizophrenia, and offering them the most effective interventions available for reducing symptoms and enhancing function, there would be no need for this kind of rhetoric; there would be no "revolution." So what does the revolutionary nature of transformation involve? What is revolutionary about it? And why is now the time for such a revolution?

Considering the perspectives of the civil rights and independent living movements, the revolution seems fairly straightforward. The various civil rights movements established that people of color did not need to be white, women did not need to be men, and lesbian/gay/bisexual/transgendered individuals did not need to be solely heterosexual to be considered, treated as, and accorded all of the rights and responsibilities of full citizenship. Similarly, as noted earlier, the independent living movement made this case for people with disabilities, insisting that it is in the presence of enduring disability that people most need to be guaranteed their rights to inclusion in community life and self-determination. Extrapolating to schizophrenia, the point would be that people living with psychosis do not need to be cured of their illness, do not need to become "normal," to pursue their lives in the community alongside everyone else. This does not mean merely that they can no longer be confined to hospitals against their will. It also means that they can make their own decisions, follow their own dreams, and participate in activities they enjoy or find meaningful in settings of their choice (within the limitations imposed by their resources or lack thereof), *as they are.*

A story may help to make this point concretely. The story of a woman, Celeste (name changed for anonymity purposes), who was 33 years old and enjoyed sewing, and who received different services from the same agency with different results, may be illustrative here.

Celeste's first clinician viewed her difficulties in managing her illness, obtaining employment, and having a social life as being due primarily to her mental illness. Although Celeste expressed an interest in working, the case manager believed that she could not yet work, because she still experienced the hallucinations and paranoia associated with her psychiatric condition. Thus, the case manager focused on trying to get Celeste to take her medication as prescribed and to attend a skills group for people who were interested in employment, hoping to address the sources of her difficulties before pursuing seriously Celeste's stated desires to work. If Celeste's disability had been related to her mobility or vision, it is obvious that she would not have acquired a job until she no longer needed to use a wheelchair or regained her vision. As it was, Celeste was soon discharged from case management due to her failure to attend scheduled meetings and her refusal to be evaluated by the agency psychiatrist. From her perspective, the case manager was indifferent to her needs and wants, and saw no change in her condition. Celeste began to feel that the agency was simply trying to drug her into a state of passivity and hopelessness; evidence for which she unfortunately found in the agency's waiting room among some of the older, more "chronic" clients. She did not want to become one of them.

After refusing these services but showing up repeatedly in hospital emergency rooms due to persistent, harassing voices, Celeste was then approached by an outreach worker from the same agency, who suggested that she *could* in fact work despite her disability. This clinician encouraged Celeste's desire to work, offering her several options of treatments and supports from which to choose in pursuing her goal most effectively. With frequent support and assistance with transportation, Celeste chose to get a job working at a fabrics store. She then found, however, that hearing voices and feeling paranoid made it difficult to be comfortable at work, and she asked whether the clinician could do anything to help. The clinician described both pharmacological and psychosocial approaches to symptom management, and suggested that Celeste discuss these concerns with her family and with a psychiatrist or nurse practitioner at the agency, who might be able to suggest medications that could help with these difficulties.

After some reluctance, Celeste eventually chose to describe her situation to a nurse, who, based on Celeste's concerns about being "drugged," initially suggested a low dose of an antipsychotic medication, explaining to Celeste that this would not make her too tired to work. With the medication Celeste found some relief and, less harassed by the voices, began to feel more comfortable at the store. As she began to bring in some of her sewing projects and to make friends with a few of her coworkers, Celeste's paranoia significantly decreased. In her case, work served several functions, giving her a reason to utilize treatment and helping to offset and/or reduce her symptoms.

Celeste's second clinician did an important thing that the first had failed to do: she listened. Now it certainly is not a revolutionary idea that clinicians need to listen, or that they should be trained to listen in a disciplined and respectful way. The practice of psychotherapy grew out of a conviction that listening should be valued. But in psychoanalytic and psychodynamic psychotherapies, listening has an additional purpose, to cultivate insight and understanding that might eventually lead to behavioral change. Celeste neither wanted to change nor was she asked by the second clinician to do so. She neither was seen as lacking, nor was she offered, insight. In fact, the problem to be addressed was not situated within Celeste at all, but in the poor fit between her disability and her environment. When Celeste wanted to work, the clinician helped Celeste to get a job that she would like and that was consistent with her interests. When Celeste was bothered by the voices brought on by the schizophrenia, the clinician suggested a few options that might make the voices less bothersome. When Celeste was concerned that her coworkers and employer would not like her, her clinician encouraged her to find out by actually trying to socialize and to share with them her interests and skills.

Against the historical backdrop of stigma, discrimination, and society's demand that people be restored to "normality," what appears to be revolutionary is that this approach assumes from the start that Celeste is a competent adult doing her best to manage a disabling condition that she neither asked for nor deserved as punishment for some earlier misdeeds. It assumes that Celeste *can and will* figure out how best to live with her disability, and that she has many areas of health and competence alongside her disability. It assumes, most importantly, that Celeste knows what is best for Celeste, and that the role of the clinician is to offer knowledge, expertise, and resources for Celeste's consideration and benefit.

From a theoretical point of view, then, this approach assumes that schizophrenia is an illness like other illnesses, for which a range of effective interventions are available for people. It also recognizes that adults with schizophrenia are autonomous, and that ultimately the choice—in concert with their loved ones, if they so choose—of which interventions they agree to try, under what conditions, in what circumstances, and with what intended outcomes, is theirs. In addition to serving people with schizophrenia, who have demanded this kind of care over the last decade, this model of collaborative decision making is taking over other domains of medicine as well. What is revolutionary about it in mental health is that it requires us to treat psychiatry more broadly, primarily as a form of medicine or health care. This is the nature of the revolution that people with psychiatric disabilities have brought about and one from which they vow not to turn back; that is, the consumer/survivor movement has established that people with serious mental illnesses such as schizophrenia remain citizens of their communities, with all of the rights and responsibilities associated with citizenship, unless, until, and only for as long as clear and compelling evidence of extenuating circumstances (e.g., serious and imminent risk) obligates society to interfere with their personal sovereignty. In all other circumstances, the illness is theirs to manage, as are their lives.

IMPLICATIONS FOR ASSESSMENT AND TREATMENT: WHAT MAKES CARE "RECOVERY ORIENTED"?

So what must be done differently in the delivery of mental health services to make them legitimately recovery-oriented? Is it enough that services be offered respectfully, and maintain the client's dignity and worth? Although this certainly would be a welcome improvement from much of current practice, it falls well short of the aim of promoting recovery. What is missing? In defining *transformation*, as noted earlier, the Federal government's *Action Agenda* spoke of "new sources of power" that needed to emerge, and "new competencies" that need to be developed. Let's begin here.

What are the new sources of power that emerge in recovery-oriented care? It is primarily the power of the person with the psychiatric disability that is tapped and brought into the process—a process that currently affords the person an almost entirely passive and subordinate role. In a recovery-oriented system of care, recovery is not something that he or she might "help" along by being compliant. Recovery is the responsibility of the person with the serious mental illness. Recovery must be pursued; it does not occur simply in response to medication or other treatments. Recovery, in this sense, refers primarily to what the person with the psychiatric disability does to manage his or her illness and to reclaim his or her life in the presence of enduring disability. Thus, the major source of power driving this process is the person's own efforts, energies, and interests.

This brings us to the second question, which pertains to the emergence of "new competencies" in transformation that belong primarily to mental health providers. Similar to progressive educators, midwives, and orchestra conductors, the recovery-oriented clinician must become competent in eliciting, encouraging, and supporting the client's interests, assets, talents, energies, and efforts. Midwives catalyze the mother's own natural processes and her efforts to facilitate the baby being born (as opposed to "delivered"). Conductors bring out the unique contributions of their musicians to create a whole that is greater than the sum of its parts. Recovery-oriented clinicians likewise focus on identifying and maximizing the person's own interests and abilities in laying the foundation for the work of recovery.

A recovery-oriented clinician identifies and builds upon each person's strengths and areas of health and competence to help him or her achieve a sense of mastery over his or her condition, while regaining a meaningful, constructive sense of membership in the community. Furthermore, when engaging in evaluation and treatment, recovery-oriented clinicians place as much, or possibly even more, emphasis on clients' personal narratives and quality of life as on their symptoms and diagnosis. In other words, in addition to attempting to reduce and/or contain the symptoms and impairments associated with the illness, practitioners focus on ways to promote their clients' functioning and help them reclaim a meaningful and gratifying life in the presence of enduring disability. As we saw with Celeste's second clinician in the case presented earlier, the key components of this process involve active and disciplined listening, and the cultivation of a trusting relationship, which then provides the basis for enhancing the client's access to various opportunities to pursue his or her own interests and gifts. Finally, recovery-oriented practitioners also stand together with their clients in the forefront of the struggle for a society more accommodating of those individual differences that make each of us unique.

KEY POINTS

- There are many different meanings of *recovery* related to serious mental illnesses such as schizophrenia.
- *Recovery* is variously used to refer to a cure, the absence of symptoms, the resumption of normal functioning and more recently, the assumption of fundamental rights and responsibilities, as well as the promotion of the kinds of institutional change that guarantee these rights and responsibilities will be respected by society.
- The most confusing, but also perhaps the most important, meaning of recovery, which is addressed in a number of recent Federal policy documents, is that being in recovery does not require being cured, diminution of symptoms, or restoration of previous level of functioning.
- This notion of being in recovery is grounded in a civil rights movement that seeks to restore to people with schizophrenia their fundamental rights and responsibilities as citizens, including most centrally the rights to self-determination and full inclusion in community life.
- Mental health services, education, and training oriented to this sense of recovery emphasizes identifying and building on people's strengths, and areas of health and competence to support their management of the condition, while they regain a meaningful and constructive sense of membership in the community.

REFERENCES AND RECOMMENDED READINGS

Anthony, W. A. (1993). Recovery from mental illness: The guiding vision of the mental health service system in the 1990s. *Psychosocial Rehabilitation Journal, 16*(4), 11–23.

Davidson, L. (2003). *Living outside mental illness: Qualitative studies of recovery in schizophrenia.* New York: New York University Press.

Davidson, L., Harding, C. M., & Spaniol, L. (2005). *Recovery from severe mental illnesses: Research evidence and implications for practice.* Boston: Center for Psychiatric Rehabilitation of Boston University.

Deegan, P. E. (1993). Recovering our sense of value after being labeled. *Journal of Psychosocial Nursing, 31*(4), 7–11.

Hopper, K., Harrison, G., Janca, A., & Sartorius, N. (2007). *Recovery from schizophrenia: An international perspective.* Oxford, UK: Oxford University Press.

Liberman, R. P., & Kopelowicz, A. (2005). Recovery from schizophrenia. A concept in search for research. *Psychiatric Services, 56*(6), 735–742.

Noordsy, D., Torrey, W., Mueser, K., Mead, S., O'Keefe, C., & Fox, L. (2002). Recovery from severe mental illness: An intrapersonal and functional outcome definition. *International Review of Psychiatry, 14,* 318–326.

Onken, S. J., Craig, C. M., Ridgway, P., Ralph, R. O., & Cook, J. A. (2007). An analysis of the definitions and elements of recovery: A review of the literature. *Psychiatrist Rehabilitation Journal, 31,* 1–9.

Ralph, R., & Corrigan, P. (Eds.). (2004). *Recovery in mental illness: Broadening our understanding of wellness.* Washington, DC: American Psychological Association.

Roe, D. (2001). Progressing from "patienthood" to "personhood" across the multi-dimensional outcomes in schizophrenia and related disorders. *Journal of Nervous and Mental Disease, 189*(10), 691–699.

U.S. Department of Health and Human Services. (1999). *Surgeon General's report on mental health.* Rockville, MD: Substance Abuse and Mental Health Services Administration.

U.S. Department of Health and Human Services. (2003). *Achieving the promise: Transforming mental health care in America.* Rockville, MD: Substance Abuse and Mental Health Services Administration.

U.S. Department of Health and Human Services. (2005). *Federal action agenda.* Rockville, MD: Substance Abuse and Mental Health Services Administration.

CHAPTER 56

GENDER

MARY V. SEEMAN

Gender effects are important to schizophrenia. Why is that so? First, they are important because of the many differences between men's and women's experience of schizophrenia. Clinicians need to learn to recognize these differences and to assess, treat, and, support men and women with schizophrenia in somewhat different ways to optimize the quality of their lives. Researchers, too, need to study these differences to determine whether they offer clues to the etiology and pathogenesis of schizophrenia.

GENETICS

Although a positive family history has been claimed in the past to be more common in women than in men patients with schizophrenia, there is no good evidence that this is the case. Genetic risk seems identical in the two sexes, which suggests that the expression of schizophrenia-prone genes is not affected by biological sex or steroid hormones. That being said, it is possible that in the future some schizophrenia risk genes may still be found that are transmitted at higher rates in one sex than in the other. The enzyme catechol-O-methyltransferase (COMT), for instance, has been the object of extensive investigations as a risk gene because of its major role in dopamine metabolism. In several older studies, a reported gender-specific association of COMT polymorphisms with schizophrenia had given rise to speculations on transmission ratio distortions, but the most recent studies have found no gender differences.

ENVIRONMENTAL RISK FACTORS

Known environmental risk factors for schizophrenia, such as prenatal infection, obstetric complications, early rearing environments, and adolescent cannabis use impact the two genders differently and probably contribute to the reported differences in morbidity risk. The association between prenatal exposure to influenza and later onset of schizophrenia is stronger in females, but obstetric complications have been reported to be more strongly associated with schizophrenia in men than in women (although this is controversial),

575

whereas adolescent substance abuse, particularly cannabis, is more prevalent in the premorbid histories of males.

Because the pace of cerebral development is slower in males than in females, the male fetal brain is considered more susceptible to environmental adversity than the female brain, due at least in part to estrogen. By activating common intracellular signaling pathways and initiating "cross-talk" with neurotrophins, the female hormone estrogen is known to play an influential role in promoting neuronal survival after environmental insult. More symmetrical brain organization in females is also considered protective, in that the other side of a symmetrical brain can compensate for functions unilaterally disrupted. During adolescence, sex-specific (hormonally induced?) reductions in synaptic density may additionally contribute to the extra vulnerability of the male brain at that critical time.

INCIDENCE RATES

Recent meta-analyses of incidence risk report a mean ratio of 1.42 for men over women, an excess for males that is only slightly reduced when studies of lower quality are excluded. This sex difference in incidence is significantly smaller in studies conducted prior to 1980. This suggests that the broader diagnoses prevalent before 1980 (at that time, the diagnosis of schizophrenia would have included schizoaffective disorder and perhaps bipolar disorder with psychotic features) tended to flatten the sex ratio. No significant sex differences in incidence have been reported in studies from developing countries. The high death rate of vulnerable children and adolescents in developing countries might offer a partial explanation. Because more women than men first become ill with schizophrenia after age 55 (the frequent cutoff age for epidemiological studies), these older women may be lost to incidence analysis. But studies with an age cutoff of 64 years or older also yield a higher mean risk ratio for men (1.32). On the other hand, no sex differences have been found in prevalence rates of schizophrenia (whether point, period, lifetime, or lifetime morbid risk prevalences). The discrepancy between incidence and prevalence sex ratios could be accounted for by better male recovery (doubtful), higher rates of male incarceration (i.e., epidemiological unavailability) or higher male death rates, particularly from suicide.

CHILDHOOD DEVELOPMENT

Adult-onset schizophrenia is preceded in childhood by mild neuromotor, cognitive, and behavioral anomalies that occur with the same frequency in boys and girls during early childhood. But from school age on, behavioral anomalies in children who later go on to develop schizophrenia appear to be more severe, and to be more frequent in boys than in girls. Boys exhibit more hyperactivity, physical and verbal aggression, and failure of behavioral inhibition, whereas girls exhibit more shyness, social withdrawal, depression, and anxiety. This is not specific to those predisposed to schizophrenia but reflects childhood development in general: little behavioral sex difference initially, but, by late childhood, more evidence of externalizing behaviors and attention deficits in boys and more anxiety in girls.

PRODROME

Girls who later develop schizophrenia, as a group, are apt to be shy, reserved, insecure, and relatively isolated. In contrast, boys who later develop schizophrenia tend toward irritability and defiance. Men with schizophrenia have consistently reported more premorbid deficits in social and occupational functioning than do women with schizophrenia. The precipitants to full-blown illness also differ between the sexes. In boys, illness is frequently triggered by substance abuse or head trauma; in girls, common antecedents include social isolation and childbirth.

AGE OF ONSET

In Germany, Häfner (2005) showed that boys develop schizophrenia 3–4 years earlier than do girls. This finding has been replicated around the world, although a few studies have found no difference. The onset distribution across the lifecycle differs in men and women. The peak age of onset in males is between 21 and 25 years, whereas the peak age in females ranges from 25 to 30 years. More men first become ill in late adolescence; women show a second peak of incidence around menopause. Women have a two to three times greater relative risk of developing late-onset (after age 45) schizophrenia. In familial cases, however, age-of-onset gender differences are not significant. Women with a family history first become ill at the same mean age as do men. The difference in age at onset between familial and nonfamilial schizophrenia (older onset age in nonfamilial cases) is significantly greater in women than in men, suggesting that the effect of genetic loading on onset age overcomes what has been described as women's natural "neuroprotection" against adolescent breakdown.

Women's later onset age in nonfamilial schizophrenia holds true for all definitions of *onset*: the first sign of any disorder, the first negative symptom, and the first positive symptom. All these milestones differ by 3–4 years between men and women and are not, as far as can be ascertained, attributable to gender-specific delays in seeking help.

BRAIN ABNORMALITIES

On magnetic resonance imaging (MRI) scans, reduced cortical brain areas, small left hippocampal formations, and enlarged lateral ventricles are present more often in male than in female patients with schizophrenia. There may also be sex differences within the affected brain areas. Compared to men, women with schizophrenia have better preserved gray matter in the hippocampus, frontal cortex, caudate nucleus, and temporal gyrus—all regions involved in higher functions such as thinking, attention, language, and working memory. But women's brains show more gliosis and focal damage in the brain areas associated with emotional processing.

NEUROPSYCHOLOGICAL DIFFERENCES

Although social cognition is more impaired in men than in women with schizophrenia, it is not clear whether other cognitive deficits are more pronounced in one sex than in the other.

SYMPTOMS

Self-neglect, reduced interest in a job, social withdrawal, and deficits of communication occur significantly more frequently in men than in women at first presentation. The prevalence of drug and alcohol abuse is significantly higher in men. Women in the general population (and also women with schizophrenia) compared to men show more emotional reactivity to the stresses of everyday life. They also have higher rates of positive psychotic symptoms (delusions and hallucinations). These findings agree with what is known about the role of emotional processes in the cognitive biases that lead to positive symptoms. Negative emotional states may contribute to a "psychotic" appraisal of experience, thus provoking psychotic symptoms. Higher levels of depression, such as those found in women with schizophrenia compared to men, may induce biases in logical reasoning that contribute to positive symptoms.

COURSE AND OUTCOME TRAJECTORY OF ILLNESS IN MEN AND WOMEN

Men have a poorer short- and medium-term course of schizophrenia than do women. This is true whether one looks at relapse rate, rehospitalization, time to relapse, duration of hospital admission, response to treatment, or social adjustment and occupational functioning. Prison rates and suicide rates are also lower in women. In a review of short- (2–5 years) and medium- (5–10 years) term follow-up studies, Angermeyer, Kuhn, and Goldstein (1990) found that about half of the studies indicated a more favorable outcome in women. The other half found no sex differences. It is the social course of the illness, rather than symptom scores, that is significantly associated with gender. Women's general tendencies toward prosocial behavior, cooperativeness, and compliance might be a key influence here. Long-term prognosis (13–40 years), however, appears to be the same for women and men. The improved earlier course for women is perhaps a result of a later start to their illness; the seeming deterioration after menopause may be secondary to the loss of the neuroprotective effects of estrogens or to the problems that women generally experience when they grow old: loneliness, poverty, age-related health problems, loss of social supports.

SOCIAL ROLE EFFECTIVENESS

Female patients with schizophrenia, more often than men, are able to enter into and maintain social roles. For instance, at first occurrence of illness, roughly one-third of women are married, compared to less than one-fifth of men. Comparable figures for the general population show that three-fourths of women and over one-half of men are married. With respect to parenting roles, approximately half of all women with schizophrenia have children. However, because blunted affect and paranoid thinking can severely impair maternal competence, women with schizophrenia are frequently unable to rear their children. About one-third lose custody of their children to family members, ex-partners, foster care, or to adoption. Single motherhood adds to the stresses of mothers with schizophrenia, and this is usually exacerbated by partner violence, poverty, and substance abuse.

TREATMENT RESPONSE

Women appear to require lower doses of antipsychotic drugs than do men to achieve equal improvement. This may be due to the attainment of higher blood levels (partly accounted for by women smoking less than men), to the fact that women are generally more compliant with prescribed medications, and to their greater fat stores, which extend the half-life of lipophilic drugs. It may also result from estrogen action at receptor target sites, such as brain dopamine receptors. Women's relatively superior response appears to be lost after menopause.

CLINICAL IMPLICATIONS

Assessment

Textbook descriptions of schizophrenia are of male-type schizophrenia. When assessing women, clinicians may miss a first episode of schizophrenia, because the woman may seem too old for a first episode or may have too many affective symptoms. When assessing women, clinicians can also mistake the following for schizophrenia: posttraumatic stress, eating disorder with starvation, psychotic depression, or a short-lived psychosis in the context of a personality disorder. When assessing women, clinicians should ascertain the influence of hormones on symptoms (e.g., contraceptive pill use, time of the month, pregnancy, postpartum period, menopause).

Treatment

Effective antipsychotic drug doses in women are generally lower than those in men (in both genders, it is important to inquire about cigarette smoking, coffee drinking, and concomitant medication). Depot medications can be given at longer intervals in women. Many women require relatively higher doses premenstrually and postmenopausally, and when pregnant may need only very small doses. Women are generally more emotionally involved with their friends and families than are men, and effective treatment must take interpersonal stressors into greater account. It is essential to inquire about the presence of children and to ensure that children under the care of women with schizophrenia are being cared for adequately. Comorbid depression is more prevalent in women than in men and usually needs to be treated.

Advocacy

There is an urgent need for family-centered services with therapeutic day care for mothers and children, including parent coaching and support services. Advocacy for individual patients is needed to convince child care agencies that it is generally preferable to provide support for the mother with schizophrenia at home than to take children away to foster care.

KEY POINTS

- Differential diagnosis in women includes mood disorder, and posttraumatic stress disorder, and starvation secondary to anorexia; in men, substance use disorders need to be ruled out.
- Hormonal triggers are important in women with schizophrenia (e.g., premenstrual period, postpartum period, menopause, contraceptive use).
- Depending on the antipsychotic used, women often require lower doses than do men.
- Heavy smoking lowers antipsychotic drug levels in both sexes.

- Because antipsychotic drugs are stored in adipose tissue, sudden gain or loss of weight affects efficacy and side effects of these drugs. This is a special issue for women.
- Women are especially vulnerable to weight gain and to disturbances of glucose and lipid metabolism secondary to long-term use of antipsychotics.
- No drugs are fully safe for the fetus in the first trimester, but the mother's safety and well-being must take priority.
- Parenting is difficult for women with schizophrenia. Extra supports are needed for prevention of mental health problems in children.
- Exacerbation of psychotic symptoms after menopause is not unusual in women.

REFERENCES AND RECOMMENDED READINGS

Aleman, A., Kahn, R. S., & Selten, J. P. (2003). Sex differences in the risk of schizophrenia: Evidence from meta-analysis. *Archives of General Psychiatry, 60,* 565–571.

Angermeyer, M. C., Kuhn, L., & Goldstein, J. M. (1990). Gender and the course of schizophrenia: Differences in treated outcomes. *Schizophrenia Bulletin, 16,* 293–307.

Cho, J. J., Iannucci, F. A., Fraile, M., Franco, J., Alesius, T. N., & Stefano, G. B. (2003). The role of the estrogen in neuroprotection: Implications for neurodegenerative diseases. *Neuroendocrinology Letters, 24,* 141–147.

Goldstein, J. M., Seidmann, L. J., O'Brien, L. M., Horton, N. J., Kennedy, D. N., Makris, H., et al. (2002). Impact of normal sexual dimorphisms on sex differences in structural brain abnormalities in schizophrenia assessed by magnetic resonance imaging. *Archives of General Psychiatry, 15,* 154–164.

Häfner, H. (2005). Gender differences in schizophrenia. In N. Bergemann & A. Riecher-Rössler (Eds.), *Estrogen effects in psychiatric disorders* (pp. 53–94). Wien New York: Springer.

Könnecke, R., Häfner, H., Maurer, K., Löffler, W., & an der Heiden, W. (2000). Main risk factors for schizophrenia: Increased familial loading and pre- and peri-natal complications antagonize the protective effect of oestrogen in women. *Schizophrenia Research, 44,* 81–93.

Kulkarni, J., de Castella, A., Downey, M., White, S., Taffe, J., Fitzgerald, P., et al. (2002). In H. Häfner (Ed.), *Risk and protective factors in schizophrenia: Towards a conceptual model of the disease process* (pp. 271–284). Darmstadt, Germany: Steinkopff-Verlag.

Myin-Germeys, I., Krabbendam, L., Delespaul, P. A., & van Os, J. (2004). Sex differences in emotional reactivity to daily life stress in psychosis. *Journal of Clinical Psychiatry, 65,* 805–809.

Riecher-Rössler, A. (2003). Oestrogens and schizophrenia. *Current Opinion in Psychiatry, 16,* 187–192.

Sand, P., Stortebecker, P., Langguth, B., Hajak, G., & Eichhammer, P. (2004). [No evidence for gender-specific sharing of COMT alleles in schizophrenia.] *Psychiatrische Praxis, 31*(Suppl. 1), S58–S560.

Seeman, M. V. (1982). Gender differences in schizophrenia. *Canadia Journal of Psychiatry, 27,* 107–112.

Seeman, M. V., & Lang, M. (1990). The role of estrogens in schizophrenia gender differences. *Schizophrenia Bulletin, 16,* 185–194.

Seeman, M. V. (2004). Schizophrenia and motherhood. In M. Göpfert, J. Webster, & M. V. Seeman (Eds.), *Parental psychiatric disorder* (2nd ed., pp. 161–171). Cambridge, UK: Cambridge University Press.

CHAPTER 57

QUALITY OF LIFE

STEFAN PRIEBE
WALID K. H. FAKHOURY

This chapter introduces the concept and methods to measure quality of life in schizophrenia, and explains the difference between objective and subjective indicators of quality of life in patients with schizophrenia. It also outlines the various uses of quality-of-life measures, and the way quality-of-life assessments may be applied in research and in routine care.

THE CONCEPT

Quality of life has become a popular measure in psychiatric research since the 1980s. It was introduced and promoted in psychiatry for patients with severe mental illness, particularly schizophrenia, because clinicians felt that symptom reduction through medication would not be sufficient for the management of these patients' illness, and that a wider concept was required to guide and evaluate care programs. The concept itself can be traced to the World Health Organization's (WHO) definition of health in general in 1948 as "a state of complete physical, mental and social well-being and not merely the absence of disease or infirmity." Since then, the many attempts to delineate what defines quality of life have led to the concept being defined in different ways and within various theoretical frameworks.

In the literature on quality of life in general, at least 12 different concepts are identified. Of these, two directly apply to psychiatry: the "social indicators approach" and the "psychological indicators approach." In the social indicators approach, quality of life is a measure in which only objective information is collected, with a focus on external conditions such as education, income, housing, and neighborhood. In the social indicators approach, many indicators are used to reflect psychological well-being, despite the fact that they have no basic anchor in the human meaning of social events.

In the psychological indicators approach, the focus is on how people view their own lives. Examples of models in this approach are the "schizophrenic needs" and the "competency" models. In the former, the quality-of-life concept is based on the needs of the recovering patient with schizophrenia: medical care, human relationships, material quality of life, communication and transport services, work and work conditions, safety, knowledge, education, leisure and recreation, and inner experience (May, 1986). Competency models, on the other hand, view people as active agents who govern their own lives. The core variables of competency models are personal autonomy (Mercier & King, 1994), and self-esteem and self-efficacy (Arns & Linney, 1993).

At least two further concepts of quality of life found in the psychiatric literature can be summarized as the "combined approach" and "adaptive functioning models." In the combined approach, both social and psychological indicators are taken into account. The best-known combined approach model was designed by Lehman (1983) and considered quality of life a subjective matter, reflected in a sense of global well-being. In this model, quality-of-life experience is reflected by personal characteristics (e.g., age and sex), objective indicators in various domains of life, and subjective quality of life in the same life domains. The objective indicators are external life conditions, such as income, housing, and access to the community; whereas subjective quality of life represents the individual's appraisal of these conditions and uses mostly satisfaction constructs. The domains included in the combined approach are living situation, family, social relations, leisure, work, law, safety, finances, and health.

In adaptive functioning models, importance is given to individual satisfaction in relation to social expectations; a reasonable or high quality of life is dependent on the degree to which patients can meet the demands of life and achieve fulfillment of needs and find satisfaction. An example of an adaptive functioning model is that of Baker and Intagliata (1982), in which quality of life is a measure of the environmental system (social indicators), the experienced environment (psychological indicators), the biopsychological system (health, well-being, and needs), and behavior (self-management and adaptation). Both the experienced environment and the biopsychological system are within the person, and comparisons (against standards/levels of adaptation) are made between both these foci.

Different concepts of quality of life exist, and no universally accepted unitary concept has emerged in the last two decades of extensive research in psychiatry. This helps keep the construct of quality of life open, with lively debate on the issue. The consensus, however, is that quality of life is multidimensional, and that it encompasses objective and subjective indicators, as well as health- and non-health-related domains. It is this combination of indicators and domains that makes quality of life a measure both useful and challenging as a specific health outcome.

OBJECTIVE AND SUBJECTIVE INDICATORS

Over the last two decades, the trend has moved from more objectively defined quality-of-life concepts toward understanding quality of life as largely determined by the patient's subjective experiences of life and life conditions. Patients' subjective perceptions of their quality of life appear linked to their personal subjective evaluation of life events and circumstances, and to the inevitable psychological burden imposed by the often-debilitating consequences of schizophrenia. An understanding of the relationship between the objective and subjective indicators may, however, be required to make an informed decision, when necessary, on which quality-of-life measure to choose.

Although objective and subjective indicators reflect aspects of quality of life, the association between the objective and subjective indicators is reported to be weak to moderate at best, with correlations ranging from .04 to .57, suggesting that they measure different concepts of quality of life (Lehman, Ward, & Linn, 1982). International comparisons indicated that differences in subjective quality-of-life domains did not correspond with differences in the objective data. However, this is not always the case, and substantial differences in objective living situations were found to be related to differences in subjective quality of life. Evidence exists of congruence at a group level between unemployment and homelessness, and their corresponding subjective domains, whereby those employed and those with housing stability were found to have higher satisfaction scores in the subjective quality-of-life domains of employment (Priebe, Warner, Hubschmid, & Eckle, 1998) and accommodation (Lehman, Kernan, Deforge, & Dixon, 1995), leading to higher general satisfaction with life. Also, dramatic changes in the living situation, such as discharge into community care after long-term hospitalization, can have a positive effect on patients' subjective quality of life (Priebe, Hoffmann, Isermann, & Kaiser, 2002).

From an anthropological perspective, Warner (1999) suggested that the subjective–objective distinction in quality-of-life research is similar to the difference between Pike's (1967) emic and etic units of data. For Pike, an anthropological linguist, an *emic* unit of data is something that insiders in a culture regard as being the same entity regardless of variation, whereas an *etic* unit of data is one that an outsider can objectively observe and verify. It has been postulated that "emic statements are those referring to logical systems whose discriminations are real and significant to the actors themselves, while etic statements depend on distinctions judged appropriate by scientific observers" (Harris, 1968). Therefore, based on this, there is a difference between what the patient perceives is his or her quality of life (subjective indicators) and what researchers can objectively measure to assess what they believe is that patient's quality of life (objective indicators). Researchers have indicated that whereas objective data are of immense importance for the prediction of change over time, psychological adaptation, or "response shift," can happen in chronic illnesses such as schizophrenia, resulting in a shift in the patient's appraisal of his or her current state; thus, the patient's responses to subjective well-being questions can change significantly, reducing the strength of the association between subjective assessment and objective conditions. Psychological adaptation can also occur in the general population, for quality of life tends to be relatively stable over time and not greatly affected in the long term by dramatic changes in life conditions. Some have argued that the most practical information for portraying outcomes of mental health services may indeed be etic (e.g., does the person have accommodation?); however, to understand such data and develop an intervention to change the outcome, emic data are needed (e.g., does the person wish to spend his or her income on rent?). In research, subjective indicators have become dominant, but in clinical practice, data on both objective and subjective indicators of quality of life are important, because they are used to provide services tailored to patients' specific needs.

ASSESSMENT INSTRUMENTS

A spectrum of scales, checklists, and structured and semistructured interviews assess quality of life among psychiatric patients. Measures can be classified into two groups: (1) proxy and (2) specifically designed.

Proxy measures of quality of life are established psychiatric rating scales used to assess the patient's symptom levels, particularly symptoms of depression. Such scales have been used in the screening and surveillance of psychiatric disorders, particularly in studies mapping psychiatric disorders in the community (e.g., the General Health Questionnaire;

Goldberg, 1972) and in the evaluation of various interventions in clinical samples. Although scores on these scales have frequently been taken as indicators of quality of life, these scales are not specific to quality of life and do not capture its objective and subjective indicators.

Specifically designed health-related quality-of-life instruments are developed with the multidimensionality concept of the quality of life in mind. Table 57.1 summarizes some of the established instruments. Measures such as the Quality of Life Scale (QLS), the Quality of Life Interview (QLI), and the Oregon Quality of Life Scale (OQLS) are popular in the United States, whereas instruments such as the Lancashire Quality of Life Profile (LQOLP), the Manchester Short Assessment of Quality of Life Scale (MANSA), and the European Quality of Life 5-Dimensional Format (EuroQol-5D) are more widely used in Europe. However, despite differences in their geographical use, some of these instruments are related (e.g., the MANSA was based on the LQOLP, which in turn was based on the QLI).

TABLE 57.1. Specifically Designed Quality-of-Life Instruments

Title	Author(s)	Number of items	Number of domains	Estimated completion time
Client Quality of Life Interview	Mulkern et al. (1986)	65	8	30 min
EuroQol-5D	EuroQol group (1990)	15	5	5 min
Index of Health-Related Quality of Life	Rosser et al. (1992)	107, 225	3	Not known
Lancashire Quality of Life Profile (LQOLP)	Oliver (1991)	100	11	30–50 min
Manchester Short Assessment of Quality of Life (MANSA)	Priebe et al. (1999)	25	12	10–15 min
Munich Quality of Life Dimensions List	Heinisch et al. (1991)	20	4	10 min
Oregon Quality of Life Scale (OQS)	Bigelow et al. (1991)	146	14	45 min
Quality of Life Checklist	Malm et al. (1981)	93	11	60 min
Quality of Life Interview (QLI)	Lehman (1988)	143	8	45 min
Quality of Life Scale (QLS)	Heinrichs et al. (1984)	21	21	45 min
Satisfaction with Life Domains Scale	Baker and Intagliata (1982)	15	15	10 min
Schizophrenia Quality of Life Scale (SQLS)	Wilkinson et al., 2000	30	3	5–10 min
SmithKline Beacham Quality of Life	Dunbar et al. (1992)	78	23	Not known
Subjective Well-Being Under Neuroleptics Scale (SWN)	Naber (1995)	38	5	Not known
Well-Being Project Client Interview	Campbell et al. (1989)	151, 76, and 77	60	Not known
World Health Organization Quality of Life Instrument—Brief (WHOQOL)	World Health Organization (1996)	26	4	5–10 min

Specifically designed quality-of-life measures can be generic, health-related, or disease-specific. Generic scales are not specific to illness, treatment types, or patient characteristics, and they contain health-related quality-of-life concepts pertaining to both patients and the general population. These scales allow comparison of quality-of-life results across interventions, diagnostic conditions, and groups of the population. Examples are the Sickness Impact Profile (SIP), the Nottingham Health Profile, QLI, LQOLP, and MANSA.

Health-related quality-of-life measures are designed to describe the health problems of populations across several dimensions of health, but not specifically mental health. They are classified under generic scales, with the term *generic* referring to all nondisease-specific measures. Examples are the Medical Outcome Study (MOS) questionnaire (which was modified to the 36-item Short-Form General Health Survey (SF-36; Ware & Sherbourne, 1992) and the EuroQol-5D.

Generic scales are, however, not specific enough to capture the quality-of-life problems of patients with specific illnesses; hence, there is a need for disease-specific quality-of-life scales. Disease-specific measures may have greater clinical appeal due to the specificity of content and an associated increased responsiveness to specific change in condition. Perhaps the best-known disease-specific quality-of-life measure is the QLS, a clinician-rating scale that was designed to assess patients' symptoms and functional status in the course and treatment of schizophrenia, and that has acceptable psychometric properties. The scale items reflect the manifestations of the deficit syndrome in schizophrenia, and are classified into four subscales: Intrapsychic Foundations, Interpersonal Relations, Instrumental Roles, and Common Object and Activities. Other, newer disease-specific quality-of-life scales exist but have not been as widely used as the QLS, such as the Subjective Well-Being Under Neuroleptics Scale (SWN) and the Schizophrenia Quality of Life Scale (SQLS). However, whereas disease-specific quality-of-life scales may be useful to explain symptoms directly and the experience of medication side effects, quality-of-life constructs may become blurred and overlap with other constructs, most notably symptomatology, a problem that some of the disease-specific scales share with proxy measures.

Selection of Measures

Specifically designed quality-of-life measures are multi-item scales. Some of these scales, such as the OQLS and the LQOLP, are lengthy and time-consuming to complete. Lengthy scales covering the different domains of subjective quality of life may be preferable to short ones, which may be less sensitive. However, length may become a problem if the scale is used as a part of a battery of instruments (too many long scales to complete) and/or yields various scores for which there is no clear method of analysis. Regarding the use of self-administered or interviewer-administered quality-of-life scales, it has been argued that self-administered scales (e.g., the Quality of Life Index for Mental Health; Becker, Diamond, & Sainfort, 1993) should not be administered to people with severe mental illness, because these patients' negative symptoms, such as apathy and withdrawal, might make completion of the questionnaires difficult, and various aspects of thought disorder and auditory hallucinations can diminish patients' ability to concentrate and may affect the reliability of their answers. As far as psychometric properties are concerned, quality-of-life instruments have to be reliable, valid, and sensitive to changes in patients' conditions over time. Several measures have been used with acute patients (e.g., after admission to the hospital), and there is no evidence that the findings lack validity, although such concerns have repeatedly been expressed. Thus, quality-of-life instruments may also be administered in acute states of schizophrenia, as long as it is feasible and not too burdensome for the patient. There is a symptom level above which a reasonable response to the quality-of-life scale questions becomes increasingly unlikely. However, research has not yet established the maximum symptom level to gain valid responses to quality-of-life questions, and the exact level may vary among individuals.

The decision on which measure to use therefore depends on striking a balance among factors such as clinical time spent administering the instrument, practicalities related to ways of collecting the information (e.g., whether through face-to-face interviews, postal questionnaires, etc.), and psychometric properties of the instrument. The purpose of data collection should also be considered. If the measure is used to help clinicians in individual patient care, a detailed measure may be needed to provide comprehensive information on areas of dissatisfaction in the patient's life that need to be addressed. On the other hand, if it is used to evaluate a service at a group level, then a shorter measure with good psychometric properties may be more appropriate. A further criterion for selecting an instrument may be the availability of data to compare results. With respect to patients with schizophrenia, various studies providing such data have been published using the QLS, QLI, LQOLP, MANSA and WHO Quality of Life Instrument—Brief (WHOQOL), and these scales have become established in schizophrenia research.

ASSOCIATION WITH OTHER CONSTRUCTS

There is a tendency in psychiatry to use several instruments to describe the subjective experience of patients with schizophrenia. While subjective quality of life reflects the patient's appraisal of the current life, self-ratings of needs and symptoms, as well as treatment satisfaction, are also used as research criteria to assess the outcomes of interventions, and are intended to assess distinct constructs. Is subjective quality-of-life independent of other constructs reflecting subjective experience, and should it be measured along with other constructs in the same study? Evidence indicates moderate to strong correlations between subjective quality of life and ratings of symptoms, needs, and treatment satisfaction, with correlations ranging from .5 to .7 (Fakhoury, Kaiser, Röder-Wanner, & Priebe, 2002; Priebe, Kaiser, Huxley, Röder-Wanner, & Rudolph, 1998). A single subjective appraisal factor—reflecting negative subjective quality of life, more symptoms, and more needs—explained 48–69% of the variance of all these patient-rated outcomes (Fakhoury et al., 2002; Priebe, Kaiser, et al., 1998). All this indicates that subjective criteria are all interrelated and do not really capture distinct constructs. Thus, scales to assess several of these constructs should not be used as outcome criteria, unless a specific hypothesis justifies the use of separate scales to assess patient-rated outcomes.

Research also suggests a significant association between subjective quality of life and the Antonovsky's Sense of Coherence instrument. Sense of Coherence measures the personal orientation toward life that determines one's health experience. Individuals with a strong sense of coherence believe that the world around them is structured, explicable, and predictable; that the resources needed to meet the demands of the world are available to them; and that these demands are worthy of investment. There are three domains within the construct: comprehensibility, manageability, and meaningfulness. In a sample of patients with schizophrenia it was found to be significantly associated with quality of life. Increased Sense of Coherence score over time was found to be significantly associated with improvements in overall subjective quality of life (Bengtsson-Tops & Hansson, 2001). Finally, a significant positive association between psychosocial functioning and subjective quality of life in patients with schizophrenia has also been reported. This association was moderated by the executive functioning of the patient, independent of patient psychopathology, suggesting the need to incorporate executive capacity in models of quality of life (Brekke, Kohrt, & Green, 2001).

FACTORS INFLUENCING QUALITY OF LIFE

Studies have shown that patients with schizophrenia are frequently more satisfied with their lives than clinicians would objectively expect them to be given their poor living situation, and that they are also no more dissatisfied than members of other groups with physical illnesses or social disadvantages. Schizophrenia often is a persistent condition that lasts for several decades. A high subjective quality of life despite poor living conditions may be explained by the relatively long duration of illness, which has given the patients time to accept their chronic condition; to adjust their expectations of life, their state of health, and their available resources; and to compare themselves to other patients rather than to people from preillness peer groups. Yet, in addition to the length of illness, a number of other factors associated with subjective quality-of-life scores may be grouped into sociodemographic and clinical domains.

Sociodemographic Factors

Lower quality of life is more likely to be reported by male patients with schizophrenia who are younger, have a high level of education, live alone, live in a less restrictive environment, and are not employed. However, these characteristics are not strong predictors of subjective quality of life in clinical populations.

Clinical Factors

Symptom level is the most important factor influencing subjective quality of life of patients with schizophrenia. The higher symptom level is consistently associated with lower subjective quality of life, explaining up to 30% of the variance (Kaiser et al., 1997). The association is dominated mostly by mood, especially anxiety and depression symptoms. Indeed, depression is the strongest variable associated with life satisfaction in psychiatric patients. On the individual-patient level, changes over time in subjective quality of life were found to correlate with changes in anxiety and depression, suggesting that changes in depressive symptoms need to be considered when interpreting changes in satisfaction with life (Fakhoury et al., 2002). The significant impact of mood on subjective quality of life suggests that any intervention to improve psychopathology may need to consider patients' affective state, which is significantly related to their subjective quality of life. However, the direction of the influence can be questioned: Does depression influence the appraisal of life and lead to less favorable subjective quality-of-life scores? Or does the reverse occur, with a negative view of life leading to more depressive symptoms? Or is the association more complex, so that both depression and subjective quality of life are determined by similar underlying cognitive and emotional processes? Research has not yet answered these questions. Clinical characteristics such as subclass of schizophrenia (e.g., paranoid schizophrenia), early onset of symptoms, previous hospitalization, and age at first hospitalization are negatively associated with subjective quality of life of patients with schizophrenia.

QUALITY OF LIFE AS AN OUTCOME CRITERION

The current prominence of quality of life stems from its frequent use as an outcome in clinical trials. However, it is a rather "distal" outcome, because the effect of most therapeutic interventions on quality of life is likely to be indirect and evidenced at a later time. This is in contrast to "proximal" outcomes, such as symptoms, whose effect is likely to be direct and immediate. Thus, the time it takes for an intervention to impact on quality-of-life measures needs to be considered by the clinician using the concept as an outcome criterion. Another issue is the sensitivity of these measures in capturing changes over time. Some measures reported significant changes in objective, but not subjective, indicators over time, whereas others reported congruent changes in objective indicators and their corresponding subjective domains. This mixed picture highlights the importance of examining the different effects of well-defined interventions on the objective and subjective indicators of quality of life.

Use in Pharmacological Interventions

The questions of whether neuroleptics—directly or indirectly—improve patients' quality of life, and whether the impact varies between typical and atypical neuroleptics, are of obvious clinical relevance and, subsequently, of marketing interest to pharmaceutical companies sponsoring major drug trials. Quality-of-life measures have therefore been used frequently to assess the outcome of antipsychotic medication.

Pioneering conceptual work in this area has been provided by Awad, Vorauganti, and Heselgrave (1997), who developed the *integrative conceptual model for quality of life of patients with schizophrenia on neuroleptics*. In this model, *quality of life* is defined as the patient's own perception of the outcome of an interaction among psychotic symptom severity, medication side effects, and the level of psychosocial performance. Personality characteristics, premorbid adjustment, values and attitudes toward health and illness, and resources and their availability are all sets of variables that may modulate the interaction and are therefore considered in the model. The model also specifies requirements that the measure must meet to assess properly the quality of life of patients on neuroleptics. Based on these variables, the 136-item SIP was identified as the most suitable scale to discriminate the effects of medication. However, although this model is innovative, it ignores the objective indicators of quality of life, and requires more validation in research and practice.

With respect to the potential effect of different neuroleptics on quality-of-life measures, empirical evidence from 31 published randomized clinical trials involving more than 12,000 individuals indicates that, compared to typical neuroleptics, the effect of atypicals on patients' quality of life is not consistently more favorable; only about half of the studies reported significant improvements (Corrigan, Reinke, Landsberger, Charat, & Tombs, 2003). Some evidence suggests that patients on olanzapine may have more positive quality-of-life scores than patients on other atypical (Taylor et al., 2005) or typical (Silva De Lima et al., 2005) neuroleptics.

Use in Psychosocial and Other Interventions

Psychosocial interventions have a documented positive impact on the clinical outcomes of patients with schizophrenia. However, their influence on quality of life has not always been measured, and in studies that assessed quality of life as an outcome, a nonsignificant effect has often been found. Interventions such as art therapy, standard case management, and client-focused case management have not been found to have a significant effect on patients' quality of life. However, intensive case management, hallucination-focused integrative treatment—which incorporates an element of cognitive-behavioral therapy (CBT), and discharge into community after long-term hospitalizations have all been associated with significant improvements in quality of life. More evidence is required to establish which psychosocial interventions impact on quality of life, their mediating processes, and expected effect sizes.

Use in Treatment

Since 2000, quality-of-life measures have increasingly been used to improve individual treatment processes in mental health services, mostly in forms of outcome management in which data are assessed regularly and individually—and later possibly aggregated on the levels of groups and services. The results are fed back to clinicians, managers, and patients to inform their decisions on care and service management (McCabe & Priebe, 2002). There have been attempts to implement outcomes management in routine practice, with a view toward improving quality and outcome of treatment, although there is no consistent evidence for its effectiveness in mental health care.

An example of outcome management is the Quality of Life Profiling Project that was developed around the LQOLP. The project used a computerized system to assess quality of life with results fed back to patients through graphs. In a randomized controlled trial (Slade et al., 2006), researchers assessed patients' quality of life and other outcome criteria, and reported the results to clinicians in community mental health care teams. The intervention was associated with lower care costs but did not lead to an improvement of patients' quality of life. Another trial conducted in six European countries incorporated quality-of-life assessments in the routine sessions between patients and clinicians in community mental health care teams. Computer-mediated procedures were used to display results, including comparisons with previous ratings, and results were expected to feed into the therapeutic dialogue between clinicians and patients (Priebe, McCabe, et al., 2002). Compared with a control group receiving treatment as usual, patients in the intervention group showed a small but significant improvement in subjective quality of life after 1 year.

KEY POINTS

- There is no universally agreed-upon concept of quality of life.
- In clinical practice, data on both objective and subjective indicators of quality of life are used, and the importance of subjective indicators reflecting the views of patients has increased over time.
- Quality of life in patients with schizophrenia is measured by generic and disease-specific scales; whereas the former have concepts pertaining to both patients and the general population, the latter have greater clinical appeal due to the specificity of content.
- The selection of a quality-of-life scale depends on its psychometric properties, the clinical time to administer it, and practicalities related to collecting the data.
- Symptom level, particularly depression, is the most important factor negatively influencing subjective quality of life of patients with schizophrenia.
- Quality of life is a distal outcome criterion to evaluate the effects of all types of therapeutic interventions, particularly long-term treatment.
- Quality-of-life measures are used to improve individual treatment processes in mental health services in the form of outcomes management.

REFERENCES AND RECOMMENDED READINGS

Arns, P. G., & Linney, J. A. (1993). Work, self and life satisfaction for persons with severe and persistent mental disorders. *Psychosocial Rehabilitation Journal, 17,* 63–69.

Awad, A. G., Vorauganti, L. N. P., & Heslegrave, R. J. (1997). A conceptual model of quality of life in schizophrenia: Description and preliminary validation. *Quality of Life Research, 6,* 21–26.

Baker, F., & Intagliata, J. (1982). Quality of life in the evaluation of community support systems. *Evaluation and Program Planning, 5,* 69–79.

Becker, M., Diamond, R., & Sainfort, F. (1993). A new patient focused index for measuring quality of life in persons with severe and persistent mental illness. *Quality of Life Research, 2,* 239–251.

Bengtsson-Tops, A., & Hansson, L. (2001). The validity of Antonovsky's sense of coherence measure in a sample of schizophrenia patients living in the community. *Journal of Advanced Nursing, 33,* 432–438.

Bigelow, D. A., McFarland, B. H., & Olson, M. M. (1991). Quality of life of community mental health programme clients: Validating a measure. *Community Mental Health Journal, 27,* 43–55.

Bowling, A. (1995). *Measuring disease: A review of disease-specific quality of life measurements.* Buckingham, UK: Open University Press.

Brekke, J., Kohrt, R., & Green, M. (2001). Neuropsychological functioning as a moderator of the relationship between psychosocial functioning and the subjective experience of self and life in schizophrenia. *Schizophrenia Bulletin, 27,* 697–708.

Campbell, J., Schraiber, R., Temkin, T., & Ten Tuscher, T. (1989). *The Well-Being Project: Mental health clients speak for themselves.* Sacramento: California Department of Mental Health.

Corrigan, P. W., & Buican, R. (1995). The construct validity of subjective quality of life for the severely mentally ill. *Journal of Nervous and Mental Disease, 183,* 281–285.

Corrigan, P. W., Reinke, R. R., Landsberger, S. A., Charat, A., & Tombs, G. (2003). The effects of atypical antipsychotic medication on psychosocial outcomes. *Schizophrenia Research, 63*(1), 97–101.

Dunbar, G. C., Stroker, M. J., Hodges, T. C., & Beaumont, G. (1992). The development of the SBQOL: A unique scale for measuring quality of life. *British Journal of Health Economics, 2,* 65–74.

Euroqol Group. (1990). EuroQol: A new facility for the measurement of health-related quality of life. *Health Policy, 16,* 199–208.

Fakhoury, W. K. H., Kaiser, W., Röder-Wanner, U. U., & Priebe, S. (2002). Subjective evaluation: Is there more than one criterion? *Schizophrenia Bulletin 28*(2), 319–327.

Fakhoury, W. K. H., & Priebe, S. (2002). Subjective quality of life: Its association with other constructs. *International Review of Psychiatry, 14,* 219–224.

Goldberg, D. P. (1972). *The detection of psychiatric illness by questionnaire* (Maudsley Monograph No. 21). London: Oxford University Press.

Harris, M. (1968). The rise of anthropological theory. *Current Anthropology, 9*(5), 519–533.

Heinisch, M., Ludwig, M., & Bullinger, M. (1991). Psychometrische testung der "Münchner Lebenqualitäts-Dimensionen-Liste (MLDL)." In M. Bullinger, M. Ludwig, & N. von Steinbuchel (Eds.), *Lebenqualität bei Kardiovaskulären Er-Krankungen.* Gottingen: Hogrefe.

Heinrichs, D. W., Hanlon, T. E., & Carpenter, W. T. (1984). The Quality of Life Scale: An Instrument for rating the schizophrenia deficit syndrome. *Schizophrenia Bulletin, 10,* 388–398.

Kaiser, W., Priebe, S., Barr, W., Hoffmann, K., Isermann, M., Röder-Wanner, U. U., et al. (1997). Profiles of subjective quality of life in schizophrenic in- and out-patient samples. *Psychiatric Research, 66,* 153–166.

Katschnig, H., Freeman, H., & Sartorius, N. (Eds.). (1997). *Quality of life in mental disorders.* Chichester, UK: Wiley.

Lehman, A. F. (1983). The well-being of chronic mental patients: Assessing their quality of life. *Archives of General Psychiatry, 40,* 369–373.

Lehman, A. F., Kernan, E., Deforge, B. R., & Dixon, L. (1995). Effects of homelessness on the quality of life of persons with severe mental illness. *Psychiatric Services, 46,* 922–926.

Lehman, A. F., Ward, N. C., & Linn, L. S. (1982). Chronic mental patients: The quality of life issue. *American Journal of Psychiatry, 139,* 1271–1276.

Malm, U., May, P. R., & Dencker, S. J. (1981). Evaluation of the quality of life of schizophrenic outpatients: A checklist. *Schizophrenia Bulletin, 7,* 477–487.

May, P. R. A. (1986). Some research relating to the treatment of Bleuler's disease (schizophrenia). *Psychiatric Journal of the University of Ottawa, 11,* 117–126.

McCabe, R., & Priebe, S. (2002). Focusing on quality of life in treatment. *International Review of Psychiatry, 14,* 225–230.

Mercier, C., & King, S. (1994). A latent causal model of the quality of life of psychiatric patients. *Acta Psychiatrica Scandinavica, 89,* 72–77.

Mulkern, V., Agosta, J. M., Ashbaugh, J. W., Bradley, V. J., Spence, R. A., Allein, S., et al. (1986).

Community support programme client follow up study (Report to NIMH). Rockville, MD: National Institute of Mental Health.

Naber, D. (1995). A self-rating to measure subjective effects of neuroleptic drugs, relationships to objective psychopathology, quality of life, compliance and other clinical variables. *International Clinical Psychopharmacology, 10,*(3), 133–138.

Oliver, J. P. J. (1991). The social care directive: Development of a quality of life profile for use in community services for the mentally ill. *Social Work and Social Sciences Review, 3*(1), 5–45.

Oliver, J. P. J., Huxley, P. J., Bridges, K., & Mohamad, H. (1996). *Quality of Life and Mental Health Services.* London: Routledge.

Pike, K. L. (1967). *Language in relation to a unified theory of structure of human behavior* (2nd ed.). The Hague: Mouton.

Priebe, S., Hoffmann, K. N., Isermann, M., & Kaiser, W. (2002). Do long-term hospitalised patients benefit from discharge into the community? *Social Psychiatry and Psychiatric Epidemiology, 37*(8), 387–392.

Priebe, S., Huxley, P., Knight, S., & Evans, S. (1999). Application and results of the Manchester Short Assessment of Quality of Life (MANSA). *International Journal of Social Psychiatry, 45*(1), 7–12.

Priebe, S., Kaiser, W., Huxley, P., Röder-Wanner, U. U., & Rudolph, H. (1998). Do different subjective evaluation criteria reflect distinct constructs? *Journal of Nervous and Mental Disease, 186,* 385–392.

Priebe, S., McCabe, R., Bullenkamp, J., Hansson, L., Rossler, W., Torres-Gonzales, F., et al. (2002). The impact of routine outcome measurement on treatment processes in community mental health care: Approach and methods of the MECCA study. *Epidemiologia e Psichiatria Sociale, 11,*(3), 198–205.

Priebe, S., Oliver, J. P., & Kaiser, W. K. (Eds). (1999). Quality of life and mental health care. *Quality of life and mental health care.* Hampshire, UK: Wrightson Biomedical Publishing.

Priebe, S., Warner, R., Hubschmid, T., & Eckle, I. (1998). Employment, attitude towards work, and quality of life among people with schizophrenia in three countries. *Schizophrenia Bulletin, 24*(3), 469–477.

Renwick, R., Brown, I., & Nagler, M. (Eds.). (1996). *Quality of life in health promotion and rehabilitation: Conceptual approaches, issues, and applications.* Thousand Oaks, CA: Russell Sage Foundation.

Silva De Lima, M., De Jesus Mari, J., Breier, A., Maria Costa, A., Ponde De Sena, E., & Hotopf, M. (2005). Quality of life in schizophrenia: A multicenter, randomized, naturalistic, controlled trial comparing olanzapine to first-generation antipsychotics. *Journal of Clinical Psychiatry, 66,*(7), 831–838.

Slade, M., McCrone, P., Kuipers, E., Leese, M., Cahill, S., Parabiaghi, A., et al. (2006). Use of standard outcome measures in adult mental health services: Randomised controlled trial. *British Journal of Psychiatry, 189,*(4), 330–336.

Taylor M., Turner, M., Watt, L., Brown, D., Martin, M., & Fraser, K. (2005). Atypical anti-psychotics in the real world—a naturalistic comparative outcome study. *Scottish Medical Journal, 50*(3), 102–106.

Ware, J. E., & Sherbourne, C. D. (1982). The MOS 36-Item Short-Form Health Survey (SF-36) I: Conceptual framework and item selection. *Medical Care, 30,* 473–483.

Warner, R. (1999). Quality of life assessment: An anthropological perspective. In S. Priebe, J. P. J. Oliver, & W. Kaiser (Eds.), *Quality of life and mental health care.* Hampshire, UK: Wrightson Biomedical Publishing.

Wiersma, D., Jenner, J. A., Nienhuis, F. J., & Van De Willige, G., (2004). Hallucination focused integrative treatment improves quality of life in schizophrenia patients. *Acta Psychiatrica Scandinavica, 109,* 194–201.

Wilkinson, G., Hedson, B., Wild, D., Cookson, R., Farina, C., Sharma, V., et al. (2000). Self-report quality of life measure for people with schizophrenia. *British Journal of Psychiatry, 177,* 42–46.

World Health Organization. (1996). *WHOQOL-BREF: Introduction, administration, scoring, and generic version of the assessment.* Geneva: Author.

CHAPTER 58

SPIRITUALITY AND RELIGION

ROGER D. FALLOT

In the larger sociocultural context, as well as in behavioral health settings, several factors in recent years have converged to make attention to spirituality and religion more prominent in mental health and other supportive services for people diagnosed with schizophrenia. Social, political, and cultural movements have offered reminders of the importance of religion and spirituality at individual and collective levels. Sociologists, who as recently as the late 1980s were convinced of the inevitable and progressive secularization of the modern world, now increasingly recognize the tenacity with which many people and cultures maintain strong religious commitments. In recent years, numerous controversies have heightened the frequently contentious discussion of the place of religion in public and political spheres. In the United States, polls consistently find both widespread and intensive commitment to religious beliefs and activities; identifying oneself as a "religious" person is extremely common. Many other people, including those whose involvement in formal, institutional religion may be minimal, understand themselves as "spiritual" people who engage in spiritually oriented, though not necessarily religious, activities. This increasingly noted distinction between spirituality and religion implies a difference in emphasis that I adopt in this chapter. *Spirituality* refers primarily to an individual's or group's sense of connection to sacred, transcendent, or ultimate reality. *Religion*, by contrast, carries a primarily institutional or organizational meaning; religions have a more or less identifiable community of believers who share rituals, practices, and beliefs. Understood in this way, religion may provide the most meaningful avenue for spiritual experience for some individuals, whereas it may be virtually irrelevant to spirituality for others. In different areas, then, both religion and spirituality have proven to be more central in most cultures than secularization theory predicted.

In the narrower context of mental health services and allied disciplines, discussion of spirituality and religion has also taken on greater relevance and urgency. In addition to renewed examination of the relationships between psychotic and spiritual experiences from both philosophical and neurobiological perspectives, several trends in clinical work with people diagnosed with schizophrenia bear directly on the importance of spirituality and religion. First, there has been a growing recognition of the value of *holistic approaches*, those that integrate biological, social, psychological, and spiritual perspectives, in both assessment and service delivery. Spirituality is increasingly seen not as a domain separate from the rest of consumers' lives, but as an integral part of whole-person functioning. From this point of view, spirituality directly affects and is in turn affected by other life dimensions. In addition, the necessity and value of incorporating *cultural competence* into service models have led to calls for greater awareness of the important role religious expression plays in many cultures. Being attuned to a culture's characteristic range of religious views is essential to accurate assessment and to services that take into account cultural dynamics and norms. In a related way, there has been renewed attention to the significance and meaning of the *subjective experiences* of people diagnosed with schizophrenia. Alongside advances in biological psychiatry have stood studies of the ways in which individuals experience mental distress and disorganization, construct meaning, and renew a sense of self; these qualitative approaches have contributed substantially to a more comprehensive understanding of psychotic experience and of healing. Finally, led by many consumers and advocacy groups, enhanced awareness of the possibility of recovery from schizophrenia has grown into seeing *recovery* as a key, orienting value in many mental health service systems. Many individuals understand and describe their recovery as most fundamentally a spiritual process or journey, one that relies heavily on a sense of meaning and purpose. Each of these clinically derived emphases—holism, cultural competence, subjective experience, and a recovery orientation—has contributed to a heightened attentiveness to spirituality and religion in relationship to schizophrenia and other severe mental disorders.

The research literature has provided an additional set of reasons for attending to religion and spirituality. Focusing directly on numerous potential connections between religion and health—physical and social health, as well as mental health—these studies initially emphasized broad measures of religion (e.g., religious affiliation, organizational involvement, religious or spiritual practices) and of well-being and illness. Numerous reviews of this literature have noted a growing consensus that, on the whole, religiousness is related positively to many measures of mental health and, conversely, to lower levels of distress. However, such findings are not at all unequivocal. In fact, other work has suggested that certain types of religious involvement or spiritual coping may be related to poorer mental health and lower levels of overall functioning. Recently, researchers have begun to move into a second phase of more specific questions, asking, for example, about how specific aspects or styles of religiousness or spirituality may affect particular life domains for particular people at particular times. This line of research has also begun to address questions about the potential role of religion or spirituality in coping with symptoms of schizophrenia and in the process of recovery. Thus, from both clinical and research perspectives, spirituality and religion have emerged as increasingly important avenues for exploration in understanding the lives and experiences of people diagnosed with schizophrenia.

EXPRESSION OF RELIGION AND SPIRITUALITY IN PSYCHOSIS

People diagnosed with psychotic spectrum disorders frequently express religious content in delusions or hallucinations. Two questions related to this observation are especially important for clinicians. The first concerns the relationship between religious delusions and the cultural context. Both the frequency and the content of religious delusions seem to vary significantly from culture to culture. Not surprisingly, since religious/spiritual beliefs and practices may be understood as basic expressions of a culture's meaning-giving structure, the centrality and prevalence of religious practice in a given culture appear to be related to the frequency with which religious delusions are expressed in severe mental disorders. Those cultures in which religious self-understanding and ritual practices are more prominent (e.g., the United States) seem to have higher rates of religious content in delusions. Religious content also varies with the predominant religious context and the commitments of the individual. In short, religious content in psychotic experience reflects to a significant degree the cultural context and the extent to which the individual participates in and is shaped by that culture. For clinicians, then, interpreting religious content accurately and helpfully rests on an understanding of the person's broader cultural setting and its characteristic beliefs—especially those regarding mental and physical health and illness, and their relationships to spiritual realities.

Second, research has begun to examine whether the presence of religious delusions or hallucinations predicts an individual's likely response to treatment. Clinicians have frequently noted the especially high stakes associated with religious language and experience in psychosis. Often highly publicized are reports of people who mutilate themselves (e.g., by self-castration or by removing the eye that has "offended"), or who attempt suicide or murder in response to command hallucinations (e.g., hallucinatory voices that tell the person to kill a child labeled "evil" or "demon-possessed"). Some researchers have found that those individuals who identify themselves as strongly religious, or whose delusions or hallucinations are overtly religious, have poorer treatment outcomes. Others, however, have not found this to be the case, indicating no difference in treatment response. Still others suggest that the positive role religiousness or spirituality may play in recovery is neglected in many, especially shorter-term outcome studies, and that the longer-term impact of religion is on the whole a positive one.

The implication of these perspectives for the practicing clinician is to highlight the importance of a culturally attuned, individualized, functional assessment of the role specific religious or spiritual activities and beliefs play in the person's life at a specific time. It may be the case, for example, that someone who is strongly involved in a religious community, and who understands religion to be especially important to his or her self-concept, may in the midst of a psychotic episode voice religious delusions or be especially distressed by religiously based perceptions of guilt or sinfulness. However, this individual may also be able to draw on religiously based resources in recovering from these acute symptoms. Understanding these possibilities is a task for spiritual assessment.

ASSESSMENT OF SPIRITUALITY AND RELIGION IN SCHIZOPHRENIA

Cultural competence in assessment is particularly relevant for life domains such as religion and spirituality, precisely because these domains are so closely tied to cultural concerns. The meaning of religious beliefs and practices depends on an understanding of the larger context in which they are expressed. DSM-IV has explicitly noted the dangers of pathologizing behavior and thoughts that, in the cultural setting of the consumer, may not be out of the ordinary and/or may have clearly prescribed meanings and responses that differ from those of Western medicine. Some of these are especially germane to diagnostic judgments related to schizophrenia. For example, in some communities, people hold strong beliefs in the capacity of individuals to influence others from a distance. Sometimes the influence is exercised by concrete means such as "working roots" or manipulating sacred likenesses or effigies; at other times, immaterial demons or spirits are the media by which control is exerted. Insensitivity to the culture-specific implications of such beliefs may easily lead to premature, pathologizing clinical judgments, such as erroneously labeling the beliefs as delusional symptoms of schizophrenia or paranoia.

Though this is a fairly straightforward example of the dangers that follow from a lack of cultural awareness, similar dynamics occur in many situations in which cross-cultural differences are not as evident. It may in practice be more difficult for clinicians to appreciate subtle distinctions regarding religious activities that are common in their own experience or background. The phenomenon of prayer provides a pertinent example. Prayer may appear to carry a meaning that is readily shared. When someone using services says that she or he will pray about a concern, clinicians may end the conversation, thinking they have an adequate understanding of the person's way of coping with that problem. Yet there are wide variations in the practice and understanding of prayer among faith communities in a single religious tradition, and even greater individual differences in prayer expectations. Understanding these individual meanings is essential to adequate clinical assessment. When someone says she will pray about a problem, does she mean that solving the problem is then up to God or a higher power who is the presumed hearer of the prayer? Or that she is talking in a way that facilitates her collaboration with a higher power? Or that she is expressing her priorities in an ultimate context so that she can act on her own, independent of divine assistance? Or does she expect to achieve a calm or peacefulness that will enable her to choose wisely? Or a literal answer from an external reality to the prayer, an answer that will inform her of the right course to take? Is praying the only response she will make to the problem, or is it one element in a larger problem-solving agenda? Does the praying help or hurt other problem-solving attempts? Or does this individual have yet another idea or carry a number of these expectations simultaneously? What are the implications of these various beliefs and expectations for assessments of mental health and psychosocial functioning? In short, how does the person's understanding and practice of prayer function in her life as a whole? How does it affect her overall well-being?

Adequate judgments about the meaning of such religious or spiritual beliefs and practices, then, can usually be made only following an exploratory conversation devoted to an interpretation of the *function* of spirituality in the overall life structure of the individual. These conversations and judgments do not require clinicians to develop special expertise about myriad spiritual and religious practices—though additional education in those most relevant for the people being served is necessary. Functional assessment of spirituality requires, first of all, openness on the part of clinicians to hearing about the diversity of religious experiences. For mental health workers, who frequently identify themselves as more spiritual than religious, this stance entails careful listening to discern the place and role of not only spiritual but also more structured and traditional religious involvements. Such discussions also require clinicians who are willing to be informed, often most helpfully by the consumer himself, about the customs and norms of any faith community involved, and about the consumer's perspective on spiritual commitments in his life. By discussing in an accepting way the role a particular spiritual belief or activity plays, *and* its consequences for the person's overall well-being, the clinician is engaging in an inquiry that is similar to that involving other life domains (e.g., discussing the role of a specific relationship and its implications). This approach to spiritual assessment, then, involves applying many standard approaches—empathic questioning and listening, a functional perspective on behavior, exploration of motives and meanings—to spirituality and religion.

Beyond this, though, a clinically useful spiritual assessment is built on an understanding of certain key content areas. The assessment needs to take into account multiple dimensions: the individual's spiritual *history* (including any significant changes that led to more or less intense commitments); the individual's characteristic *beliefs*, and sense of purpose and meaning; the overall *emotional tone* of the person's spiritual or religious life; regular religious *activities or rituals*; and the extent to which a *community* of others is involved in the individual's spiritual practice. Gaining an understanding of these dimensions of spirituality enables the clinician to see more clearly the ways in which an individual's spiritual life is related to his or her overall goals and well-being.

SPIRITUALITY AND RELIGION IN RECOVERY

As noted earlier, there is growing evidence that many aspects of religious or spiritual involvement are related to positive mental health and to lower levels of distress. The ways in which religion may be related to recovery from schizophrenia and other severe mental disorders have been examined in both qualitative and quantitative reports. Several findings emerge with some consistency from these studies.

Religion and Spirituality as Resources for Recovery

Substantial numbers—the vast majority in some surveys—of people diagnosed with schizophrenia and other severe mental disorders report that religious and spiritual *activities* offer them important resources for coping with life stressors, including psychiatric symptoms. Importantly, both activities that are often done alone and those that involve other people have been among the most commonly reported: prayer, meditation, reading scripture or other inspirational writings, listening to religious music, participating in formal religious services or spiritually oriented groups, and talking with religious professionals. Furthermore, these activities are seen as both generally helpful and specifically useful in dealing with distressing symptoms. Self-reported benefits range from lessening of troubling symptoms (e.g., listening to religious music as a uniquely helpful way to deal with upsetting auditory hallucinations) to a broad array of recovery-oriented strengths (e.g., enhanced inner calm and strength). It is not surprising, then, that some reports indicate an increase in faith after a psychotic episode. One plausible explanation is that acute psychotic symptoms set in motion both specific, sometimes spiritual, attempts to minimize distress and, subsequently, more general efforts to give meaning and structure to those experiences, to weave them into a coherent life narrative with purpose and direction.

This kind of coping involves not only activities but also ways of *thinking* about and understanding life events. Much of what has been described as "religious coping" in fact revolves around various interpretive schemas that a person may adopt in dealing with life problems. "Positive" religious coping, demonstrably related to better mental health outcomes, frequently entails, for example, affirming that the person sees himself as part of a larger spiritual force or that she works together with God as a partner is dealing with stressors. "Negative" coping and religious strain, linked to poorer outcomes, are reflected in concerns that God is punishing or has abandoned the individual or, conversely, that the individual is angry and distancing from God. Religion and spirituality characteristically offer much more than a set of activities and ritualized disciplines. These activities grow out a comprehensive interpretive frame that directs a person's attention to certain events as more important and meaningful than others, provides a way of understanding life's complexities, and proffers guidelines for how life is to be lived in response to this understanding. For clinicians who want to grasp the place of religion or spirituality in a person's life, this larger interpretive approach is a key.

Three themes warrant special attention in considering the positive place of religion and spirituality in recovery for people diagnosed with schizophrenia. First, people in recovery from the often devastating reality of, and profound stigma associated with, schizophrenia need to construct and reconstruct a sense of *meaning and purpose* in their lives. Severe mental disorders, and the social isolation and conflict that often accompany them, frequently raise "ultimate" questions—about the nature of reality, about the trustworthiness of other people, about good and evil, about the role of the divine in human suffering, and about sources of hope and a meaningful personal future. At a psychosocial level, the importance of establishing valued day-to-day goals—involving, among others, meaningful work, relationships, housing, leisure—has become increasingly understood as central to recovery. At a spiritual or religious level, however, these goals depend on a larger understanding of self that makes a meaningful future possible and worth pursuing. For many, spirituality offers a way to piece together and make sense of what has happened to them; to place these experiences and events in context; to gain a sense of perspective; and to develop hopefulness about the future. As an example, in some religious traditions, people frequently recount what they refer to as "wilderness" experiences: difficult periods of struggle and pain that must be endured before reaching a more sanguine state. Placed in this sort of interpretive frame, psychotic experiences may be seen not as permanently disabling, but as temporary states through which one passes on the way to a more positive future. Very importantly, in such stories, the power of the divine is on the side of helping the individual (and often the community) to find their way through the wilderness; there is good reason to be hopeful. For individuals who find meaning in these narratives, religious and spiritual realities may bolster recovery.

Second, spirituality and religion often provide vivid reminders of a robust and complex *personal identity*, that people diagnosed with schizophrenia are "whole people." In this way, spiritual understandings and practices serve as antidotes to a reductionism that narrows a person's identity to a psychiatric diagnosis. Many individuals report that one of the most painful, angering, and still all too common, experiences in dealing with a diagnosis of schizophrenia is professional overemphasis on the labeling of pathology, symptoms, and deficits. Furthermore, this overidentification of the person with his or her problem-defined label is often reinforced by socially stigmatizing communities. Spiritually and religiously informed identities, though, are characteristically both more holistic (involving strengths and skills, as well as weaknesses) and more positively toned (each individual has unique worth and value). Especially for those who have frequent and longstanding contact with the mental health service system, it is difficult to overstate the importance of the reminder that they are not to be identified with their illness label. Spiritual and religious perspectives often offer powerful countermessages in two ways. First, they offer direct, alternative identities. Metaphors of being a "child of God," or more generally, a valued and full-fledged member of the human race, are common. In addition, these identities may be reinforced by spiritual practices that deepen an individual's sense of wholeness and self-acceptance. Religious communities can also reinforce this more expansive sense of self, going far beyond illness-based identity to that of valued member of a caring community. Taking on a meaningful role in a faith community is one means of cementing more positive self-understanding.

The third theme is somewhat more concrete and often closer to the immediate experiences of people diagnosed with schizophrenia. Spirituality and religion may helpfully bolster the emotional life by offering *energy* for engagement with life and, at other times, *calmness* in the face of chaotic disruption. In terms of the usual categorization of positive and negative symptoms, then, spiritual activities and beliefs may offer resources for coping with both. In response to withdrawal and constricted emotion, spirituality may encourage hopefulness, enthusiasm, and even joy; it may enhance motivation for (re)involvement with other people and the world at large. Beliefs that emphasize the possibility of emotionally and spiritually "uplifting" moments and activities that provide direct experience of such moments provide an illustration of such possibilities. For example, for many African American consumers, traditions of gospel singing and expressive worship offer avenues for vigorous and lively self-expression, a tangible antidote to wary social withdrawal.

In dealing with positive symptoms, the capacity of spiritual and religious practices to cultivate a "calm mind" is particularly noteworthy. Meditating, focusing, grounding, centering, praying—all of these activities can offer stark alternatives to the often threatening internal chaos that attends psychosis. Like relaxation more generally, this kind of calmness is incompatible with anxiety. However, spiritual and religious practices often go beyond simply facilitating a relaxation response. Sometimes the practice is embedded in a larger, purposeful discipline, so that it is not merely an "exercise" but a core expression of spiritual devotion. Sometimes the practices involve content—images, holy words or phrases, sacred texts—that reflects unique meanings of a religious tradition, thus deepening ties to a faith community and its self-understanding. Sometimes the practice is consciously intended to bring the whole person to a particular state of well-being. In any case, the peacefulness or calm that spiritual practices and beliefs may engender offers a distinct contrast to the intrusive and often threatening experiences characteristic of psychotic states.

Some Dilemmas of Religion and Spirituality in Recovery

Historical bias against religion and spirituality is common in psychology and psychiatry, especially in certain psychodynamic traditions and other theoretical frameworks. As the preceding discussion has indicated, it would be an error to allow such theoretical blinders to lead clinicians to minimize the importance of possible roles for religion and spirituality in recovery from schizophrenia. Most people diagnosed with severe mental disorders report that spirituality has a valuable place in support of their recovery. On the other hand, it would be erroneous to permit enthusiasm for this potentially positive role of religion to obscure its difficulties. Spiritual and religious involvements are complex and can be related in correspondingly complex ways to recovery stories. Negative religious coping and experiences of "religious strain" frequently carry negative outcomes in terms of mental health: heightened depression, anxiety, and posttraumatic stress disorder (PTSD) symptoms, among others. It is helpful to consider some paradoxes related to spirituality and religion, especially as these dilemmas may be experienced and described by people recovering from diagnosed psychotic disorders.

Inclusion and Exclusion

In recovery from schizophrenia and other severe mental disorders, experiences of stigmatization and exclusion are common. Correspondingly, the importance of being *included*, being a part of, being accepted, or simply "let in" has been noted by many people in recovery and by advocates as key values supporting recovery. On the positive side, spiritual groups and religious communities may provide welcoming and caring havens in the midst of what can be a rejecting and indifferent society. Many individuals report the positive impact of being invited to join faith communities as full participants, without a focus on their deficits or problems. Such groups at their best can offer unconditional acceptance and create places where hospitality is extended beyond initial contacts, where active reaching out creates spaces for the whole person to be involved in ongoing community life. One woman reported that joining such an accepting church offered her a way to reestablish contact with the larger society, convincing her that she was capable of meaningful relationships just when she had thought she "would never be able to be with people again."

Religious communities, however, can be as rejecting and closed as they are accepting and open. In fact, organized religious groups are not infrequently built around dynamics that emphasize certain qualifications for full membership and, equally important, characteristics that lead to disqualification and exclusion. For people with severe mental disorders, this can lead to painful feelings of rejection—because of the group's expectations about ideas, behaviors, or dress that may be impossible for the individual to meet, because of implicit or explicit demands for financial support beyond the person's means, or because of principles that rule out acceptance of the whole person. One woman reported, for example, that she was under tremendous pressure from her faith community to change her sexual orientation. Though she had been accepted in many ways by this group, their understanding of homosexuality made it impossible for them to include her in this area that was basic to her identity. Her painful dilemma was, on one hand, to leave this church and relinquish its supports to be able to accept her own sexual orientation, or on the other hand, to remain in the church but try to relinquish her homosexuality. Both alternatives involved difficult losses and threatened her recovery.

Empowered Self and Devalued Self

Spirituality and religion often acknowledge the richness and complexity of human life, and place individuals in relationship to their own greatest potential. They frequently emphasize the inherent goodness of humanity, or at least the possibility of its amelioration. Spiritual and religious practices can lead to a sense of empowerment, of not only having certain strengths but also of being invited to develop and use those strengths for self-improvement and for the well-being of others. As with other aspects of spiritual reality, this kind of empowerment is rooted in ultimate or sacred contexts; the divine or transcendent or higher power is supportive of self-actualization (as this is understood in each tradition). This ultimate sense of being known by, important to, and valued by the divine or transcendent supports recovery by creating a strong basis for self-valuing. For example, people who so often report a sense of their own diminished worth can find an effective countermessage in reminders that God loves them and sees their potential for full and meaningful lives.

In contrast, though, individuals with severe mental disorders sometimes draw on religious language that devalues the self. This is certainly evident in acute episodes of psychosis that may incorporate images of the self as irredeemably sinful, damaged, or cursed. But even in recovery, individuals report that some religious convictions, frequently reinforced by faith communities, contribute to self-denigration. One of the more common themes in this regard is a belief that symptoms of mental disorder or distress reflect an underlying lack of personal faith or discipline. When people diagnosed with schizophrenia are told, and come to believe, that mental or emotional problems are primarily a result of their spiritual deficiencies, religion becomes a one-sided obstacle to recovery. Whether by seeing the use of mental health services, especially psychotropic medication, as a sign of moral failure or by setting goals that are unattainable by spiritual means alone (e.g., "simply" praying harder to lessen psychiatric symptoms), religion can undermine an individual's sense of self-esteem and reinforce images of deficiency.

Expressive Self and Constricted Self

Many spiritual and religious practices facilitate self-expression and creativity. Via traditionally expressive means such as music, ritual, journaling, and art, spiritually based activities call for the enactment of basic beliefs and convictions about both self and world. These activities can be especially powerful for individuals whose emotional or social life may be otherwise narrowed and limited. Certain strains in the Christian tradition, for example, emphasize a core value of life being lived "to the full" or "abundantly," understood as a full expression of followers' self-understanding as faithful disciples. For many religious communities, the ultimate "self-expression" involves this kind of authentic life lived out in keeping with the most fundamental tenets of the faith. Each individual may discover a unique purpose for his or her life, a "vocation" or "calling" that brings together one's own strengths and weaknesses, and orients the self toward meaningful goals.

However, faith communities may be just as powerfully experienced as rigid sources of rules and regulations that more frequently limit self-expression than facilitate it. In recovery from schizophrenia, some have reported the appeal of highly structured and clear expectations and routines. At times of personal confusion, especially, there may be psychological and social advantages in relying on a community with very explicit behavioral guidelines. Even in less stressful or challenging periods, such clarity can be helpful in giving shape to a person's life structure. The more negative impact of this dynamic becomes obvious in narrowly judgmental attitudes and practices often institutionalized in publicly or privately humiliating sanctions. Individuals report that involvement in certain communities may come to revolve around fear of being chastised by other members or of being shamed by those more senior in the faith. For individuals struggling with interpersonal sensitivity to criticism and rejection, this process can deepen withdrawal and constriction.

Autonomy and External Control

In a related vein, consumers and advocates have often noted that autonomy is one of the core principles of recovery. Rather than relying automatically or unnecessarily on professionals or other supports, increasing autonomy for those in recovery involves making increasingly independent decisions and taking action to meet their own goals. Spirituality and religion may offer both a rationale (genuineness, dignity, human rights, freedom of conscience, and attendant responsibility for one's own life) and specific resources (including the positive coping methods described earlier) for recovery. One survey reported that people found spiritual or religious activities that they did by themselves to be especially valuable in their recovery. One plausible explanation is that people have more control and choice over these activities than over those that involve others. Thus, self-determination is supported in many religious traditions and in numerous spiritual practices.

Just as a very strong emphasis on rules for living, especially when backed by shaming and humiliation, can lead to a constricted sense of self, so can these rules lead to a sense of external rather than internal control. The culture, beliefs, and rituals of virtually every faith community reflect elements of both individualism and belonging; indeed, this two-sided reality has been described as a fundamental tension in human life, as well as in faith communities. For people diagnosed with schizophrenia and other severe mental disorders, though, experiences with professionals and family are likely to stress their need to "comply" with treatment recommendations or to follow physicians' "orders." In short, traditional clinical approaches often overemphasize external control and minimize autonomy. When faith communities directly or indirectly similarly stress compliance at the expense of individual choice and decision making, they may undermine the possibility of recovering persons' exploring their options fully and experiencing support for their autonomous actions and chosen goals.

Hopefulness and Despair

People frequently find in spirituality deep reservoirs of hopefulness. Many spiritual and religious settings and activities paint a hopeful vision of the future. In this kind of orientation, the future is more likely to be seen as open, and one's valued place in it is more likely to find affirmation. Spiritually speaking, hopefulness is built into the nature of reality, because there are forces for good, whether these are seen as divine or not, that are influentially active in the world. Religious faith often carries the conviction that things—from the broadest perspective, at least—will work out for the best, and even more frequently expresses the certainty that individuals have divine allies when striving to live faithfully. For people in recovery, the sense that there are real options in the future, that life can change for the better, that healing and growth are both possible and supported by ultimate powers, is a comforting set of convictions and provides energy for the recovery journey.

Alternatively, of course, spirituality and religion can be sources of discouragement and despair. Especially when they emphasize guilt and sinfulness, and make the possibility of redemption remote, faith communities can deepen depression and despair. Theologically, when they stress the tremendous difficulty of attaining salvation (or, in psychosocial terms, health and well-being), they place additional obstacles in the way of people who all too often experience themselves as broken and damaged. Even, perhaps especially, for those who grew up with positive and hope-engendering contacts with a faith community or spirituality, discouraging messages can lead to demoralization. Particularly when these messages emphasize punishment and ostracism for "falling short," or for not fitting the mold of an idealized adherent, and when the community portrays the ideal in a way the person in recovery is very unlikely to meet, hopelessness is not a surprising outcome.

RECOMMENDATIONS

Clinicians often underestimate the importance of spirituality to the people they serve and may be unaware of the ways in which religion and spirituality function in the lives of consumers. There are several implications of recognizing a more central role for spirituality. First, for those individuals who report that spirituality is important to their self-understanding or recovery, a functional spiritual assessment—attention to the role spirituality plays for a particular individual at a particular time—is fundamental. Such an assessment is far more complex than simply noting a person's religious affiliation (or lack thereof). It takes seriously the value of exploring the relationship between the individual's spiritual practice or understanding and his or her overall functioning. Recognizing the complexity of religion's role allows the clinician to listen carefully for ways in which spirituality may foster or hinder recovery.

Second, if the consumer wishes to discuss the implications of spirituality for the services he or she receives, clinicians can follow through on this assessment by discussing with the consumer a range of options. A further conversation might usefully explore ways to enhance the role of spirituality that is primarily supportive of recovery, and to examine possible alternatives to spiritual dynamics that undermine well-being. For these conversations to be most helpful, though, clinicians need to be willing to learn from the consumer about the specifics of his or her spiritual life and choices. Clinicians also need to be knowledgeable about common religious and spiritual expressions among the people they serve, so that they place individuals' experience in appropriate cultural and social contexts. After individuals' personal and cultural commitments are clear, the conversation can meaningfully turn to ways in which mental health services can take more fully into account individuals' spirituality.

Some mental health agencies have begun to offer group or individual counseling and psychoeducation that explicitly focuses on spirituality. Religious or spiritual discussion groups that provide a safe place for people to explore the potentially positive and negative roles of spirituality have become more common. Peer-led discussions frequently address spirituality. Even in those programs that do not wish to offer such formal, spiritually focused services, clinicians can be aware of the larger community's resources for responding to the spiritual needs of consumers and include these resources appropriately in their discussion of recovery planning. Knowing, for example, those faith communities or spiritual groups that have been open to and supportive of people diagnosed with severe mental disorders is key in helping consumers sort through their options for connecting their recovery with their spiritual lives.

Spirituality and religion are frequently controversial topics, no less in mental health than in the larger public contexts. Both positive and negative generalizations about the role of religious or spiritual involvements may become overstated and inaccurate. Though it is certainly true that the preponderance of evidence supports the potentially supportive role of spirituality and religion in recovery, there are also pitfalls in these domains that may make recovery more difficult. Clinicians do well to adopt a stance of empathic listening and openness to understanding the complexity of spirituality as it may be expressed at a specific time by a particular individual. By approaching spirituality in the same kind of collaborative, conversational exploration that characterizes other topics of interest, clinicians create a space for meaningful discussion of the important and often minimized place of spirituality in the lives of people diagnosed with schizophrenia.

KEY POINTS

- Very substantial numbers of people diagnosed with schizophrenia report that spiritual and religious resources are helpful to them in dealing with their mental health difficulties.
- These supportive resources include a wide range of spiritual *activities,* as well as specific ways of *understanding* the individual's life circumstances.
- Among the positive roles spirituality and religion may play in a person's life are strengthening a sense of meaning and purpose; enhancing personal identity; and bolstering emotional well-being.
- On the other hand, certain kinds of spiritual or religious activities and beliefs (e.g., negative religious coping) may undermine recovery.
- Some key themes of religious and spiritual experience present both positive and negative possibilities in relationship to recovery from schizophrenia: inclusion–exclusion, empowered self–devalued self, expressive self–constricted self, autonomy–external control, and hopefulness–despair.
- Clinicians should familiarize themselves with the religious and spiritual expressions, as well as the personal and organizational spiritual resources, that are common among the people they serve, with special attention to their social and cultural contexts.
- Clinicians should have a culturally attuned, individualized conversation—a functional "spiritual assessment"—to understand the role of spirituality or religion in the person's life.

- With consumers who are interested in exploring the implications of spirituality or religion for their services, clinicians should engage in a collaborative discussion of the ways spirituality may be supportive of recovery.
- Service programs should consider ways to make spiritual or religious resources more accessible for people in recovery, either by offering appropriate spiritual discussion options—individual or group, professional- or peer-led—or by referral to knowledgeable and supportive spiritual communities and their representatives.

REFERENCES AND RECOMMENDED READINGS

Blanch, A., & Russinova, Z. (Eds.). (2007). Spirituality and recovery [Special issue]. *Psychiatric Rehabilitation Journal, 30*(4).

Bussema, K. E., & Bussema, E. F. (2000). Is there a balm in Gilead?: The implications of faith in coping with a psychiatric disability. *Psychiatric Rehabilitation Journal, 24*(2), 117–124.

Corrigan, P., McCorkle, B., Schell, B., & Kidder, K. (2003). Religion and spirituality in the lives of people with serious mental illness. *Community Mental Health Journal, 39*(6), 487–499.

Exline, J. J. (2002). Stumbling blocks on the religious road: Fractured relationships, nagging vices, and the inner struggle to believe. *Psychological Inquiry, 13*(3), 182–189.

Fallot, R. D. (Ed.). (1998). *Spirituality and religion in recovery from mental illness* (New Directions for Mental Health Services, Vol. 80). San Francisco: Jossey-Bass.

Koenig, H. G. (Ed.). (1998). *Handbook of religion and mental health.* San Diego, CA: Academic Press.

Pargament, K. I. (1997). *The psychology of religion and coping: Theory, research, practice.* New York: Guilford Press.

Pargament, K. (2002). The bitter and the sweet: An evaluation of the costs and benefits of religiousness. *Psychological Inquiry, 13*(3), 168–181.

Phillips, R. S., Lakin, R., & Pargament, K. (2002). Development and implementation of a spiritual issues psychoeducational group for those with serious mental illness. *Community Mental Health Journal, 38*(6), 487–496.

Russinova, Z., Wewiorski, N., & Cash, D. (2002). Use of alternative health care practices by persons with serious mental illness: Perceived benefits. *American Journal of Public Health, 92*(10), 1600–1603.

Tepper, L., Rogers, S. A., Coleman, E. M., & Malony, H. N. (2001). The prevalence of religious coping among persons with persistent mental illness. *Psychiatric Services, 52*(5), 660–665.

CHAPTER 59

SEXUALITY

ALEX KOPELOWICZ
ROBERT PAUL LIBERMAN
DONALD STOLAR

Sexual functioning and its consequences should be a clinically important concern for practitioners and programs serving the needs of persons with schizophrenia. Unfortunately, sexuality is rarely on the radar screen of the vast majority of mental health professionals. By default, the normal and natural sexual interests, needs, and abilities of persons with schizophrenia are sadly neglected in this area of human experience. For the silent chorus of psychiatrists, psychologists, social workers, and allied mental health workers, it is as though persons with schizophrenia are asexual. Awareness and concern by mental health professionals about sexuality in schizophrenia emerge only in the context of its inappropriate occurrence in hospitals or when sexually transmitted diseases or unwanted pregnancies arise as consequences of uninformed sexual activity. As long as the sex lives of individuals with schizophrenia lie deeply buried beneath other clinical priorities of mental health professionals, a vital and normalizing life aspect is suppressed, thereby disenfranchising thousands of individuals with schizophrenia from the potentialities of recovery.

The lack of substantive and systematic interest in the sexuality of their patients should not be surprising given the stigma and prevailing views of schizophrenia as a disorder of despair, deficit syndrome, neurodevelopmental abnormalities, and enduring cognitive impairments. For most providers of mental health services, the sex lives of those with schizophrenia are preferably out of sight and out of mind. Being blind and silent to the sexual needs, desires, and capacities of men and women with schizophrenia perpetuates the myth that schizophrenia is a monolithic, lifelong disorder that separates its victims from the rest of "normal" humanity. One might obtain some interesting responses from mental health practitioners if one were to ask, "Is there sex after schizophrenia?"

But under the ashes, some embers still burn. With the voices of the seriously mentally ill consumers increasingly being heard, there may be an awakening to the sexuality of persons with schizophrenia, with its attendant pleasures and problems. In this chapter, we summarize what is known about the following:

- Sexual activity of persons with schizophrenia.
- Sexual dysfunctions that they experience, including those resulting from side effects of their long-term use of antipsychotic drugs.
- Vulnerability of this population to sexually transmitted diseases.
- Psychoeducational programs that have been developed for this population to prevent unwanted pregnancies and sexually transmitted diseases.
- Development of a *Friendship and Intimacy Module* designed to teach safe and satisfying sex to persons with schizophrenia and other mental disabilities.

Because mental health professionals have little experience, knowledge, or clinical competence in mounting treatment and education on sex, they are often embarrassed, awkward, and self-conscious when trying to address this topic with their patients in clinical settings. Practitioners require special training experiences and self-awareness exercises if they undertake the important task of teaching individuals with schizophrenia how to make decisions about sexual relations and to engage in safe and satisfying sex. Therefore, this chapter also contains suggestions about the organization and curriculum for professional training in this area.

SEXUAL ACTIVITY OF INDIVIDUALS WITH SCHIZOPHRENIA

Although limited data are available on sexuality in persons with schizophrenia, a few studies have been published in the past decade. For instance, in comparison with representative samples of non-mentally-ill persons in the United States, men with schizophrenia and mood disorders had approximately the same number of lifetime sexual partners. Both non-mentally-ill and seriously mentally ill males reported three to four times as many sexual partners as women. In terms of sexual precocity, there were no differences between the mentally ill and non-mentally-ill cohorts. The average age of first reported sexual intercourse was 16–18 for men and women. It is interesting to note that similar surveys of physically disabled individuals—such as those with spinal cord injuries—have revealed a strong interest in sex, sexual activity of various types, and a mature response to educational programs on sexuality relevant to paraplegics.

SEXUAL DYSFUNCTION AFFECTING PERSONS WITH SCHIZOPHRENIA

Despite a healthy interest in sex, many people with schizophrenia report a progressive deterioration of their sexual and sociosexual function beginning in young adulthood, closely paralleling the age of onset of their illness. Indeed, there appears to be a complex yet definite relationship between sexuality and schizophrenia. For example, estrogen, a key hormone for sexual functioning, is lower than normal in females with schizophrenia at the onset of illness. Similarly, lower levels of gonadotropins and testosterone have been observed in unmedicated males with schizophrenia. Together these findings suggest that these hormonal disturbances contribute to the sexual dysfunction associated with the disorder.

Sexual dysfunctions may also result directly or indirectly from symptoms of the disorder and their functional consequences. For example, individuals with schizophrenia may have low self-confidence, few personal relationships, loss of impulse control, and negative or deficit symptoms, such as lack of interest and loss of pleasure, all of which may result in sexual problems. Given their anhedonia, limited social initiative, social anxiety, and deficits in social perception, sexual dysfunctions can be the source of their demoralization and discouragement in seeking sex with appropriate partners. Because of these barriers, many individuals with schizophrenia seek hazardous sex from prostitutes or workers in massage parlors.

Perhaps most importantly, the antipsychotic and antidepressant medications commonly prescribed and used to treat symptoms of the disorder effectively may actually cause or contribute to the sexual dysfunctions experienced by persons with schizophrenia. Rates of sexual dysfunction associated with the use of these medications range from 50 to 90% for the older, conventional antipsychotics and 10 to 30% for the newer, atypical antipsychotics. Sedation and weight gain may lead to diminished interest in sex. Alternatively, extrapyramidal side effects and tardive dyskinesia may reduce mobility, which in turn adversely affects sexual functioning. Finally, the neural systems and neurotransmitters affected by the drugs themselves may have a direct impact on sexual functioning. Serotonin, cholinergic antagonism, alpha-adrenergic blockade, calcium channel blockade, and dopamine blockade at the pituitary level (resulting in increased prolactin levels) can cause sexual dysfunctions, including loss of libido, orgasmic dysfunction, ejaculatory difficulty, and menstrual disturbances. Most importantly, sexual dysfunction has been implicated as one of the major factors contributing to noncompliance with antipsychotic medication regimens.

VULNERABILITY TO SEXUAL VICTIMIZATION AND SEXUALLY TRANSMITTED DISEASES

Compared to normal controls, people with schizophrenia have significantly less knowledge about reproduction and contraception. Moreover, deficits in social cue perception and social judgment put individuals with schizophrenia at heightened risk of being sexually victimized. Compared to non-mentally-ill women, women with schizophrenia report being more likely to have been pressured into unwanted sexual intercourse and less likely to use contraception, resulting in higher rates of sexually transmitted diseases and unwanted pregnancies.

Men with schizophrenia are also at high risk. In one study, sexual activity of men with schizophrenia often occurred with homosexual or bisexual individuals known to be infected with human immunodeficiency virus (HIV). Half of the men with schizophrenia were involved in sex exchange behavior; that is, sex bought or sold for money, drugs, or goods. In addition, condom use was low, with fewer than 10% utilizing protective measures. Other investigators have reported that the risk for HIV is much higher in the schizophrenia population, and rates of infection have increased substantially in recent years.

PSYCHOEDUCATIONAL PROGRAMS FOR TEACHING SAFE SEX

During the past two decades, a relatively small number of sexual education programs designed for mentally disabled persons have been described in the literature. They have almost exclusively focused on safe sex, not on helping patients to learn about the process of considering and deciding whether or not to have sexual relations. Nor have these programs taught patients how to go about having mutually satisfying sex with a partner. Extant educational programs primarily have been discussion groups. Typically the discussion leader follows an outline and distributes printed handouts for patients to read and refer to in the future.

Given the problems with verbal learning and memory, "talk groups" and printed assignments go about as far as the next hour in the mind/brain processing of persons with schizophrenia. Nonetheless, programs have been presented that touch on increasing patients' knowledge and comfort about sexual physiology, identifying and clarifying values and attitudes about sexuality, overcoming medication-related sexual dysfunctions, and basic HIV education and proper condom use. In some programs, graphics have been emphasized to compensate for the cognitive impairments of individuals with schizophrenia.

One such program, *Choices: An AIDS Prevention Curriculum*, is a program for high-risk, seriously mentally ill persons subject to sexual exploitation and ignorance about sexual practices. Designed to be taught to small groups in four 1-hour sessions, *Choices* follows a psychosocial education model guided by the emotional and attentional responsiveness of the patients. This educational package presents information and encourages discussion and learning through multimedia sources: videos and audiotapes, illustrations and photographs, printed brochures, games, role plays, quizzes, and problem-solving and question-and-answer segments. Extensive experience in outpatient, inpatient, and residential settings has shown *Choices* to be effective, tolerable, and enjoyable for a wide variety of patients.

Sex Education Course for Young Adults with Schizophrenia at UCLA

At the UCLA Neuropsychiatric Hospital and Behavioral Health Service, an eight-session sex education course was devised and offered by the Aftercare Clinic, a program devoted to young persons within 2 years of the onset of their schizophrenia. The aims of the course were to help participants gain more knowledge and comfort about their own sexuality and that of others; to identify and clarify their values and attitudes about sexuality; and to acquire decision-making skills regarding sexual relations. The curriculum of the course is presented in Table 59.1.

When the course was first proposed to the interdisciplinary mental health staff at a team meeting of the Clinic, there was a collective "gulp and gasp" at the explicitness of the material and format. The team members described discomfort at having patients discuss topics such as their previous sexual experiences, number of partners, and sexual dysfunction. In contrast, the course leaders did not discern discomfort among the patients in open discussion of these topics. As would be expected with low assertive and socially withdrawn young persons with schizophrenia, active verbal participation had to be specifically elicited during the group meetings. The exercises were an excellent means of "warming up" the group to facilitate the sharing of experiences and exploration of attitudes. None of the participants objected to participating, and none avoided answering relevant questions about their sexuality. Over the course of the seminar, the atmosphere in the group became lighter with appropriate joking, sharing of personal sexual frustrations and desires, and asking questions. With regular, biweekly ratings made routinely in this research-oriented setting, it was possible to determine that the presented material did not lead to any exacerbations of symptoms.

FRIENDSHIP AND INTIMACY MODULE

Although few psychiatric rehabilitation programs have comprehensively addressed the friendship and intimacy needs of seriously mentally ill persons, the studies conducted to

TABLE 59.1. UCLA Sex Education Course

Session	Exercise
1. Your sexual identity and self-esteem	Make a collage of your sexual identity (magazines, including *Playboy* and other sexually explicit magazines, were made available for cutting and pasting), then present your collage and discuss it in terms of how your feel about your sexual self.
2. Think of your sexual partner as a person	List and share three characteristics of someone you would like to date and role-play introducing yourself to such a person.
3. Male and female reproductive anatomy and physiology	Slide shows with questions, answers, and discussion of reproductive anatomy and physiology.
4. Your strengths as a partner and date	Share personal experiences of dates and any sexual feelings or experiences that occurred. Write a classified ad about your positive qualities to attract a dating partner.
5. Pleasure, not performance, as the focus of sex	Sensate focus by using talcum powder and having participants rub each other's hands while guiding their partner with positive and corrective feedback.
6. Birth control and the prevention of sexually transmitted diseases	Assignment to go to a pharmacy, write down the different types of contraception available, and bring the list back to the next group session.
7. Open communication with sexual partners	Educational video showing communication between sexual partners about what they did and did not like in a previous sexual encounter. Participants then discuss the communication skills they see.
8. Human sexual response and sexual dysfunctions	Educational video on human sexual response as it is affected by adverse effects of physical diseases, medication, stress, or anxiety. Participants then discuss the video.

date have demonstrated the feasibility of their use and participants' enthusiasm for the subject matter. Given the apparent need for this type of material, practitioners' difficulties with expressing sexual material cannot fully explain the relative rarity of such programs. Perhaps another contributing factor is that deficiencies in vital areas of social functioning of many individuals with serious mental illness potentially obscure from the clinician's view the importance of their sexuality. It is not surprising, therefore, that sexuality issues frequently arise in the context of social skills training, because this modality is geared toward eliciting the goals and desires of participants. As such, skills training technology is a place to start when constructing a program to provide explicit instructions to individuals with serious mental illness in the realms of friendship, dating, intimacy, and sexuality.

Skills training closes the gap between the individual's current skills and those needed for improved functioning. The methods used to teach friendship, and safe and satisfying sex are based on motivational enhancement and behavioral learning principles:

- Ensure that patients "buy into" the module through identifying its relevance to their own personal goals.
- Understand the benefits to patients of learning the skills from a personal frame of relevance.
- Specify the know-how and skills to be trained; check for understanding.
- Demonstrate the skills. Learn by watching videotaped models and answering patients' questions to ensure that they have internalized the skills.
- Have patients practice the skills until they can perform them competently. Provide

abundant positive reinforcement for patients who approximate criteria of competence.

- Teach patients to employ the skills in everyday life and gain reinforcement from the group, the trainer, and people in the natural environment.

Developing the curricula to teach friendship and intimacy skills is neither quick nor easy. Moreover, the instructional techniques must compensate for individuals' cognitive dysfunctions that might interfere with learning. Liberman and colleagues (1993) addressed this difficulty by producing a series of eight "modules" that teach community living skills with thoroughly specified curricula and highly structured training steps: *Medication Self-Management, Symptom Self-Management, Substance Abuse Management, Recreation for Leisure, Basic Conversation, Workplace Fundamentals, Community Reentry* and, most recently, *Friendship and Intimacy*. All use the same behavioral learning activities and problem-solving exercises to train each skill in each module. Only the content varies among modules, and the repetition of the learning activities provides a predictable teaching environment that enables trainers to conduct the modules and individuals to acquire the skills.

The *Friendship and Intimacy* module uses a plot line that follows a couple whose relationship develops from friendship and dating to the considerations and problem solving regarding the pros and cons of engaging in sex. In the context of a maturing relationship, the partners demonstrate appropriate communication skills with each other, with trusted friends and relatives, and with health care professionals. After evaluating their relationship and how it might change if they engaged in sexual intimacy, they decide gradually to engage in physical affection and ultimately sexual intercourse.

It is important to note that the latter skills areas of the module contains sexually explicit material, thus requiring trainers to obtain essential education and supervision as a means of becoming confident, assertive, and comfortable in discussing intimate sexual matters with patients. The earlier skills areas are organized in one videocassette, trainer's manual, and participants' workbook, whereas the more sexually explicit skills areas that teach how to engage in mutually satisfying sex are presented as a second volume, with its own videocassette, trainer's manual, and participants' workbook. Thus, it is possible to use the initial volume to teach dating and friendship skills, safe sex, and how to consider the advantages and disadvantages of having sexual relations, without including the more physically explicit skills areas that teach participants how to have satisfying sex and overcome sexual problems.

In Skills Area 1, *Establishing a Friendship*, the focus is on teaching participants how to begin friendships. Participants learn how to meet people with similar interests, while practicing and polishing their conversational skills. They are taught how to express feelings about the importance of a relationship, and how to ask someone out on a date. Skills Area 1 ends with a demonstration of a typical date, including how to begin, maintain, and end a conversation. There are also scenes that present problems depicting awkward moments in conversations on a date and the dilemma of whether or not to kiss a date goodnight.

Skills Area 2, *Obtaining Information about Safe Sex*, introduces the participant to some basic information about sexuality. This skills area includes four vignettes that focus on conception, contraception, sexual desire, and sexually transmitted diseases. In the first vignette, the main characters, Jim and Katie, visit a physician to elicit the information they need prior to including sex in their relationship. The next vignette features three young people, like the main characters, who have their own discussion about contraception and the notion of shared responsibility between partners in a loving relationship.

This second vignette reinforces the use of contraception as the means of avoiding unwanted pregnancy and maintaining good health. Abstinence from sex is also included as a viable option.

The third and fourth vignettes in Skills Area 2 demonstrate how the knowledge presented earlier can be used in a practical and realistic situation. In the third vignette, Jim goes to a pharmacy to purchase condoms. A pharmacist reminds him why condoms are recommended: "to prevent pregnancy and to avoid sexually transmitted diseases." In the fourth vignette, the scene is repeated, except that Katie goes by herself to the pharmacy to purchase condoms.

Skills Area 3, *Identifying the Benefits and Risks of Having Sex*, follows the protagonists as they discuss the consequences of including or not including sex in a relationship. These conversations elaborate on both the positive and negative aspects of the physical, financial, familial, employment, relationship, and emotional consequences of engaging in sexual behavior. Sexual decision making is demonstrated in seven vignettes, including conversations between two male friends, two female friends, Jim and Katie (a couple in a serious relationship), and between Jim and Katie and a second couple with a young child. This final vignette places sexual decision making in a real-life context as unmarried partners discuss the consequences of having a child whom they both love, but who was not planned. The parents discuss, and at times argue about, the pressures they face. From losing sleep, having to take a second job, and lack of support from the baby's grandparents, to relapse of psychiatric symptoms and increased alcohol use by one of the parents, both acknowledge that "having sex just one time without a condom" can have significant adverse consequences.

Skills Area 4, *Sharing Concerns, Consequences, and Cautions about Sexuality*, introduces the very contemporary and vitally important topic of giving one's own history and eliciting a sexual history from a partner. Jim and Katie exchange information about their previous sexual contacts. Emphasis is placed on self-disclosure, particularly with respect to past and current partners, and the recognition that one cannot safely assume the absence of sexually transmitted disease because of a current lack of symptoms. Jim and Katie acknowledge that they are both willing to be tested for sexually transmitted diseases and agree to make their relationship monogamous.

Skills Area 5, *Sexual Decision Making*, uses nine brief interactions between Jim and Katie to introduce an essential set of communication skills. These so-called "go/no-go" signals include the subtle and not so subtle cues that people use to indicate interest in a two-way conversation or an exchange of information. Go/no-go signals are used by the partners to communicate a lack of interest in pursuing sexual activity or to reinforce a partner's sexual advances. Acquiring the skill to accurately read a partner's go/no-go signals is a prerequisite to good communication and to achieving a satisfying sexual relationship.

By this point in the plot, Jim and Katie have made a well-reasoned decision about having sex, they have been tested for sexually transmitted diseases, and they have a supply of condoms. Thus, they proceed to the next step. In Skills Area 6, *Learning Appropriate Sexual Behavior*, a range of sexual behaviors is modeled, including appropriate touching, communication skills preceding sexual relationships (e.g., asking permission), and communication skills while engaged in a sexual encounter (e.g., attending to the needs of one's partner). Limit setting and respectful compliance are demonstrated in the opening vignette. The vignettes that follow all include full nudity.

To desensitize viewers' to the discomfort caused by the explicit nature of their behavior, Katie and Jim are first seen nude individually, each at his or her own apartments, preparing for the date that will culminate in their first sexual encounter. In the next few vignettes, explicit sexual behavior, including intercourse, is graphically depicted. Jim and Katie meet in their friend's apartment. They acknowledge both their eagerness for sexual intercourse and their nervousness about adding that new dimension to their relationship. Safe and appropriate use of a condom and spermicidal jelly is modeled as this series of vignettes is concluded. The final vignette of this skills area focuses on Jim and Katie after their sexual relationship has matured for a few months. They acknowledge their initial awkwardness and the importance of communicating their sexual needs. This skills area closes with a sexual encounter that "puts it all together" as Jim and Katie demonstrate the skills they have learned. The component skills (giving and receiving permission, assertive requests, guided hands) are combined into a free flowing, loving, and tender sexual encounter.

Skills Area 7, *Communication Skills after Sexual Intercourse*, involves two brief vignettes. In both, Jim and Katie engage in appropriate verbal and nonverbal communication after they have had intercourse. They mutually reinforce each other for their decision making, for being able to give specific instructions about how they like to be touched, and for pleasing each other.

Skills Area 8, *Sexual Problems: Desire, Arousal, and Orgasm*, uses a number of vignettes to present common problems related to the phases of sexual response, namely, desire, arousal, and orgasm. The purpose for including this section is to provide education about sexual functioning; to normalize problems of desire, arousal, and orgasm; and to teach effective problem-solving methods when sexual dysfunctions occur. Vignettes include scenes of Jim and Katie talking with their respective male and female friends/confidants, and Jim and Katie alone.

The training methodology comprises the seven learning activities detailed in Figure 59.1. The introduction sets the stage for the learning; it tells the learners the "payoff" they can expect from their investment of time and energy. The demonstration videotape provides a clear presentation of the skills that can be easily and consistently presented across diverse staff and settings. The videotape's periodic stops and the questions to assess viewers' comprehension are essential to ensure that the training achieves its instructional objectives. The role-play practice is similarly critical, because learning is not just comprehension; it is ultimately the enactment of a skill. Furthermore, the more often participants practice enacting the skill, the more polished their performances when the actual opportunities arise.

The problem-solving activities are the first steps in helping participants to transfer their skills to their natural, living environments. Two types of problems are considered: how to obtain the resources required to perform a skill, and how to overcome the obstacles inherent in situations and environments when others do not respond as expected. The final two activities—*in vivo* and homework assignments—extend training into the real world. Participants complete the *in vivo* assignments accompanied by a trainer or support person. Once they demonstrate their facility in using the skills in a protected environment, they are asked to complete homework assignments on their own. The sequences of gradually learning more skills, success using the skills, and taking more responsibility for reaching personal goals combine to move the patient further along the pathway to empowerment, self-efficacy, and recovery.

Each module is packaged with a trainer's manual, participant's workbook, and demonstration videotape. The manual specifies exactly what the trainer is to say and do to teach all of a module's skills; the videotape demonstrates the skills; and the workbook provides written material, forms, and exercises that help the individual learn the skills. A module can be easily conducted by one trainer with one to eight participants. More than eight, however, reduces the opportunities for each participant to answer the questions,

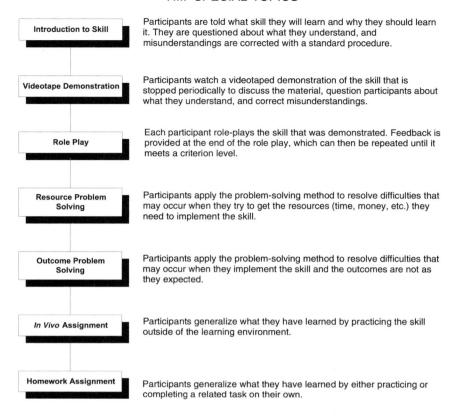

Introduction to Skill — Participants are told what skill they will learn and why they should learn it. They are questioned about what they understand, and misunderstandings are corrected with a standard procedure.

Videotape Demonstration — Participants watch a videotaped demonstration of the skill that is stopped periodically to discuss the material, question participants about what they understand, and correct misunderstandings.

Role Play — Each participant role-plays the skill that was demonstrated. Feedback is provided at the end of the role play, which can then be repeated until it meets a criterion level.

Resource Problem Solving — Participants apply the problem-solving method to resolve difficulties that may occur when they try to get the resources (time, money, etc.) they need to implement the skill.

Outcome Problem Solving — Participants apply the problem-solving method to resolve difficulties that may occur when they implement the skill and the outcomes are not as they expected.

***In Vivo* Assignment** — Participants generalize what they have learned by practicing the skill outside of the learning environment.

Homework Assignment — Participants generalize what they have learned by either practicing or completing a related task on their own.

FIGURE 59.1. Seven learning activities.

and practice the skills and the problem-solving exercises. Therefore, larger groups require a cotherapist or cotrainer. This module can also be used effectively and for a briefer time with individuals or couples.

Of course, the teaching must be modified to fit and to compensate for the large variations in people's functioning, symptoms, and capabilities to benefit from training. The modules' repetitive, "tight" structures provide a completely reproducible starting point for these modifications. Experienced trainers can experiment with a variety of alterations, and inexperienced trainers can return to the structure should their modifications prove ineffective. The repetitive structure and social learning principles intrinsic to the modules compensate for most symptomatic and cognitive limitations, and form a constant background of psychosocial treatment against which the effects of other treatments (e.g., medications) can be determined.

Clinical Experience with the Friendship and Intimacy Module

The module has been in active use for the past 2 years at the Hollywood Mental Health Center's Psychosocial Rehabilitation Program, the San Fernando Mental Health Center's Wellness Program, the UCLA Psychiatric Rehabilitation Program, and the UCLA Neuropsychiatric Partial Hospital Program. It has been well received by patients; however, the caveat mentioned earlier regarding careful selection of professionals who are comfortable teaching the subject matter of the module in an active/directive mode is important. A variety of individuals from various mental health disciplines have led the module, including recovered consumers who have "graduated" from the module and serve as coleaders.

Susan was a 36-year-old, single woman with schizophrenia who lived with her parents. Her symptoms of psychosis had been in remission for over 6 years, and she faithfully took her medication. After more than 5 years as a volunteer, Susan subsequently was hired by a local charity that valued her work highly. She was sociable and extremely attractive, well-dressed and -groomed, and sexually active. Her pattern was to meet men in bars and have frequent "one night stands," much to the chagrin and worry of her parents. Many of the men she met took advantage of her naivete, and her desire to have a boyfriend and be involved in a close relationship. She had several episodes of sexually transmitted diseases; fortunately, each was treatable and did not produce long-term sequelae.

Susan was referred to the UCLA Psychiatric Rehabilitation Program by her psychiatrist to help her acquire better judgment in her choice of sexual partners. Although initially querulous about how the Friendship and Intimacy Module might assist her, Susan became highly motivated after attending the sessions on making friends and dating. When the group got to the skills area on "go/no-go" sex signals, Susan realized that she had been inadvertently encouraging men she met in bars by allowing them to touch her hand and by leaning toward them with her face in close proximity to theirs soon after beginning a conversation. She also realized that there were nonverbal no-go signals she could give that would limit her contacts with new male acquaintances to more mundane, nonflirtatious conversation. As a result of participating in the module, Susan became much more discriminating in her contacts and relationships with men, and developed a long-term, intimate relationship with a man who genuinely cared about her and understood that she had schizophrenia.

The skills she learned in the module enabled Susan to improve her social judgment, interpersonal communication regarding romantic interests, and assertiveness in taking control of interactions with men. After employing the friendship and dating skill for 6 months, Susan met a man through a mutual friend and developed a companionable relationship with him. They had much in common, and the conversation and friendship skills Susan had learned enabled her to maintain and enjoy their time together in the activities they had in common. Gradually, over a number of months, steady dating and then a long-term relationship ensued. This time, Susan and her boyfriend gave serious consideration before initiating a sexual relationship. Their successful interaction was made possible by Susan's continuing contacts with her therapist, who offered refresher training on a number of the skills areas in the module.

TRAINING THE TRAINERS

One of the great therapeutic accomplishments of the second half of the 20th century was the establishment of legitimacy and efficacy in interventions exclusively targeting sexual difficulties. Despite the availability of empirically validated techniques for helping patients with sexuality, there remains a significant training challenge, namely, convincing mental health professionals that such treatment is appropriate, safe, and necessary for this population. Some clinicians fear that people with schizophrenia, by definition, cannot "tolerate" such explicit discussion and graphic illustration of sex, and assume that such exposure will cause patients to regress psychotically and/or engage in inappropriate sexual behavior.

To overcome this limitation in clinicians' knowledge base and comfort level, clinical training workshops in sexuality have been developed. At UCLA, such workshops have been conducted for over 20 years. These workshops are taught in two intensive training weekends by clinicians trained and experienced in human sexuality and sex therapy. Some elements of these training workshops include the following:

1. Education in the anatomy and physiology of sex.
2. Learning the effects of illness and certain medications on sexuality.
3. Dispelling sexual myths and misinformation.
4. Exploration of the concepts of "normal" and "abnormal" sex.
5. Becoming fully knowledgeable about safe and unsafe sexual practices.
6. Learning specific behavioral programs for treating both genders' sexual difficulties (e.g., knowing how and when to initiate appropriate sexual activity, and how to deal with problems of desire, arousal, and orgasm).
7. Learning to individualize these programs to a patient's specific behavioral, cognitive, affective, and cultural profile.
8. Creating an environment in which discussing sexual feelings, behaviors, fantasies, and experiences feels emotionally safe.

The weekend workshops are followed by ongoing weekly seminars that include (1) didactic teaching, (2) viewing sexually explicit training media, (3) exercises in verbal sexual self-disclosure, (4) role playing by patient and therapist, and (5) case presentations. Ideally, once trainees begin seeing patients specifically for sex education training, concurrent weekly supervision is provided. The great majority of participants in the workshops and seminars report feeling more comfortable openly discussing their own sexual feelings, fantasies, and experiences, which in turn leads them to experience greater willingness and facility when teaching sexually explicit material to their patients.

KEY POINTS

- Despite stereotypes to the contrary, people with schizophrenia are as likely as individuals without a serious mental disorder to engage in sexual activity.
- However, people with schizophrenia are susceptible to sexual dysfunction, because of both the symptoms of their disorder and the side effects of their medications.
- Cognitive deficits and lack of social support lead individuals with schizophrenia to be particularly vulnerable to sexually transmitted diseases (including HIV/AIDS) and unwanted pregnancies.
- Psychoeducational programs that provide information on sexuality to people with schizophrenia can increase their knowledge and encourage behavior that is consistent with safe and satisfying sex.
- Mental health practitioners require special training to undertake the task of teaching people with schizophrenia how to make informed decisions about sexual relations.

REFERENCES AND RECOMMENDED READINGS

Assalian, P., Fraser, R. R., Tempier, R., & Cohen, D. (2000). Sexuality and quality of life of patients with schizophrenia. *International Journal of Psychiatry in Clinical Practice, 4,* 29–33.

Coverdale, J. H., & Turbott, S. H. (2000). Risk behaviors for sexually transmitted infections among men with mental disorders. *Psychiatric Services, 51,* 234–238.

Crenshaw, T. L., & Goldberg, J. P. (1996). *Sexual pharmacology: Drugs that affect sexual functioning.* New York: Norton.

Friedman, S., & Harrison, G. (1984). Sexual histories, attitudes and behavior of schizophrenic and "normal" women. *Archives of Sexual Behavior, 13,* 555–567.

Goisman, R. (2001). *Choices: An educational program for AIDS prevention.* Boston: MMH Reseach Corporation.

Grassi, L., Biancosino, B., Righi, R., Finotti, L., & Peron, L. (2001). Knowledge about HIV transmission and prevention among patients with psychiatric disorders. *Psychiatric Services, 52,* 679–681.

Liberman, R. P., Wallace, C. J., Blackwell, G., Ekman, T. A., Vaccaro, J. V., Mintz, J., et al. (1993). Innovations in skills training for the seriously mentally ill: The UCLA Social & Independent Living Skills Modules. *Innovations and Research, 2,* 43–60.

Lukoff, D., Gioia-Hasick, D., Sullivan, G., Golden, J. S., & Nuechterlein, K. H. (1986). Sex education and rehabilitation with schizophrenic outpatients. *Schizophrenia Bulletin, 12,* 669–677.

Miller, L. J. (1997). Sexuality, reproduction and family planning in women with schizophrenia. *Schizophrenia Bulletin, 23,* 623–635

Psychiatric Rehabilitation Consultants. (2006). *Friendship and Intimacy Module.* (Available from Psychiatric Rehabilitation Consultants, P.O. Box 2867, Camarillo, CA 93011, *www.psychrehab.com*)

Rowlands, P. (1995). Schizophrenia and sexuality. *Sexual and Marital Therapy, 10,* 47–61.

CHAPTER 60

SCHIZOPHRENIA IN AFRICAN AMERICANS

WILLIAM B. LAWSON

Schizophrenia is considered the most severe psychiatric disorder. It has a poor prognosis, an unknown etiology, and an age of onset in the late teens and early 20s, when many individuals finish their education and begin their careers. Current treatments are mostly palliative, with uncertain recovery and rarely substantiated cures. Individuals and their families often face a lifetime of illness that is associated with individual and societal morbidity, shortened lifespan, and high suicide rates. Recent advances have led to improved diagnostic accuracy, a better understanding of genetic risks and psychosocial stressors, and improved treatment that has made recovery an attainable goal. This chapter indicates that race and ethnicity impact the diagnosis, course, and treatment of this illness through biopsychosocial factors that are only beginning to be appreciated. The focus is on African Americans, for whom there is a more extensive literature than for other ethnic minorities.

EPIDEMIOLOGY

African Americans have always been viewed as being overdiagnosed with schizophrenia. Even recent clinical reports show that African Americans are at as much as a tenfold increased risk over other ethnic minorities despite improved diagnostic accuracy and widespread use of the DSM-III and DSM-IV. Lawson, Hepler, Holladay, and Cuffel (1994) reported that African Americans in both inpatient and outpatient settings were diagnosed with schizophrenia at higher percentage rates than African Americans in the overall population. Rates of mood disorder for African Americans, and both schizophrenia and affective disorders for European Americans were the same as rates in the general population. Strakowski and colleagues (2003) reported higher rates of schizophrenia for African Americans in inpatient and outpatient settings. The higher rates were often associated with correspondingly lower rates of affective disorders.

The findings have generally been assumed to reflect affective disorders misdiagnosed as schizophrenia. These differences often disappeared with the use of structured interviews, which presumably minimize bias. Large-scale, door-to-door epidemiological surveys have tended to support this interpretation as well. The Epidemiologic Catchment Area study, which sampled five major cities and oversampled ethnic minorities, found no difference between African Americans and other ethnic groups when socioeconomic class was controlled. The National Cormobidity Survey and the more recent National Comorbidity Survey Replication found that African Americans were less likely to have nonaffective psychosis, which is primarily schizophrenia.

Nevertheless, recent clinical studies continue to report an overdiagnosis of schizophrenia in African Americans despite controls for a variety of settings. Table 60.1 summarizes reports comparing rates of schizophrenia by race. These findings show that the overdiagnosis occurs in juvenile facilities, in the Veterans Administration, and in public and private facilities. The overdiagnosis occurs despite the use of structured interview instruments. The development of DSM-III has certainly improved validity and diagnosis of psychiatric disorders. However, consistent use of DSM-III and now DSM-IV often does not prevent the misdiagnosing of African Americans. Strakowski and colleagues (2003) showed that the misdiagnosis was not the consequence of the misapplication of diagnostic criteria (i.e., variance in criteria). Rather, information variance (failure to obtain adequate information) was more of a factor. In addition, African Americans with affective disorders are more likely to have prominent first-rank psychotic symptoms than European Americans, which uninformed clinicians often interpret as evidence for schizophrenia, while overlooking affective symptoms. Other factors include clinician bias based on preconceived notions about the presence of affective disorders in African Americans, lack of familiarity with culture-based idioms of distress, and social distance.

Patient factors may also be involved. The increased likelihood of diagnosing psychotic symptoms in African Americans may be a result of misinterpretation of other intrapsychic experiences. African Americans without schizophrenia are more likely to report dissociative symptoms. Paranoia, which is often reported, is frequently seen on older versions of the Minnesota Multiphasic Personality Inventory (MMPI). A cultural reticence to disclose inner feelings to strangers of a different ethnicity is often reported and has been referred to as a "healthy paranoia." African Americans often delay or do not seek mental health treatment until symptoms are severe, thereby making diagnosis difficult. Clearly, the diagnosis of schizophrenia in African Americans should be made only after other, alternative diagnoses are considered.

In summary, in diagnosing African Americans and other ethnic groups as well, all sources of information should be included. Family members, caretakers, and past medical records should be consulted. Premature closure should be avoided when a patient presents with psychotic symptoms. It is important to remember that hallucinations may occur in affective and anxiety disorders, especially when treatment has been delayed. Close adherence to DSM-IV criteria should be encouraged, with the recognition that DSM-IV does not exclude mood or anxiety disorders when psychotic symptoms are present. Certainly awareness of cultural issues, such as specific idioms of distress, should be recognized. It is difficult to know the nuances of every culture, which is why sources other then the patient must be consulted. Whatever the case, the diagnosis of schizophrenia should be presumptive for African Americans only when other diagnoses are excluded.

GENETIC FACTORS

Throughout much of the 20th century, schizophrenia was thought to be the result of family pathology. A diathesis–stress model is now prevalent. Schizophrenia clearly has a genetic risk, since a heavy loading of biological relatives increases the risk.

TABLE 60.1. Reports Comparing Rates of Schizophrenia by Race

Reference	Results	Setting
Delbello et al. (2001)	African Americans are more likely to be diagnosed with schizophrenia than European Americans.	Inpatient adolescent facility
Blow et al. (2004)	African Americans are four times more likely to be diagnosed with schizophrenia than European Americans.	Veterans Administration database
Barnes (2004)	African Americans are four times more likely to be diagnosed with schizophrenia than European Americans.	State psychiatric hospitals
Neighbors et al. (2003)	African Americans are more likely to be diagnosed with schizophrenia than European Americans when semistructured interviews are used.	Private and public inpatient facilities
Strakowski et al. (2003)	African Americans are more likely to be diagnosed with schizophrenia than European Americans despite use of structured interviews.	Inpatient, outpatient county mental health system
Minsky et al. (2003)	African Americans are more likely than Latinos or European Americans to be diagnosed with schizophrenia.	Behavioral health service system in New Jersey

Several studies have reported putative gene associations for African Americans when findings in other ethnic groups have been negative. Polymorphisms of the *synapsin III* and *NOTCH 4* genes were associated with schizophrenia in African Americans but not European Americans. One possibility is that schizophrenia may have a different genetic etiology in African Americans. A more likely explanation is that individuals of African ancestry have older genetic variations, since they have ancestry genes and greater haplotype diversity. As a result, genetic differences that may exist are easily identified.

The Caspi Study reminded us that for psychiatric disorders, genes should only be considered in the context of environmental factors. In that study, major depression was associated with the number of lifetime episodes of childhood abuse, but only in the presence of a certain allele of the serotonin receptor. Family members often ask about their risk for schizophrenia. A simple statement of known risk could be misinterpreted. It is also important to inform families that ethnicity probably does not increase risk, and that family environment does not cause schizophrenia. Nevertheless, risk is not conferred by genetic factors alone. Environment, in a broad sense, is also important.

SOCIOCULTURAL FACTORS

African American families face the challenge of having limited resources. The direct costs of schizophrenia often exceed the median family income of African Americans. Moreover, African Americans are more likely to believe that mentally ill individuals are violent. Yet African American families are more likely to retain schizophrenic members in their midst despite limited resources. Part of the reason is that African Americans are more tolerant of the often unconventional and unpredictable behavior of a family member with schizophrenia. African Americans are less likely than European Americans to believe that individuals with schizophrenia should be blamed and punished for violent behavior. European American families are more likely to feel burdened and rejecting toward the family member with schizophrenia. Cultural factors may therefore be more important then socioeconomic status in determining whether family members will be caretakers.

Although the idea that family dynamics "cause" schizophrenia has been discredited, family relationships can certainly affect the course of the illness. However, factors that contribute to poor outcome differ in European American and African American families. High emotionality and family intrusiveness have been shown consistently to predict poor outcome in European Americans with schizophrenia. This does not appear to be the case in African Americans. Critical comments by relatives that were perceived as expressed criticism by European American and Latino family members with schizophrenia were not perceived consistently as criticism by African Americans with schizophrenia. Moreover, in European Americans, family intrusiveness and critical comments, elements considered important in families with high emotionality, showed no association with outcome. Presumably, such behavior was interpreted as displaying more concern in African American families.

The take-home message is that family factors do play an important role in outcomes of African Americans with schizophrenia. African Americans tend to be supportive and to continue family involvement, but they tend to be fearful of the mentally ill. Moreover, the relationships seen in family dynamics and schizophrenia in European Americans may be very different in African Americans. Behavior that is considered toxic in other cultures may be protective in African American cultures. In conclusion, culture is important in family interactions. However, findings about the relationship between schizophrenia and family members in European American families simply may not apply to African Americans and other ethnic minorities.

TREATMENT AVAILABILITY

African Americans have more illness burden, because they do not have the same access to services and often receive suboptimal treatment. African Americans are more likely to be homeless or in prison, settings in which treatment is suboptimal. Hospitalization is more common, especially involuntary admissions, and the disposition after discharge is often medication-only or emergency room care. Preferential treatment such as day treatment or case management are less likely to be available.

Racial differences in income may contribute to the lack of treatment access. Although African Americans have 60% of the income of European Americans, they have only 10% as much family wealth because of slavery and later job discrimination. Only recently has wealth accumulation become widely available. As noted earlier, direct costs for the treatment of schizophrenia exceed the median family income of African Americans. Yet African Americans with schizophrenia are more likely to be cared for within the family. Without disposable income, patients sometimes have to choose between necessities and medications. Family members can access only the most rudimentary care.

Although income is important, other factors play a part. As noted earlier, issues such as misdiagnosis persisted even when income was controlled. The Surgeon General's Report noted that when income was taken into account, ethnic disparities still persisted. Moreover the National Comorbidity Study Replication also reported less access to care for ethnic minorities, even when income was controlled. When we look closely at pharmacotherapy we find similar provider and patient issues that contribute to misdiagnosis.

PHARMACOTHERAPY

Although psychosocial support is important in managing schizophrenia, pharmacotherapy remains essential for maintenance and recovery. Unfortunately, the treatment of ethnic minorities is often inappropriate. African Americans often receive excessive doses of medication, whereas Hispanics and Asians receive lower medication doses, when treated by ethnic providers. Moreover African Americans are more likely to receive first-generation rather than second-generation or atypical medications, higher doses of medication, and more depot medication. Table 60.2 summarizes findings about the medicating of African Americans. Please note that some of the studies involved Medicaid or Veterans Administration hospital patients, and income presumably should not have affected the difference. Also note that some of the typical agents and high doses may have been a consequence of the use of depot medication, for which only one atypical agent is now available, and no atypical form was available at the time of many of the studies. Yet when the use of depot medication was controlled, the high dosing of typical medication persisted.

The biological evidence, if anything, supports lower dosing for ethnic minorities. Ethnic differences have been found in the way many psychotropic agents are metabolized through the cytochrome P450 family of liver isoenzymes. The CYP450 2D6 isoenzyme in particular shows ethnic variation. Relative to the majority of European Americans, Asians, Hispanics, and African Americans show reduced activity in this enzyme, whereas many Ethiopians show increased activity. Reduced activity means that a drug is metabolized more slowly, therefore having higher plasma levels. Individuals with CYP450 2D6 alleles associated with reduced or no activity who are given standard medication doses are more likely to have extrapyramidal side effects on antipsychotics and to discontinue

TABLE 60.2. Reports on Pharmacotherapy for African Americans

Reference	Setting	Medication
Opolka et al. (2004)	Texas Medicaid	African Americans are less likely than European Americans to receive risperidone or olanzapine.
Daumit et al. (2003)	National outpatient database	African Americans are less likely to receive atypical antipsychotics.
Kreyenbuhl et al. (2003)	Outpatient study of two states	African Americans are less likely to receive atypical antipsychotics, and more likely to receive depot medication.
Olpolka et al. (2003)	Medicaid population	African Americans are less likely to receive olanzapine or risperidone.
Mark et al. (2003)	Schizophrenia Care and Assessment Program	African Americans are more likely to receive depot medication, and less likely to receive second-generation antipsychotics even after controlling for the use of depot medication.
Herbeck et al. (2004)	American Psychiatric Institute Practice Research Network	African Americans are less likely to receive second-generation antipsychotics when clinic, socioeconomic status, and health system are controlled.
Olpolka et al. (2004)	Medicaid population	African Americans are less likely to receive olanzapine or risperidone.
Valenstein et al. (2001)	Veterans Administration hospital	African Americans are more likely to be on depot medication, first-generation antipsychotics, and higher doses.

treatment, whereas those with increased activity may not show any response at all. Thus, there is no biological reason for the excessive dosing of African Americans.

Pharmacological studies provide some support for prescribing atypical antipsychotics to African Amerians. Second-generation, or atypical antipsychotics, are less likely to cause extrapyramidal side effects and are believed to cause less tardive dyskinesia. Moreover, some of the newer antipsychotic agents are not predominately metabolized through the CYP450 2D6 system and are instead metabolized through CYP450 1A2, with CYP450 2D6 as a minor pathway. Asians and Hispanics are more likely than European Americans to experience movement disorder side effects, such as acute dystonic reactions, when given typical or first-generation antipsychotics. African Americans are twice as likely as European Americans to develop tardive dyskinesia on typical antipsychotics. African Americans are also more likely than European Americans to experience acute extrapyramidal symptoms with typical antipsychotics, but these differences disappear with atypical agents.

For ethnic minorities, especially African Americans, the atypical antipsychotics appear to offer a decided advantage when movement disorder side effects are considered. However some of the atypical agents have been associated with unacceptable metabolic consequences, such as diabetes and metabolic syndrome. These disorders are more common in African Americans and Latinos. The Clinical Antipsychotic Trials of Intervention Effectiveness (CATIE), a naturalistic federally funded study that compared the atypical agents to each other and to a typical agent, showed that the atypical agents did not provide a great advantage. The CATIE study had 40% African American participation, so insufficient numbers of minorities cannot be used as an argument against it. Nevertheless, the study excluded those with tardive dyskinesia, limited the dosing range, and involved a limited time period. Regarding ethnic minorities, although better than most studies, CATIE must be considered in the context of differing ethnic needs.

The atypical agent clozapine has consistently shown superior efficacy and fewer movement disorder side effects compared to other antipsychotics. Like other atypical antipsychotics, it is also less available to African Americans, but for different reasons. Its side effects include the metabolic side effects seen in atypical agents, but this is not the limiting factor. The difficulty is its greater risk for agranulocytosis, which requires regular blood monitoring. Before taking clozapine, minimal leukocyte counts are recommended despite the lack of evidence that preexisting white counts predict agranulocytosis. However, African Americans are known to have normal leukocyte counts whose range may extend well below listed normal values (i.e., a "benign leukopenia"). As a result, the overly cautious clinician may choose not to start otherwise healthy African American patients on clozapine.

Since pharmacological factors do not explain the differing prescribing patterns seen with African Americans, what does? As noted earlier, provider attitudes and eithic minorities' perceptions of the mental health system are extremely important. The view that African Americans are more hostile than they actually are may be confounded by poor communications and social, economic, and ethnic distance. Patients who become suspicious and hostile to the system either choose other alternatives or are less compliant, as shown by the high rate of noncompliance. The solution appears to be straightforward. African Americans must be made to feel welcome in the mental health system. When physicians are more willing to consider patients' ethnic differences, excessive dosing disappears.

To summarize, ethnic minorities receive older antipsychotics. African Americans receive higher doses and more depot medication, probably due more to attitudinal factors than to socioeconomic or biological factors. These treatment differences ignore biological differences that may require lower doses and a greater concern for movement disorder side effects. The prudent clinician should individualize treatment. The patient should be considered a partner in developing a reasonable dosing plan. Culture, ethnicity, and the patient's individual risk profile must be considered. Family history and family members must be consulted. As much as possible, rapport should be established regardless of ethnicity.

CONCLUSION

Schizophrenia is a devastating disorder for anyone, but especially for ethnic minorities. Limited access to treatment increases illness burden for economically depressed families. When treatment is available, misdiagnosis is common; other disorders, mislabeled as schizophrenia, are treated inappropriately. Genetic factors are important in schizophrenia, as is the family environment. Consideration of cultural factors means that findings about family environment in European American families do not apply to ethnic minorities. Suboptimal treatment of African Americans with schizophrenia is not simply a consequence of socioeconomic factors. Excessive dosing with older medications is common and cannot be accounted for by biological factors. The physician–patient relationship, willingness of the physician to engage the patient, and individualized treatment are crucial to optimal pharmacotherapy. Race and ethnicity, their cultural determinants, and their interaction with socioeconomic and biological factors must be considered in the diagnosis and treatment of schizophrenia.

KEY POINTS

- Overdiagnosis of schizophrenia is common among African Americans, with affective disorders often misdiagnosed as schizophrenia, mainly due to a failure to get adequate information, clinician bias, and cultural factors.
- For a proper diagnosis of schizophrenia in African Americans and other ethnic groups, all sources of information should be considered, including adherence to DSM-IV criteria, and taking cultural issues into account.
- Several studies have shown putative gene associations for schizophrenia in African Americans (e.g., polymorphisms of the *synapsin III* and *NOTCH 4* genes); however, genes should only be considered in the context of environmental factors.
- Despite limited resources, African American families are more likely than European American families to become caregivers for family members with schizophrenia.
- High emotionality and family intrusiveness have been shown to predict poor outcome in European Americans with schizophrenia, but not in their African American counterparts.
- African Americans have less access to health care (even after income is controlled), a greater rate of involuntary hospitalizations, and lower use of preferential treatments, such as day treatment or case management, than European Americans.
- African American patients are more likely to receive first-generation antipsychotics, *higher* doses of medications, and more depot medication than European Americans, whereas Hispanics and Asians receive lower dosages.
- African Americans, Asians, and Hispanics show reduced activity of the cytochrome P450 isoenzyme CYP450 2D6 compared to a majority of European Americans; this suggests higher plasma levels of the antipsychotic drugs, and thereby a *need for lower* dosages in the ethnic minority groups.
- Asians and Hispanics are more likely to develop antipsychotic-induced movement disorders such as acute dystonia, whereas African Americans have a greater risk of developing tardive dyskinesia with first-generation antipsychotics than do European Americans.
- To reduce mental health care disparity, African Americans (as well as other ethnic minority groups) should be made to feel welcome in the mental health system; treatment should be individualized, and cultural factors should be considered.

REFERENCES AND RECOMMENDED READINGS

Barnes, A. (2004). Race, schizophrenia, and admission to state psychiatric hospitals. *Administration and Policy in Mental Health, 31,* 241–252.

Blow, F. C., Zeber, J. E., McCarthy, J. F., Valenstein, M., Gillon, L., & Bingham, C. R. (2004). Ethnicity and diagnostic patterns in veterans with psychoses. *Social Psychiatry and Psychiatric Epidemiology, 39,* 841–851.

Daumit, G. L., Crum, R. M., Guallar, E., Powe, N. R., Primm, A. B., Steinwachs, D. M., et al. (2003). Outpatient prescriptions for atypical antipsychotics for African Americans, Hispanics, and whites in the United States. *Archives of General Psychiatry, 60,* 121–128.

DelBello, M. P., Lopez-Larson, M. P., Soutullo, C. A., & Strakowski, S. M. (2001). Effects of race on psychiatric diagnosis of hospitalized adolescents: A retrospective chart review. *Journal of Child and Adolescent Psychopharmacology, 11*(1), 95–103.

Herbeck, D. M., West, J. C., Ruditis, I., Duffy, F. F., Fitek, D. J., Bell, C. C., et al. (2004). Variations in use of second-generation antipsychotic medication by race among adult psychiatric patients *Psychiatric Services, 55*(6), 677–684.

Kreyenbuhl, J., Zito, J. M., Buchanan, R. W., Soeken, K. L., & Lehman, A. F. (2003). Racial disparity in the pharmacological management of schizophrenia. *Schizophrenia Bulletin, 29*(2), 183–193.

Lawson, W. B. (1986a). The black family and chronic mental illness. *American Journal of Social Psychiatry, 6,* 57–61.

Lawson, W. B. (1986b). Clinical issues in the pharmacotherapy of African-Americans. *Psychopharmacology Bulletin, 32,* 275–281.

Lawson, W. B. (1990). Biological markers in neuropsychiatric disorders: Racial and ethnic factors. In E. Sorel (Ed.), *Family, cultures, and psychobiology.* New York: Levas.

Lawson, W. B. (2002). Mental health issues for African Americans. In B. Guillermo, J. E. Trimble, A. K. Burlow, & F. T. I. Leong (Eds.), *Handbook of racial and ethnic minority psychology.* Thousand Oaks, CA: Sage.

Lawson, W. B., Hepler, N., Holladay, J., & Cuffel, B. (1994). Race as a factor in inpatient and outpatient admissions and diagnosis. *Hospital and Community Psychiatry, 45,* 72–74.

Lawson, W. B., & Kennedy, C. (2002). Role of the severely mentally ill in the family. In F. Lewis-Hall, T. S. Williams, J. A. Panetta, & J. Herrera, (Eds.), *Psychiatric illness in women: Emerging treatments and research.* Washington, DC: American Psychiatric Association Press.

Lawson, W. B., Yesavage, J. A., & Werner, R. D. (1984). Race, violence, and psychopathology. *Journal of Clinical Psychiatry, 45,* 294–297.

Mark, T. L., Palmer, L. A., Russo, P. A., & Vasey, J. (2003). Examination of treatment pattern differences by race. *Mental Health Services Research, 5*(4), 241–250.

Minsky, S., Vega, W., Miskimen, T., Gara, M., & Escobar, J. (2003). Diagnostic patterns in Latino, African American, and European American psychiatric patients. *Archives of General Psychiatry, 60,* 637–644.

Neighbors, H. W., Trierweiler, S. J., Ford, B. C., & Muroff, J. R. (2003). Racial differences in DSM diagnosis using a semi-structured instrument: The importance of clinical judgment in the diagnosis of African Americans. *Journal of Health and Social Behavior, 44,* 237–256.

Opolka, J. L., Rascati, K. L., Brown, C. M., & Gibson, P. J. (2004). Ethnicity and prescription patterns for haloperidol, risperidone, and olanzapine. *Psychiatric Services, 55*(2), 151–156.

Strakowski, S. M., Keck, P. E., Jr., Arnold, L. M., Collins, J., Wilson, R. M., Fleck, D. E., et al. (2003). Ethnicity and diagnosis in patients with affective disorders. *Journal of Clinical Psychiatry, 64,* 747–754.

Valenstein, M., Copeland, L. A., Owen, R., Blow, F. C., & Visnic, S. (2001). Adherence assessments and the use of depot antipsychotics in patients with schizophrenia. *Journal of Clinical Psychiatry, 62*(7), 545–551.

CHAPTER 61

ETHICS

ABRAHAM RUDNICK
CHARLES WEIJER

Health problems and health care frequently raise ethical issues of various types. The discipline that addresses such ethical issues is currently called *bioethics*, a field of practice, research, and education that influences public policymaking and legislature, as well as clinical research and care. It is grounded in philosophy, law, and social sciences, as well as in health care sciences, such as medicine and nursing. Contemporary bioethics involves social institutions such as bioethics committees, bioethics consultants, professional codes of bioethics, associations of bioethics, and texts of bioethics (Beauchamp & Childress, 2001).

Ethics in general, including bioethics, addresses moral problems, sometimes called *ethical dilemmas*. Moral problems primarily comprise conflicts of accepted principles or values that arise in particular situations. In health care, such situations are frequently related to the end of life, such as in euthanasia (mercy killing for people with terminal illnesses), when the value of preserving life conflicts with the value of reducing suffering, or to the beginning of life, such as in abortion, when the conflict is commonly stated as pro-life (protecting the fetus) versus pro-choice (protecting the pregnant woman). Moral problems are commonly resolved by applying ethical theories, as well as moral intuitions, preferably by engagement in a process of deliberation and dialogue with the parties involved (Rudnick, 2002b). Well-known ethical theories used in bioethics include *utilitarianism*, which addresses the consequences of actions; *deontology*, which addresses duties; and *virtue ethics*, which addresses character traits and intentions. Perhaps the most commonly used bioethical approach is *principlism*, which combines some of these well-known theories while balancing the principle of respect for persons (addressing autonomy or self-determination of the patient), the principle of beneficence and nonmaleficence (addressing maximal benefit and minimal harm to the patient), and the principle of justice (addressing fairness to the patient and to others).

Mental health problems and care raise various ethical issues or moral problems, as reflected in areas such as involuntary commitment and substitute decision making. Some of these issues have been addressed in other chapters in this book. This chapter focuses on two important ethical issues that are not directly addressed by other chapters in this book, and that are important enough to deserve separate consideration. These are the issues of the ethics of client-centered care for people with schizophrenia and of research on people with schizophrenia. The section on client-centered care is primarily authored by Rudnick, and the section on research is primarily authored by Weijer.

ETHICS OF CLIENT-CENTERED CARE IN SCHIZOPHRENIA

Client-centered care, also termed *patient-centered care* and *person-centered care*, is now considered a mainstay of acceptable health care, both in mental health care and in physical health care (Stewart et al., 2003). It is commonly characterized as health care that serves the goals and the needs of the patient. It guides health care in the sense that clinical assessments and interventions are directed by the goals and needs of patients, rather than by those of others, including caregivers such as family members and clinicians. Thus, client-centered care clearly manifests the principle of autonomy or self-determination. Indeed, the recent rising of the recovery movement in mental health largely revolves around client-centeredness and self-determination. Yet schizophrenia challenges the notion of (purely) client-centered care and the underlying principle of self-determination, and requires the consideration of additional ethical principles in the provision of care.

People with schizophrenia demonstrate various psychiatric symptoms and cognitive impairments, some of which undermine self-determination. For instance, impaired insight into illness, which is common in schizophrenia, disrupts decision-making capacity, leading to the determination of incompetence to consent to or refuse treatment (Grisso & Appelbaum, 1998). Another example is that of delusions, which are very common in schizophrenia and by definition disrupt reality testing, leading to involuntary commitment if risk of harm to self or others is also involved. Both examples illustrate how impairments and symptoms of schizophrenia undermine self-determination. So how does this impact on client-centered care for people with schizophrenia?

The mental health care area that attempts to be most client-centered is psychiatric rehabilitation (Anthony, Cohen, Farkas, & Gagne, 2002). Psychiatric rehabilitation aims to improve the functioning and quality of life of individuals with severe psychiatric disorders, so that they achieve and maintain lives that are satisfactory and meaningful to them, thus facilitating recovery. It consists of enhancing the living skills and environmental supports of individuals with mental illness, enabling them to achieve goals that, preferably, they set themselves. Yet such individuals may set goals reflecting values that conflict with those held by mental health practitioners or by society at large, and that are induced by mental impairment, such as stalking another person due to erotomanic delusions (i.e., the mentally ill individual thinking that the other person is infatuated with him or her). Psychiatric rehabilitation practitioners have reported difficulty, due to this problem, in working toward goals set by their clients (Hendrickson-Gracie, Staley, & Morton-Neufeld, 1996). Goals set by individuals with mental illness that involve harm to self or to others are suspect, such as in the case of the stalker with erotomanic delusions. In such cases, a client-centered approach that endorses patient goals at all cost runs into ethical trouble, because it rigidly compromises acceptable values such as preservation of life and fairness to others. If so, others—such as legally appointed guardians or substitute decision makers—may be required to set goals for individuals with mental illness. Yet rehabilitation goals set by others are problematic, because if the goals of the individual prior to the psychiatric disorder are not known (as frequently occurs), then best interests, not patient goals, are considered. This may preserve an aspect of the client-centered approach in that best interests can be claimed to address patient needs. But this is conceptually problematic, because there is no—and probably cannot be—consensus on what a person needs to achieve and maintain a satisfactory and meaningful life and, arguably, that is so subjective that it can only be determined by the person, mentally ill or not.

Thus, client-centered mental health care, at least in the area of psychiatric rehabilitation, may not be ethically and conceptually sound in some cases. In such cases, alternative approaches may be required, with the recognition that forced or coerced psychiatric rehabilitation may not be ethically acceptable with regard to achievement of goals, and to maintenance of goals (the latter would probably require continuous and possibly increased coercion or force). An alternative could be a dialogical approach, where all involved parties engage in structured dialogue to establish mutually acceptable goals in an ethically sound manner (Rudnick, 2002a). Schizophrenia, with its various symptoms and impairments, may challenge this approach, but there may be ways to overcome this challenge within a dialogical approach by facilitating communication and accommodating for such psychiatric symptoms and cognitive impairments (Rudnick, 2007). For instance, impairments in executive functions may disrupt the ability to predict consequences of actions, and hence to discuss relevant utilitarian considerations, but cognitive rehabilitation and support strategies (Twamley, Jeste, & Bellack, 2003) may be helpful in overcoming this challenge, therefore facilitating such dialogue with cognitively impaired individuals who have schizophrenia. Future study may explore this approach in detail.

ETHICS OF CLINICAL RESEARCH IN SCHIZOPHRENIA

Research ethics is concerned with the moral principles and rules that govern the conduct of scientific study involving human subjects. Clinical research is essential to further our understanding of the causes of schizophrenia and the development of safe and effective treatments. But these ends cannot be pursued legitimately by any means. Clinical research must be conducted in a manner that protects the liberty and welfare interests of research subjects. Standards for the conduct of clinical research are set out in federal regulations and are enforced by institutional review boards. Clinicians who conduct research, or whose patients may be enrolled in such research by others, need an understanding of the regulation of clinical research, ethical principles and rules, and issues of special importance to psychiatric research.

The need for regulation of research by the State is often traced to unethical practices in the past. Unfortunately, medical history is replete with examples of research that fails to take adequate account of the rights and welfare of subjects (Moreno, 2001). For instance, at the Allen Memorial Institute in Montreal, Canada, in the 1950s and 1960s, Dr. Ewan Cameron used a variety of experimental techniques on psychiatric patients, including electric shocks; "psychic driving," in which taped messages would be repeated for days at a time; and sensory deprivation. Later, experiments funded by the Central Intelligence Agency involved the administration of LSD (lysergic acid diethylamide) to patients. The ethical failings of these experiments were multiple: informed consent was either not obtained or was inadequate; the interventions lacked a scientific basis; and patients were subjected to serious risks.

To protect research subjects, the State has established a system of oversight for clinical research in which the keystone is the institutional review board (IRB). IRBs are local committees that review research on human subjects for ethical acceptability. IRB approval is required for such research to be conducted. The first IRBs were federally mandated in 1966 and, by current estimates, there are 3,000–5,000 IRBs at universities, hospitals, and research institutions in the United States. The IRB must have at least five members, and include researchers, one or more community representatives, an ethicist or a lawyer, and in some cases a statistician. The IRB reviews the research protocol, the investigator's brochure related to any study drugs, and the informed consent form to determine study acceptability. While the purview of the IRB includes both ethical and scientific issues, the review of scientific issues may be delegated to another more qualified body (e.g., an NIH [National Institutes of Health] Study Section).

In its review, the IRB ensures that the study complies with relevant regulations and guidelines (Emanuel, Wendler, & Grady, 2000). In the United States, all human subject research funded by the Federal government, or conducted at an institution that receives Federal funds, must comply with the Federal *Common Rule* (Title 45 *CFR* Part 46). Other regulations define additional protections for pregnant women (referred to as Subpart B regulations), prisoners (Subpart C), and children (Subpart D). Despite repeated calls over the last 20 years, Federal regulations do not define additional protections for incapable adults, including those incapacitated by mental illness (Karlawish, 2006). Other relevant guidelines for clinical research include the World Medical Association's *Declaration of Helsinki*, the Council for International Organizations of Medical Sciences' *International Ethical Guidelines for Biomedical Research Involving Human Subjects*, and the International Conference on Harmonization's *Good Clinical Practice* guidelines. Relevant regulations and guidelines, guidance, and educational materials are found at the website of the Office for Human Research Protection (*www.hhs.gov/ohrp*).

Clinical research is governed by three ethical principles: respect for persons; beneficence; and justice (Table 61.1). The principle of *respect for persons* means that the wishes of autonomous individuals ought to be taken seriously, and that persons incapable of autonomous choice are entitled to protection. It grounds requirements for free and informed consent from research participants and confidentiality of research information. The principle of *beneficence* signifies that one must protect people from harm and, where possible, promote their benefit. It underpins the requirement that the benefits and harms of research participation stand in reasonable relation. The principle of *justice* implies that one must treat people fairly. It is the basis for the requirement that study selection procedures must be fair, neither unduly advantaging nor disadvantaging any relevant group of potential study participants.

The free and informed consent of research subjects must generally be sought prior to study participation. Prospective subjects must be informed of the purpose of the study, duration of participation, procedures to be administered, the benefits and harms of study participation, alternatives, and their rights as research subjects. A distinction may be drawn between the *consent process* and the consent form. The consent process is the ethically mandated dialogue between the clinical investigator and the prospective study par-

TABLE 61.1. Moral Principles and Rules for Clinical Research

Moral principle	Moral rule
Respect for persons	• Obtain the free and informed consent of prospective research subjects. • Protect the confidentiality of private information.
Beneficence	• Therapeutic procedures must satisfy clinical equipoise. • Risks of nontherapeutic procedures must be (1) minimized and (2) reasonable in relation to knowledge to be gained.
Justice	• Subject selection procedures must be fair.

ticipant regarding study participation. The conversation may take place over one or more sessions, during which time the investigator must disclose relevant information, answer questions, and ensure that the prospective subject understands the information presented. The *consent form* is mandated by Federal regulation and is a written summary of the information to be conveyed in the consent process. The mere provision of a consent form to a prospective participant does not constitute an adequate consent process. As may not infrequently be the case in schizophrenia research, when a prospective subject is incapable of providing free and informed consent, consent must be sought from the subject's legally authorized representative in accord with State law (Dunn, 2006). Finally, both the consent process and the consent form must detail adequate protections for the research subject's data.

The benefits and harms of research participation must stand in reasonable relation (Weijer & Miller, 2004). Clinical research often contains a mixture of study procedures. Therapeutic procedures are interventions, such as antipsychotic drugs or counseling administered on the basis of therapeutic warrant, that is, on the basis of evidence that makes it reasonable to believe that they may benefit the research subject. Therapeutic procedures in research must meet the standard of *clinical equipoise*; that is, they must be consistent with competent medical care. Formally, clinical equipoise requires that there exist a state of honest, professional disagreement in the community of expert practitioners as to the preferred treatment. Nontherapeutic procedures, such as additional blood tests or questionnaires not a part of routine clinical practice, on the other hand, are not administered with therapeutic warrant and are given solely to answer the scientific question at hand. The risks of nontherapeutic procedures must be minimized by using procedures that are consistent with sound scientific design and reasonable in relation to the knowledge expected to be gained from the study. Only if ethical requirements for both therapeutic and nontherapeutic procedures are fulfilled may one conclude legitimately that the benefits and harms of study participation are reasonable.

Study selection procedures must be fair. Study eligibility criteria must be clearly stated and ought to be accompanied by a clear justification. Research subjects ought not to be wrongfully included in, or excluded from, research. It is generally accepted that research ought to be carried out on the least vulnerable study population possible, consistent with the scientific goals of the study. Therefore, a study ought to include only subjects capable of providing informed consent, unless the scientific ends of the study require the inclusion of incapable subjects. Having said this, it is also recognized that patient populations (e.g., women, children, and older adults) may be deprived of important benefits if not included in clinical research. Thus, the exclusion of these groups requires adequate justification.

Schizophrenia research raises a considerable number of ethical questions for investigators and clinicians alike. Here we consider two of these briefly. First, what are the obligations of the clinician to the patient in research? Second, when may placebo controls be used ethically?

What are the obligations of the clinician to the patient in research? In clinical practice, the clinician has a broad range of fiduciary duties to the patient, including a *duty of care*. The duty of care requires that the clinician act and advise in the best medical interests of the patient. But how can the clinician do this when the patient is a research subject? The research protocol may involve a detailed regimen for treatment of the research subject. Beyond this, the study itself has been approved by the IRB as being scientifically and ethically sound. Finally, changing the management of a patient in a clinical study may interfere with the scientific ends of the study. What role is there then for clinician judgment in clinical research?

Despite these seeming obstacles, clinical judgment is a critical protection for research subjects (Miller & Weijer, 2006). IRB approval of a research study means that it has determined that the benefits and harms of study participation are acceptable. But in making this determination the IRB can appeal only to population-level evidence. The circumstances of individual research subjects are not in view at the time of IRB approval; hence, such approval does not imply the acceptability of enrollment or continued participation of particular patients. It remains for the clinician to meet his or her obligations to the research subject through the exercise of clinical judgment that takes into account the circumstances of the research subject. If the clinician judges study participation to be medically irresponsible based on evidence that ought to be convincing to colleagues, the clinician is obliged to decline to offer enrollment or to recommend to the patient or to the legal guardian withdrawal of the patient/subject from the study.

When may placebo controls be used ethically? Placebo is a nonactive intervention, such as a sugar pill. In standard clinical trials, subjects (and clinicians) are blinded to whether they are receiving placebo or active treatment. The use of placebo controls in psychiatric research has proven controversial. Proponents of the routine use of placebo controls have argued that good science and ethics require their use (Temple & Ellenberg, 2000). Scientifically, the placebo control provides a clinical trial with a "benchmark" according to which investigators may ensure that conclusions derived from study results are sound (i.e., that the new intervention/medication being studied is indeed beneficial). Proponents argue that free and informed consent provides sufficient moral grounds for placebo studies, provided that research subjects are not exposed to a risk of death or permanent disability. Critics of this view point out that the design of the study ought to depend on the scientific question, and not on unsubstantiated claims regarding the special properties of placebo controls (Weijer, 1999). Clinically relevant scientific questions usually regard the comparative effectiveness of treatments and require designs that employ a standard therapy control. Although often permissible ethically, the use of placebo controls is problematic when therapeutic procedures in a study are not consistent with clinical equipoise, as may be the case for schizophrenia, where there are evidence-based beneficial interventions such as various antipsychotic medications.

Given the contentious nature of placebo use in clinical research currently, how ought the clinician approach the issue? It is a well accepted maxim in research ethics that the medical care of a patient ought not to be disadvantaged by research participation. In considering decisions to refer, enroll, or continue a patient in a clinical trial, the clinician ought to act accordingly. The use of a placebo control is generally agreed to be unproblematic when there is no treatment for a condition, when nontreatment is consistent with competent medical care, or when all patients receive standard care and the study is concerned with the efficacy of the addition of a treatment to the standard regimen. This may not be the case for clinical research on schizophrenia using placebo-only controls. Hence, such research on subjects with schizophrenia may not be ethically justified. As discussed earlier, clinical judgment must also take into account the circumstances of each patient.

KEY POINTS

- Bioethics addresses conflicts of values that arise in health care situations.
- Mental health care such as psychiatric rehabilitation for individuals with schizophrenia is not ethically and conceptually sound if it is (purely) client-centered at all costs.
- A dialogical approach to the mental health care of individuals with schizophrenia may pro-

vide an ethically and conceptually sound alternative to a purely client-centered approach when the latter fails ethically or conceptually.
- Research ethics considers the moral principles and rules that govern the conduct of scientific studies on human beings.
- Clinical research is governed by Federal regulations that are implemented through an upfront review of research by IRBs.
- Whereas obligations of the State to protect the research subject are fulfilled by IRB review, clinicians have an obligation to use clinical judgment to protect patients in research from harm.
- Placebo-only controlled clinical research on subjects with schizophrenia may be ethically justified only under special circumstances, such as when evaluating the effects of medications on treatment-refractory patients or the effects of ancillary medications on associated symptoms (e.g., cognitive impairment).

REFERENCES AND RECOMMENDED READINGS

Anthony, W. A., Cohen, M., Farkas, M., & Gagne, C. (2002). *Psychiatric rehabilitation* (2nd ed.). Boston: Center for Psychiatric Rehabilitation.

Beauchamp, T. L., & Childress, J. F. (2001). *Principles of biomedical ethics* (5th ed.). New York: Oxford University Press.

Dunn, L. B. (2006). Capacity to consent to research in schizophrenia: The expanding evidence base. *Behavioral Sciences and the Law, 24,* 431–445.

Emanuel, E. J., Wendler, D., & Grady, C. (2000). What makes clinical research ethical? *Journal of the American Medical Association, 283,* 2701–2711.

Grisso, T., & Appelbaum, P. S. (1998). *Assessing competence to consent to treatment: A guide for physicians and other health professionals.* New York: Oxford University Press.

Hendrickson-Gracie, K., Staley, D., & Morton-Neufeld, I. (1996). When worlds collide: Resolving value differences in psychosocial rehabilitation. *Psychiatric Rehabilitation Journal, 20,* 25–31.

Karlawish, J. (2006). Alzheimer's disease—clinical trials and the logic of clinical purpose. *New England Journal of Medicine, 355,* 1604–1606.

Miller, P. B., & Weijer, C. (2006). The trust-based obligations of the state and physician–research to patient–subjects. *Journal of Medical Ethics, 32,* 542–547.

Moreno, J. D. (2001). *Undue risk: Secret state experiments on humans.* New York: Routledge.

Rudnick, A. (2002a). The goals of psychiatric rehabilitation: An ethical analysis. *Psychiatric Rehabilitation Journal, 25,* 310–313.

Rudnick, A. (2002b). The ground of dialogical bioethics. *Health Care Analysis, 10,* 391–402.

Rudnick, A. (2007). Processes and pitfalls of dialogical bioethics. *Health Care Analysis, 15,* 123–135.

Stewart, M., Brown, J. B., Weston, W. W., McWhinney, I. R., McWilliam, C. L., & Freeman, T. R. (2003). *Patient-centered medicine: Transforming the clinical method* (2nd ed.). Oxon, UK: Radcliffe.

Temple, R., & Ellenberg, S. S. (2000). Placebo-controlled trials and active-control trials in the evaluation of new treatments: Part 1. Ethical and scientific issues. *Annals of Internal Medicine, 133,* 455–463.

Twamley, E. W., Jeste, D. V., & Bellack, A. S. (2003). A review of cognitive training in schizophrenia. *Schizophrenia Bulletin, 29,* 359–382.

Weijer, C. (1999). Placebo-controlled trials in schizophrenia: Are they ethical? Are they necessary? *Schizophrenia Research, 35,* 211–218.

Weijer, C., & Miller, P. B. (2004). When are research risks reasonable in relation to anticipated benefits? *Nature Medicine, 10,* 570–573.

INDEX